D0138912

The Continuum of
Long-Term Care

This book is dedicated to my young son, Tom.
May long-term care be better organized by the time
his generation needs it—and may he never have to use it.

The Continuum of Long-Term Care

Third Edition

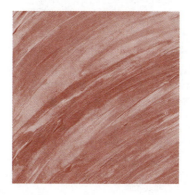

Connie J. Evashwick, ScD

Professor
Health Care Administration Program
California State University Long Beach
Long Beach, California

THOMSON

DELMAR LEARNING

Africa Australia Canada Denmark Japan Mexico New Zealand Philippines
Puerto Rico Singapore Spain United Kingdom United States

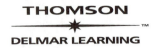

THOMSON

™

DELMAR LEARNING

The Continuum of Long-Term Care, 3rd Edition
by Connie J. Evashwick, ScD

Vice President,
Health Care Business Unit:
William Brottmiller

Editorial Director:
Cathy L. Esperti

Acquisitions Editor:
Maureen Rosener

Editorial Assistant:
Elizabeth Howe

Marketing Director:
Jennifer McAvey

Marketing Coordinator:
Chris Manion

Production Editor:
Jennifer Luck

Production Coordinator:
Mary Ellen Cox

Art and Design Coordinator:
Christi DiNinni

Library of Congress Cataloging-in-Publication Data

ISBN 1-4018-9637-5

NOTICE TO THE READER

Publisher does not warrant or guarantee any of the products described herein or perform any independent analysis in connection with any of the product information contained herein. Publisher does not assume, and expressly disclaims, any obligation to obtain and include information other than that provided to it by the manufacturer.

The reader is expressly warned to consider and adopt all safety precautions that might be indicated by the activities described herein and to avoid all potential hazards. By following the instructions contained herein, the reader willingly assumes all risks in connection with such instructions.

The publisher makes no representations or warranties of any kind, including but not limited to, the warranties of fitness for particular purpose or merchantability, nor are any such representations implied with respect to the material set forth herein, and the publisher takes no responsibility with respect to such material. The publisher shall not be liable for any special, consequential, or exemplary damages resulting, in whole or part, from the readers' use of, or reliance upon, this material.

INTRODUCTION TO THE SERIES

This Series in Health Services is now in its second decade of providing top quality teaching materials to the health administration/public health field. Each year has witnessed further strengthening of the market position of each of the principal books in the Series, also reflecting the continued excellence of the products. Each author, book editor, and contributor to the Series has helped build what is widely recognized as the top textbook and issues collection of books available in this field today.

But we have achieved only a beginning. Everyone involved in the Series is committed to further expansion of the scope, technical excellence, and usability of the Series. Our goal is to do more for you, the reader. We will add new books in important areas, seek out more excellent authors, and increase the physical attributes of the books to make them easier for you to use.

We thank everyone, the authors and users in particular, who have made this Series so successful and so widely used. And we promise that this second decade will be dedicated to further expansion of the Series and to enhancement of the books it contains to provide still greater value to you, our constituency.

Stephen J. Williams
Series Editor

THOMSON DELMAR LEARNING SERIES IN HEALTH SERVICES ADMINISTRATION

Stephen J. Williams, ScD, Series Editor

Ambulatory Care Management, third edition
Austin Ross, Stephen J. Williams, and Ernest J. Pavlock, Editors

The Continuum of Long-Term Care, third edition
Connie J. Evashwick, Editor

Health Care Economics, sixth edition
Paul J. Feldstein

Health Politics and Policy, third edition
Theodor J. Litman and Leonard S. Robins, Editors

Introduction to Health Services, sixth edition
Stephen J. Williams and Paul R. Torrens, Editors

Motivating Health Behavior
John P. Elder, E. Scott Geller, Melbourne F. Hovell, and Joni A. Mayer, Editors

Really Governing: How Health System and Hospital Boards Can Make More of a Difference
Dennis D. Pointer and Charles M. Ewell

Strategic Management of Human Resources in Health Services Organizations, second edition
Myron D. Fottler, S. Robert Hernandez, and Charles L. Joiner, Editors

Financial Management in Health Care Organizations
Robert A. McLean

Principles of Public Health Practice, second edition
F. Douglas Scutchfield and C. William Keck, Editors

The Hospital Medical Staff
Charles H. White

Essentials of Health Services, second edition
Stephen J. Williams

Essentials of Health Care Management
Stephen M. Shortell and Arnold D. Kaluzny, Editors

Essentials of Human Resources Management in Health Services Organizations
Myron D. Fottler, S. Robert Hernandez, and Charles L. Joiner, Editors

Health Services Research Methods
Leiyu Shi

Supplemental Reader:
Contemporary Issues in Health Services
Stephen J. Williams, Editor

CONTRIBUTORS

William E. Aaronson, PhD
Fox School of Business and Management
Temple University
Philadelphia, PA

Laurence G. Branch, PhD
College of Public Health
University of South Florida
Tampa, FL

Judith Connell, DrPH
Institute for Healthcare Advancement
La Habra, CA

Stephen R. Connor, PhD
National Hospice and Palliative Care Organization
Alexandria, VA

Nancy J. Cox
Wake Forest University School of Medicine
Partners in Caregiving
Winston-Salem, NC

Leslie A. Curry, PhD, MPH
University of Connecticut
Health Center
Farmington, CT

Marie F. Denis, MSPH, MPH
Division of HIV/AIDS Prevention
Centers for Disease Control
Atlanta, GA

Connie J. Evashwick, ScD
Health Care Administration Program
California State University Long Beach
Long Beach, CA

Richard H. Fortinsky, PhD
Center on Aging
University of Connecticut Health Center
Farmington, CT

Janice E. Frates, PhD
Health Care Administration Program
California State University Long Beach
Long Beach, CA

Susan L. Hughes, DSW
Center for Research on Health and Aging
University of Illinois at Chicago
Chicago, IL

Kathryn Hyer, MPP, PhD
Center on Aging
University of South Florida
Tampa, FL

Jung Kwak, MSW
Aging Studies Program
University of South Florida
Tampa, FL

Margaret A. Lampe, RN, MPH
Division of HIV/AIDS Prevention
Centers for Disease Control
Atlanta, GA

Mark R. Levinstein, MD
Veterans Affairs Health Care System
Long Beach, CA

Ann Sheck McAlearney, ScD
Health Services Management and Policy
Ohio State University
Columbus, OH

Galen Miller, MD
National Hospice and Palliative Care Organization
Alexandria, VA

Deborah M. Mullen
Health Partners
Minneapolis, MN

Christy M. Nishita, PhD
Andrus Gerontology Center
University of Southern California
Los Angeles, CA

Linda S. Noelker, PhD
Margaret Blenkner Research Institute of Benjamin Rose
Cleveland, OH

Edward jj Olson, MS
Ed Olson and Associates
Milwaukee, WI

Marcia Ory, PhD, MPH
School of Rural Public Health
Texas A&M University System
College Station, TX

Deborah L. Paone, MHSA
Paone and Associates, LLC
Bloomington, MN

Ruth B. Pickard, PhD
Department of Public Health Sciences
Wichita State University
Wichita, KS

Jon Pynoos, PhD
Andrus Gerontology Center
University of Southern California
Los Angeles, CA

Megan E. Renehan
Center for Research on Health and Aging
University of Illinois at Chicago
Chicago, IL

Louis Rubino, PhD
Department of Health Sciences
California State University Northridge
Northridge, CA

Thomas G. Rundall, PhD
School of Public Health
University of California Berkeley
Berkeley, CA

Amber Schickedanz
School of Rural Public Health
Texas A&M University System
College Station, TX

Debra J. Sheets, RN, PhD
Department of Health Services
California State University Northridge
Northridge, CA

Lisa Shugarman
RAND Corporation
Santa Monica, CA

Alek A. Sripipatana, MPH
UCLA Center for Health Policy Research
Los Angeles, CA

Roberta M. Suber, MSW
Health Science Department
California State University Northridge
Northridge, CA

James H. Swan, PhD
Department of Applied Gerontology
University of North Texas
Denton, TX

Kathleen T. Unroe
Health Services Management and Policy
Ohio State University
Columbus, OH

Terrie Wetle, PhD
Public Health and Public Policy
Brown University
Providence, RI

Monika White, PhD
Center for Healthy Aging
Santa Monica, CA

Carol J. Whitlatch, PhD
Margaret Blenkner Research Institute of Benjamin Rose
Cleveland, OH

Rick T. Zawadski, PhD
RTZ Associates
Oakland, CA

CONTENTS

P A R T

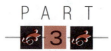

Integrating Mechanisms / 185

P A R T

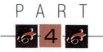

Continuums for Special Populations / 293

PREFACE

Long-term care is one of the greatest challenges facing the health care delivery system. In terms of population need, consumer demand, resource consumption, financing, and system organization, long-term care will be a dominant issue during the coming decades. The components of long-term care each have grown during the past decades. Service availability has increased; integration is beginning to occur. For the limited available resources to meet the increasing demand, the system that currently exists—an ad hoc, distinct arrangement for each individual—must evolve into a well-organized, efficient, client-oriented continuum of care.

To accomplish the cost-effective goals currently being promoted in the acute care and health care financing arenas, long-term care must be dealt with as an essential complement to acute care. Most clients' problems cannot be bifurcated into acute and long-term needs. Thus, for health care providers and payers to accomplish their market and financial goals, long-term care will be needed. Conversely, long-term care providers will not enjoy the same market niche over time unless they affiliate at some level with broader health care delivery systems. In the future, no service or payer will be able to function totally independently and succeed in capturing a market or sustaining financial viability.

Thus, administrators in acute care, payer systems, or any segment of long-term care must understand at least the basics of the other components of the continuum of care. As providers and payers negotiate contracts and try to manage client care efficiently,

administrators will not be able to function in isolation. They must know the strengths and weaknesses of other services and how to use them appropriately and cost-effectively. They must know how to link services and guide clients over time through changing needs. They must be able to merge private and public funding streams and regulations.

The purpose of this book is to proffer a conceptual framework for thinking about the ideal organization of an integrated continuum of care and to provide concrete information about the components of the continuum as they exist today. At minimum, it is hoped that administrators can learn enough about the basics of each component of the continuum of care to manage client flow effectively, despite the current fragmentation of long-term care services. At best, it is possible that administrators may gain insights about how to design and develop a comprehensive, integrated system of care for the future.

In Part One, Chapter 1 defines long-term care and the continuum of care and gives the rationale for the organization of the book. Chapter 2 describes the range of clients needing long-term care. Chapter 3 elaborates on caregivers—critical partners to both clients and providers.

A continuum comprises both services and integrating mechanisms. Part Two is devoted to the services. Although ideally the services will be integrated, the reality of the present is that each service has its own distinct clients, financing, staffing, and other features. Except for the single exclusion of the physician, these chapters present detailed information about the services that are the most fundamental to long-term care. The "Service Snapshot" for many chapters enables the reader to compare and contrast the services easily, and thus highlights the challenges to achieving integration.

Part Three covers integrating mechanisms. Each of the four essential integrating mechanisms of the continuum is discussed: organization, care coordination/case management, information systems, and financing. Public policy and ethical issues pertaining to long-term care are also described in this section.

Part Four describes continuums of care that are designed for special populations: those with HIV/AIDS, the aged, those with disabilities, those with mental illness, veterans, those needing rehabilitation, and children with special needs.

Throughout, the book attempts to be pragmatic, giving administrators the information they need to know to interact with the organizations that are involved in providing or paying for long-term care. Case studies and examples have been included whenever possible. "Where to Go for Further Information" sections include professional and trade associations and government agencies, complete with Web site

addresses. Appendix A is a list of major federal legislation pertaining to long-term care. Appendix B lists contact information for many national organizations that are helpful to professionals concerned with the continuum of care.

We assume that any administrator who intends to specialize in one aspect of long-term care will seek in-depth information about the area of interest. The purpose of this book is to present an overview in sufficient depth to give administrators the management information they need to develop successful organizational relationships and the perspective they need to assist clients in getting the services they need, when they need them, with efficiency and quality.

ACCOMPANYING INSTRUCTOR SUPPORT

An accompanying Online Companion, including an Instructor's Manual and PowerPoint presentation, can be downloaded from the following website: *www.delmarhealthcare.com.* Select *Allied Health* and then select *Online Companions.*

ACKNOWLEDGMENTS

The authors who contributed chapters to this book are among the nation's leaders in a relatively small field. Through their writings and day-to-day practice, they have helped shape the evolution of the long-term care field. All have great demands on their professional time. It is a tribute to their dedication to the field that they would devote time and energy to writing for this book. Most have also been my personal friends for many years, and the collegiality within this field is one of the compelling reasons that most of us have remained in what might otherwise be a frustrating and heart-wrenching arena. This edition also adds several new young authors, whom we welcome to the field with hopes that they will remain to contribute their expertise to the next generation. My great thanks to all of the contributing authors.

That this book came to be is due to Dr. Stephen Williams, editor of Delmar's Health Services Administration Series and a longtime friend from graduate school. Without his suggestion, the original idea of a textbook on long-term care would not have come up. Without his encouragement at a number of points along the way when the magnitude of the task seemed overwhelming, the project would have been abandoned. He is the exemplary editor—initiating, inspiring, and supporting his authors.

Without Patricia Fabian, this book would never have been completed. Her dedication to detail, extreme patience, and unfailing optimism, plus 12 months of daily effort, brought the book from table of contents to full text.

My thanks to all of my colleagues who participated in this endeavor and to the others in our field who have taught me to understand and appreciate long-term care. Collectively, those who have dedicated their professional lives to long-term care are the hope that the system of the future may indeed make it easy for all of us in our personal lives to give and receive long-term care in an easy, affordable, positive way.

The author would like to acknowledge the following reviewers:

Amelia Broussard
Assistant Professor
Department of Health Care Management
Clayton College and State University
Morrow, GA

Robert E. Burke, PhD
Interim Chair, Department of Health Services
Management and Leadership
Director, Wertlieb Educational Institute for Long-Term Care Management
School of Public Health and Health Services
The George Washington University
Washington, DC

James Ciesla
Associate Professor and Program Coordinator
School of Allied Health Professions
Northern Illinois University
DeKalb, IL

Janet C. Frank, DrPH
Assistant Director for Academic Programs
Multicampus Program in Geriatric Medicine and
Gerontology
The David Geffen School of Medicine at UCLA
Los Angeles, CA

Cynthia Massie Mara, PhD
Associate Professor of Health Care Administration
and Policy
School of Public Affairs
Penn State University Harrisburg
Middletown, PA

Mary Helen McSweeney, PhD
Assistant Professor
Department of Health Care Programs
Iona College
New Rochelle, NY

Nancy Persily, MPH
Clinical Professor, Department of Health Policy,
Management and Behavior
Associate Dean for Academic Programs,
University at Albany School of Public Health
Assistant Provost, University at Albany, State
University of New York
Albany, NY

Louis Rubino, PhD, FACHE
Associate Professor
Department of Health Sciences
California State University, Northridge
Northridge, CA

Amanda Grant Smith, MD
Geriatric Psychiatrist
Suncoast Gerontology Center
University of South Florida
Tampa, FL

Kathleen Wilber, PhD
Mary Pickford Foundation Professor of
Gerontology
Professor of Health Services Administration
Andrus School of Gerontology
University of Southern California
Los Angeles, CA

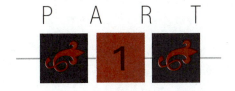

P A R T

1

The Continuum of Long-Term Care

The continuum of long-term care is all-encompassing, including healthy seniors, chronically ill children, and middle-aged adults with disabilities. It does not exclude acute care, but rather incorporates and extends it. *A continuum is more than a collection of services: it is an integrated system of care in which the services are linked together by integrating mechanisms.* No two continuums of care are identical: each is unique to its community, its institutions, and the needs of its target populations. A given community or organization may have several continuums operating in parallel.

Part One presents a definition of the continuum of care that an organization can use as a framework for shaping and evaluating its own service delivery system. It also describes the range of target audiences that benefit from an integrated continuum of long-term care, both care recipients and caregivers.

CHAPTER 1

Definition of the Continuum of Care

Connie J. Evashwick

An 87-year-old woman who is too frail to shop and cook receives meals daily from Meals on Wheels, which is run by a local social service agency and funded by the federal government under the Older Americans Act.

A 21-year-old man who is recovering from multiple fractures sustained in a severe automobile accident is visited by a home health nurse and a physical therapist twice a week until he is strong enough to go to therapy at the physical therapy clinic. Services are paid for by his private insurance, with a co-pay out of pocket.

A 63-year-old man with advanced Alzheimer's disease resides in a nursing home. His care is paid for by the state Medicaid program because he has already depleted all of his own personal financial resources.

A 34-year-old woman with controlled schizophrenia lives in a group home and visits her mental health center monthly to have her medication level and mental status checked. Her medications, residential care, and medical care are paid for through the state and local mental health departments, but she is unable to earn an income.

A 51-year-old veteran of the Vietnam war who sustained spinal cord injuries receives adult day services at the Veterans Affairs Medical Center on a daily basis at no charge.

A 10-year-old child who has cerebral palsy, and her 75-year-old grandmother, who has heart trouble and arthritis, are cared for in the home by the child's mother, with medical costs paid for by the family's private insurance and a combination of government programs.

All of these are examples of long-term care. This book distinguishes between long-term care—the provision of services by one individual to another—and the continuum of care—the formal organizational arrangements that orchestrate the provision of care.

The focus of this book is on the formal organizational arrangements for providing long-term care. The book seeks to describe the services and their relationships as they exist at present, and to describe what needs to be done to improve the currently fragmented organization of long-term care to achieve an integrated continuum of care for the future. Examples of continuums orchestrated for different client groups show the variety of ways a continuum of care can play out.

DEFINITION OF LONG-TERM CARE

Long-term care is defined as a wide range of health and health-related support services provided on an informal or formal basis to people who have functional disabilities over an extended period of time with the goal of maximizing their independence.

The recipients may be people of any age who have one or more functional disabilities, ranging from children with congenital anomalies, to young adults with lengthy recovery periods from trauma, to frail seniors with chronic diseases and the multifaceted changes associated with aging.

Functional disabilities are the primary reason for long-term care, not a specific disease or condition. The ability to perform the Activities of Daily Living (ADLs) and the Instrumental Activities of Daily Living (IADLs) (see Chapter 2) is the key. If a person can take care of himself, regardless of physical or mental health status, he does not need long-term care. Conversely, if a person cannot take care of herself because of any type of physical or mental problems, she will require care.

Over an extended period of time usually means for 90 days or longer. Ninety days is the number the U.S. Public Health Service uses to denote a "chronic condition." For some, long-term care occurs for a finite period of time—perhaps while they are recovering from an accident. The total period of time may be relatively short, e.g., four to six months, and may end when the person recovers, achieves functional independence, or dies. For others, long-term care goes on indefinitely, perhaps for years.

The goal of long-term care is to enable a person to maintain the maximum level possible of functional independence. Unlike acute care, for which the goal is cure, long-term care recognizes that a person's condition may be irreversible and may possibly deteriorate over time. Realistically, care is directed not with the expectation of cure, but for the purpose of enabling the person to do the most he can for himself, given his condition, within the least restrictive setting.

Currently, most long-term care is provided by friends and family (see Chapter 3). Long-term care services in the United States are arranged on an ad hoc basis. The formal system of providing long-term care has no single structure or financing. Each community has its own combination of available resources, funding sources, and organizations. Indeed, most communities have a vast number of organizations engaged in providing specific long-term care services. Multiple tracks of long-term care exist— sometimes parallel, sometimes intersecting. A person with a permanent mental health condition and a person with a hip fracture may use entirely separate services, yet each is receiving long-term care. In general, a unique arrangement is made for each individual.

DEFINITION OF THE CONTINUUM OF CARE

The *ideal* system of long-term care is referred to throughout this book as the "continuum of care." A **continuum of care** is defined as

> a client-oriented system composed of both services and integrating mechanisms that guides and tracks clients over time through a comprehensive array of health, mental health, and social services spanning all levels of intensity of care (Evashwick, 1987).

The continuum of care concept extends beyond the traditional definitions of long-term care. A continuum of care is a comprehensive, coordinated *system of care* designed to meet the needs of people with complex and/or ongoing problems efficiently and effectively. *A continuum is more than a collection of fragmented services. It includes mechanisms for organizing those services and operating them as an integrated system.*

A continuum of care is *client-oriented,* not

provider- or payer-oriented. The orientation is to organize services according to a client's needs, not according to a provider's convenience or a payer's rigid guidelines.

The ideal continuum takes *a holistic approach,* considering the health, mental health, social, and financial aspects of a person's situation. The dynamic interactions of these arenas are considered, and services provided, in a coordinated rather than disjointed way.

A continuum also emphasizes *wellness rather than illness.* Ideally, once a person engages with a continuum, the continuum guides and tracks the client over time, through spells of illness and wellness. The continuum of care concept does not imply that a person must be sick to be part of a continuum. Rather, if persons do become ill, they will be assured of easy access to the services needed. In the interim, they participate in wellness and health promotion activities.

The *comprehensive array of health, mental health, and social services* need not be owned by a single entity. The key is to be able to give clients *access* to the services they need when they need them. The organizational arrangements among providers may be ownership, contracts, affiliations, or even informal but strong relationships.

All levels of intensity of care refers to the range of services—from acute, high-technology interventions to ongoing support services, such as housekeeping. The continuum incorporates both acute and long-term services, intertwining the two with common integrating mechanisms, rather than creating two separate systems of care.

The goal of the continuum of care is to facilitate the client's access to the appropriate services quickly and efficiently. Ideally, a continuum of care:

- Matches resources to the client's condition, avoiding duplication of services and use of inappropriate services
- Takes a multifaceted approach to the client's and family's situation
- Monitors the client's condition and modifies services as needs change

- Coordinates the care of many professionals and disciplines
- Integrates care provided in a range of settings
- Streamlines client flow and facilitates easy access to services needed
- Maintains a comprehensive record incorporating clinical, financial, and utilization data across settings
- Pools and negotiates comprehensive financing

A true continuum of care should (1) enhance quality and client satisfaction through appropriateness, ease of access, shared information, and ongoing continuity of care; (2) increase provider efficiency; and (3) achieve cost-effectiveness by maximizing the use of resources.

The most effective continuums are designed as service configurations appropriate for specific client groups. Several continuums of care may exist simultaneously, even within the same organization. For example, a major medical center may have a rehabilitation center, a cancer center, a heart center, a women's health center, and a Program of All-Inclusive Care for the Elderly (PACE). Each one may have a core set of services used by its clients, and each may be organized as its own continuum, with its own case management, information system, and organizational arrangements. The continuums may overlap in their use of select services. For example, all centers might use the parent organization's home health agency or refer to the same senior housing complex.

Once an organization has set up one continuum of care, creating additional continuums targeted at specific populations is much easier. The integrating mechanisms are the most challenging part and, once in place, may be used for multiple continuums. Or, if separate integrating mechanisms are necessary, at least the organization will have experience with the principles and techniques of establishing structural integration.

The continuum of care concept implies that a person will remain part of an organized continuum of care. It further implies that, rather than having the consumer decide on the provider of each separate service, the organization will arrange the services based on preestablished relationships, formal or informal. A continuum may not preclude a client or family from selecting an alternative provider, but it could eliminate the necessity of doing so. The consumer's participation may be ongoing (as in a managed-care arrangement) or time-limited (as in a terminal chronic illness).

Services

More than 60 distinct services can be identified in the complete continuum of care. For simplicity, the services and settings are grouped into seven categories: extended care, acute inpatient care, ambulatory care, home care, outreach, wellness, and housing (Evashwick, 1982). Table 1.1 lists the major services within these categories. To attain the integration of services, managers must understand the distinct operating characteristics of each of the separate services. The chapters in Part Two of this book describe the major services in detail.

In brief, the seven categories represent the basic types of health and health-related assistance that a person might need over time, through periods of both wellness and illness. In addressing the needs of specific target populations, additional services could be included, such as legal counseling, retirement planning, or guardianship.

Extended inpatient care is for people who are so sick or functionally disabled that they require ongoing nursing and support services provided in a formal health care institution, but who are not so acutely ill that they require the technological and professional intensity of inpatient hospitalization. The majority of extended care facilities are referred to throughout this text as nursing homes, although this is a broad term that includes many levels and types of programs.

Acute inpatient care is hospital care for those who have major and acute health care problems. For most people, a typical hospital stay of five to eight days is the intensive aspect of a longer spell of illness,

preceded by diagnostic testing and succeeded by follow-up care or the flareup of a chronic condition.

Ambulatory care is provided in a formal outpatient health care facility, whether a physician's office or the clinic of a hospital. It encompasses a wide spectrum of preventive, maintenance, diagnostic, and recuperative services for people who manifest a variety of conditions, from those who are entirely healthy and simply want an annual checkup, to those with major health problems who are recuperating from hospitalization, to those who require ongoing monitoring for chronic conditions.

Home care represents a variety of nursing, therapy, and support services provided to people who are homebound and have some degree of illness but whose needs are satisfied by bringing services into the home setting. Home health programs range from formal organizations providing skilled nursing care to relatively informal networks that arrange housekeeping by friends and family members.

Outreach programs make health services and social services readily available in the community rather than inside the formidable walls of a large institution. Health fairs in shopping centers, senior membership programs, and emergency response systems are all forms of outreach. These are often targeted at the healthy or mildly ill to keep them connected with the health care system. Those who are severely ill and homebound may also be reached by community organizations that extend their services into the home, such as Meals on Wheels.

Wellness programs are provided for those who are basically healthy and want to stay that way by actively engaging in health promotion. Wellness programs include health education, exercise programs, and health screenings.

Housing for frail populations increasingly includes access to health and support services and, conversely, recognizes that the home setting affects

Table 1.1 Categories and Services of the Continuum of Care*

Extended
___ Skilled nursing facilities
___ Step-down units
___ Swing beds
___ Nursing home follow-up
___ Intermediate care facility for the mentally retarded

Acute
___ Medical/Surgical inpatient unit
___ Psychiatric inpatient unit
___ Rehabilitation inpatient unit
___ Interdisciplinary assessment team
___ Consultation service

Ambulatory
___ Physicians' offices
___ Outpatient clinics
  • Primary care
  • Specialty medical care
  • Rehabilitation
  • Mental health
___ Psychological counseling
___ Alcohol and substance abuse
___ Day hospital
___ Adult day services

Home Care
___ Home health—Medicare
___ Home health—Private
___ Hospice
___ High-technology home therapy
___ Durable medical equipment
___ Home visitors
___ Home-delivered meals
___ Homemaker and personal care
___ In-home caregiver

Outreach and Linkage
___ Screening
___ Information and referral
___ Telephone contact
___ Emergency response system
___ Transportation
___ Senior membership program
___ Meals on Wheels

Wellness and Health Promotion
___ Educational programs
___ Exercise programs
___ Recreational and social groups
___ Senior volunteers
___ Congregate meals
___ Support groups
___ Disease management

Housing
___ Continuing care retirement communities
___ Independent senior housing
___ Congregate care facilities
___ Adult family homes
___ Assisted living

SOURCE: Evashwick, C. (1987). Definition of the continuum of care. In C. Evashwick & L. Weiss (Eds.), *Managing the continuum of care: A practical guide to organization and operations*. Rockville, MD: Aspen Publishers.

* Lists of services within each category are not exhaustive.

health. Housing that incorporates health care ranges from independent apartments affiliated with a health care system that sends a nurse to do weekly blood pressure checks to assisted living with on-site personal care and social services.

The categories are for heuristic purposes only. Figure 1.1 shows the services schematically. The order of the categories and the services constituting them can vary. The categories can be reordered on the basis of select dimensions: duration of stay, intensity of care, stage of illness, disciplines of professionals, type of physical plant, and availability of informal support. Within each category are health, mental health, and social services, potentially provided by professional clinicians and by various provider organizations.

Rather than a list of services, a more accurate diagram would be a multidimensional matrix showing the interrelationship of all of these factors in caring for a single individual and family. Such a matrix would be *dynamic*, not static, for the relationships would be different for each individual client and would change over time as the client's needs changed.

Within the categories, as well as between them, the services in the continuum are distinct. This is due primarily to the wide array of federal, state, and local laws and regulations, as described in Chapter 15. Each service has different regulatory, financing, target population, staffing, and physical requirements. Each has its own admission policies, client treatment protocols, and billing system. Each organization has its own referral and discharge networks. Table 1.2 highlights the operating characteristics of several of the major services of the continuum and

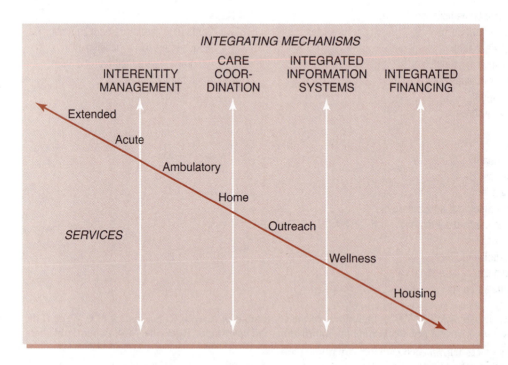

Figure 1.1   Services and Integrating Mechanisms

SOURCE: Evashwick, C. (1987). Definition of the continuum of care. In C. Evashwick & L. Weiss (Eds.), *Managing the continuum of care: A practical guide to organization and operations.* Rockville, MD: Aspen Publishers.

shows the array of differences across services on almost all dimensions.

A primary reason for organizing services into a continuum is to achieve integration of care; yet the operational differences among services make unified planning and management difficult. A major challenge faced by administrators in the initial creation of a continuum of care is that each service must be dealt with separately and then all the services collectively must be brought into a cohesive whole.

INTEGRATING MECHANISMS

By definition, a continuum of care is more than a collection of fragmented services. It is an integrated *system* of care. The full continuum of care is so extensive that it is unlikely that any single organization can offer a complete continuum of services for all of its clients. The goal of the provider should be to facilitate *access* for clients to the services they need.

To gain the system benefits of efficiencies of operation, smooth client flow, and quality of service, structural integrating mechanisms are essential. Whether within a single large organization or across several organizations in the community, formal structures are needed to manage coordination. The four fundamental integrating management systems are: interentity organization and management, care coordination, information systems, and financing. These are briefly outlined here and described in more detail in Part Three.

Interentity organization and management means that arrangements and operating policies are in place to enable services to coordinate care, facilitate smooth client flow, and maximize use of professional staff and other resources. Examples include product line management, centers of excellence, joint planning committees, transfer arrangements, and contracts that delineate client flow procedures as well as financial arrangements.

Care coordination refers to the coordination of the clinical components of care, usually by a com-

bination of a dedicated person and established processes that facilitate communication among professionals of various disciplines across multiple sites and services.

Integrated information systems refers to a single client record that combines financial, clinical, and utilization information to be used by multiple providers and payers across multiple sites, or to an information system that permits access and use of data from multiple distinct data sources.

Integrated financing removes barriers to continuity and appropriateness of care by having available adequate and flexible financing for long-term care as well as acute care; care is not limited based on externally defined eligibility criteria.

CLIENT EXAMPLE

Long-term care services are intended for people who require multiple and ongoing health, mental health, and support services over an extended period of time, and whose needs are likely to change over time. A case study illustrates the complexity of the service delivery system for long-term care and highlights some of its important problems.

Current System

Mr. Jackson is a 66-year-old successful businessman who lives alone in a third-story suburban walk-up apartment. He is generally healthy, but has mild hypertension and diabetes. One night during the winter, he slips on the ice while carrying groceries up the front steps of his building and breaks his hip. A neighbor calls the 911 emergency number and eventually an ambulance arrives. The ambulance takes Mr. Jackson to the emergency room of the nearest hospital, where he is examined and scheduled for surgery to repair his hip fracture. After surgery, Mr. Jackson spends two weeks in the hospital, one on the surgical floor and one on a step-down unit.

Table 1.2 Operating Characteristics of Major Health Services

Service	Number (rounded)	Admissions per year	Average Length of Stay	Accreditation	Major Payers	Unit Cost
Hospitals[a]	5,800	36 million	5–8 days	JCAHO	Medicare; commercial insurance	$1,500/day
Nursing homes[b]	18,000	2.5 million		JCAHO	Medicaid; individual	$3,000–5,000/ month
Home health agencies[c] (Medicare-certified)	7,747	2.7 million	42 visits	CHAP JCAHO	Medicare; commercial insurance	$93/RN visit
Home health agencies (private)	12,250 (est.)	5.1 million (est.)	NA	NHC NLN ACHC	Medicaid; private pay; commercial insurance; government	$90/RN hour
Hospice[d]	3,200	885,000	51 days mean 26 days median	JCAHO CHAP ACHC	Medicare; Medicaid; commercial insurance	$113/day
Adult day services[e]	3,400	85,000 clients each weekday	1–2 years	CARF	Medicaid; private pay; government	$56/day

NOTE: JCAHO is the Joint Commission for the Accreditation of Healthcare Organizations; CHAP is the Community Health Accreditation Program; CARF is the Commission for the Accreditation of Rehabilitation Facilities; NHC is National Homecaring Council; NLN is National League of Nursing; ACHC is Accreditation Commission for Home Care.

[a] American Hospital Association, 2003. Copyright 2003 Edition of Hospital Statistics™, Health Forum, LLC, an American Hospital Association Company.

[b] Jones, A. (2002). The National Nursing Home Survey. 1999 Summary. *Vital and Health Statistics* 13(152). Hyattsville, MD: National Center for Health Statistics (NCHS).

[c] National Association of Home Care. Basic Statistics on Home Health, 2002.

[d] National Hospice and Palliative Care Organization, 2003.

[e] Partners in Caregiving (2003).

Mr. Jackson's physician recommends that he go to a rehabilitation hospital. However, the nearest one is in the next town. Instead, Mr. Jackson agrees to go to a nursing home for rehabilitation.

Even after two weeks in the nursing home, Mr. Jackson is unable to ambulate easily. Because of his diabetes, he is not recovering as quickly as expected. He develops pneumonia and is readmitted to the hospital 29 days after the initial admission. To minimize costs, the hospital keeps him only long enough to ensure that he is fully recovered from the acute exacerbation. Mr. Jackson then returns to the nursing home, but he has regressed somewhat and has to restart the process of regaining independent ambulation.

Eventually Mr. Jackson returns to his home, but he needs assistance walking up and down the stairs, as well as with many activities such as grocery shopping and traveling to the doctor for checkups. A neighbor who is a nurse arranges for a homemaker from a local agency to come in three days a week for two hours to help him. A colleague from work offers to stop by the pharmacy and pick up a prescription for him. Another friend arranges for Meals on Wheels to deliver a hot lunch and a cold dinner Monday through Friday. However, no food comes on the weekends.

Meanwhile, bills begin to flood in from the emergency room, the hospital, the nursing home, several physicians, and the home health agency. Mr. Jackson is not sure what his private insurance will pay, what Medicare will pay, and what he must pay himself. He is trying to conduct his business by constant telephone calls with his staff, but as the owner, his presence is missed for overall direction. Anxiety over his business adds to Mr. Jackson's stress.

Mr. Jackson returns to the hospital outpatient department for rehabilitation therapy, but he must depend on one of his neighbors being at home to help him get up and down the stairs. He cannot drive, so he calls a cab, which does not always come to his neighborhood on time and is expensive. (He received taxi vouchers from the hospital. However, he lives just over the line of jurisdiction, so the taxi for which he has vouchers does not come to his home.)

The therapists at the outpatient department are not the same ones who treated him at the hospital or at the nursing home, and Mr. Jackson feels as though no one quite knows what has happened to him clinically. Medicare Part B covers the major cost of these services, but Mr. Jackson still has to pay the co-pay.

Mr. Jackson struggles along for several weeks and eventually is able to return to work at his office, after nearly 100 days lost to disability. He believes that the medical care and therapy he received were of good quality. However, he also comes out of the experience with huge bills and negative feelings about the fragmented services and the frustrating inability of health care professionals to mobilize the resources necessary to facilitate the simple functions of daily living.

To treat and rehabilitate his broken hip, Mr. Jackson had to coordinate services from an ambulance provider, emergency room, hospital, nursing home, homemaker agency, pharmacy, Meals on Wheels program, outpatient clinic, transportation services, and numerous doctors, nurses, physical therapists, and other caregivers. The task was so overwhelming that an informal care network of friends and neighbors had to make many of the arrangements for Mr. Jackson's care. All the while, Mr. Jackson lived in fear of being driven into bankruptcy by his injury. Ultimately, Medicare and his Medicare Supplemental policy paid for much of his care, but deciphering the bills to determine the remaining portion that was his responsibility was highly confusing.

Unfortunately, Mr. Jackson's experience is all too common. Each of the providers, organizations, and individuals involved in his care did a responsible job. However, they acted independently. For millions of individuals, the effectiveness of the long-term care system depends on the client's own expertise and informal relationships. Although exceptions can be found in various communities, for the most part, the long-term care system is not formally organized; is underfunded, highly regulated, and costly; and, most of all, frequently fails to meet the needs of consumers or providers.

In most communities the current structure of the

long-term care system does not approach the ideal. Each community has its own combination of services, and in each community there are numerous formal and informal arrangements by which clients enter the system and navigate its complex array of programs and resources. The case example illustrates what frequently occurs.

Moreover, most people in need of long-term care are unaware of the range of services that are available. They are subjected to repeated intake assessments and enrollment procedures for each service they use, and then they receive services in an uncoordinated way. The clients themselves, albeit lacking clinical or administrative expertise, are likely to serve as the information conduit across the different service providers about the services they are receiving and the treatment plan each provider may have for the future.

Financing is highly fragmented. A variety of government programs cover some long-term care services completely, and some, not at all. Commercial insurance and health plan coverage is equally varied. Much long-term care is paid for by clients directly out of pocket. Ultimately, the client—the person who is ill—must manage the multiple potential payers.

Ideal Continuum of Care

The goal for long-term care in the twenty-first century is to be organized as an efficient, coordinated continuum of high-quality care. Such a system might alter Mr. Jackson's experience in the following ways.

When Mr. Jackson falls and breaks his hip, the lifeline system automatically calls 911. The emergency response team finds Mr. Jackson's Health Smart Card on his refrigerator door. The Health Smart Card, which is provided by the personal health information system to which Mr. Jackson subscribes, contains vital information that Mr. Jackson uses repeatedly during his recovery period. It connects to an integrated information system that gathers information throughout the Preferred Provider Organization (PPO) network of providers to which Mr. Jackson belongs.

The emergency response team takes Mr. Jackson

by ambulance to the closest hospital. His Health Smart Card is used to process his admission papers, while Mr. Jackson goes directly to be treated. The Health Smart Card provides the name, phone number, and e-mail address of Mr. Jackson's primary care physician, who is alerted by e-mail that his patient has been admitted to the hospital; as well as information about Mr. Jackson's Medicare Supplemental insurance company, which is also sent an e-mail notifying it of the emergency care received by Mr. Jackson.

Meanwhile, when Mr. Jackson transfers to the skilled nursing facility, his rehabilitation records are transmitted in detail to the physical and occupational therapists at the nursing home. The Minimum Data Set (MDS), required to be completed by the nursing facility on admission, is filled in partially by information from the Health Smart Card, with supplements from electronic records transmitted by the hospital. Core data from Mr. Jackson's acute hospital and skilled nursing stays are transmitted and stored in the master client record maintained by the secured personal health information service.

While Mr. Jackson is receiving inpatient care, the case manager from the PPO arranges home health, durable medical equipment, Meals on Wheels, homemaker, and prescription delivery by mail services, to take effect as soon as his stay in the skilled nursing facility ends. The Health Smart Card is used once again to transmit preadmission information to each of the providers, who use it to initiate their own admissions records. Once service has begun, each person providing care logs into a master client calendar maintained by the personal health information service to schedule visits to complement and not interfere with other providers. Each also e-mails to the client's master client record a notice of attendance and activities. Transportation to Mr. Jackson's physician's office is arranged by the case manager as well. A van with a lift arrives according to schedule and returns Mr. Jackson when he has completed his visit.

Much of Mr. Jackson's treatment is paid for by Medicare, because his fracture was an acute episode.

However, Medicare Supplemental insurance covers co-pays, deductibles, and select other expenses. Mr. Jackson has long-term care insurance through a small group policy he purchased for his business, and this covers the homemaker and private van service. The personal health information service also compiles all bills, transmits them to the correct insurers, monitors payment, and sends Mr. Jackson a consolidated statement once a month, noting clearly how much, if anything, he is to pay directly. The explanation of benefits and payments are screened for outliers and errors.

Mr. Jackson is given a list of pertinent health Web sites to consult while he is homebound. He is also linked to a chat room of those recovering from broken hips and those with diabetes and hypertension.

FRAMEWORK FOR THE FUTURE

In the coming decades the demand for long-term care will increase. As the population ages, with twice as many people age 65 and older expected by the year 2030 (see Chapter 3), the nation will have many more frail seniors who require functional assistance over a long period of time. As technology increases medicine's ability to keep those with trauma and degenerative diseases alive longer, the nation will also have more younger people with disabilities and chronic conditions who need long-term care. As medical care moves steadily from the acute care hospital to an outpatient setting, the role of the acute care hospital will become less dominant, and care for those residing at home and in community settings will expand. As managed care links providers, payers, and patients formally in an ongoing relationship, the concerns of providers and payers will expand beyond acute care to the long-term needs of their clients.

The challenge is to develop an approach to long-term care that is efficient, affordable, and appropriate for the individual and family, and simultaneously affordable and cost-effective for society. The concept of the continuum of care presented here, and elaborated on throughout this book, is a framework for thinking about how to organize health and related services to achieve these goals.

FACTS REVIEW

1. Define "long-term care."
2. Define "continuum of care."
3. How many services constitute the continuum of care?
4. What are the seven basic categories of continuum services?
5. What are the four essential integrating mechanisms?
6. Why are integrating mechanisms necessary?

REFERENCES

Evashwick, C. (1982). Hospitals and older adults: Current actions and future trends. *Monograph in series on aging, Office on Aging and Long-Term Care.* Chicago: Hospital Research and Educational Trust.

Evashwick, C. (1987). Definition of the continuum of care. In C. Evashwick & L. Weiss (Eds.), *Managing the continuum of care: A practical guide to organization and operations* (pp. 23–43). Rockville, MD: Aspen Publishers.

CHAPTER 2

Clients of the Continuum

Laurence G. Branch, Connie J. Evashwick, and Jung Kwak

The clients who can benefit from the continuum of care encompass a broad range of individuals who require formal and/or informal care (health, mental health, or social support) over an extended period of time because they are unable to function on their own. These individuals range from people who employ wellness measures to control chronic conditions to those who have suffered an acute episode of illness and require a complex array of services designed to promote recovery.

Those who use the continuum of care represent a mosaic of subgroups, including those who have multiple chronic conditions, health problems complicated by advancing age, birth defects or congenital abnormalities, degenerative neurological conditions, strokes, major debilitating trauma or permanent disability from accidents, mental illness, and recent episodes of acute illness that require complex post-episode care. This chapter serves as an introduction to the clients of the continuum; subsequent chapters in Part Four of this book deal with specific subgroups. Caregivers have dual roles as providers of

care and as clients of the continuum. Caregivers are discussed in detail in Chapter 3.

Projecting the total demand for the continuum of care is like constructing an intricate jigsaw puzzle, with overlapping colors but separate pieces. The magnitude of aggregate need and potential demand provides the rationale for public attention to long-term care. The diversity of users of long-term care provides partial explanation for the diffuseness of long-term care services and the challenges of creating an integrated continuum.

DEFINITIONS AND NATIONAL PROFILE

Although there is no single "long-term care population," various definitions categorize those who use the continuum of long-term care.

Chronic is defined by the National Health Interview Survey, conducted by the federal government, as a condition that has a duration of more than

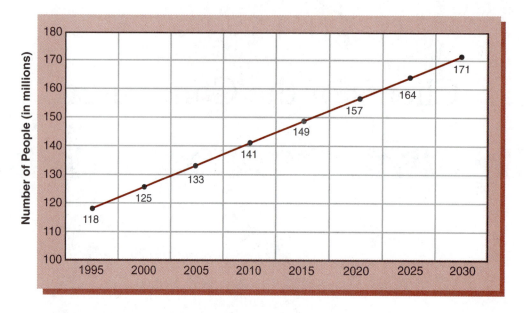

Figure 2.1   The Number of People with Chronic Conditions is Rapidly Increasing

SOURCE: Wu, Shin-Yi, and Green, Anthony. *Projection of chronic illness prevalence and cost inflation.* RAND Corporation, October 2000.

three months (NCHS, 1995). This definition does not imply any level of severity or the nature of the condition, merely duration. This three-month definition is somewhat arbitrary, but nevertheless useful as a common reference point.

Chronic conditions may be as life-threatening as coronary artery disease or as minimal as arthritis, which may be painful or inconvenient but is not life-threatening. Although most chronic illnesses are permanent, the definition also includes conditions from which clients might recover over a prolonged period, such as stroke disabilities that resolve over six months due to rehabilitation and recovery. Figure 2.1 shows the current and projected prevalence of chronic illness in the United States. Of the 280 million U.S. citizens in 2000, an estimated 125 million have some type of chronic condition (Wu and Green, 2000). Over time, this number is projected to grow to 170 million.

Chronic conditions affect people of all ages, but are more common among older people. Table 2.1 shows the prevalence of select chronic conditions and demonstrates the rise in prevalence with age. Chronic illness also affects people of all ethnic and racial groups, although some conditions are more prevalent in some groups than in others.

Impairment is defined as "a chronic or permanent defect, usually static in nature, that results from disease, injury, or congenital malformation" (NCHS, 1995). Impairments cause a decrease in the ability to perform various functions. Musculoskeletal and sensory deficits, such as, respectively, an amputated leg or blindness, are examples.

Disability refers to "any long-term or short-term reduction of a person's activity as a result of an acute or chronic condition" (NCHS, 1995, p. 5). Disabilities are wide-ranging in the types of limitations they impose. Almost one in five people in the United States has a disability (NIDRR, 1996). Figure 2.2 shows the aggregate number of people in the United States with disabilities according to level of severity.

Table 2.1 Selected Chronic Health Conditions Causing Limitation of Activity among Adults by Age: United States, 1998–2000

Type of Chronic Health Condition	Number of Persons with Limitation of Activity Caused by Selected Chronic Health Conditions per 1,000 Population			
	18–44 Years	45–64 Years	65–74 Years	75 Years and Older
	Rate	*Rate*	*Rate*	*Rate*
Mental illness	10.4	18.6	11.4	10.7
Diabetes	2.6	18.5	38.4	42.5
Fractures/joint injury	6.8	15.9	25.4	48.6
Vision/hearing	4.2	13.8	31.2	82.5
Heart/other circulatory	5.4	45.5	110.8	170.9
Arthritis/other musculoskeletal	22.0	73.2	117.8	193.1

NOTES: "Heart/other circulatory" includes heart problem, stroke problem, hypertension, and other circulatory system conditions.

SOURCE: Pastor, P. N., Makuc, D. M., Reuben, C., & Xia, H. (2002). *Chartbook on trends in the health of Americans. Health, United States (2002).* Figure 17, p. 64. Hyattsville, MD: National Center for Health and Statistics.

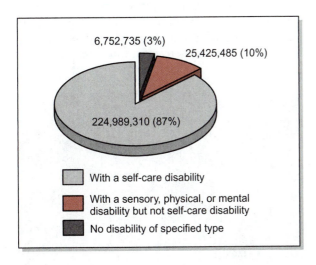

Figure 2.2 Selected Types of Disability for the Civilian Noninstitutionalized Population 5 Years and Over by Age: 2000

SOURCE: U.S. Census Bureau. (2004). *Disability status of the civilian noninstitutionalized population by sex and selected characteristics for the United States and Puerto Rico: 2000.* Retrieved September 23, 2004 from *http://www.census.gov/population/cem2000/phc-t32/tab01-USpdf.*

Functional status is the primary consideration that makes an individual appropriate for long-term care. Functional status is different from health or illness. If one is functioning at an independent and robust level, the services of a comprehensive long-term continuum of care are rarely required. If functional status is compromised, then the formal and informal services of the continuum are essential for the individual to maintain his or her well-being.

Functional ability has multiple dimensions: physical, cognitive, emotional, and social. Each can be measured or operationally defined in a variety of ways. Functional ability may be influenced by concomitant health, mental health, or environmental, social, or economic circumstances. Hence, people with the same chronic (or acute) condition may function at different levels.

The most commonly used measure of physical function is the assessment of basic activities of daily living (ADLs) scale. This was developed in the 1960s by Katz and his colleagues (Katz et al., 1963), initially for monitoring the rehabilitation of stroke survivors. The basic activities necessary for a person to perform on a daily basis are bathing, dressing,

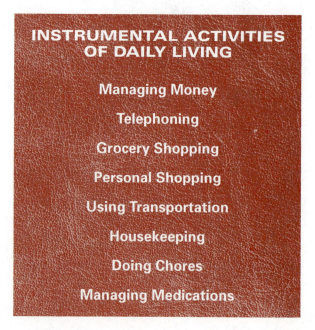

ACTIVITIES OF DAILY LIVING

Bathing

Dressing

Toileting

Transferring

Continence Control

Eating

SOURCE: Katz et al., 1963.

Instrumental activities of daily living (IADLs) comprise basic activities that one must be able to perform to live independently in the community (Lawton & Brody, 1969). Less standardized than the ADLs, they include functions such as managing money, telephoning, shopping for groceries, doing personal shopping, using transportation, housekeeping, doing chores, and managing medications (see box). Whereas ADLs involve use of large motor skills, IADLs are more likely to involve use of fine motor skills. IADLs also tend to require greater cognitive ability.

The groups of individuals with chronic illness, impairments, disabilities, or functional limitations intersect; however, they do not overlap completely, nor is a single pattern of progression always predictable. Moreover, some people with the same conditions may be users of formal continuums of care, whereas others rely solely on informal support or assistive devices.

Numerous paths lead to the need for long-term care because of inability to function independently. Figure 2.3 shows the multiple ways that a person might ultimately come to need long-term care from

toileting, transferring, continence control, and eating (see box). In the original construct, a person's ability to perform each activity was assessed according to one of four categories:

1. totally independent
2. requiring mechanical assistance only
3. requiring assistance from another person, or
4. unable to do the activity at all

The abilities to carry out these activities are typically acquired during the first years of life in a defined hierarchical order (i.e., eating, continence, transferring, toileting, dressing, bathing) (Katz & Akpom, 1976). Independence in these skills is often lost in the reverse order; that is, bathing tends to be the first loss of independent functioning, and eating, the last.

In subsequent years, a number of approaches to measuring ADLs have been offered, including altering some of the dimensions (such as adding ambulation or grooming) (Branch et al., 1984) and changing the metric from independence/dependence to degree of difficulty (Fitti, Kovar, & National Center for Health Statistics, 1987). However, ADL assessment has become a standard part of determining a person's need for long-term care.

INSTRUMENTAL ACTIVITIES OF DAILY LIVING

Managing Money

Telephoning

Grocery Shopping

Personal Shopping

Using Transportation

Housekeeping

Doing Chores

Managing Medications

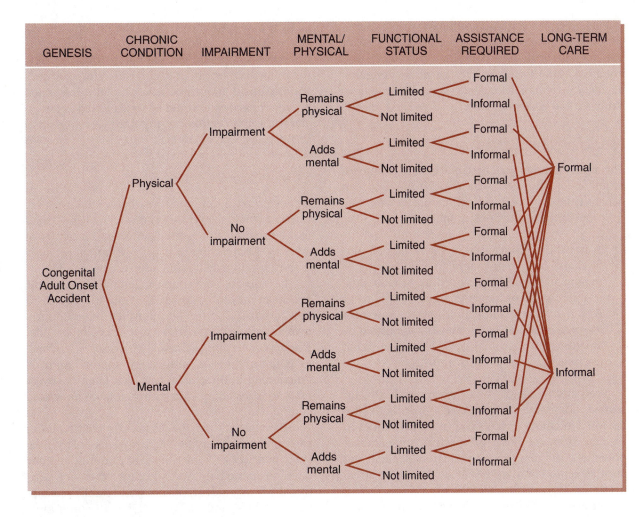

Figure 2.3 Progression of Chronic Illness

SOURCE: Evashwick, C. (1998). Progression of chronic illness. In S. Williams & P. Torrens (Eds.), *Introduction to health services* (5th ed.), Figure 11.2, p. 303. Clifton Park, NY: Thomson Delmar Learning.

formal or informal sources. As the figure shows, there is a multistage pathway from pathology (disease or condition), to impairment (at the organ or organ system level), to functional limitations (at the level of the whole person), to disabilities (at the level of societal roles) (Nagi, 1965). In another construct, the current World Health Organization (WHO) stages are labeled impairments (same as Nagi's), activity limitations (similar to Nagi's func-

tional limitations), and limitations in participation (akin to Nagi's disability) (WHO, 1997).

As Figure 2.3 shows, the paths to needing help with daily functioning start with different etiologies and progress with varying iterations. People of all ages and with a variety of conditions may eventually need formal or informal long-term care to assist them with performing the basic functions of daily living.

Each person's condition will have a unique progression, so patterns of service use may be similar, but not identical. This complex progression and potential variation in service use make designing payment systems for long-term care challenging to structure and costly to insure.

Need versus Demand

The distinctions between need and demand influence estimates of the size of the populations that can benefit from an integrated continuum of care. The concepts have been defined as follows:

- A **need** is considered to be the result of a professional judgment that a specific service or treatment should be provided to an individual to improve his or her condition.
- A **demand** is an individual's overt request for a service or treatment, presumably stimulated by a perceived deficit and a belief in the benefits of the requested service or treatment.

Need and demand are not always perfectly correlated. Sometimes the clinician's process of professional judgment is too stringent, other times too lenient. From the other perspective, sometimes a potential client may express premature demand and at other times fail to appreciate or recognize a real need.

The need-versus-demand distinction is particularly important in long-term care because needs are multidimensional and may not be manifested by acute episodes. It is thus often difficult for providers to recognize the need. From the client's perspective, demand may be weak or missing because people do not want to admit a loss of independence and because functioning may decline gradually and informal accommodations are made along the way.

In the context of fee-for-service (FFS) health care delivery, the financial incentives are to stretch the boundaries. If there is lack of concordance between need and demand, the FFS system incentives are to err in the direction of enrolling or admitting clients who are in ambiguous circumstances.

In a managed care system, the financial incentives with these ambiguous cases would be in the direction of watchful waiting before initiating service delivery. In an era of health care reform, organizations positioning themselves to offer integrated continuums of care would be well advised to understand the implications of the need-versus-demand distinctions.

Dynamic versus Static

At any point in time a subset of potential users are in fact *actual current users* of a formal integrated continuum that spans time, place, and intensity of services. Another group is using informal services. A third group may be using no services at all.

The popular conception that frail older people are on an inevitably downward trajectory is a myth that is not supported by published literature. Approximately one out of three people age 65 or older who report needing assistance with basic ADLs, such as bathing, dressing, and eating, report improved functioning in these areas one year later. Recovery rates are substantial and important in an integrated continuum.

At any given time, the clients of a continuum of care may reflect varying degrees of need. From the static perspective, some clients of a continuum may have no immediate needs because they are functionally independent, have a well-established support network, and have stable health conditions. Others may have modest needs at a particular time because of relatively complicated problems that require more assistance than their informal networks can provide. Still others may experience severe needs because of more complicated ongoing problems or acute flareups of otherwise manageable problems.

From the dynamic perspective, an individual client's needs can range over time from no need, to moderate need, to acute need—and back again. Both the individual client and the care managers who recognize the underlying fluctuating continuum of needs of the individual will tend to seek the efficiencies and advantages of a comprehensive integrated continuum of care.

Short-Term Long-Term Care versus Long-Term Long-Term Care

The clients of an integrated continuum fall into two categories: those whose complex problems likely will require multifaceted care over an extended or indefinite interval, and those whose complex problems are rapidly changing and who require care for a short period of time but with greater coordination than the client or family can be expected to handle without formal or professional assistance.

The first group tends to have chronic, persistent, multiple problems, with etiologies that are permanent. Their functional abilities may vary over time, but tend to decline rather than improve. The majority of these people who are able to remain in their homes with specific types of assistance have worked out informal relationships with friends or family to provide the assistance they need. Some depend on the formal system and pay out of pocket for help on a regular or intermittent basis. A relatively small proportion—about 5 percent—have health conditions and/or functional disabilities so great, or support systems so minimal, that they cannot remain in their homes, and must reside instead in institutions (i.e., nursing homes or adult group homes). The individuals in this first group are the classic *long-term care users.*

The short-term long-term care users are also in need of an integrated continuum because of functional disabilities. However, their use of formal services is finite. They are characterized by their rapidly changing pattern of needs, by an expectation of recovery or rehabilitation, and by their shorter reliance on an integrated continuum. These individuals may be recovering from strokes, hip replacements, or spinal cord injuries. The etiologies of their present conditions are specific and of short duration—a recent stroke, surgery, accident, or change of family situation that causes temporary dysfunctioning. Some of these may indeed become members of the first long-term care group, with expectations of extended or indefinite complex care. The majority, however, require the long-term care services of the continuum for only a short period of time. Nonetheless, once engaged with the comprehensive continuum of care, they may remain a part of the same continuum and use the acute services as episodic needs occur.

From the provider perspective, many providers serve both short-term long-term care and long-term long-term care clients, as well as acute clients. A Medicare-certified home health agency is a good example. Providers may or may not distinguish among long-term, short-term long term, and acute clients. The reasons for making such distinctions include staffing assignments (for long-term clients, one would try to get continuity of staff), reimbursement policies (a long-term care client might be eligible for Medicaid, a short-term care client might be eligible for Medicare), and efforts to educate client and family about self-care.

Clients of the long-term continuum of care therefore are both the traditional long-term care clients and complex short-term clients. The proper focus of an integrated continuum of care spanning time and place in providing intensive and complex care is on those subgroups that have complex problems, functional disabilities, and an inability to meet their own needs but yet cannot depend entirely on the informal support network available to them. The goal is to help these individuals access the type of support they need to achieve the highest possible level of health and functional independence, either by regaining temporarily lost function or by minimizing subsequent functional loss.

Institutional versus Community-Based Setting

The majority of people who have functional disabilities and are unable to maintain 100 percent of their independence reside in the community. A small percentage reside in institutions. Long-term care was once equated with nursing home care. After years of education, the connotation of the term has finally been changed. It is now widely recognized that people with similar medical and functional conditions may be found in either the community or an institution. Similarly, those within institutions may be more physically or mentally functional than those residing in their homes.

The factors that determine setting of residence are complex. They include family support and social structure, marital status, homeowner status, and financial situation. State and federal regulations about institutional admissions and payment also affect options for residence. For administrators, it is important to note that the type and location of care a long-term care recipient gets can be codified to only a limited degree. The array of factors involved varies for each individual.

Long-term care services can be provided to people regardless of their location of residence. A nursing home resident may receive home health care from an independent home health agency; people who reside in their homes may receive adult day services at nursing homes. A resident of a nursing home may receive care from a family member, such as a spouse who comes to help feed her at dinner. People who reside in their own homes may go to nursing homes to recover from acute episodes of illness or for family respite, but then return home. In brief, long-term care can be provided in either institutional or home settings, and the exchange between the two is ongoing.

SUBGROUPS OF LONG-TERM CARE CLIENTS

Select subgroups of the total population are more likely than others to require help from the formal long-term care continuum. In addition to distinguishing physical and mental conditions, continuum of care clients are differentiated by the array of federal, state, and local policies that provide, authorize, fund, and regulate services. Chapter 15 discusses how public policy pertaining to long-term care is formed and how it affects clients' use of services. Because of the disjointed funding and regulatory policies, the continuum of care varies for each subgroup.

Select subgroups of the long-term care client population and the continuums that serve them are covered in Part Four of this textbook. Subgroups likely to use long-term care services include the following.

Older Adults

Of all the subgroups, those who are age 65 and older are most likely to need and use the services of the continuum of long-term care. Older adults are also differentiated because they are the primary group eligible for Medicare. The older population is projected to grow dramatically during the coming decades, increasing from about 35 million in 2000 to 70 million by 2030 (see Figure 2.4), which will dramatically increase the need and demand for long-term care services.

The majority of older adults have one or more chronic conditions. They range from potentially life-threatening heart problems to conditions that produce functional disabilities, such as hearing impairments and arthritis. As a result of both chronic conditions and acute episodes, older adults are high users of all types of health care services.

Functional limitations also increase with age. Figure 2.5 shows the percentage of older people who have difficulty performing physical activity, ADLs, and IADLs. As is evident, those age 75 and older are twice as likely as those age 65 to 74 to have difficulty performing ADLs and IADLs. Whereas those seniors age 65 to 85 may have chronic conditions, the conversion from independence despite a chronic condition to need for assistance increases markedly once a person reaches the mid-80s.

Chapter 18 describes the services of the Aging Network, which are designed to help older adults with their myriad of health and health-related social support needs.

Children with Special Health Care Needs

Approximately 13 percent of the nation's 70.4 million children have a chronic condition that causes them to need special health care. The continuum of care for children includes the added dimension

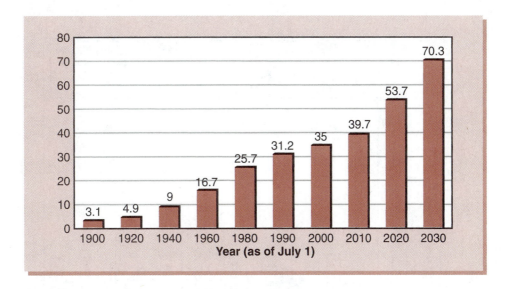

Figure 2.4   Number of Persons Age 65 and Older, 1900-2030 (in millions)
SOURCE: Retrieved October 1, 2003 from *http://research.aarp.org/general/profile97*

of schools and school health services. Chapter 23 discusses the continuum of care for children with special health care needs.

People with Disabilities

Disabilities affect about 13 percent of noninstitutionalized residents of the United States, or about 32 million people (U.S. Census, 2004). One fifth of these people have a severe disability that limits their self-care ability. Disability is a broad-ranging construct that encompasses people with many types of conditions, both mental and physical. Many of those with disabilities also suffer from other chronic conditions that exacerbate or are exacerbated by their disability. Disability is discussed in detail in Chapter 17.

People with Mental Disorders and Mental Retardation

In any given year, millions of people experience a mental disorder (President's New Freedom Commission on Mental Health, July 2003). These range from short-term depression and anxiety disorders to severe schizophrenia. A distinct continuum of care has evolved for those with mental disorders, including separate services, public funding streams, and professionals. In addition, about 1 percent of the noninstitutionalized population, or about 2.7 million people, is classified as mentally retarded. Chapter 20 discusses services for those with mental health disorders.

Informal Caregivers

Informal caregivers are family members and friends who volunteer their time and resources to assist a frail person who is unable to live independently due to functional limitations. According to a national survey of caregivers, at least 22 million informal caregivers provide care to adults so that they can stay in community settings. Caregivers provide help with a variety of daily demands, including ADLs and IADLs. Caregivers are discussed in detail in Chapter 3.

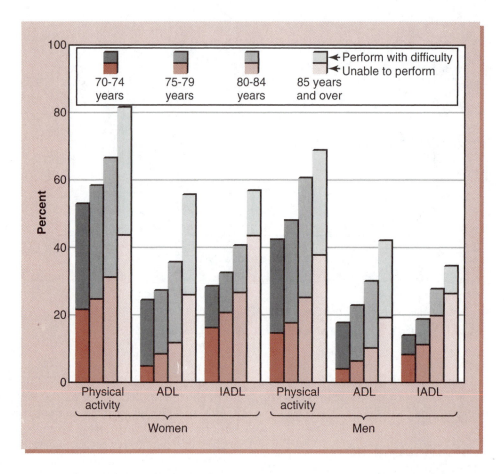

Figure 2.5 Difficulty Performing Physical Activity, ADLS and IADLS, by Age
SOURCE: Centers for Disease Control and Prevention, National Center for Health Statistics, 1994 National Health Interview Survey, Second Supplement on Aging.

Others

Various other subgroups of populations use long-term care services, and, in some instances, have unique continuums of care. Veterans, as discussed in Chapter 21, have their own set of services, funded and managed by the U.S. Department of Veterans Affairs. People suffering from HIV/AIDS may access services that are organized and funded by the provisions of the federal Ryan White Act, as described in Chapter 19. People with relatively short-term disabilities, such as those recovering from strokes or broken hips, may use the rehabilitation continuum (see Chapter 22).

As noted in Chapter 1, an ideal continuum of care is orchestrated around the needs of a specific client group. A given individual may fall into more than one category and may use services from more than one continuum. However, integration of services for the individual client remains the goal of the continuum, and this is easier to achieve when client needs, services, funding streams, accreditation standards, and regulatory provisions are aligned.

CONCLUSION

The clients of the continuum of long-term care represent a wide spectrum of health status and personal characteristics. Chronic conditions, impairments, disability, and functional disability are related but separate. Those actually using the continuum of long-term care services at any given time span all ages and have a wide variety of disabling conditions. They all share the characteristics of functional disability, which makes both independent living and customary medical care problematic. In designing a continuum of care, an organization must relate the services to the specific subgroup; a generic continuum is unlikely to meet the needs of a distinct target audience.

In aggregate, the number of people in the United States suffering from chronic conditions and disabilities is large and growing larger. The population projections are that the highest users of long-term care will grow in numbers and proportion of the U.S. population during the early part of the twenty-first century. For the acute-oriented health care system to meet the current and future demands of all those needing long-term care, major restructuring along the lines of an integrated continuum of care is essential.

CLIENT EXAMPLE

The ability to maintain functional independence may be inhibited by physical, mental, emotional, and social conditions, or even by economic circumstances. Which continuum of care a person uses, as well as which specific services within that continuum, depends on the nature of the problem. Consider the following example. An older woman is suffering from malnutrition, which is causing mental dysfunc-

tion, apathy, and physical lethargy. The woman may not be independent in eating because she has:

- A major physical condition affecting her digestive system that must be treated surgically to enable her to regain the ability to eat without indigestion
- Severe arthritis that makes it difficult for her to use a knife or fork
- Dementia, which makes her forget to eat or not remember how to do so
- Lack of transportation to get to the grocery store to buy food
- Not enough money to buy an adequate supply of food
- A stroke that leaves her with partial paralysis that makes it difficult for her to cook or prepare food

The woman's needs may be short-term or permanent. She may or may not recognize the problem.

For this woman, the role of the continuum of care would be to identify the correct cause of the eating problem, clinical or otherwise, and to ensure that the woman has access to the appropriate services. The services may be surgery, case management, high-technology home therapy, occupational therapy, telephone contact, home-delivered meals, transportation, application for Supplemental Security Income (SSI), or going to live with her daughter—depending on what causes her to be unable to function.

WHERE TO GO FOR FURTHER INFORMATION

Agency for Healthcare Research and Quality
540 Gaither Road
Rockville, MD 20850
(301) 427-1364
http://www.ahrq.gov

Centers for Disease Control and Prevention (CDC)
1600 Clifton Road

Atlanta, GA 30333
(404) 639-3534 / (800) 311-3435
http://www.cdc.gov

National Center for Health Statistics (NCHS)
6525 Belcrest Road
Hyattsville, MD 20782-2003
(301) 458-4636
http://www.cdc.gov/nchs

U.S. Census Bureau
4700 Silver Hill Road
Washington, DC 20233-0001
(301) 457-4608
http://www.census.gov

U.S. Department of Education
National Institute on Disability and Rehabilitation
Research
400 Maryland Avenue, SW
Washington, DC 20202-0498
(202) 205-5465
http://www.ed.gov/offices/list/osers/nidrr/index

FACTS REVIEW

1. What is the definition of "chronic"?
2. Name five common chronic conditions.
3. What is the difference between "impairment" and "disability"?
4. What do ADL and IADL stand for? Give examples of each.
5. Why is functional status more important than diagnosis in orchestrating the services of the continuum of care?
6. What factors determine whether a person with functional deficits uses formal long-term care services?

REFERENCES

Branch, L. G., Katz, S., Kniepmann, K., & Papsidero, J. A. (1984). A prospective study of functional status among community elders. *American Journal of Public Health, 74*(3), 266–268.

Centers for Disease Control and Prevention, National Center for Health Statistics, 1994 National Health Interview Survey, Second Supplement on Aging.

Evashwick, C. (1998). Progression of chronic illness. In S. Williams & P. Torrens (Eds.), *Introduction to health services* (5th ed.), Figure 11.2, p. 303. Clifton Park, NY: Delmar Learning.

Fitti, J. E., Kovar, M. G., & National Center for Health Statistics. (1987). *The supplement on aging to the 1984 National Health Interview Survey.* Hyattsville, MD: U.S. Department of Health and Human Services, Public Health Service, National Center for Health Statistics.

Katz, S., & Akpom, C. A. (1976). A measure of primary sociobiological functions. *International Journal of Health Services, 6*(3), 493–508.

Katz, S., Ford, A., Moskowitz, R., Jackson, B., & Jaffe, M. (1963). Studies of illness in the aged. *Journal of the American Medical Association, 185,* 914–919.

Lawton, M. P., & Brody, E. M. (1969). Assessment of older people; self-maintaining and instrumental activities of daily living. *The Gerontologist, 9,* 179–186.

McNeil, J. (1997). Americans with disabilities; 1997. *U.S. Bureau of the Census, Current Population Reports,* pp. 70–73. Washington, DC: U.S. Government Printing Office.

Nagi, S. Z. (1965). Some conceptual issues in disability and rehabilitation. In M. B. Sussman (Ed.), *Sociology and rehabilitation,* pp. 100–113. Washington, DC: Columbus Mershon Center, Ohio State University.

National Center for Health Statistics (NCHS). (1995). *Current estimates from the National Health Interview Survey, 1994* (U.S. Department of Health and Human Services, PHS Series 10, No. 193, p. 5). Washington, DC: U.S. Government Printing Office.

National Institute on Disability and Rehabilitation Research (NIDRR). (1996). *Chartbook on disability in the United States.* Washington, DC: U.S. Government Printing Office.

Pastor, P. N., Makuc, D. M., Reuben, C., & Xia, H. (2002). Chartbook on trends in the health of Americans. *Health, United States,* Figure 17, p. 64. Hyattsville, MD: National Center for Health and Statistics.

President's New Freedom Commission on Mental

Health (2003). Retrieved September 23, 2004 from *www.mentalhealthcommission.gov/reports/reports.htm*

Rice, D., & Hoffman, C. (1996). *Chronic care in America: A 21st century challenge.* Princeton, NJ: Robert Wood Johnson Foundation.

U.S. Census Bureau. (2003). *Disability Status: 2000.* Census 2000 Brief.

World Health Organization (WHO). (1997). *ICIDH-2: International classification of impairments, activities, and participation* (Beta-1 draft for field trials). Geneva, Switzerland.

CHAPTER 3

Informal Caregiving

Linda S. Noelker and Carol J. Whitlatch

Informal care is defined as ongoing assistance with a broad range of tasks, such as personal care, household help, and activities of daily living, from family, friends, and others who generally are unpaid. Family members, primarily immediate kin, assume most responsibility for the care of chronically disabled adults, typically with limited or no help from service agencies or other paid providers.

Most people with severe chronic disabilities could not continue to live outside of institutional settings without help from informal caregivers. According to a national survey of noninstitutionalized persons with chronic disabilities, 83 percent of those under age 65 had help exclusively from family members and friends, compared to 73 percent of those age 65 and older (Stone, 1995). Only 9 percent of disabled adults relied exclusively on care from professionals and other paid helpers. Clearly, the burden of long-term care for disabled adults falls squarely on informal caregivers. The economic value of this help far exceeds the economic value of help from

formal service providers. In 1997, for example, the estimated economic value of informal care was $196 billion, compared to a total of $115 billion for formal care, with $83 billion spent on nursing home care and $32 billion spent on home health care (Arno, Levine, & Memmott, 1999).

Should large numbers of family members and other informal helpers become unwilling or unable to fill this role in the future, the burden would shift to the formal long-term care sector, making the demands on this sector as it currently exists untenable. Due to social and demographic changes occurring in the United States, such a shift may occur in future decades. Current trends include a growing number of employed women, families with no or few children, blended families, families with geographically dispersed members, and a decline in the number of women age 25 to 54 (who typically serve as caregivers). As a result of these trends, and in recognition of the central role played by informal caregivers throughout the continuum of long-term care, more public attention and resources are being directed to services and interventions that support caregiver efforts.

PREVALENCE OF CAREGIVING AND TYPES OF CARE PROVIDED

The most recent survey of U.S. households indicates that 25 percent included an informal caregiver (Table 3.1). Estimates about the prevalence of caregiving vary in relation to the breadth or narrowness of the definitions used for *caregiving, caregiver,*

and *care recipient.* According to the U.S. Census, 18.6 percent (33.2 million) of the population ages 16 to 64 had a disability, compared to 41.9 percent (14 million) of those age 65 and over (Figure 3.1).

The types of disabilities affecting older adults include sensory (14.2 percent or 4.7 million), physical (28.6 percent or 9.5 million), mental (10.8 percent or 3.6 million), self-care (9.5 percent or 3.2 million), or difficulty going out of the home (20.4 percent or 6.8 million). In contrast, employment disability affects the largest number of those under age 65 (21.3 million or 11.9 percent).

Estimates indicate that more than 7 million of the 33.3 million adults age 65 and older in the

Table 3.1   Studies Documenting Prevalence of Informal Caregiving

Survey	Year	Prevalence
Survey of Income and Program Participation	1990	83 percent of disabled persons under age 65 relied exclusively on informal care; 72.7 percent of elderly 65+ relied solely on informal care
National Survey of Families and Households	1987–1988, 1992	52 million Americans (31 percent of the adult population ages 20 to 75) provide informal care to a family member or friend who is ill or disabled at some point during the course of a year
National Health Interview Survey, Supplement on Aging	1994	34 percent of those age 70+ received assistance from 12 million caregivers, of whom 73 percent are informal caregivers
National Health Interview Survey, Disability Supplement	1994	86 percent of those ages 18 to 64 received informal care only; 66 percent of those age 65+ received informal care only
National Long-Term Care Survey	1994	90 percent of chronically disabled elders living in the community receive some informal care; two-thirds rely exclusively on informal care
National Alliance for Caregiving Survey	1996	23 percent of all U.S. households with telephones contain at least one caregiver who is currently providing informal care or who has provided informal care within the past 12 months to a relative or friend ages 50+
National Survey of Long-Term Care from the Caregiver's Perspective	2002	25 percent of U.S households sampled by telephone contained a person who in the previous year provided unpaid help or arranged help for a friend or relative with an illness or disability

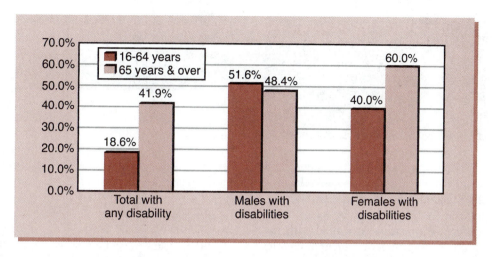

Figure 3.1   Civilian Noninstitutionalized Population with Any Disability by Age and Gender
SOURCE: U.S. Census Bureau, Census 2000.

United States require assistance with personal care or instrumental tasks, such as bathing, dressing, preparing meals, and housekeeping. About 70 percent of this long-term care is provided in the community, mostly by family and friends, who are estimated to number 5.8 to 7 million people (U.S. Department of Health and Human Services, 1998; Spector, Fleishman, Pezzin, & Spillman, 2000). In comparison, only 14 percent of home-based long-term care is supplied by paid professionals. When younger disabled persons or those age 20 and older are included, the estimated number of informal caregivers rises to 52 million (U.S. Department of Health and Human Services, 1998).

The increasing prevalence of Alzheimer's disease and other memory-impairing disorders accompanying the "graying" of the population is of concern because of the intensity and length of caregiving and related costs. Of the households involved in caregiving for an older adult, 5 million (22 percent) are assisting people with some form of dementia or cognitive impairment (National Alliance for Caregiving & AARP, 1997). An additional 1.69 million informal caregivers continue to provide some level of assistance to a relative once that person is insti-

tutionalized. These prevalence figures and changing demographic trends suggest that the number of people in need of assistance will grow dramatically in the twenty-first century. By the year 2007, households that care for people age 50 and older could reach 39 million (National Alliance for Caregiving & AARP, 1997).

FACTORS AFFECTING THE PROVISION OF INFORMAL CARE

The type of assistance from informal sources varies greatly depending on characteristics of both caregiver and care recipient. Pivotal factors for the care recipient are the type of debilitating disease and the extent of functional impairment. Care needs of cognitively impaired adults differ from those of physically impaired but cognitively intact adults. For example, caregivers of adults with physical impairments (e.g., stroke, traumatic brain injury, multiple sclerosis) report providing substantial assistance with self-care activities such as bathing, eating, dressing, and walking. In contrast, caregivers of people suffering from

> "I love him as much as the day I took his name, but I find myself wishing he were his old self. I realize it's not his fault he had a stroke and can't speak, but it can be tough. And I refuse to put him in a nursing home."
> —72-year-old caregiving wife

dementia or Alzheimer's disease report spending a great amount of time dealing with their relative's problem behaviors, such as agitation, wandering, and perseveration.

Other care recipient factors associated with the type and amount of informal care include characteristics of the social network (e.g., size, composition) in which the caregiving dyad is embedded, household income, and access to community services. It is often assumed that formal services will be used only after all sources of informal assistance are exhausted. Although this is true for some families, income level exerts a strong influence on service use, because most community- and home-based long-term care is paid for out-of-pocket. Thus, income and network characteristics are interrelated and instrumental for accessing services (Whitlatch & Noelker, 1996).

The characteristics of individuals that influence whether they become caregivers, and the types and amounts of care provided, include relationship to the care recipient; health status; residential proximity to the care recipient; and competing demands, such as full-time employment and parenting of young children.

> "My mother's becoming more forgetful. Thank God for the next-door neighbor. But she won't be able to help if my mother puts herself in danger. And I work full time and have my kids. There are only so many hours in a day. There must be help available somewhere." —51-year-old caregiving daughter

Table 3.2 Distribution of Caregivers by Relationship to Care Recipient

Relationship to Care Recipient	Percent of all Caregivers
Wife	13.4 percent
Husband	10.0 percent
Daughter	26.6 percent
Son	14.7 percent
Other female relative	17.5 percent
Other male relative	8.6 percent
Other female non-relative	5.7 percent
Other male non-relative	1.8 percent

SOURCE: Data drawn from Spector et al., 2000.
Percentages do not total 100 percent due to rounding.

The immediacy of the kin relationship to the care recipient influences if and when a family member serves as a primary caregiver. Spouses are first to take on the role and typically do not regard it as a responsibility distinct from marital responsibilities—a phenomenon also common among adult-child caregivers. Should the spouse caregiver die or become disabled, an adult child, usually a daughter or daughter-in-law, takes up the role (Table 3.2). When immediate relatives are absent or unable to serve, other kin, such as a sibling, are likely to become the major caregivers.

GRANDPARENTS RAISING GRANDCHILDREN

A related issue concerns older generations caring for younger generations. Though it is common for older parents to care for their chronically ill children, the prevalence of grandparents raising grandchildren is growing and now approaches nearly 5.5 million children (U.S. Census 2000). Differences in prevalence are evident by cultural group: 12 percent of African American children live with grandparents, compared to 5.8 percent of Hispanics and 3.6 percent of whites. Within the African American community, increasing numbers of mid-life and older women have primary responsibility for their grandchildren and great-grandchildren. Typically, a family crisis related to substance abuse, incarceration or unemployment and impoverishment precipitates grandparents' assuming the care of grandchildren. The conditions under which grandparents in general, and grandmothers in particular, become caregivers often reflect the broader context within which these caregivers live. Factors such as low or nonexistent child support, low income, legal entanglements to gain custody, and inadequate social support, as well as their own age-related health problems, place grandparents at greater risk of experiencing caregiver stress, and further complicate the caregiving situation. Grandparents are especially challenged as caregivers when the children for whom they care suffer from disabilities or chronic illnesses, such as inherited drug addiction or attention deficit disorder.

FACTORS AFFECTING THE EXPERIENCES OF INFORMAL CAREGIVERS

Gender

The caregiver's gender has a major influence on the caregiving process and its effects. An estimated 59 percent to 75 percent of caregivers are women, and the annual value of their provided care ranges from $148 to $188 billion (Arno, 2002). Female caregivers, whether employed or not, spend as much as 50 percent more time providing care than male caregivers (U.S. Department of Health and Human Services, 1998). The tasks undertaken by female caregivers also differ from the tasks of their male peers. Women are more likely to provide personal care assistance, whereas men are more likely to take on more instrumental tasks such as financial management. Moreover, women often have multiple roles in addition to their caregiving responsibilities, including hands-on health care provider, care manager, companion, surrogate decisionmaker, and ad-

vocate (Navaie-Waliser, Feldman, Gould, Levine, Kuerbis, & Donelan, 2002).

Caregiving women report greater personal distress than men, regardless of the care recipient's diagnosis and level of impairment. This finding is consistent regardless of caregiver employment status or the type of chronic health condition affecting the care recipient. However, in general, women score higher than men on indicators of stress and distress.

Ethnicity

Within the United States, recent research focusing on ethnic diversity among caregivers indicates both similarities and differences. For the age cohort between the ages of 45 and 55, Asian Americans are more likely to provide care for older relatives than other ethnic groups (AARP, 2001; National Alliance for Caregiving & AARP, 1997). Yet, across all ethnic groups, family care is the most preferred and relied-upon source of assistance. Extensive and supportive kin networks have been documented in Americans of all ethnic backgrounds, including Hispanic Americans (27 to 34 percent), African Americans (28 to 29 percent), Asian Americans (32 to 42 percent), and Euro-Americans such as Italian, Polish, and Irish (19 to 24 percent).

Employment

As noted, many caregivers have responsibilities related to their own careers and employment, in addition to caregiving responsibilities. Indeed, approximately 25 percent of employed adults provide some type of elder care (Bond, Galinsky, & Swanberg, 1998). Many who give care to people age 50 and older are employed full-time (52 percent), with an additional 12 percent employed part-time (National Alliance for Caregiving & AARP, 1997). For informal employed caregivers of persons age 65 and older, two-thirds report rearranging their work schedules, decreasing the hours they work, or taking unpaid leave to fulfill the caregiving role (U.S. Department of Health and Human Services, 1998, cited by Family Caregiver Alliance, 2001).

Transitions in the Caregiving Career

Caregiving can be viewed as "an evolving set of circumstances" that are long-term and continually changing (Aneshensel, Pearlin, Mullan, Zarit, & Whitlatch, 1995). The experience of caregiving reaches across a trajectory that includes demands and situations that can move from in-home care to institutional care through bereavement and, finally, adjustment and reintegration when caregiving ends. Because of the length of the caregiving role and changes over time, caregiving can be defined as a "career" with multiple stages and transitions, not a fixed set of experiences. Each stage within the career presents both distinct (e.g., relocation) and parallel stressors (e.g., time spent providing care) and taps unique resources as the caregiver copes with progressive change.

Caregivers spend a great deal of time providing care, ranging from an average of 18 hours per week when caring for people age 50 and older, to 20 hours per week when caring for people age 65 and older (U.S. Department of Health and Human Services, 1998). About 20 percent of caregivers spend more than 40 hours per week giving care, while a smaller portion provides constant or round-the-clock care (National Alliance for Caregiving & AARP, 1997). The long hours and demanding tasks of long-term care have a wide range of adverse effects on the caregiver's mental and physical health, finances, employment, and social and familial activities (see the "Impact of Caregiving" section later in this chapter).

The Transition to Institutional Care and Bereavement

Institutional care often becomes an option for families if the demands of providing care in the home become too stressful for a family caregiver or if the care recipient's symptoms and needs dramatically worsen or increase. In other situations, a specific crisis precipitates placement in an institutional setting (e.g., severe illness and/or hospitalization of caregiver or care recipient). Still, the tasks and responsibilities of caregivers do not necessarily end once a care recipient is placed in an institutional setting. Caregivers continue to remain very active following the care recipient's institutional placement, visiting nearly 4 days per week and spending about 10 hours per week at the facility (Zarit & Whitlatch, 1992). Caregivers of nursing home residents perform many of the same tasks they did while giving care at home, including assistance with eating, personal care, and walking.

Once the care recipient is institutionalized, caregivers must restructure and redefine their lives and adjust to their new role. Caregiving stress is not fully alleviated by placement even though these caregivers are relieved of the day-to-day demands. In fact, although some caregivers are less distressed, many exhibit symptoms well above their preplacement levels of distress, indicating that placement alters rather than eliminates care-related stress.

Disengagement from the caregiving role is the final stage of the caregiving career. Most frequently, the death of the care recipient initiates this stage, although it is not uncommon for caregivers to exit the role because of their own severe disability or by shifting their responsibilities to another family member or formal provider. With bereavement, caregivers are faced with the emotional, physical, and often spiritual aftermath of the death, and must confront the inevitability of reestablishing or reconfiguring their precaregiver identities and lives (Aneshensel et al., 1995). As with nursing home placement, the effects of bereavement can be both short- and long-term. The adverse mental health consequences of long-term caregiving, such as de-

> "In the last three months, I have felt very strongly it is time to put her in a nursing home. It is getting much more difficult and I don't feel the guilt I used to. I used to feel she would hate us and she would die there. Now I feel she might die sooner without that kind of care." —49-year-old granddaughter caring for 80-year-old grandmother

pression and loneliness for spousal caregivers, can continue for several years after caregiving ends (Robinson-Whelen, Tada, MacCallum, McGuire, & Kiecolt-Glaser, 2001).

INTERACTIONS BETWEEN CAREGIVERS AND SERVICE PROVIDERS

Relationships that develop (or fail to develop) between informal caregivers and formal helpers or service providers have a huge impact on service use and the outcomes of care experienced by care recipients. Caregivers often function as *gatekeepers* to and from the formal care system, influencing when, where, and from whom the care recipient obtains services. They also function as *intermediaries* between the care recipient and formal helpers by providing and interpreting information about care needs and service effectiveness. Caregivers can take the place of or assist professionals by serving as *care managers,* seeking out and arranging services for the care recipient and helping monitor service quality.

Because of service gaps and fragmentation along the long-term care continuum, caregivers fill the important function of *facilitators,* smoothing transitions between care settings (such as from hospital to home or home to nursing home). Because of their long-standing and close relationship to the care recipient, they are ideal *advocates* for individualized and high-quality care and quality of life in a long-term care system not designed to ensure these outcomes. Functioning in these capacities, as well as that of direct care provider, caregivers can be essential partners with service providers in the ongoing provision of care.

Correspondingly, formal service providers can function in ways designed to benefit both caregivers and care recipients. These include assessing the assistance needs of both members of the dyad. Caregiver service needs often include respite or mental health counseling, and formal providers can ensure that these services are accessible and provided. When

case managers target the caregiver and care recipient as a dyad for service planning and delivery, outcomes are better for both (Noelker, 2002). In nursing home settings, the adjustment of both caregiver and care recipient to the institutional placement is enhanced when nursing staff are responsive to family requests for information about their relative, and are perceived as providing good care (Whitlatch, Schur, Noelker, Ejaz, & Looman, 2001).

The nature of the relationship and interaction between informal and formal caregivers, however, can have mutually negative effects. For example, verbal and physical abuse of nursing staff in skilled nursing facilities by residents' families is not uncommon (Vinton & Mazza, 1994). The stress and frustration experienced by informal caregivers in their efforts to obtain information, access services for the care recipient, and navigate the bureaucratic mazes in the long-term care sector can result in aggression and other negative behaviors toward service providers.

Models of the Relationship between Informal and Formal Caregivers

Several models have been proposed as ways to conceptualize the relationship between informal and formal caregivers (see box). The *Hierarchical Compensatory Model* posits that there is a preferred order to who provides care, and this is based on the closeness of relationships (Cantor, 1979). Informal care is expected from the closest available and capable family member, with spouses as first choice, followed by children, other kin, friends or neighbors, and lastly, formal helpers. However, when care recipients are more severely impaired and need more assistance, or when the availability of informal helpers is limited, there is more fluidity and overlap between informal and formal helpers.

A second model of the relationship between informal and formal helpers is the *Task-Specific Model* (Litwak, 1985). In this model, the type of task with which help is needed influences the appropriate source for help. Informal helpers are best suited to assisting with nontechnical tasks and tasks that

> ## MODELS OF THE RELATIONSHIP BETWEEN INFORMAL AND FORMAL CAREGIVERS
>
> Hierarchical Compensatory Model
>
> Task-Specific Model
>
> Supplementation Model
>
> Substitution Model

cannot be easily scheduled, such as toileting and transferring from chair to bed, whereas formal helpers can best manage tasks requiring specialized knowledge and training that can be scheduled, such as wound care. As a result, the allocation of tasks between informal and formal tasks reflects a clear division of labor, with "dual specialization" or task segregation occurring between the two types of helpers. This arrangement is thought to minimize the likelihood of conflict and other negative outcomes occurring between the informal and formal helpers.

The *Supplementation Model* suggests that task sharing occurs mainly between the informal and formal helpers (Edelman, 1986). Because most assistance needed by chronically ill and disabled persons is routine help with personal care and daily activities, rather than technical and specialized care, supplemental assistance from formal helpers alleviates the time-consuming and potentially exhausting demands on informal caregivers.

In contrast, an alternative conceptual model is premised on the assumption that given the option, formal care would be used by families to substitute for informal care (Greene, 1983). The *Substitution Model* gives pause to planners and policymakers who advocate expanded reimbursement for community- and home-based services because of the presumed "woodwork effect." Their concern is that if publicly funded services become more widely available, consumers will gravitate to them, and the demand will exceed the resources available. Current U.S. policy

mitigates the need for the public sector to assume the full cost of long-term care for people with functional disabilities. Empirical evidence does not support the concept that families abrogate their role as the primary source of assistance to impaired relatives when service availability is expanded.

IMPACT OF CAREGIVING

Most research on the effects of caregiving has focused on its detrimental impact on caregiver health and functioning. Substantial evidence indicates that the stress of providing long-term care has a range of adverse effects on mental and physical health, employment, social and leisure activities, and family relationships (see Table 3.3). However, the study samples typically have included caregivers of persons with Alzheimer's disease or other forms of dementia. These disorders present the greatest challenges and stress for caregivers because of the associated memory and identity loss and behavioral problems exhibited by the care recipient. As a result, the negative effects of caregiving may be overrepresented in these samples, and thus overestimated. In recent years, more empirical attention has been given to the positive effects of caregiving, but far less is known about these outcomes than about its negative effects.

Physical Health Consequences

Caregivers typically rate their overall health more negatively than noncaregivers and do not routinely engage in good health practices, such as adhering to an exercise schedule, getting enough rest, and

> "She just won't accept anyone in the house outside of family. Pretty frustrating. I can't help her so much but she's just so stubborn, won't let anybody into the house because she's afraid of a nursing home." —69-year-old niece caring for 82-year-old aunt

Table 3.3   Summary of the Effects of Informal Caregiving

Negative Physical Health Changes	Negative Mental Health Changes
Poorer perception of health status	Depressive symptoms
Poorer health care practices	Clinical depression
Compromised immune functioning	Anxiety
Negative changes in metabolic functioning	Greater use of psychotropic medication
Obesity	Perceptions of caregiving burden
	Anger
	Insomnia
Employment and Financial Outcomes	**Declines in Social and Leisure Activities**
Absenteeism/tardiness	Reduced personal time
Decrease in hours or termination of employment	Decreased participation in social and recreational activities
Financial strain	Decreased ability to travel and take vacations
Exhaustion and lack of concentration	Less time for caregiver's own activities of daily living
	Loneliness
Negative Changes in Family Relations	**Positive Emotional Effects**
Marital discord	Increased sense of mastery
Family conflict	Caregiving satisfaction
	Positive caregiving experiences
	Enhanced sense of identity
	Personal growth

SOURCE: Adapted from Martire & Schulz, 2001.

watching their diet. About 30 percent of family caregivers of persons age 65 and older view their health as "fair to poor" (U.S. Department of Health and Human Services, 1998). There also is evidence of impaired immune function in Alzheimer's caregivers, reflected in slower wound healing compared to controls (Keicolt-Glaser, Marucha, Malarkey, Mercado, & Glaser, 1995), and impaired immune response to influenza vaccine (Kiecolt-Glaser, Glaser, Gravenstein, Malarkey, & Sheridan, 1996). Similarly, spouse caregivers of persons with dementia are more likely to be obese and have higher insulin levels than controls (Vitaliano, Russo, Scanlan, & Greeno, 1996; Vitaliano, Scanlan, Krenz, Schwartz, & Marcovina, 1996). Compared to family members who do not provide care, family caregivers are more likely to be in worse physical health (Stone, Cafferata, & Sangl,

1987), and those who feel strained with caregiving are more likely to die (Schulz & Beach, 1999). Despite these findings regarding changes in the immunologic and metabolic systems, research has not linked caregiving definitively to the onset of specific health conditions or diseases.

Mental Health Consequences

Family caregivers report being more depressed than age-matched controls in the general population (Haley, Levine, Brown, Berry, & Hughes, 1987) or family members not giving care (Dura, Haywood-Niler, & Kiecolt-Glaser, 1990; Dura, Stukenberg, & Kiecolt-Glaser, 1991; Pruchno & Potashnik, 1989; Tennestedt, Cafferata, & Sullivan, 1992). They also report more emotional strain in terms of higher

> "Physically, I am less and less able to lift her and help her when she needs full care."
> —82-year-old husband caring for 80-year-old wife

levels of depression, anger, and anxiety (Anthony-Bergstone, Zarit, & Gatz, 1988; Friss & Whitlatch, 1991; Gallagher, Rose, Rivera, Lovett, & Thompson, 1989). As a consequence, caregivers use prescription drugs for these conditions, as well as for insomnia, two to three times more often than the rest of the population.

Financial and Employment Consequences

Caregivers report financial and employment strain as a result of providing care over a long period of time, including lost income from leaving the workforce (Petty & Friss, 1987; Scharlach, 1989; Wagner & Neal, 1994). Whether the care recipient lives at home or in an institution, the cost of providing care to a disabled or demented family member can be exorbitant. In some areas of the United States, the cost of caring for an adult with Alzheimer's disease has been estimated at $52,000 per year. Compared to their same-aged peers in the general population, caregivers are more likely to report adjusted family incomes below the poverty line. Adding to this financial strain is the fact that the responsibilities of caregiving often lead to changes in work status. Caregivers often are disrupted and exhausted while at work, have trouble concentrating, lose time from work, retire early, or give up work entirely.

> "In general, I do a lot less of what I used to do. I used to be active in church, used to bowl, volunteer. Now, it's a challenge even to get to the grocery store, let alone have free time to socialize." —59-year-old caregiving daughter

Social and Leisure Consequences

A common complaint from caregivers is that they have little, if any, personal time. They also report little time to engage in social and recreational activities, to go on vacation, to go out for meals or entertainment, or to socialize with friends. As a result, loneliness, social isolation, and diminished social support also are widely reported, and may contribute to the depressive symptoms and other adverse mental health consequences of caregiving. Similarly, family conflict between caregiving children and parent(s), and between siblings, over where and how care should be given and by whom can exacerbate the stress of caregiving. Not having enough time for the spouse or marital discord for a married adult child caring for an aged parent can also have negative mental health effects.

Positive Emotional Effects

As noted earlier, far less is known about the benefits of caregiving than about the problems. This has limited the development of more balanced models of caregiving effects and interventions to promote more positive emotional effects. Caregivers report the following beneficial effects: the role is personally meaningful, an important part of their identity comes from caregiving, they gain a sense of mastery over the challenges faced, the relationship with the care recipient is enhanced, personal growth occurs, there is satisfaction with the caregiving role, and they take pride in the fact that the care recipient can remain at home and out of an institution (Hinrichsen, Hernandez, & Pollack, 1992; Kramer, 1997; Martire & Schulz, 2001; Walker, Shin, & Bird, 1990). Although these positive effects are important to caregivers, research indicates that the positives are not consistently associated with reductions in stress or negative mental and physical health outcomes. Yet, as noted by Kramer (1997), it is important for practitioners and providers to acknowledge and investigate these positive aspects for three reasons. First, caregivers seem to want to discuss their full range of experiences, not just the negative consequences. Second, clinicians and service providers may be able to work more effectively with caregivers if they have a better understanding of caregiving's positive effects. Third, these positive effects may reflect the quality of care provided to care recipients. Clearly, further inquiry into the positive effects of caregiving is warranted and has the potential to provide information and insight for use in service settings.

EFFORTS TO STRENGTHEN CAREGIVERS

The past 25 years have seen tremendous growth in caregiver services and support, as well as federal and state policy changes to benefit informal caregivers.

As Table 3.4 shows, services and interventions can be organized in relation to the area targeted for improvement (Kennet, Burgio, & Schulz, 2000). When caregivers are asked what would be most helpful to them, the most common response is information, education, and training. As a result, training programs in caregiving techniques, such as bathing, lifting, and transferring, are becoming more widely available, often through community colleges, the Red Cross, and similar organizations. National and regional associations serving older adults and caregivers make a great deal of information available through Web sites, chat rooms, and listservs, as noted at the end of this chapter. One innovative program installed computers in caregivers' homes, giving them access to a database on caregiving information while also enabling an electronic support group (Brennan, Moore & Smyth, 1995). The limited evaluation conducted on caregiver education and training programs, however, shows that such programs have little impact on health-related outcomes.

Cognitive, Behavioral, and Affective Interventions

Because of extensive reports from caregivers about burden and emotional distress, a variety of cognitive interventions have been tested to improve problem solving, time management, and coping skills; they have shown modest beneficial effects. Behavioral interventions focused on improving communication skills for caregivers of persons with dementia disorders provide evidence of increased conversation between caregiver and care recipient, caregiver self-efficacy, and positive caregiver affect. Most interventions have as one goal decreasing the caregiver's experience of negative affect and increasing positive affect. Individual and group or family counseling and caregiver support groups have been tested to determine their impact on affect and mental health. Although results are inconsistent and at times equivocal, findings have demonstrated the benefits of counseling for reducing psychiatric symptoms and caregiver burden, as well as delayed institutional placement of the care recipient.

Respite Services

Respite services are viewed as a mainstay for caregivers, allowing them a break from their responsibilities, and thereby reducing burden and providing personal time and time for social and leisure activities. Respite care is available in a variety of settings to meet the varied needs of caregivers for time away and the assistance needs of the care recipient. These include: private homes, through the use of home care workers and companions for the care recipient; adult day programs when the care recipient is capable of participating; and in nursing homes and other residential settings for short stays of a week or two. Unfortunately, many caregivers fail to take advantage of respite services altogether, wait too long in the caregiving process to access them, use too little, or do not make best use of the time away to maximize the potential benefits of respite care.

Evaluations of respite care benefits show that short-term use of in-home respite is more problematic for caregiver outcomes than ongoing respite use or no use of respite (Whitlatch, Feinberg, & Sebesta, 1997). This and other work suggest that caregivers often delay their use of respite care (Gwyther, 1994). Respite used "too little, too late"

Table 3.4   Services and Interventions to Improve Caregiver Well-Being

Targeted for Improvement	Service/ Intervention
Knowledge	Training programs in caregiving techniques
	Print and audio-video materials
	Web sites for caregivers
	Computer networks and chat rooms
Cognitive skills	Problem-solving techniques
	Time management methods
	Cognitive reframing/alteration of dysfunctional thoughts
Behavior	Communication skills training
	Cognitive-behavioral therapy
Affect	Therapeutic counseling (individual and family)
	Affect management skills training
	Coping skills training
	Support groups (peer and professionally led)
Alleviating caregiver burden	In-home respite
	Adult day program for respite
	Short-stay residential respite
Financial losses/Employment problems	Payment for caregiving
	Employee assistance programs
	Workplace interventions (job sharing, flextime, dependent care reimbursement, case management and counseling, on-site care center)
Physical environment	Home modification/remodeling
	Adaptive and assistive devices
	Safety and monitoring systems

SOURCE: Adapted from Kennet, Burgio, & Schulz, 2000.

(Deimling, 1991) may not be as beneficial as an early and consistent program of respite that is combined with other supportive services.

> "I am better able to handle things if I have some quality time to myself and know she is being cared for by people who care. That would make me feel so much better if I could have someone there I trusted. I could actually enjoy myself if I went out and someone cared for her properly." —42-year-old caregiving daughter

Financial and Workplace Interventions

To lessen the financial burdens of caregiving, support has been growing for publicly funded payments to informal caregivers. Currently, Arkansas, California, Oregon, and Washington are the only states that have large caregiver payment programs. Some programs provide small monthly stipends of $100 to $200 for caregivers; others enable the disabled person to employ and pay a person of choice, including a family member, as the caregiver. Under its initiative to promote community living for persons with disabilities, the U.S. Veterans Health Administration (VHA) offers veterans who are homebound or in need of aid and attendant services additional monetary compensation or pension to pay for home care services that can be provided by family members. The VHA also offers 30 days of respite care annually in VA nursing homes and intermediate care units, as well as contract respite care with community nursing homes. This service allows caregivers to take vacations or extended time away from caregiving. Other caregiver services available through the VA are support groups, information and education, and counseling services.

Workplace initiatives have been launched in response to the needs of employees with dependents. Most notable is the Family and Medical Leave Act (FMLA), passed in 1993. The FMLA requires employers with more than 50 employees to allow up to 12 weeks of *unpaid leave* to care for newborn or newly adopted children or family members of any age who are ill and require care. Employees' positions are protected because the law guarantees their right to return to the same or equivalent job—with certain exceptions. About 20 percent of the workforce takes family leave annually; however, less than 10 percent of these workers designate it as FMLA leave. Because FMLA leave is unpaid, most employees prefer to use paid time off under other provisions such as sick days, maternity leave, and/or vacation time (Keigher & Stone, 1994).

The number of corporations, businesses, and unions attempting to make the workplace more "family friendly" is growing. This movement is driven by an effort to recruit and retain the most capable workers by reducing conflicts between work and family responsibilities. These interventions include flexibility in work schedules, job sharing, and reduced hours with partial or full benefits. Under employee assistance programs (EAPs), information and referral services, case management, and education and support groups for caregivers are made available. Financial assistance for dependent care that is available through federal legislation to shelter tax-deferred dollars for payment are rarely used, probably because of employers' reluctance to expend the administrative time and cost of setting up and monitoring these employee accounts.

> "The [respite] money could be better used if we could hire my two sisters for $60 rather than taking her to a formal organization." —54-year-old caregiving son

Environmental Interventions

Environmental interventions are changes or alterations in the physical living environment that improve the care recipient's functioning and safety and facilitate the provision of care. The care recipient's mobility and safety can be improved through relatively modest and inexpensive changes, such as the installation of handrails in stairways and grab bars in the bathroom. Newer technological interventions include video cameras and sensors built into the floors to monitor the care recipient's movement, activity, and weight. Extensive research by Mann and his colleagues (1999) show the benefits of assistive devices and the application of new technologies for maintaining the care recipient's independence and reducing care costs. Other researchers have investigated caregivers' choices of environmental interventions that would best meet their needs from a list of possible interventions developed by a panel of experts (Pynoos & Ohta, 1991). The impact of implementation of the changes was monitored after 7 months, and 89 percent of the caregivers still found them to be very effective.

POLICY ISSUES

People with chronic disabilities, particularly the very old, disproportionately use acute and long-term health care services, whether home- and community-based or institutional (hospital, nursing home). Consequently, they and their informal caregivers are more widely affected by legislation that has significantly changed reimbursement for health care and led to corresponding changes in health care availability and delivery. In 1983, the implementation of the Medicare hospital prospective payment system dramatically altered admission and discharge patterns, effectively transferring 21 million hospital days to home and community (Estes & Associates, 1985). The "sicker and quicker" discharge of older persons from the hospital was viewed as placing a heavier burden on informal caregivers, as well as spurring the growth of hospital-based and proprietary home care agencies.

The passage of the Omnibus Budget Reconciliation Act (OBRA) in 1987 led to increased requirements for the training of nursing home staff and changes in resident care planning and review designed to improve the quality of resident care. OBRA also addressed the pressing issue of the frequent impoverishment of community-dwelling spouses of nursing home residents. Specifically, OBRA mandated policy allowing the community-dwelling spouse to retain the equity in the home and one-half of the other assets to facilitate their continued ability to live independently. The extent to which these changes actually resulted in improved care, more positive attitudes toward nursing homes, and decreased spousal impoverishment are not known.

The National Family Caregiver Support Program (NFCSP), funded through the Older Americans Act reauthorization in 2000, is the most comprehensive federal legislation supporting family caregivers. Funds are allocated to states through a congressionally mandated formula that is based on a proportionate share of the state's population age 70 years and older. As part of the NFCSP, states are expected to work with area agencies on aging (AAAs) to develop multifaceted systems of caregiver support in five areas: (1) information about available caregiver services, (2) assistance in gaining access to services, (3) counseling and the organization of support groups and caregiver training, (4) respite care, and (5) other services that complement the care provided by caregivers. These services may support caregivers of older relatives, grandparent and other relative caregivers of children age 18 and younger, and older adults caring for persons with developmental disabilities (Fox-Grage, Coleman, & Blancato, 2001).

Aging networks are currently in various stages of caregiver support service development. Many of the programs currently under development are innovative partnerships between AAAs and existing agencies that serve family caregivers. Some programs are working to ensure that direct cash payments are available to family caregivers, an option that is neither specifically included nor precluded by the NFCSP statute. Thus, direct payments may be possible for certain services as the state deems appropriate. Although there is great hope that the NFCSP will breathe new life into the caregiving service system, the potential for "reinventing the wheel" remains a real concern to many in the already existing, well-established family caregiver service delivery system. Overall, the NFCSP has the potential to provide valuable assistance and support to a variety of family caregivers, especially those not already linked to a service delivery system, as long as service replication is the exception rather than the rule.

Lastly, legislative efforts to reform U.S. health care during the Clinton administration prompted provider-initiated reengineering of hospitals and other health care organizations. Current trends indicate a move toward larger health systems in which flat fees are paid by insurers on a per capita basis to keep enrollees healthy. These changes were intended to limit the frequency and amount of service use and simultaneously contain health care costs. However, health care costs continue to rise precipitously, and growing concerns about patient safety abound. As yet, it is unclear how these dramatic changes in reimbursement and the organization of health care systems will affect patterns of formal service use and outcomes for people with chronic illnesses, or alter the role of family caregivers.

CONCLUSION

Informal caregivers are the major providers of long-term care to the millions of people with functional disabilities and chronic conditions who live outside of institutions. About one-quarter of all U.S. families report being engaged in caregiving activities, and the estimated number of caregivers to disabled persons of all ages is 52 million. Caregivers are typically immediate family members, with nearly two-thirds being spouses or adult children. Between 59 percent and 75 percent of all caregivers are women, who often have to manage multiple roles as spouse, parent, and employee in addition to their caregiving responsibilities.

Caregiving can be viewed as "an evolving set of circumstances" that are long-term and continually changing (Aneshensel et al., 1995)—that is, as a career. Major transitions or phases occur along the career trajectory, such as establishment of a shared residence, institutional placement, bereavement following the care recipient's death, and disengagement from the caregiving role.

Substantial research attention has been directed to the effects and impact of caregiving. Much of this attention has been given to the negative consequences of caregiving, such as depression, compromised immune function, social isolation, family conflict, and loss of leisure and personal time. Caregiving has a significant effect on the nation's economic productivity. Caregivers contribute thousands of hours of unpaid labor that would otherwise be required of a paid workforce. Conversely, hours spent during work time fulfilling caregiving duties reduces productivity.

Other investigations, however, that have explored the positive effects of caregiving report that caregivers enjoy an increased sense of mastery, enhanced sense of identity, and personal growth. These findings demonstrate the importance of examining the full range of caregiving outcomes in order to develop interventions that address negative consequences, as well as interventions that build on caregiver strengths.

Formal services and interventions can function in ways that benefit both caregivers and care recipients. For example, assessment of the needs of both caregiver and care recipient is essential in developing a comprehensive service plan for the dyad. In turn, caregivers act as gatekeepers to the service system, facilitators who smooth transitions across care settings, monitors of service quality, and advocates on the care receiver's behalf. Other services have been developed to target specific areas for improvement in caregiver functioning and well-being, such as respite services, education and training, support groups, and employee assistance programs.

Conceptual models of the nature of relationships between informal and formal caregivers provide a framework for understanding the primacy of various caregivers, their reciprocal roles, and the division of labor around caregiving tasks. Empirical findings from the investigation of these models have been used in the design of services for caregiving families and for policy development.

Over the years, a variety of state and federal policies have been established to support informal caregivers. Some of these include policies to prevent the impoverishment of community-dwelling spouses of nursing home residents, the use of public dollars to compensate family caregivers, and the provision of respite and other supportive services. In 2000, the National Family Caregiver Support Program was reauthorized as part of the Older Americans Act to extend the availability of information to caregivers about available services; to improve access to services; and to expand the scope of respite care, support groups, training programs, and counseling. This program reflects growing public awareness of informal caregivers' central role in long-term care. It also recognizes the importance of supporting their efforts with expanded services to ensure that caregiver health and well-being are not compromised while they continue to meet the needs of persons with chronic disabilities.

CLIENT EXAMPLE

Mrs. Johnson, age 43, is an African American daughter who has cared for her 84-year-old mother, Mrs. Saywell, for just over a year. Mrs. Saywell lives with her daughter, son-in-law, and two adolescent grandchildren in the suburbs of a midwestern metropolitan area. Mrs. Johnson continues to work full-time, but had to change her place of employment and take a substantial salary cut as a result of her caregiving responsibilities. Typically, Mrs. Johnson spends 15 hours helping her mother during the week and 8 hours on the weekend. She reports feeling very stressed because she has to manage her job responsibilities; her family's needs; the housework, shopping, and cooking; and her mother's personal care. Although helping with bathing, dressing, grooming, and medication monitoring is time-consuming, Mrs. Johnson is most frustrated by her mother's incontinence and toileting accidents.

Mrs. Saywell began showing signs of memory loss about five years ago and was diagnosed with Alzheimer's disease two years later. In addition to her memory loss, Mrs. Saywell exhibits other dementia-related behaviors. The behaviors most troubling for her daughter are the repetitive questioning, agitation, and wandering. Mrs. Johnson is bothered by her mother's irritability, which often makes her uncooperative when Mrs. Johnson tries to assist with dressing and other personal care. Mrs. Johnson feels that her brothers do not understand the severity of their mother's condition or how difficult it is to care for her; she believes that if they did, they would offer to help out and provide her with a break. She hesitates to ask her husband and children to help much beyond watching out for her mother's safety, because of her mother's resistance and uncooperativeness. Mrs. Johnson believes that she is a good daughter, but that her mother does not appreciate all she does.

At the time of her first visit with a social worker, Mrs. Johnson reported feeling very frustrated about managing all her mother's responsibilities. She also discussed her need for assistance as she began contemplating nursing home placement for her mother. Consequently, the social worker's care plan included short-term counseling, with the goal of helping Mrs. Johnson alleviate her depressive symptoms. At the same time, the social worker helped Mrs. Johnson make an informed decision about nursing home care by providing information about the many facilities near Mrs. Johnson's home and work. The social worker also encouraged Mrs. Johnson to arrange at least one family meeting with her brothers and their families; however, no meetings were held. The brothers consistently cancelled or failed to keep the appointments made with the social worker.

Three months after her first visit with the social worker, Mrs. Johnson's mother developed renal problems that affected her mobility and dramatically increased her need for care. Mrs. Johnson became increasingly exhausted. With little support from her family, she felt she had no alternative but to institutionalize her mother. Within two months of beginning her search, she found a nursing home that was acceptable and had her mother admitted. Because the nursing home was located near her home, Mrs. Johnson was able to visit several times a week. Mrs. Saywell died six months later. During this time, Mrs. Johnson continued to meet with the social worker. Mrs. Johnson experienced guilt about placing her mother in a nursing home and her mother's death there. Through discussions with her social worker, she realized that caregiving had caused her own health to deteriorate, as well as taking a serious toll on family relationships. She valued the hospice services she and her family received in the nursing home, and found them helpful in better managing the dying process and coping with the loss of her mother.

WHERE TO GO FOR FURTHER INFORMATION

The American Association of Retired Persons
601 E Street, NW
Washington, DC 20049
(202) 434-2300 / (800) 424-3410
http://www.aarp.org

For booklets on caregiving, titled *Miles Away and Still Caring: A Guide for Long-Distance Caregivers* (D12748) and *Care Management: Arranging for Long-Term Care* (D13803), write to:
    AARP Fulfillment (EE0321)
    Box 22796
    Long Beach, CA 90801-5796

Alzheimer's Association National Headquarters
919 N. Michigan Avenue

Suite 1000
Chicago, IL 60611-1676
(312) 335-8700; toll-free (800) 272-3900
http://www.alz.org

Foundation for Hospice and Home Care
228 7th Street, NE
Washington, DC 20003
(202) 547-7424
http://www.nahc.org

National Alliance for Caregiving—A National
Resource for Caregivers
4720 Montgomery Lane, 5th Floor
Bethesda, MD 20814-3425
http://www.caregiving.org

National Association of Area Agencies on Aging
927 15th Street NW, 6th Floor
Washington, DC 20006
(202) 296-8130
http://www.n4a.org

National Association of Professional Geriatric
Care Managers (NAPGCM)
1604 N. Country Club Road
Tucson, AZ 85716-3102
(502) 881-8008 (for information on how to find
geriatric care managers in particular geographic
areas)
http://www.caremanagers.org

National Association of State Units on Aging
(NASUA)
1201 15th Street NW, Suite 350
Washington, DC 20006
(202) 785-0707
http://www.nasua.org

National Center on Caregiving
Family Caregiver Alliance
690 Market Street, Suite 600
San Francisco, CA 94104
(415) 434-3388
http://www.caregiver.org

U.S. Administration on Aging
330 Independence Avenue, SW
Washington, DC 20201

Publications: (202) 619-0724
Eldercare Locator: 1-800-677-1116
http://www.aoa.gov

U.S. Department of Health and Human Services
Office of the Assistant Secretary of Planning and
Evaluation, Division of Aging, Disability, and
Long-Term Care Policy
200 Independence Avenue, SW
Washington, DC 20201
http://www.aspe.hhs.gov/daltcp/home.shtml

U.S. Department of Health and Human Services
200 Independence Avenue, SW
Washington, DC 20201
(202) 619-0257
http://www.dhhs.gov

FACTS REVIEW

1. Give three explanations for why there will be an increasing need for and decreasing availability of family caregivers over the next 25 years.
2. Briefly describe the four models that conceptualize the relationship between informal and formal caregivers.
3. List the five categories of potentially negative outcomes associated with providing ongoing care to a chronically impaired person, and give two or three examples of specific outcomes within each category.
4. What are some of the positive outcomes associated with family caregiving?
5. List four target areas for caregiver interventions, and for each area describe a service or intervention designed to result in positive benefits for caregivers.
6. How did OBRA affect the financial security and independence of caregiving spouses?

REFERENCES

AARP. (2001, July). *In the middle: A report on multi-cultural boomers coping with family and aging issues.* Washington, DC: Author.

Aneshensel, C. S., Pearlin, L. I., Mullan, J. T., Zarit, S. H., & Whitlatch, C. J. (1995). *Profiles in caregiving: The unexpected career.* New York: Academic Press.

Anthony-Bergstone, C. R., Zarit, S. H., & Gatz, M. (1988). Symptoms of psychological distress among caregivers of dementia patients. *Psychology and Aging, 3,* 245–248.

Arno, P. S. (2002, February). *The economic value of informal caregiving, U.S., 2000.* Paper presented at the annual meeting of the American Association for Geriatric Psychiatry, Florida.

Arno, P. S., Levine, C., & Memmott, M. M. (1999). The economic value of informal caregiving. *Health Affairs, 18*(2), 182–188. [Data from 1987/1988 National Survey of Families and Households (NSFH).]

Bond, J. T., Galinsky, E., & Swanberg, J. E. (1998). *The 1997 national study of the changing workforce.* New York: Families and Work Institute.

Brennan, P. F., Moore, S. M., & Smyth, K. S. (1995). The effects of a special computer network on caregivers of persons with Alzheimer's disease. *Nursing Research, 44,* 166–172.

Cantor, M. H. (1979). Neighbors and friends: An overlooked resource in the informal support system. *Research on Aging, 1,* 434–463.

Deimling, G. T. (1991). Respite use and caregiver well-being in families caring for stable and declining Alzheimer's patients. *Journal of Gerontological Social Work, 18*(1), 117–134.

Dura, J. R., Haywood-Niler, E., & Kiecolt-Glaser, J. K. (1990). Spousal caregivers of persons with Alzheimer's disease and Parkinson's disease dementia: A preliminary comparison. *The Gerontologist, 30,* 332–339.

Dura, J. R., Stukenberg, K. W., & Kiecolt-Glaser, J. K. (1991). Anxiety and depressive disorders in adult children caring for demented parents. *Psychology and Aging, 6,* 467–473.

Edelman, P. (1986). The impact of community care to the homebound elderly on provision of informal care. *The Gerontologist (special issue) 26,* 263.

Family Caregiver Alliance. (2001). *Fact sheet: Selected caregiver statistics.* San Francisco: Author.

Fox-Grage, W., Coleman, B., & Blancato, R. B. (2001, October). *Federal and state policy in family caregiving: Recent victories but uncertain future* (Executive Summary No. 2). San Francisco, CA: Family Caregiver Alliance.

Friss, L. R. & Whitlatch, C. J. (1991). Who's taking care? A statewide study of family caregivers. *The American Journal of Alzheimer's Care and Related Disorders and Research, 6,* 16–26.

Gallagher, D., Rose, J., Rivera, P., Lovett, S., & Thompson, L. W. (1989). Prevalence of depression in family caregivers. *The Gerontologist, 29,* 449–456.

Greene, V. L. (1983). Substitution between formally and informally provided care for the impaired elderly in the community. *Medical Care, 21,* 609–619.

Gwyther, L. P. (1994). Service delivery and utilization: Research directions and clinical implications. In E. Light, G. Niederehe, & B. D. Lebowitz (Eds.), *Stress effects on family caregivers of Alzheimer's patients* (pp. 293–300). New York: Springer.

Haley, W. E., Levine, E. G., Brown, S. L., Berry, J. W., & Hughes, G. H. (1987). Psychological, social and health consequences of caring for a relative with senile dementia. *Journal of the American Geriatrics Society, 35,* 405–411.

Hinrichsen, G. A., Hernandez, N. A., & Pollack, S. (1992). Difficulties and rewards in family care of the depressed older adult. *The Gerontologist, 32,* 486–492.

Keigher, S. M., & Stone, R. I. (1994, March). Family care in America: Evolution and evaluation. *Ageing International,* 41–48.

Kennet, J., Burgio, L., & Schulz, R. (2000). Interventions for in-home caregivers: A review of research 1990 to present. In R. Schulz (Ed.), *Handbook on dementia caregiving: Evidence-based interventions for family caregivers* (pp. 61–125). New York: Springer.

Kiecolt-Glaser, J. K., Glaser, R., Gravenstein, S., Malarkey, S. B., & Sheridan, J. (1996). Chronic stress alters the immune response to influenza virus vaccine in older adults. *Proceedings of the National Academy of Sciences, 93,* 3043–3047.

Kiecolt-Glaser, J. K., Marucha, P. T., Malarkey, S. B., Mercado, A. M., & Glaser, R. (1995). Slowing of wound healing by psychological stress. *Lancet, 346,* 1194–1196.

Kramer, B. J. (1997). Gain in the caregiving experience: Where are we? What next? *The Gerontologist, 37*(2), 218–232.

Litwak, E. (1985). *Helping the elderly: The complementary roles of informal and formal systems.* New York: Guilford Press.

Mann, W. C., Ottenbacher, K. J., Fraas, L., Tomita, M., & Granger, C. V. (1999, May/June). Effectiveness of assistive technology and environmental interventions in maintaining independence and reducing home care costs for the frail elderly: A randomized trial. *Archives of Family Medicine, 8.*

Martire, L. M., & Schulz, R. (2001). Informal caregiving to older adults: Health effects of providing and receiving care. In A. Baum, T. A. Revenson, & J. E. Singer (Eds.), *Handbook of health psychology* (pp. 477–493). Mahwah, NJ: Lawrence Erlbaum Associates, Publishers.

National Alliance for Caregiving & AARP. (1997, June). *Family caregiving in the U.S.: Findings from a national survey.* Bethesda, MD: National Alliance for Caregiving, & Washington, DC: AARP.

Navaie-Waliser, M., Feldman, P. H., Gould, D. A., Levine, C. L., Kuerbis, A. N., & Donelan, K. (2002). When the caregiver needs care: The plight of vulnerable caregivers. *American Journal of Public Health, 92*(3), 409–413.

Noelker, L. S. (2002). Case management for caregivers. *Care Management Journals, 3*(4), 199–204.

Petty, D., & Friss, L. (1987). A balancing act of working and caregiving. *Business and Health, 4,* 22–26.

Pruchno, R. A., & Potashnik, S. L. (1989). Caregiving spouses: Physical and mental health in perspective. *Journal of the American Geriatrics Society, 37,* 697–705.

Pynoos, J., & Ohta, R. (1991). In home interventions for persons with Alzheimer's disease and their caregivers. *Physical & Occupational Therapy in Geriatrics, 9*(3), 81–88.

Robinson-Whelen, S., Tada, Y., MacCallum, R. C., McGuire, L., & Kiecolt-Glaser, J. K. (2001). Long-term caregiving: What happens when it ends? *Journal of Abnormal Psychology, 110*(4), 573–584.

Scharlach, A. E. (1989). A comparison of employed caregivers of cognitively impaired adults and physically impaired elderly persons. *Research on Aging, 11,* 225–243.

Schulz, R., & Beach, S. R. (1999, December). Caregiving as a risk factor for mortality: The caregiver health effects study. *Journal of the American Medical Association, 282*(23), 2215–2219.

Spector, W. D., Fleishman, J. A., Pezzin, L. E., & Spillman, B. C. (2000, September). *The characteristics of long-term care users* (AHRQ Publication No. 00-0049). Rockville, MD: U.S. Department of Health and Human Services, Agency for Healthcare Research and Policy.

Stone, R. I. (1995). Foreword. In R. A. Kane & J. D. Penrod (Eds.), *Family caregiving in an aging society.* Thousand Oaks, CA: Sage.

Stone, R., Cafferata, G. L., & Sangl, J. (1987). Caregivers of the frail elderly: A national profile. *The Gerontologist, 27,* 616–626.

Tennestedt, S., Cafferata, G. L., & Sullivan, L. (1992). Depression among caregivers of impaired elders. *Journal of Aging and Health, 4,* 58–76.

U.S. Census Bureau. (2000). Retrieved September 18, 2003, from *http://www.census.gov/population/www*

U.S. Department of Health and Human Services. (1998, June). *Informal caregiving: Compassion in action.* Washington, DC: Author. Based on data from the National Survey of Families and Households (NSFH).

Vinton, L., & Mazza, N. (1994). Aggressive behavior directed at nursing home personnel by residents' family members. *The Gerontologist, 34*(4), 528–533.

Vitaliano, P. P., Russo, J., Scanlan, J. M., & Greeno, K. (1996). Weight changes in caregivers of Alzheimer's care recipients: Psychobehavioral predictors. *Psychology and Aging, 11,* 155–163.

Vitaliano, P. P., Scanlan, J. M., Krenz, C., Schwartz, R. S., & Marcovina, S. M. (1996). Psychological distress, caregiving, and metabolic variables. *Journals of Gerontology: Psychological Sciences, 51B,* P290–P297.

Wagner, D., & Neal, M. B. (1994). Caregiving and work: Consequences, correlates and workplace responses. *Educational Gerontology, 20,* 645–663.

Walker, A. J., Shin, H., & Bird, D. (1990). Perceptions and relationship change and caregiver satisfaction. *Family Relations, 39,* 147–152.

Whitlatch, C. J., Feinberg, L. F., & Sebesta, D. (1997). Depression and health in family caregivers: Adaptation over time. *Journal of Aging and Health, 9,* 222–243.

Whitlatch, C. J., & Noelker, L. S. (1996). Caregiving and caring. In J. E. Birren (Editor-in-Chief), *The encyclopedia of gerontology.* New York: Academic.

Whitlatch, C. J., Schur, D., Noelker, L. S., Ejaz, F. K., & Looman, W. J. (2001). The stress process of family caregiving in institutional settings. *The Gerontologist, 41*(4), 462–473.

Zarit, S. H., & Whitlatch, C. J. (1992). Institutional placement: Phases of the transition. *The Gerontologist, 32*(5), 665–672.

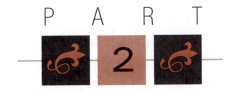

P A R T

2

Services of the Continuum

The services constituting a continuum of care number more than 60. For simplicity, these can be grouped into seven basic categories. The continuum organization need not own or operate all services; rather, it gives its clients access to them. Some services are used by many; other services are used by a relatively small proportion of those needing long-term care.

Each of the services has distinct operating characteristics. One of the foremost challenges of integrating service delivery is managing the operational differences to achieve coordination of care and efficiency of resource use. To manage client care across services, managers must have at least a basic understanding of each service.

The chapters in Part Two describe the operating characteristics and financing of the major services of the continuum of long-term care.

CHAPTER 4

Hospitals

Deborah L. Paone and Deborah M. Mullen

Hospitals are typically thought of as providing intense care to people with acute illnesses who have short inpatient stays. However, hospitals are also major providers of inpatient and outpatient care to people suffering from chronic conditions.

BACKGROUND

Hospitals in the United States have evolved from humble beginnings. Initially built as charitable institutions to house the poor and sick, they are now seen as the embodiment of high-tech medicine, offering sophisticated diagnostic methods, medications, treatments, and surgical procedures during brief stays and involving many highly trained medical professionals.

In 1872, there were only 178 hospitals in the United States (Starr, 1982). By 1920, this number had grown to 4,013 general acute care hospitals, with an average bed size of 78. The physical size and sophistication of hospitals grew, as did the number of institutions nationwide throughout the next 50 years. By 1970, there were 7,123 hospitals with an average bed size of 227 beds.

Thereafter, the number of facilities declined, as did the average number of licensed beds in each facility. During the decade of the 1990s, the United States experienced a 13 percent decline in the number of hospitals. By 2001, hospitals in the United States numbered 5,801, including short-term general community hospitals, military and federal hospitals, and specialty hospitals (American Hospital Association, 2003).

Advances in medicine during the twentieth century provided the means for curing or significantly reducing the impact of acute disease, infections, and trauma. Over that same time period, better public health measures improved water quality, air quality, food handling methods, sewage and garbage disposal, and identification and prevention of communicable diseases in the community. Given the success of medical advances and public health safeguards, as well as an increase in prosperity of the general population, the twenty-first century has witnessed a change in the nature of need for health care services in the U.S. population. A greater number of people now enter the hospital requiring care for multiple chronic health problems, rather than an acute episode of illness that can be quickly treated and cured. Today, the leading causes of morbidity and mortality are almost all related to chronic conditions (University of California, San Francisco, 1996).

Over the last 20 years, many hospitals developed services specifically targeted to older adults and those with chronic conditions or disabilities. Hospitals established both inpatient and outpatient services, such as:

- Geriatric acute care units (inpatient)—providing more extensive focus on the complex needs of older adults and attention to maintaining functional capacity
- Skilled nursing units (inpatient)—for short-term postacute care needs
- Rehabilitation units (inpatient and outpatient)—for physical and medical rehabilitation, often following an acute event
- Medicare-certified home health care agencies (outpatient)—to meet patients' needs for care in the home, following hospitalization
- Senior clinics (outpatient)—staffed with geriatricians and geriatric clinical nurse specialists, to offer a more comprehensive model of primary care, assessment, and prevention explicitly targeted to the older adult's needs.

These and other services were created in part in recognition of and in response to the growing number of older people in our society. However, certain factors have impeded the development of geriatric services by hospitals: restrictions on benefits and payment under Medicare, Medicaid, and other third-party payers; changes in regulation and marketplace characteristics; organizational culture; changes in the priorities of senior administrators; and workforce issues. These factors have acted as barriers to hospitals seeking to create a continuum of services that promote continuity of care across settings and over time. Nonetheless, hospitals remain a key component of care for people who have chronic care or long-term

care needs. By offering necessary high-technology medical care for an acute episode of a chronic disease, the care received within and following hospitalization can greatly affect both the short-term and long-term outcomes for a person with chronic care needs (Fletcher, 2000; Huckstadt, 2002).

Hospitals can ease any potential detrimental impact of hospitalization by being sensitive to the differences in the physiology and chemistry of the older body during hospitalization and by focusing on returning the older person to previous levels of function. Hospitals can also demonstrate greater awareness of their place within the continuum of care by building linkages with post-acute providers, improving post-hospitalization transition to other settings, increasing the flow of key information to other care provider(s) following hospitalization, and implementing disease management and prevention programs.

In most communities, hospitals remain a strong component of the local health care delivery system, and play a significant role in shaping the way in which health care services are provided within the community. Hospitals are thus a critical participant in the continuum of long-term care.

DEFINITION

What is a hospital? A hospital is usually a corporation, governed by a board of trustees, having organized medical and administrative staffs, that provides care for people who are sick and require acute medical care for more than 24 hours (Donabedian, 1979; Southwick, 1978). Hospitals must be licensed and may be certified. Licensure allows the institution to operate as a hospital in a given state. Certification allows the institution to provide care and receive payment for services for beneficiaries of Medicare, Medicaid, or other specified programs.

Many different types of facilities are encompassed within the definition of a licensed acute care hospital, including academic medical centers that focus on teaching, research, and clinical practice; community hospitals; and military, Veterans Affairs and government hospitals. Specialty hospitals include

SERVICE SNAPSHOT: Hospitals

Total number of all types of hospitals in 2001: 5,801

Total number of community hospitals in 2001: 4908

Average occupancy of U.S. community hospitals in 2001: 64%

Estimated average length of stay for U.S. community hospitals: 5.7 days

Number of admissions to community hospitals in 2001: 33,814,000

Number of outpatient visits to all hospitals in 2001: 538,480,378

Percentage of revenues from Medicare: 17.3%

Percentage of hospitals in multihospital systems: 46%

Accreditation: Joint Commission on Accreditation of Healthcare Organizations

SOURCE: American Hospital Association, Hospital Statistics, 2003

- Operating characteristics (e.g., average length of stay, admissions)
- Target patient population, clients served
- Services provided
- Payer mix, financial characteristics
- Marketplace characteristics

Select operating characteristics of various types of hospitals are shown in Table 4.1.

Number and Size of Hospitals

The U.S. hospital industry experienced major downsizing in the late twentieth century, both in terms of number of hospitals and number of beds (Sloan, Ostermann, and Conover, 2003). Though the number and size of hospitals have been declining since the early 1970s, this pace accelerated in the 1990s. From a peak of 7,174 hospitals with 1,513,000 beds in 1974, hospitals numbered 5,801 facilities with 987,000 beds in 2001, representing an average bed size of 170 (AHA, 2003) (Table 4.2). The average daily census for all registered U.S. hospitals in 2001 was 658,000, representing an average occupancy of 66.7 percent, although actual occupancy varied greatly from one institution to another and from one geographic area to another (AHA, 2003).

psychiatric, long-term care, rehabilitation, disease-specific, and women and children's hospitals. **Community hospitals** are any nonfederal, short-term general or specialty hospital open to the public (AHA, 2003). The definitions used to classify hospitals and the master data sets of all U.S. hospitals have been developed by the American Hospital Association (AHA), the trade association for U.S. hospitals.

HOSPITAL CHARACTERISTICS

The characteristics of the various types of hospitals differ widely, including

- Mission/purpose
- Profit/nonprofit status

Urban/Rural

The AHA defines **rural hospital** as a hospital located outside a metropolitan statistical area (MSA; in turn defined as a distinct geographic designation of an integrated social and economic unit with a total population of at least 100,000 people). *Urban hospitals* are defined as being located within an MSA. Looking at all community U.S. hospitals in 1997, 2,852 hospitals were located in urban areas, and 2,205 hospitals were in rural areas. Five years later, in 2001, there were 2,741 urban and 2,167 rural hospitals in the United States, a decline of 111 urban and 38 rural hospitals (AHA, 2003).

In general, urban areas have more hospitals and greater access to hospital beds than do rural areas. In many rural areas, there is only one hospital in

Table 4.1   Selected Operating Characteristics of Various Types of Hospitals, 2001

Hospital Type	Number of Hospitals	Annual Admissions (in millions)	Average LOS (in days)	Target Population	Average Bed Size
Total hospitals	5,801	35.6	6.7	People in need of acute, emergency and specialty care	170
General	4,880	34.1	5.8	All people in need of tertiary care	174
Psychiatric	503	0.77	36.8	People with acute psychiatric needs and the metally retarded	186
Rehabilitation	180	0.24	17.8	People with acute rehabilitation needs	85
Other special and long-term care	238	0.49	17.3	People in need of specialty care or long-term care	124

SOURCE: AHA, 2003. *Hospital statistics™ 2003 edition* (derived from Tables 1 and 2, pp. 2–7), Health Forum, LLC, An American Hospital Association Company, copyright 2003.

NOTE: Average length of stay (LOS) is computed as follows: number of inpatient days divided by the number of admissions. Average occupancy rate is computed as follows: number of inpatient days divided by the sum of the number of beds × 365.

town, and it tends to be small. In fact, 3,485 hospitals have fewer than 199 beds. About one-fifth of all community hospitals, or 1,100, have fewer than 50 beds. The majority (77 percent) of these smaller hospitals are in rural areas (AHA, 2003).

Most Americans live in hospital service areas with three or fewer hospitals, and 39 percent of Americans have only one hospital in their service area (Wennberg et al., 1996). Furthermore, the 3,436 defined hospital service areas have relatively small populations—92 percent of these hospital service areas have fewer than 180,000 people.

Pivotal work done by researchers from Dartmouth in the late 1990s revealed dramatic geographic differences in access to and use of medical care services, including services offered through hospitals (e.g., surgical procedures, inpatient admissions, physician visits). Even after adjusting for differences

Table 4.2   Number and Size of Hospitals, Selected Years

Year	Number of Hospitals	Total Beds (in thousands)	Average Number of Beds per Hospital
1955	6,956	1,604	231
1965	7,123	1,704	239
1975	7,156	1,466	205
1985	6,872	1,318	192
1995	6,291	1,081	172
2001	5,801	987	170

SOURCE: AHA, 2003. *Hospital Statistics™ 2003 edition* (derived from Table 1, p. 2–5), Health Forum, LLC, An American Hospital Association Company, copyright 2003.

in the age, sex, and race of resident populations, Wennberg and his colleagues found a greater than twofold difference in the number of hospital beds per thousand people (Wennberg et al., 1996). More recent studies have shown that more medical services do not, in and of themselves, produce better outcomes (Fisher et al., 2003).

Mission and Profit Status

Hospitals differ according to primary mission and orientation. Some hospitals and not-for-profit institutions have been established as community resources. Others are owned by shareholders as proprietary institutions. Both types of organizations have reasons to operate efficiently and provide high-quality care.

In 2001, there were 754 investor-owned community hospitals and 2,998 not-for-profit community hospitals (out of 4,908 community hospitals reporting) (AHA, 2003). The number of investor-owned hospitals increased 5 percent over the 5-year period between 1996 and 2001, whereas the number of not-for-profit community hospitals decreased by 4 percent (and the overall number of community hospitals decreased by 6 percent) (Table 4.3).

Mission statements of hospitals have continued to change and evolve as the industry and environment change. Missions have evolved from a focus on the acute care needs of those who entered the doors of the hospital to providing a continuum of care for individuals to improving the health of the community in which the hospital resides (see box). For example, Crozer-Keystone Health System, a hospital and primary care health system operating outside of Philadelphia, conducts a biennial community assessment, and the board of directors evaluates progress toward corporate goals related to community health.

For some institutions, an expanded focus on a broad continuum of community health care is difficult to maintain, as hospitals are paid only when people are sick or injured, and few sources pay for community health initiatives or services that lose money. Some organizations set aside a percentage

Table 4.3 Proprietary and Not-for-Profit Hospitals

Year	Investor-Owned Hospitals	Not-for-Profit Hospitals
1993	717	3,154
1995	752	3,092
1997	797	3,000
1999	747	3,012
2001	754	2,998

SOURCE: AHA, 2003. *Hospital Statistics™ 2003 edition* (Table 3, p. 10), Health Forum, LLC, An American Hospital Association Company, copyright 2003.

of net revenues to fund community health projects, including chronic care, while others budget for specific community health programs. Either strategy becomes very hard to maintain during tight financial times when layoffs or other operating challenges arise (Sandrick, 2001). In select states, hospitals

MISSION STATEMENT

The mission statement of Fairview Health Services, a nonprofit integrated health system of hospitals (8), clinics, and ancillary services in the Minneapolis/St. Paul area of Minnesota reads: "Fairview's mission is to improve the health of the communities we serve. We commit our skills and resources to the benefit of the whole person by providing the finest in health care, while addressing the physical, emotional and spiritual needs of individuals and their families. We further pledge to support the research and education efforts of our partner, the University of Minnesota, and its tradition of excellence" (Fairview Web site, 2003).

maintain their not-for-profit status by documenting the uncompensated care or other contributions they make to the community. Community benefit, whether imposed or mission-driven, has been a major source of continuum-of-care service development.

Development of Multihospital Systems

The trend of joining multihospital systems has caused a change in the management, control, and structure of many of the nation's hospitals. Over time, many hospitals have acquired or merged with other hospitals—a decision often driven by mission, marketplace considerations, financial situation, and competition. Some hospitals have come together voluntarily, with an interest in better serving the community by consolidating duplicate services, improving access to capital, enhancing diagnostic technology, and increasing patient volume. Other hospitals have been faced with shrinking volume and rising costs, and made the decision because of financial pressures. In 1975, about 30 percent of community hospitals were part of a multihospital system. In 1994, about 37 percent of community hospitals were in multihospital systems, and that number rose to almost 45 percent by 1997, when 2,222 community hospitals were part of a system. In 2001, 2,260, or 46 percent, of the 4,908 community hospitals reported belonging to a multihospital system (AHA, 2003) (Figure 4.1).

Some argue that hospitals that are part of multihospital systems are more likely to offer a broad scope of services of the continuums. However, evidence is mixed. The characteristics of the market, such as the proportion of Medicare enrollees, may also influence hospital service configuration.

Managed-Care Market Dynamics

Managed care was at one time purported to be a positive force that would drive providers, including hospitals, to offer a more comprehensive array of services for enrollees. Marketplace evolution varies

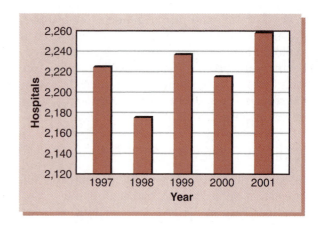

Figure 4.1   Hospitals in Multihospital Systems

SOURCE: AHA, 2003. *Hospital Statistics™ 2003* edition (Table 3, pp. 10–11), Health Forum LLC, An American Hospital Association Company, copyright 2003

widely with regard to price competition, managed-care penetration, and provider consolidation (Bovbjerg & Marsteller, 1998). *Advanced markets* are defined as those having high managed-care penetration, and major provider restructuring (e.g., as in Minnesota and California), whereas *early markets* have little managed care, particularly HMOs and organized provider groups, and are characterized by high indemnity coverage, as well as low physician supply and low-income populations (e.g., Alabama and Mississippi) (Bovbjerg & Marsteller, 1998). Managed care grew rapidly during the 1980s and 1990s. It began to fall at the end of the 1990s, and the number of Medicare managed-care plans decreased, leaving the relationship of managed care to the continuum of care uncertain.

SERVICES

Hospitals offer a mix of inpatient and outpatient services, both of which may be targeted at older adults or younger people with chronic or disabling conditions.

Inpatient Activity

Many of the operating characteristics of hospital inpatient activity reflect a history of growth through the early 1980s, followed by a decline. Shifts in inpatient volume have reflected changes in the reimbursement structure and payment levels for hospital inpatient services (especially by Medicare), as well as marketplace changes, shifts in practice patterns, and changes in standards of care due to new technology or new understanding about disease progression.

Inpatient admissions to hospitals rose steadily until about 1983 (the advent of the Medicare Prospective Payment System) and have fallen thereafter until recently. The incentives built into the Prospective Payment System (PPS), implemented in the mid-1980s, and, to a lesser extent, the effects of Peer Review Organizations (federally mandated quality review organizations in each state), combined to curtail inpatient admissions, make sure each admission was appropriate and necessary, and encourage the use of outpatient facilities. Hospitals moved from a retrospective, cost-based payment system to a prospective, diagnosis-based payment system. (Medicare PPS provides payment to hospitals for serving Medicare beneficiaries based on a classification of 467 diagnostic related groups, or DRGs. Each Medicare patient is assigned a primary DRG code, and payment is driven by historical costs for treating this condition, regardless of how long the patient stays in the hospital.) Admissions declined for most hospitals in the 1980s and 1990s. Patients' lengths of stay also declined over the same time period (Table 4.4).

Some hospitals responded to this decline by reducing acute care bed capacity and converting hospital inpatient space to other uses, including skilled nursing beds. Small, rural hospitals, in particular, created programs and services to augment shrinking acute care revenues. Many small, rural hospitals began participating in the federally designated swing-bed program, in which, for example, a given inpatient hospital bed can be used either as an acute care bed or as a skilled nursing care bed, depending on the patient's needs and the hospital's operating capacity.

Though overall occupancy for hospitals has declined since the early 1980s, wide geographical and hospital-to-hospital differences appear in occupancy rates. Hospitals in New England and mid-Atlantic regions report the highest levels (some more than 70 percent), whereas hospitals in the East and West South Central states report the lowest levels (some less than 60 percent) (AHA, 2003). Although average occupancy overall for hospitals in a given area may be reported as 64 percent, there are often peaks and valleys in admissions. Some hospitals in metropolitan areas may have a very high demand on capacity at certain times of the year and be nearly 100 percent occupied on any given day. These institutions may be forced to go on "divert status," where the trauma (emergency room) section of the

Table 4.4 Inpatient Operating Characteristics over Selected Years for U.S. Community Hospitals

Measure	1975	1985	1995	2001
Number of community hospitals	5,875	5,732	5,194	4,908
Number of beds (in thousands)	942	1,001	873	826
Admissions (in thousands)	33,435	33,449	30,945	33,814
Occupancy rate	74%	65%	63%	64%
ALOS (in days)	7.7	7.1	6.5	5.7

SOURCE: AHA, 2003. *Hospital Statistics*™ *2003 edition* (derived from Table 1, p. 4), Health Forum, LLC, An American Hospital Association Company, copyright 2003.

hospital is effectively closed to new admissions. Exacerbating this problem is a nationwide shortage of trained nurses and other workforce issues that limit hospitals' ability to operate at full, licensed bed capacity.

Outpatient Activity

Hospitals' outpatient activity has been brisk. Outpatient visits have grown steadily, reaching 612,276,000 visits in 2001 (Table 4.5). This reflects a change in the way medical care is delivered, as well as changes in payment structure. Many procedures and treatments that would have been performed exclusively in an inpatient setting 20 years ago are now done routinely on an outpatient basis. This switch from inpatient to outpatient setting has had a ripple effect on other providers, particularly home health care agencies and skilled nursing facilities. These nonacute providers have experienced a rise in the acuity level of their patients over the last three decades.

Auxiliary and ancillary services, such as laboratory, pharmacy, radiology, and other diagnostic and testing procedures, are increasingly important to hospitals' financial performance. According to the latest figures from the AHA survey, 35 percent of community hospital revenues came from outpatient services in 2001 (AHA, 2003).

The trend toward rising use of hospital outpatient services and shrinking inpatient use shifted in 1998, when inpatient days also rose. Inpatient days have increased slightly in each year since 1999. Outpatient visits continue to rise as well (Levit et al., 2003).

Patient safety in the hospital is an additional contributor to desire for fewer inpatient days and decreased lengths of stay. Iatrogenic illness (acquired while in the hospital) and hospital error are significant issues.

Emergency Department Activity

Emergency department (ED) usage appears to be climbing as well. From 1992 to 2001, ED visits rose 20 percent, even though the number of hospital emergency rooms declined. The increase in visits is attributed, in part, to the increase in the older adult population, general population growth, and a rising number of uninsured or underinsured who do not have a regular source of medical care and use the ED in place of a primary care physician. The volume of visits and the number of visits per capita are increasing. According to the Centers for Disease Control (CDC), visits per 100 people rose to 38.4 visits in 2001, from 35.7 visits per 100 in 1992, an 8 percent increase (CDC, 2003b).

Service Diversification

Hospitals have been diversifying their service mix for many decades. From the single institution focused on acute medical and surgical care needs, many hospitals developed related services, such as ambulatory and outpatient services, same-day surgery services, outpatient diagnostic and testing services, and primary care and specialty care clinic services. Many hospitals also extended their services to encompass pre- and postacute services and facilities, as well as community-based programs. Preacute services in-

Table 4.5 Hospital Outpatient Visits, Selected Years

	1975	1985	1995	2001
Outpatient visits (in thousands)	254,844	282,140	483,195	612,276

SOURCE: AHA, 2003. *Hospital Statistics™ 2003 edition* (Table 1, p. 2), Health Forum, LLC, An American Hospital Association Company, copyright 2003.

Table 4.6   Selected Special Services Offered by Hospitals, 2001

Special Service Offered	Number of Hospitals	Percent of All Hospitals
Skilled nursing care unit	1,722	36.4%
Intermediate care unit	450	9.5%
Acute long-term care	203	4.3%
Adult day services	435	9.2%
Assisted living	269	5.7%
Case management	3,376	71.4%
Geriatric services	2,006	42.4%
Home health services	1,915	40.5%
Hospice	1,118	23.6%
Palliative care	806	17%
Meals on Wheels	675	14.3%
Psychiatric-geriatric services	1,492	31.6%
Retirement housing	182	3.8%

SOURCE: AHA, 2003. *Hospital Statistics™ 2003 edition* (Table 7, pp. 151–162), Health Forum, LLC, An American Hospital Association Company, copyright 2003.

clude prevention and wellness programs. Postacute care services include skilled nursing care through short-stay, hospital-based skilled and transitional care units, home health care services, and rehabilitation units. In 1999, 58 percent of hospitals offered home health services and 45 percent had a skilled nursing care unit (AHA, 2003). Changes in reimbursement methodologies enacted by the Balanced Budget Act of 1997 caused some hospitals to close long-term care services. By 2001, about 44 percent of community hospitals offered home health services, and 39 percent of hospitals reported having a skilled nursing unit. Table 4.6 provides a breakdown of special services offered by hospitals in 2001 that may be targeted at those with long-term care needs.

Hospitals diversified into nonacute care for many reasons. In some areas, the "high-end" extended or postacute care needs were unmet by other providers in the community (particularly in rural areas, where health care resources may be scarce). Some hospitals saw this diversification as a continuation of their mission to provide service to the community.

Others saw a market opportunity, with local "baby boomers" facing care needs for their aging parents. Financial incentives to move out of what was viewed as a shrinking inpatient market and into the fertile outpatient and community-based care areas also played a part.

As discussed earlier in this chapter, Medicare's PPS had a great impact on hospital activity. Medicare PPS presented hospitals with the challenge of finding settings to discharge patients to; specifically, those patients who no longer needed the intensity of an acute inpatient setting, but still required some medical care, restorative therapies, and skilled nursing care. In addition, managed care organizations and other insurers increasingly demanded that hospitals discharge patients for recuperation in less costly settings as soon as medically possible.

Evolution of Multiorganizational Delivery Systems

Two trends in the late 1990s and early twenty-first century—consolidation of hospitals and service diversification—converged in many communities. The result was often the development of a multi-organizational entity that was described as a vertically diversified or "integrated" health care system. In the mid- to late 1990s, these larger, diversified organizations sought to offer a fuller continuum of services to address the needs of clients and the community in a more comprehensive way.

Unfortunately, two factors served as barriers to this vision of an integrated continuum of care, with the hospital providing the financial leverage and market strength to organize the continuum. First, a lack of understanding about the operating characteristics, culture, and regulatory constraints of each component of care hampered the actual connection of these separate facilities and services. The separate services (e.g., home care, nursing home care, hospital care, rehabilitation care, and community-based case management services) often continued to operate as they had before becoming part of the multiorganizational system. Common ownership, it seems, was not sufficient to integrate these large organizations. Second, payment constraints, arising from 1997 legislation governing Medicare payment to providers, affected each service segment and were compounded in the integrated delivery system, which now felt the pain in every service sector. Hospitals felt the need to return to their core business, acute inpatient care, rather than proceeding to invest in long-term care.

In the mid-1990s, in an extensive study of 11 organized delivery systems, most of which had deep hospital roots, Dr. Stephen Shortell and his colleagues looked at three aspects of integration within each delivery system: (1) functional integration, (2) physician integration, and (3) clinical integration (Shortell, Gillies, Anderson, Erickson, & Mitchell, 1996). *Functional integration* was defined as the extent to which key support functions and activities were coordinated across operating units so as to add the greatest overall value to the system. *Physician integration* referred to the extent to which physicians were integrated into the systems of care, often serving in a leadership role. *Clinical integration* was defined as the extent to which patient care services

were coordinated across people, facilities, functions, activities, and time.

Not surprisingly, the study found obstacles to each type of integration, including lack of knowledge or awareness about integration, continued commitment to individual operating units (especially the hospital), lack of geographic concentration of personnel, lack of infrastructure support (particularly information systems), comfort with the status quo, lack of aligned financial incentives, and fear among staff about what integration would mean for them. Shortell's work illustrated how difficult it is for hospital systems to operate as a seamless continuum of services organized around community need. Clinical integration, especially, was seen as "difficult, life-long work," because it involves changing so much of what is currently a standard approach to care (Shortell et al., 1996).

The movement toward developing hospital-driven, vertically integrated systems peaked in the 1990s. Fragmentation across services, which had begun to be bridged under hospital leadership, persists. It remains to be seen if at some point in the future hospitals will once again assume the charge to create integrated continuums of care for those with chronic illnesses.

CLIENT PROFILE

The general short-term community hospital serves people of all ages, with all types of diagnoses and conditions. However, hospitals increasingly serve older adults and those with an acute exacerbation of a chronic disease. People over age 65 represent about 12 percent of the U.S. population, but they typically represent 46 percent of hospitalized patients (Figure 4.2).

Older people are admitted more frequently and generally require longer lengths of stay than younger people in the hospital. The AHA's hospital panel survey reported an average length of stay of 6.0 days for older adults versus 4.6 days for people under age 65 in 2001 (data provided for selected short-term community hospitals). The number of dis-

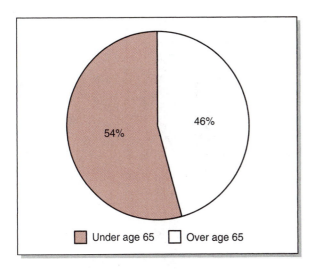

Figure 4.2 Patient Days by Age
SOURCE: AHA, Trend Analysis Group (1998–2002)
National Hospital Indicators Survey data for 1998:
4–2001:4. Reported by CMS on *http://www.cms.hhs.gov/
statistics. Hospital Statistics™ 2003* edition, Health
Forum LLC, An American Hospital Association
Company, copyright 2003.

charges per 1,000 people, a measure of the rate of
use, is also higher for people over age 65. The discharge rate per 1,000 people for those under age
65 is 89 per 1,000, versus 414 per 1,000 for those
age 65 and over (Figure 4.3).

For the older adult, hospitalization often leads to
temporary or permanent functional decline, and
can exacerbate conditions such as confusion, aggressive behavior, memory impairment, poor nutritional status, and caregiver burden. Studies have
shown that older adults perceive hospitalization as
presenting many threats to their health, quality of
life, and independence (Fletcher, 2000; Huckstadt,
2002).

Consistent with the differences in hospital type,
hospitals differ in the profile of patients they treat.
For example, the average age of the patients treated
and key admitting diagnoses vary according to hospital type (e.g., long-term care hospital, children's
hospital, women's hospital, academic medical cen-

ter). The leading diagnoses upon discharge for all
patients are:

Men	Women (excluding delivery)
1. Disease of the heart	1. Disease of the heart
2. Mental illness/substance abuse	2. Malignant neoplasm
3. Cerebral vascular disease	3. Cerebral vascular disease
4. Malignant neoplasm	4. Injury
5. Injury	5. Mental illness/substance abuse
6. Pneumonia	6. Pneumonia

SOURCE: *Health, United States, 2002,* Table 93
(National Center for Health Statistics, 2002).

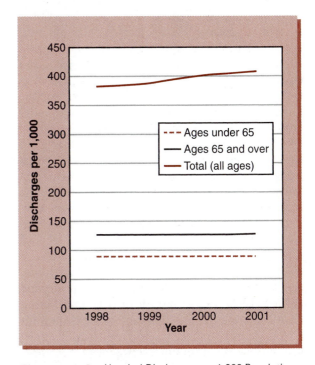

Figure 4.3 Hospital Discharges per 1,000 Population,
by Age Group, for Selected Community Hospitals
SOURCE: AHA, Trend Analysis Group (1998–2002)
National Hospital Indicators Survey data for 1998:
4–2001:4. Reported by CMS on *http://www.cms.hhs.gov/
statistics. Hospital Statistics™ 2003* edition, Health
Forum LLC, An American Hospital Association
Company, copyright 2003.

FINANCING

Expenditures for hospital services represent a significant proportion of total health care spending. In 2001, expenditures for hospital care were $451 billion, or nearly 32 percent of the total national health expenditures for the year (Centers for Medicare and Medicaid Services, 2003a).

Sources of Payment

The typical short-term community hospital relies heavily on governmental sources of payment, particularly Medicare and Medicaid. In 2001, approximately 17 percent of hospital revenues were from Medicare, and 16 percent from Medicaid. Other sources of payment include managed care (an average of 34 percent), other third-party payer, direct out-of-pocket payments by patients (self-pay), and other (see Figure 4.4). The distribution of payer type varies widely from one facility to another. A public inner-city hospital, for example, would rely more heavily on Medicaid as a primary payment source, whereas a hospital located in a second-tier affluent suburb would likely have more patients with third-party insurance offered through an employer. Similarly, average cost per discharge varies across the nation by as much as 20 percent for the same condition (U.S. Department of Health and Human Services, 1998).

Medicare changes in payment methods and rates over the last three decades have had a profound impact on hospitals and the spectrum of acute and long-term services they provide. In 1984, the Health Care Financing Administration (now the Centers for Medicare and Medicaid Services, or CMS) implemented the Medicare Prospective Payment System for hospitals. The effect on inpatient activity of this payment restructuring was described previously in this chapter. Changes in payment methods or rates by Medicare are often followed by other third-party payers. Therefore, the impact of modifying the Medicare program extends throughout the health care system.

In the late twentieth century, hospitals experi-

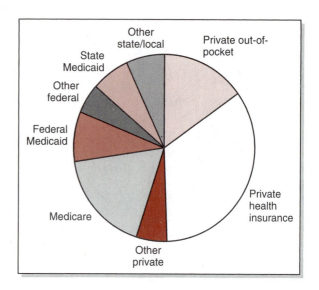

Figure 4.4 Sources of Hospital Revenue, by Payer, 2000

SOURCE: AHA, Trend Analysis Group (1998–2002) National Hospital Indicators Survey data for 1998: 4–2001:4. Reported by CMS on *http://www.cms.hhs.gov/ statistics. Hospital Statistics™ 2003* edition, Health Forum LLC, An American Hospital Association Company, copyright 2003.

enced provider payment changes due to the Balanced Budget Act of 1997 (Public Law No. 105-33, known as the BBA). This legislation was especially difficult for the hospital or health system that had diversified into many settings or programs of care, as the act resulted in budget cuts in each program. Many hospitals closed their home health care agencies and skilled nursing units, thus reducing continuity of care for individuals making the transition from acute to postacute care. The fallout from BBA 97 was still being felt in the first few years of the twenty-first century.

Financial Performance

Financial performance of hospitals nationwide has risen and declined over the years, particularly in conjunction with payment or regulatory changes in the Medicare program. In 2001, high-performing hospitals had a total margin of 8.6 percent, compared to low-performing hospitals, which had a margin of –2.3 percent. This gap has widened over the last several years. In addition, the overall profitability of hospitals declined from 1998 through 2003 due to the BBA of 1997. The majority of the impact from this legislation on hospitals is thought to have occurred by 2002, and hospital financial performance was expected to stabilize over the next few years (CHIPs, 2003). Nonetheless, the financial trauma caused by the BBA negatively affected hospital initiatives in establishing comprehensive continuums of care (Evashwick & Smith, 2000).

LICENSURE, CERTIFICATION, AND ACCREDITATION

Licensure and Certification

Hospitals are licensed according to the requirements established by the state in which they are located. Certification requirements to participate in Medicare are implemented by the Centers for Medicare and Medicaid Services. CMS reported 6,002 Medicare-certified hospitals as of 2001 (CMS, 2003b). Medicaid and other government and private payers tend to follow Medicare certification requirements, but may add their own criteria.

Accreditation

Most hospitals are accredited by the Joint Commission on Accreditation of Healthcare Organizations (JCAHO). This accreditation provides "deemed status" for hospitals; that is, a hospital that meets or exceeds JCAHO accreditation standards is "deemed" to have met the federal Medicare certification standards for hospitals. These accredited institutions may then provide care to people covered under the Medicare (and usually Medicaid) programs and receive payment for these services from the federal government. The JCAHO reports that there were 4,765 accredited U.S. hospitals in 2002 (JCAHO, 2003).

Quality

In recent years, both external evaluators of quality of care and payers (including federal agencies, health plans, and employers) have demonstrated greater interest in assessing the outcomes of care, rather than focusing only on the structure and processes of care. Through the development of standardized assessment and data collection instruments, as well as outcomes measures, greater comparability across organizations on a variety of indices is possible (Paone, 2001).

The interest in improving outcomes of care was particularly enhanced by a seminal Institute of Medicine report, *To Err Is Human,* which estimated that medical errors in hospitals account for as many as 98,000 deaths per year in the United States (Kohn, Corrigan, & Donaldson, 1999). Multiple studies have estimated that the rate of adverse events (injuries caused by medical interventions) is between 2.9 and 3.7 percent of all hospitalizations (Kohn, Corrigan, & Donaldson, 1999). Each day of hospitalization is estimated to increase a patient's chances of experiencing an adverse event by 6 percent (Kohn, Corrigan, & Donaldson, 1999). Adverse patient events also include approximately 2 million nosocomial (hospital-acquired) infections annually, according to the Centers for Disease Control (CDC, 1992).

In an attempt to improve the quality of care, hospitals are increasing their use of technology to integrate information used by clinicians involved in care of hospital patients. Electronic medical records (EMRs) systems vary in level of sophistication and capabilities. Quicker access to patient information and reduced need for employees to track paper files are two of the largest benefits of EMRs. Included in many EMRs are pharmaceutical checks and care pathways protocols. These checks and protocols warn providers of potential risks of treatments and offer resources that the provider can utilize to decrease a patient's length of stay. National criteria sets can also be loaded into EMRs to enable providers to compare their lengths of stays with national and regional best practices.

INNOVATIONS IN CARE

National Demonstrations. Over the last 20 to 30 years, many hospitals have played an important role as innovators in care for older adults and those with chronic conditions or disabilities. These forward-thinking institutions have participated in national demonstrations or pilots to test new models of care. For example, hospitals have been active in the On Lok/PACE replication demonstration (see Chapter 8) and the development of permanent PACE sites, now that this program has permanent provider status. Hospitals have also participated in national demonstrations such as the Robert Wood Johnson Foundation's Hospital Initiatives in Long-Term Care, the Community Nursing Organization demonstration, the Medicare Alzheimer's Disease Demonstration, and others.

Disease Management and Redesign of Care. Many hospitals have embraced disease management as a strategy to better manage care for targeted patients with specific chronic diseases that are known to lead to high health care utilization and high costs. Diseases such as congestive heart failure, diabetes, and COPD/asthma are often chosen as the focus of disease management programs, since these diseases offer potential for better clinical care management and for improved patient self-care support. They are also potentially high-cost, chronic conditions that can result in hospitalization if the patient fails at self-management in the community. Keys to success for disease management programs include: appropriate targeting of patients, early contact (prior to extensive decline), a defined set of indicators for monitoring effectiveness, health education and support for patient self-care and prevention behaviors, regular follow-up, effective documentation, information sharing and feedback, and ongoing collaboration with other providers involved in the person's care (see Chapter 10).

Many hospitals have developed their own approaches to disease management for select conditions, often drawing on national evidence-based guidelines that serve as the centerpiece for their care processes and management approaches. In particular, those hospitals that have extensive ambulatory or primary care services and participate in some kind of risk arrangement for a defined population group have had an incentive to manage beyond the inpatient setting. Similarly, many managed-care organizations have a financial interest in managing the care of high-risk enrolled members more effectively, and so have developed their own approaches to disease management in conjunction with hospitals and physicians. CMS also launched a number of demonstrations in the early twenty-first century around disease management, and has advocated this approach as a promising strategy for providing better care to Medicare beneficiaries with chronic conditions.

Hospitals also have recognized the need to modify or redesign clinical processes of care. In a 1998 survey of 601 hospital executives, 53 percent of the executives said that they planned to implement disease management programs, and more than 70 percent reported that they would reengineer clinical processes and develop outcome measurement programs (Deloitte & Touche, 1998).

Hospitalists. U.S. hospitals currently have 7,000 to 8,000 hospitalists (physicians that practice at the hospital, typically trained in internal medicine or pediatrics) practicing in them. In the next 10 years, that number is expected to grow to 20,000. Traditionally, upon admission, a patient was cared for by either the principal (primary care) physician or a specialist who would come to the hospital once or twice daily to make rounds. Hospitalists, because of their continuous presence at the hospital, are more easily able to facilitate patient care and increase the speed with which a patient is treated and released. Studies have found a 15 percent decrease in the length of stay and need for care when a hospitalist directs a patient's care (Diamond et al., 1998; Wachter et al., 1998).

Geriatric Evaluation Units (Inpatient). A few hospitals have developed units within their medical/surgical wings that exclusively admit older people who meet specific criteria (e.g., related to frailty or multiple chronic conditions and ADL limitations). Geriatric acute care units, often called geriatric evaluation and management units (GEUs), are inpatient units in hospitals specifically designed for older patients who could benefit from a more comprehensive model of care. Usually a geriatrician oversees an interdisciplinary or multidisciplinary team comprised of clinical nurse specialists, therapists and other rehabilitation specialists, social workers, and other specialists from such fields as pharmacy, nutrition, psychology, and audiology. Evidence from several trials of these units suggests that they can be moderately more effective than standard hospital care in maintaining older patients' functional status and in avoiding nursing home placement after hospital discharge (Agostini, Baker, & Bogardus, 2003). Model GEUs are found in the Veterans Affairs Health System (see Chapter 21).

The Health Insurance Portability and Accountability Act of 1996 (HIPAA). HIPAA included provisions for the privacy and confidentiality of consumers' health-related information. These regulations first took effect in 2003 and will continue to affect the way health information is used and how or whether it is exchanged between providers in the health care continuum. Hospitals were among the first health care entities to enact HIPAA provisions. Data exchange policies, such as billing and reporting, have become more restrictive. The most obvious changes in hospitals due to HIPAA have been tighter controls on information. For example, to protect an individual patient's confidentiality, hospitals are changing who has access to information, how patients' charts are maintained (no longer left in public view), how conversations about a patient's care are to be held (out of the public's hearing), and when patients must provide written approval for information sharing. Although HIPAA was intended to promote client well-being, the restrictions on information sharing run counter to the needs of clients with chronic, multifaceted conditions who receive care from multiple providers either simultaneously or sequentially.

ADMINISTRATIVE CHALLENGES

Hospital administrators seeking to improve services for older adults and those with chronic conditions face many challenges to reduce fragmentation, increase continuity, and improve hospital environments to better meet the needs and match the characteristics of those with functional limitations and physical impairments. Major administrative challenges in providing a hospital-organized continuum of care include:

- Restrictions on payment, especially for long-term care services, after OBRA 1997
- Lack of aligned incentives among different providers
- Inadequate information sharing across service settings, both within and external to the hospital
- Quality measurement that focuses on inpatient activity only
- Workforce constraints, and the isolation of each health care discipline, where education, training, and supervision are separate

Except for a few demonstration projects, hospitals have not had strong incentives to reorganize their care to connect more effectively with other disciplines or settings and to act as a health care team along a continuum. Little attention is paid to longitudinal cumulative care outcomes—outcomes that could be achieved only through coordination of care across disciplines and settings and over time. The need is great to bring together people and data sets to provide a whole picture of a person's extended needs over a long time horizon (e.g., several years).

Despite many ongoing obstacles, some progress is being made. Continuity of care, though not a reality for the masses, is a more recognized concept throughout the field. Care/case management services have proliferated. Many hospitals have some form of case management service to help patients transition successfully out of the hospital and to help them access needed postacute care services. Some would argue, however, that care management services are needed only because of the fragmented system that exists, and may not be a final solution for adequately connecting settings of care.

CONCLUSION

Hospitals have evolved in many ways, coming to embody the marriage of science and medical arts with highly advanced technology. As science and medicine continue to evolve, diseases that were once thought to be fatal may become tomorrow's chronic conditions.

In the early twenty-first century, many hospitals appear to be strongly focused on what they call their "core business": providing technologically sophisticated medicine in an inpatient setting. If this is the role that hospitals continue to choose to play, their challenge will be to make strong connections with other providers who help persons with chronic disease to manage over the long haul, after the brief episode of acute need is over, or to prevent inpatient episodes altogether. In the future, chronic care needs will increasingly dominate the health care landscape, and hospitals need to adapt to this context.

CLIENT EXAMPLE

Mr. Williams, a 29-year-old male, is a construction worker working on the renovation of a 30-story building. Because of an equipment error, he falls and sustains severe injuries, including several broken bones and potential brain injury. After being rushed to the emergency room at the nearest hospital, he undergoes surgery for his compound fractures, and then is transferred to intensive care. After five days, he is stabilized medically but is in a coma. He spends two weeks on a regular med-surg floor, then is officially discharged and admitted to the long-term-stay hospital on the same campus. For three weeks, he remains in a coma. Then, miraculously, he opens his eyes and begins a long process of recovery. After another two weeks, he is much better mentally and is physically able to tolerate rehabilitation. He is again discharged and admitted to the rehabilitation hospital. He remains there for six weeks receiving intensive rehabilitation. He is then declared well enough to go home and continue treatment on an outpatient basis.

Mr. Williams lives alone and is not convinced that he is well enough to function on his own. His physician gives him the option of spending another two to three weeks in a skilled nursing facility, which is owned by the hospital, although the physician is uncertain about whether worker's compensation will pay for that stay. Mr. Williams recognizes that he may have to pay out of pocket, but because the majority of his care has been covered, he has paid little to date. The skilled nursing facility meets Mr. Williams's needs for periodic nursing care and also ensures that he continues with his rehabilitation, most of which is done on site. The nursing home transports him to the hospital's outpatient rehabilitation clinic twice a week for access to specialty equipment.

After three weeks, Mr. Williams returns home, with the hospital's Medicare-certified home health agency providing rehabilitation to him at home. The hospital's private home care service sends a homemaker twice a week to help him bathe and prepare a bank of meals. Finally, after another four weeks, Mr. Williams is able to walk on his own out of his house and drive his car. Home care is discontinued, and Mr. Williams continues rehabilitation therapy on an outpatient basis. After nearly seven months of recovery, Mr. Williams feels well on his way to complete recovery—but he is not eager to climb up three flights of scaffolding again!

Mr. Williams realizes that, despite the severity of his injuries, he has been most fortunate. The medical center to which he was initially taken had a broad spectrum of specialty services. He received several levels of care, and was officially discharged and admitted several times to distinct organizational entities while remaining on the same physical campus. His care was coordinated across settings, his records were transferred, and his care plan was consistent, because the medical center had instituted processes to streamline transitions for just such complicated cases as his. Moreover, because his accident occurred at work, Worker's Compensation, a rather generous payer—covered almost all of his medical expenses. In addition to a positive recovery, he was grateful for a positive experience orchestrated by the hospital.

WHERE TO GO FOR FURTHER INFORMATION

American Association of Health Plans (AAHP)
1129 20th Street NW, Suite 600
Washington, DC 20036-3421
(202) 778-3200
http://www.aahp.org

American Association of Retired Persons (AARP)
601 E Street NW
Washington, DC 20049
(202) 434-2300 / (800) 424-3410
http://www.aarp.org

American Hospital Association (AHA)
One North Franklin
Chicago, IL 60606
(312) 422-3000 / (800) 424-4301
http://www.aha.org
http://www.hospitalconnect.com

American Medical Association
515 North State Street
Chicago, IL 60610
(312) 464-5000
http://www.ama-assn.org

American Public Health Association (APHA)
800 I Street NW
Washington, DC 20001-3710
(202) 777-2742
http://www.apha.org

Centers for Medicare and Medicaid Services (CMS)
7500 Security Boulevard
Baltimore, MD 21244-1850
(877) 267-2323
http://www.cms.gov

Joint Commission on Accreditation of Healthcare Organizations (JCAHO)
1 Renaissance Boulevard
Oakbrook Terrace, IL 60181
(630) 792-5000
http://www.jcaho.org

National Center for Health Statistics (NCHS)
6525 Belcrest Road
Hyattsville, MD 20782-2003
(301) 458-4636
http://www.cdc.gov/nchs/about/major/nhhcsd

FACTS REVIEW

1. What is a hospital? Name three different types of hospitals.
2. Approximately how many hospitals are there in the United States?
3. What are the primary payment sources for hospitals?
4. Over the last two decades, what have been the trends in inpatient and outpatient services?
5. Name two factors that have significantly influenced many hospitals' provision of services to their communities.
6. In a general, short-term community hospital, what proportion of the hospital's patients are over age 65? Identify several specialty services that target older adults and represent diversification for hospitals.

REFERENCES

Agostini, J., Baker, D., & Bogardus, S. (2003). Geriatric evaluation and management units for hospitalized patients. Retrieved June 13, 2003 from http://www.ahcpr.gov/clinic/psafety/chap30.htm

American Hospital Association (AHA), Health Forum, LLC. (2003). *Hospital statistics, 2003 edition* (Tables 1, 2, 4, 7). Chicago: American Hospital Association.

Bovbjerg, R., & Marsteller, J. (1998, November). *Health care market competition in six states: Implications for the poor* (Occasional Paper No. 17). Washington, DC: The Urban Institute.

Centers for Disease Control (CDC). (1992). Public health focus: Surveillance, prevention and control of nosocomial infections. *MMWR, 41,* 783–787.

Centers for Disease Control. (2003, June). Retrieved from *http://www.cdc.gov/nchs*

Centers for Medicare and Medicaid Services (CMS). (2003a). Office of the Actuary, National Health Statistics Group.

Centers for Medicare and Medicaid Services (CMS). (2003b). Data retrieved from *http://www.cms .hhs.gov/statistics* and *http://www.cms.hhs.gov* "Frequently Asked Questions" section.

CHIPs (Center for Healthcare Industry Performance Studies). (2003). *2003 Almanac of hospital financial and operating indicators.* Columbus, OH: Author.

Deloitte & Touche, LLP. (1998). *U.S. hospitals and the future of health care: A continuing opinion survey* (7th ed.). Philadelphia: Deloitte.

Diamond, H. S., Goldberg, E., & Janosky, J. E. (1998). The effect of full-time faculty hospitalists on the efficiency of care at a community teaching hospital. *Annals of Internal Medicine, 129,* 197–203.

Donabedian, A. (1979). Aspects of medical care administration: *Specifying requirements for health care.* Cambridge, MA: Harvard University Press.

Fairview Health Systems. (2003, June). Retrieved from *http://www.fairview.org*

Fisher, E. S., Wennberg, D. E., Stukel, T. A., Gottlieb, D. J., Lucas, F. L., & Pinder, E. L. (2003). The implications of regional variations in Medicare spending, part 1: The content, quality, and accessibility of care. *Annals of Internal Medicine, 138,* 273–287.

Fletcher, K. (2000). Acute care. In A. G. Lucckenotte (Ed.), *Gerontological nursing* (2d ed.) (pp. 757–770). St. Louis: Mosby.

Huckstadt, A. (2002). The experience of hospitalized elderly patients. *Journal of Gerontological Nursing, 28*(9), 24–29.

JCAHO (Joint Commission on Accreditation of Healthcare Organizations). (2003, June). Personal communication.

Kohn, L., Corrigan, J., & Donaldson, M. (1999). *To err is human: Building a safer health system.* Washington, DC: Institute of Medicine, National Academy Press.

Levit, K., Smith, C., Cowan, C., Lazenby, H., Sensening, A., & Catlin, A. (2003, January/February). Trends in U.S. health care spending, 2001. *Health Affairs, 22*(1), 154–164.

National Center for Health Statistics. (2002). *Health, United States, 2002.* Retrieved from *www.cdc.gov/nchs*

Paone, D. (2001). *Quality methods and measures.* Technical Assistance Paper No. 9 of the Robert Wood Johnson Foundation Medicare/Medicaid Integration Program, directed by the University of Maryland Center on Aging. Bloomington, MN: National Chronic Care Consortium.

Sandrick, K. (2001, March). No margin, big mission. *Trustee,* 6–10.

Shortell, S., Gillies, R., Anderson, D., Erickson, K. M., & Mitchell, J. (1996). *Remaking health care in America.* San Francisco: Jossey-Bass.

Sloan, F., Ostermann, J., & Conover, C. (2003, Spring). Antecedents of hospital ownership conversions, mergers, and closures. *Inquiry, 40,* 39–56.

Southwick, A. F. (1978). *The law of hospital and health care administration.* Ann Arbor, MI: Health Administration Press.

Starr, P. (1982). *The social transformation of American medicine.* New York: Basic Books.

University of California, San Francisco, Institute for Health and Aging. (1996). *Chronic care in America, a 21st century challenge.* Princeton, NJ: The Robert Wood Johnson Foundation.

U.S. Department of Health and Human Services, Health Care Financing Administration. (1998). *Health care financing review: Medicare and Medicaid statistical supplement.* Baltimore: Centers for Medicare and Medicaid Services.

Wachter, R. M., Katz, P., Showstack, J., Bindman, A. B., & Goldman, L. (1998). Reorganizing an academic medical service: Impact on cost, quality, patient satisfaction, and education. *JAMA, 279,* 1560–1565.

Wennbert, J., McAndrew-Cooper, M., & members of the Dartmouth Atlas Health Care Working Group. (1996). *The Dartmouth atlas of health care in the United States.* Chicago: American Hospital Publishing/The Trustees of Dartmouth College.

CHAPTER 5

Nursing Homes

Edward jj Olson

Nursing homes are essential components of the continuum of long-term care. In response to dramatically changing demographics and modifications in federal and state funding, they offer an increasingly broad range of services, and fill several distinct and critical niches in the continuum of care. The characteristics of nursing homes vary widely, as do the types of patients they serve. The purpose of this chapter is to highlight the unique characteristics of nursing homes, profile their clients and spectrum of services, discuss financing and regulatory requirements, and review evolving integrating mechanisms and models of care.

DEFINITION

Nursing home is a broad term that encompasses a wide spectrum of facilities, including 3-bed family-owned facilities, 20-bed units in acute community hospitals, 99-bed homes owned by multifacility corporations, and 1,000-bed government-operated institutions. For data collection purposes, the National Center for Health Statistics (NCHS) defines

nursing homes as "facilities with three or more beds that routinely provide nursing care services. Facilities may be certified by Medicare or Medicaid (or both) or not certified, but licensed by the State as a nursing home. These facilities may be freestanding or a distinct unit of a larger facility" (Jones, 2002).

The terms **Extended Care Facility (ECF), Intermediate Care Facility (ICF), Intermediate Care for the Mentally Retarded (ICF-MR),** and **Skilled Care Nursing Facility (SNF)** have each been defined by the federal government within the context of levels of institutional care certifiable for reimbursement by Medicare. Commonly used terms such as **convalescent home, long-term care facility, care center,** and other similar terms have no standard meanings. Currently Medicare pays for care only in facilities that meet Medicare requirements. Some states, however, continue to use other designations, such as intermediate care facilities and **subacute.**

Nursing homes may be either freestanding facilities, units of hospitals, or integral components of multilevel centers. Many nursing facilities have a

SERVICE SNAPSHOT:
Nursing Homes

Number of facilities	18,000
Number of beds	1.9 million
Number of residents (census)	1.6 million
Charges*	$3,000–6,000/month
Major payers	Medicaid Private out-of-pocket Medicare
Licensure	State department of health
Certification	Medicare Medicaid
Accreditation**	JCAHO

SOURCE: 1999 National Nursing Home Survey, 2002
*Does not apply to subacute units.
**See text for full name.

combination of beds designated for residents requiring skilled nursing care, those needing specialty care, and others needing personal care services. The common feature is that people who are not able to remain at home alone, because of physical health problems, mental health problems, or functional disabilities, reside at the facility and receive some level of nursing care, ranging from personal care to intensive skilled care, under medical direction.

NUMBER OF NURSING HOMES

The most recent population survey of nursing facilities nationwide was performed in 1999 by the National Center for Health Statistics (Jones, 2002). This survey reported 18,000 freestanding nursing homes with more than 1.9 million beds. Occupancy averaged 87 percent, with more than 1.6 million people residing in nursing homes at any given time. The data did not include step-down units of hospitals, intermediate care facilities for the mentally retarded, board and care facilities, or supportive living residences licensed by some states.

Table 5.1 presents select characteristics of nursing homes. Sixty-seven percent of nursing homes are proprietary facilities, 27 percent are nonprofit, and 6 percent are owned and operated by federal, state, or local governments. More than half of all nursing homes (60 percent) belong to multifacility system chains, while the remainder function independently. Though the size of nursing homes may vary widely, from fewer than 50 to more than 200 beds, the majority, or approximately 81 percent, range from 50 to 199 beds. The average size during 1999 was 105 beds. Eight percent of homes operate 200 beds or more; less than 12 percent operate fewer than 50 beds. Government-operated nursing homes have a slightly higher average number of beds than proprietary and voluntary nonprofit facilities.

Clients

Those who are cared for in nursing facilities are referred to as *residents* rather than patients. Table 5.2 characterizes nursing home residents at the time of the most recent national survey for which data were available, in 1999 (Jones, 2002). Nursing homes primarily serve the very old and frail. In 1999, more than 78 percent of the then approximately 1.6 million nursing home residents were age 75 years and older; more than 46 percent were age 85 and older. Seven out of ten residents were women, and nearly nine out of ten were white.

The primary diagnoses of nursing home residents are circulatory system disorders (25 percent), mental disorders (18 percent), and diseases of the nervous system (16 percent) (Jones, 2002). Nearly one-half of all nursing home residents (47 percent) have multiple major diagnoses, with two out of five (40 percent) having three or more diagnoses.

Previous surveys of nursing home residents (Marion Merrell Dow, 1993) found that about one-half are incontinent, nearly one-half are wheelchair-bound, approximately 20 percent require intensive nursing, and nearly 10 percent are bedridden.

Mental deficiencies due to dementia, stroke, Alzheimer's disease, or other mental conditions affect

Table 5.1 Characteristics of Nursing Homes, 1999

	Nursing Homes								
	Number	Percent	Number	Percent	Beds/home	Number	Percent	Number	Percent
Total	18,000	100.0	1,879,600	100.0	104.5	1,628,300	100.0	2,522,300	100.0
Ownership									
Proprietary	12,000	66.5	1,235,800	65.7	103.3	1,049,300	64.4	1,655,500	65.6
Nonprofit	4,800	26.7	499,500	26.6	103.9	445,600	27.4	751,800	29.8
Government	1,200	6.7	144,300	7.7	119.4	133,300	8.2	115,100	4.6
Certification									
Medicare and Medicaid	14,700	81.8	1,624,300	86.4	110.4	1,415,400	86.9	2,244,300	89.0
Medicare only	*600	*3.5	46,800	2.5	73.6	37,100	2.3	158,700	6.3
Medicaid only	2,100	11.9	169,900	9.0	79.5	143,100	8.8	98,600	3.9
Not certified	*500	*2.8	38,600	2.1	76.7	32,700	2.0	20,700	0.8
Bed Size									
Less than 50 beds	2,100	11.5	69,300	3.7	33.4	58,600	3.6	214,000	8.5
50–99 beds	7,000	38.7	484,500	25.8	69.7	414,200	25.4	585,200	23.2
100–199 beds	7,500	41.8	952,400	50.7	126.1	827,800	50.8	1,296,900	51.4
200 beds or more	1,400	8.0	373,500	19.8	259.6	327,700	20.1	426,100	16.9
Census Region									
Northeast	3,200	17.8	412,800	22.0	129.1	383,400	23.5	524,200	20.8
Midwest	6,000	33.2	598,400	31.8	100.1	498,200	30.6	709,700	28.1
South	6,000	33.2	614,900	32.7	103.0	531,500	32.6	714,800	28.3
West	2,800	15.8	253,500	13.5	89.3	215,200	13.2	573,600	22.7
Affiliation									
Chain	10,800	59.9	1,128,300	60.0	104.7	978,800	60.1	1,581,300	62.7
Independent	7,200	39.8	747,600	39.8	104.5	646,100			

*Figure does not meet standard of reliability or precision due to sample size.

SOURCE: Jones, 2002

a large proportion of nursing home residents. Although fewer than one in five residents has a primary diagnosis of mental disorder (Jones, 2002), it is estimated that 33 to 40 percent suffer from some type of mental impairment (Hing, Sekscenski, & Strahan, 1989). As the population of the nation ages, the number of people with Alzheimer's disease is expected to increase dramatically. Many of these individuals will ultimately move into a nursing home.

Functional dependence is high among nursing home residents. Table 5.3 presents the dependency status of nursing home residents in 1995 and 1999

Table 5.2 Nursing Home Residents by Age, Sex, and Race, 1999

	Number*	Percent
All Ages	**1,628,300**	**100.0**
Under 65 years	158,700	9.8
65–74 years	194,800	12.0
75–84 years	517,600	31.8
85 years and older	757,100	46.5
Unknown		
Gender		
Male	457,900	28.1
Female	1,170,400	71.9
Race		
White	1,394,400	85.6
Black	178,700	11.0
Other	37,200	2.3
Unknown	17,400	1.1

*Numbers not in bold are derived from percent distribution.

SOURCE: Jones, 2002.

(NCHS, 1997; Jones, 1999). During 1999, more than 88 percent had 2 or more functional dependencies. Fully 47 percent required assistance to eat. The average number of functional dependencies was 3.1.

Aggregate numbers mask the wide variation in resident acuity levels and functional status. Typical residents include:

- 72-year-old male undergoing rehabilitation for physical and mental stroke-related impairments
- 63-year-old woman convalescing from a diabetes-related partial leg amputation
- 88-year-old woman with heart disease requiring assistance with ADLs
- 25-year-old male suffering from head trauma as a result of a motorcycle accident
- 56-year-old male receiving hospice care during the end stages of AIDS

Individuals are admitted to nursing homes on a long-term basis for functional dependencies as well as specific diagnoses. Night wandering, incontinence, and mental deterioration are three problems that frequently stress families beyond their caregiving capacity and result in their loved ones being admitted to a nursing home. People who are single and do not have strong social support systems are also more likely to be in a nursing home.

Predictors for nursing home placement include age, ethnicity, socioeconomic status, functional status, subjective perception of health, the presence of cognitive impairment or behavioral problems, and the status of the caregiver's physical and mental health (Gaugler, Kane, Kane, Clay, & Newcomer, 2003). The availability of support systems, financial resources, cultural attitudes, geographic location,

TABLE 5.3 Dependency Status of Nursing Home Residents, 1995 and 1999

Type of Dependency (requires assistance with)	1995[1] Percent	1999[2] Percent
Bathing	96.3	93.8
Dressing	86.6	86.5
Using bathroom	57.8	56.0
Difficulty with bowel/ bladder control	43.6	48.7
Eating	45.1	47.0
Number of Dependencies		
None	3.1	5.0
One	8.5	6.7
Two	13.8	13.6
Three	33.1	31.6
Four	32.9	32.0
Five	8.6	11.1
Average	**3.1**	**3.1**

[1]SOURCE: NCHS, 1997.
[2]SOURCE: Jones, 2002.

and a host of other individual conditions are additional factors.

In general, nursing home admissions tend to be one of three types: (1) short-term recovery and rehabilitation from surgery or acute episodes of illness; (2) terminal or hospice care; and (3) long-time residency based on physical and/or mental inability to function independently. Nearly half of nursing home residents (46 percent) are admitted directly from hospitals. Conversely, nursing homes transfer a significant proportion of residents to hospitals. Nearly one-third (29 percent) of all nursing home discharges are admitted directly to hospitals (Jones, 2002).

The lifetime chance of ever being in a nursing home is approximately one in three (36 percent) at age 45 and more than one in two (56 percent) at age 85 (Murtaugh, Kemper, Spillman, & Carlson, 1997). More than half of women and one-third of men age 65 and older will require a nursing home stay (Murtaugh, Kemper, & Spillman, 1990). Contrary to popular belief, most people do not spend many years in a nursing home. The average length of stay nationally is 272 days, or approximately 9 months. More than two-thirds of those admitted to

a nursing home (68 percent) are discharged within 90 days, while an additional 15 percent are discharged within one year. Fewer than 4 percent of discharges represent a stay of 5 years or more (Jones, 2002).

SERVICES

Nursing homes provide a range of services, from assistance with ADLs; to supervision for those with memory loss or other mental deficiencies, such as Alzheimer's disease; to sophisticated technological care, such as ventilator care and infusion therapy; to palliative care, such as hospice. In addition to basic nursing care and supervision, nursing homes offer social services, rehabilitation therapies, nutrition counseling and dietary assistance, dental care, and pastoral care. Homes also administer medications, provide meals, and conduct recreational and social activities on a daily basis to keep people physically occupied and mentally stimulated. Homes are beginning to expand their services to include services for individuals who are living independently, such as adult day care, outpatient clinical and rehabilitation services, and assisted living accommodations. State and federal regulations govern the provision of some services; others are at the discretion of the home. Table 5.4 summarizes the basic and specialty services, as well as distinct programs currently offered by nursing homes.

The trend for nursing home residents during the past decade has been toward increasing levels of acuity and functional dependency. Individuals with mild functional dependencies who would probably have been admitted to a nursing facility in the past are now moving into assisted living and congregate care facilities, or remaining at home with the assistance of community-based care services. As a consequence, the services offered by nursing homes tend to be increasingly complex and sophisticated, but continue to build on a base of solid nursing care.

Subacute refers to beds in either hospitals or nursing homes that are licensed as nursing home beds; these receive higher-intensity care than standard

PREDICTORS FOR NURSING HOME PLACEMENT AMONG GENERAL OLDER POPULATION

- Demographic characteristics (age, ethnicity, socioeconomic status, etc.)
- Living arrangement
- Functional status (dependency in ADLs and/or IADLs, subjective health, cognitive impairment)
- Behavior problems (wandering, agitation, or physical aggression)
- Caregiver characteristics (burden, depression, or impaired health)

SOURCE: Gaugler et al., 2003. Copyright © The Gerontological Society of America. Reproduced by permission of the publisher.

TABLE 5.4 Nursing Facility Services

Basic Service Package	Special Services	Special Programs
Nursing care	Ventilator care	Adult day care
Personal care	Alzheimer's care	Assisted living
Meals and dietary consultation	Rehabilitation therapies	Congregate living
Medication delivery & monitoring	Wound care	Home health
Social services counseling	Infusion nutrition	Outpatient medical and rehabilitation clinics
Dental care	Pastoral care	Independent living
Recreational & social activities	Respite care	
Physician oversight	Hospice care	

skilled beds. Assisted living (discussed in Chapter 8) has recently evolved as a distinct level of supportive housing that provides personal care. In brief, the terminology applied to nursing homes has evolved over time. The only terms that have precise meaning are those tied to regulations and reimbursement; specific definitions may vary by state.

During the last decade, changes in patient mix, tightening of state and federal reimbursement, increased competition, and other environmental challenges have prompted nursing homes to expand their continuums of care. Nursing facilities now offer specialized Alzheimer's/dementia care units, more intensive rehabilitation therapies, and respite care services. Entire multifacility systems have arisen that specialize in ventilator care, traumatic brain injury, and other specialty services.

Subacute Care

Subacute care, mentioned earlier, emerged as a major growth area in the late 1990s. Although some states have a subacute category, the term does not have specific universal criteria.

Adopting Modern Medical and Management Technology

Nursing home operation is so prescribed by federal and state regulations that many homes have diffi-

culty pursuing creative and innovative programming. Although many nursing facilities continue to operate the same way they did several years ago, the world of geriatrics and gerontology has changed dramatically, with large advances in clinical care and management techniques. New information systems, knowledge about how environmental design affects patient care and staff productivity, daily activity programs specifically designed for Alzheimer's patients, use of case management, and contracting with managed care organizations all have influenced both the quality and outcomes associated with nursing home care. The challenge for nursing home administrators is to create a strategic plan that allows the implementation of creative programming to provide innovative care, thus positioning the home to play a key role in the evolution of a coordinated continuum of care for skilled care populations.

STAFFING

On average, nursing homes employ 0.81 full-time staff per bed (Jones, 2002). The majority of nursing home employees are unskilled or low-skilled nurse's aides, housekeeping personnel, and maintenance and food service workers. Aides and orderlies usually represent nearly half of all nursing home staff. In skilled nursing facilities that meet Medicare and Medicaid requirements, a registered nurse (RN) is required to be on duty at least eight consecutive hours per day, seven days per week. On evening and night shifts, the highest level professional staff may be a licensed practical nurse (LPN) or licensed vocational nurse (LVN).

In an effort to help nursing homes to control costs, the Centers for Medicare and Medicaid Services (CMS) promulgated a rule allowing the employment of part-time personnel to aid in the feeding of residents who cannot feed themselves. The concern by many is that facilities will pay for these minimally trained "feeding assistant" positions by replacing trained certified nursing assistants, thus adversely affecting the quality of care.

The senior management of a 100- to 200-bed nursing home typically consists of an administrator and a nursing director. Larger homes, or those that are part of hospitals, multifacility systems, or multiple health care systems, may have additional full- or part-time senior management positions. In general, however, nursing homes have very shallow management structures.

Other health care professionals who work with or in nursing homes include:

- Physicians
- Pharmacists
- Psychologists
- Occupational and physical therapists
- Speech and respiratory therapists
- Dentists and dental hygienists
- Clergy
- Medical social workers
- Case managers
- Nurse practitioners
- Dietitians

Except in very large homes, these professionals work on a part-time or on-call basis. They may be available for only a few hours per week or month. Typically they are paid on a contract basis rather than as employees. Medicare requires certain professionals to work at the home for a minimum number of hours per month; individual state regulations may require a broader array of professionals and/or available hours.

Physician Involvement

Regulations require that nursing home residents be visited by a physician at least once every 30 days during the first 90 days after admission, and then at least once every 60 days thereafter, or more often when medically necessary. Because the payment to physicians who care for nursing home residents is so low, many doctors find it difficult to take the time to go to nursing homes to make visits, particularly if they must travel some distance. Some facilities have a medical director who becomes the physician of record for many of the home's residents, particularly for those whose stay is indefinite.

Attracting and Maintaining Staff

Attracting and maintaining high-quality staff is a challenge for all nursing homes. The work in nursing homes is emotionally and physically demanding, and the pay scales allowed within the constraints of Medicaid reimbursement are quite low. As noted earlier, most staff have minimal skills and are typically paid at or slightly above minimum wage. The result is high turnover rates. More than 71 percent of nurse assistant positions and approximately 50 percent of nursing positions turn over within one year (American Health Care Association [AHCA], 2003); however, turnover rates as high as 100 percent are not unknown.

High turnover requires that nursing homes constantly recruit and train new staff. Although necessary, training diverts resources that otherwise might be put into other areas. The disruption in continuity of personnel poses a threat to quality care and to residents' comfort level with staff.

Administrators must be as sensitive to the needs of their staff as they are to the needs of residents. Creative ways have been found to recruit and reward staff that do not necessarily involve increasing pay. Homes have offered educational scholarships, sponsored child day care programs, set up internal banks for short-term loans, promoted "Employee of the Month" awards, invited families to join residents for a free weekly dinner, and offered English language classes.

Recruiting professional staff also poses an ongoing problem. Pay scales for professionals are higher in hospitals and other health care settings than in nursing homes. Particularly in rural areas, nursing homes may struggle to employ the full-time professional staff and consultants they need to meet minimum licensing or certification requirements. Those who work in nursing homes on a long-term basis tend to be motivated by personal commitment rather than by financial remuneration.

EVOLUTION TO HIGH-TECHNOLOGY NURSING HOMES

Basic space requirements for nursing homes are governed by the federal Life Safety Code, although individual states may add physical plant requirements for licensure. Beyond the basic requirements, nursing homes comprise a wide range of types of facilities with varying physical environments. The space, equipment, and environmental requirements of a 3-bed, privately owned family home vary tremendously from those of a 1,000-bed government-operated institution. Needs will also vary according to the types of services delivered. Even within a single facility, different levels or types of care may require different spatial arrangements. For example, a residential facility specializing in Alzheimer's care might have a wanderer's path; a step-down unit in an acute care hospital is likely to use extra space for monitoring and other technological equipment; a facility emphasizing rehabilitation might have a large therapy room and pool.

The physical plant of the nursing home of the future is likely to be much different from those that exist now. Institutional designs of the past, based on hospital layouts, are quickly being replaced by settings that convey a better sense of home to nursing home residents. Because long-term care populations will spend significant time in a nursing home,

facilities must provide all the amenities of a traditional home, in addition to spaces that accommodate socialization and individual and group therapies. Contemporary nursing home design focuses on the importance of developing homelike settings that promote resident health, privacy, dignity, safety, and security. Movement toward emphasizing 12- to 20-bed household clusters for common care populations eliminates the long corridors currently found in many nursing homes, allows efficient provision of care services, and provides a relaxed environment for social interaction among residents, staff, and family members.

Many nursing homes currently in operation were built during the 1960s and 1970s. These plants are rapidly becoming obsolete, in terms of both useful lifespan and modern concepts for the design of long-term care facilities. Technology has advanced, regulations have become more stringent, and patient care requirements have become more intense and more demanding. The return on capital investment, which was high during the early period of nursing home expansion, has been reduced by decreasing state and federal funding. The combination of all these factors often means that such facilities are unprofitable, and will likely be replaced or purchased by larger health systems. Newly designed nursing homes will be safer, more efficient, more specialized, and resident focused.

FINANCING

The average cost of care in a nursing home ranges between $3,000 and $6,000 per month, depending on geographic location, type of facility, level of care, services received, and other factors. During 2001, nursing home expenditures nationally totaled $98.9 billion, and are projected to approach $120 billion during 2005 (CMS, Office of the Actuary, 2003). During 1999, the average daily charge for nursing home care was $146 for skilled care, $114 for intermediate care, and $100.95 for residential care. The average daily charge for Medicare-certified residents was $213. For Medicaid-certified residents, the average daily charge was $105 (Jones, 2002).

As shown in Figure 5.1, the primary sources of payment for nursing home care are Medicaid (59 percent) and private individuals and families (24 percent) (Jones, 2002). Although Medicare accounts for approximately one-third of primary payments at the time of admission, the program pays for only 15 percent of the costs of nursing home care at any point in time. All other payers account for only 3 to 4 percent of all payments for nursing home care. The heavy dependence on Medicaid as a payment source poses significant financial challenges for nursing homes. In some states, expenditures for Medicaid nursing home costs are the largest single expense in the budget. As states look for ways to control their budgets, funding for nursing home care is heavily scrutinized. States have used Certificate of Need au-

thorities to limit the number of nursing home beds allowed in the state and thereby limit state spending. Many states have developed community-based care alternatives to nursing home placement, through the Medicaid Home and Community Based Services (HCBS) waiver program.

Medicaid regulations and payment policies vary widely from state to state. Three basic payment methods are used: cost-reimbursement, prospective cost-based payment, and per diem contractual arrangements. Rates may be modified by residents' level of severity (case mix systems). Under all methods, costs may be grouped into clinical care (mostly nursing and aide time), ancillary services (housekeeping, dietary, maintenance, etc.), and administration. Reimbursement for the costs of capital and an allowable return on investment, which were quite generous during the late 1960s and 1970s, have

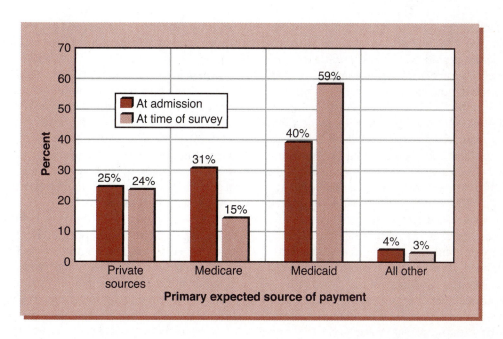

Figure 5.1   Percent Distribution of Primary Expected Source of Payment at Admission and at Time of Survey (National Nursing Home Survey)

SOURCE: Jones, A. (2002). *The national nursing home survey: 1999 summary* (National Center for Health Statistics). *Vital Health Statistics, 13*(152).

been severely curtailed and even eliminated in some states. Return on investment is not available for not-for-profit facilities.

Medicare covers certain nursing home care that is provided on a short-term basis of up to 100 days. If a person is to be admitted and covered by Medicare, he or she must have a three-day inpatient stay in an acute hospital, be admitted to a nursing home within 30 days of discharge from an acute hospital, require nursing services related to the condition for which he or she was hospitalized, and have the prognosis of improvement (CMS, 2003). Medicare does not cover maintenance-level care for those who have no potential to regain greater functional independence.

Medicare-certified nursing homes must comply with a host of stringent federal regulations, such as high staffing ratios, use of electronic billing systems, and use of specialized assessment systems. By definition, Medicare patients are more acutely ill than long-term patients. They tend to require more intensive skilled care and/or rehabilitative services, and tend to be admitted and discharged within a relatively short period of time. Though Medicare payments account for a relatively small share of all revenues, the vast majority (86 percent) of nursing homes are either Medicare or dually Medicare/Medicaid certified. Those that are dually certified tend to have some, but not all, of their beds certified. Many skilled care facilities that are Medicare certified have dedicated Medicare rehabilitation units of from 10 to 30 beds located in a designated area of the facility. These units often include dedicated staff who are trained to address the health and restorative needs of Medicare patients.

The Balanced Budget Act of 1997 required Medicare to establish a Prospective Payment System (PPS) for skilled nursing facilities (SNFs). Payments to nursing homes under PPS are resident-specific, with the amount varying based on a resident assessment utilizing the Minimum Data Set (MDS) tool and classification within the Resource Utilization Groups (RUGs) classification system. The RUGs III classification system consists of 44 groups divided into

7 categories: rehabilitation, special care, extensive services, clinically complex, impaired cognition, behavior, and reduced physical function. Each of the 44 RUGs III groups has an assigned billing code, or Health Insurance PPS Rate (HIPPS), with a separate per diem rate for each code.

Implementation of the PPS reduced the amount of payment that nursing homes receive for care provided to Medicare residents and resulted in significant operating deficits for many facilities. Many providers (an estimated 10 percent) ultimately filed for Chapter 11 bankruptcy protection. In an effort to soften the cuts enacted in 1997, Congress approved funds for nursing homes in 1999 and 2000.

Although the Medicare Prescription Drug Improvement and Modernization Act of 2003 centered on the provision of a prescription drug benefit for seniors, the implications for nursing homes include significant increases in Medicare reimbursement for certain RUGs groups, and a moratorium on Medicare reimbursement caps for therapy services (see Chapter 22). The Act increased per diem payments for the care of nursing home residents afflicted with acquired immune deficiency syndrome (AIDS), and removed Medicare reimbursement limits for occupational therapy and for physical and speech therapy combined. An additional mandate required a review of the standards of practice for pharmacy services provided to nursing home residents, and paved the way for the development of policy to ensure the provision of prescription drugs to Medicare beneficiaries residing in nursing homes.

Even with various federal budget refinements and program reforms, today's nursing homes continue to operate on a very tight margin. High occupancy rates are critical to the ongoing viability of operations. Compared to hospitals, which may have occupancy rates of less than 60 percent, the vast majority of nursing homes must stay at or above 90 percent occupancy to maintain financial viability.

Administrators must know their state reimbursement policies thoroughly, must be able to operate within financial constraints, and must maintain scrupulous records. Very little financial flexibility exists, particularly for nonprofit homes with large Medicaid populations. Nonprofit homes often have significant volunteer programs and fundraising initiatives, both of which provide additional resources. Government-operated facilities are often subsidized with local tax dollars, whereas nursing homes that are part of larger multiorganization health care systems may have access to corporate resources.

Capitated Financing

Capitation, or managed care, is an evolving model of financing for skilled care. Nursing homes across the country are entering into contracts with managed care companies or state Medicaid programs. Nursing homes are also joining together in networks to negotiate better terms with managed care plans and build the capacity to serve a plan's members. A requisite for managed care is to implement cost accounting so that expenses can be projected accurately when negotiating a contract rate.

Long-Term Care Insurance

Private individuals and families are increasingly turning to long-term care insurance in an effort to protect their assets against the high cost of quality long-term care. The long-term care insurance market grew an average of 18 percent each year from 1987 to 2001, with 137 companies selling more than 1.4 million policies during 2000–2001 alone. By the end of 2001, some 8.26 million policies had been sold nationally (Health Insurance Association of America [HIAA], 2003).

Long-term care insurance policies are sold in three ways: individual and group association plans, employer-sponsored plans, and long-term care as a rider on a life insurance policy. The majority of policies (80 percent) are sold as individual or group plans in which the average buyer is age 62. Together, employer-sponsored plans and life insurance policy riders comprise approximately 21 percent of the long-term care insurance market, with an average buyer aged 46 for employer-sponsored plans and

66 for life insurance policy riders. During 2001, the individual and employer-sponsored markets accounted for 75 percent of total market growth, while the long-term care life insurance rider market remained relatively stagnant. More than 4,700 employers currently offer long-term care insurance to employees and/or retirees (HIAA, 2003).

LICENSURE, CERTIFICATION, AND ACCREDITATION

Nursing homes are highly regulated at both the federal and state levels. Each state licenses nursing homes, and each has its own licensing requirements, reimbursement policies, governing regulations, classification systems, and terminology. As part of the regulatory process, each state establishes its own definitions of what constitutes nursing homes and other long-term care institutions. The licensing authority is usually the state equivalent of the Department of Health. If a nursing home also operates an assisted living unit, an adult day care program, a rehabilitation outpatient clinic, and a mental health clinic, it may be subject to the licensing requirements of four other departments of the state. Licensing requirements include staffing and physical plant compliance with federal Life Safety Codes.

To be reimbursed by Medicare or Medicaid, a nursing home must be certified. This means that the facility must meet the requirements (referred to as "Conditions of Participation") established by the federal government for Medicare, which also pertain to the federal portion of Medicaid. Typically, a state accepts a home that meets federal criteria as meeting state criteria. However, some states have additional requirements for a home to be certified to be eligible for reimbursement by Medicaid or other state programs. If a home is found remiss in any area, it is given a finite period of time to correct the deficiencies or lose its certification, and consequently, payment for Medicaid residents.

Homes may be licensed by the state and operate as private pay, in which case certification by Medicare

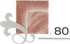

and/or Medicaid is not necessary. Skilled nursing units that are part of hospitals (i.e., subacute units) are all certified for Medicare reimbursement.

Concern about quality is juxtaposed with the limited budgets of Medicaid and private families. The 1987 Nursing Home Reform Act, incorporated into the Omnibus Budget Reconciliation Act of 1987 (OBRA 1987), made significant changes in how nursing homes operate and how they are evaluated (Coleman, 1991). The survey process was changed from one that focused on physical and task criteria to one that focuses on the quality of care, resident rights, and patient care outcomes.

Nursing homes may also be accredited by the Joint Commission on Accreditation of Healthcare Organizations (JCAHO). JCAHO has set up criteria and a separate survey process specifically for nursing homes. Compared with hospitals, the majority of which are JCAHO accredited, relatively few nursing homes apply for JCAHO accreditation, for two reasons. First, the survey is expensive. Second, unlike hospitals, accreditation is not automatically accepted by Medicare/Medicaid as a substitute for the certification process.

INTEGRATING MECHANISMS

Historically, the majority of nursing homes have functioned in isolation from other community organizations, except the hospitals with which they exchange patients. Conversely, a few nursing homes have been heavily involved in multiple levels of care, multi-health care systems, and assumed leadership in their community agency networks. In the future, the homes that survive and thrive will be the ones that become part of community-wide networks or systems, whether formal or informal.

Case Management

Most freestanding nursing homes do not have a distinct case management system. Some larger not-for-profit homes may have a social worker who assists families with alternative placement options. Nursing homes that are part of multilevel continuums are more likely to have a case manager or a system for helping residents transfer from one level of care to another. Nursing homes that contract with managed care companies may have a case manager assigned to them by the managed care entity; that person coordinates care of the managed care patients and expedites their discharge to less intensive levels of care.

Information Systems

The majority of nursing homes have stand-alone computer systems for billing. The regulations of OBRA 1987, requiring a minimum patient data set (the MDS), motivated homes to implement computerized patient care systems. However, few homes have a totally integrated financial and patient care data system. Multilevel facilities may have detailed and even computerized records for one set of residents, such as those of the skilled nursing unit, but not for others, such as those in the assisted living unit.

When nursing homes are part of hospitals or multi-health care systems, the nursing home information is almost always maintained separately. Aggregation of financial data may be done for a corporate-level report. The exception, in response to federal requirements, is step-down units of hospitals that are technically licensed and reimbursed by Medicare as skilled nursing home beds but are an integral part of the hospital's daily operation.

Recent modifications in federal payment methods have made it important for nursing homes to become well versed in the Medicare PPS and the RUGs III classification system. It is advantageous to have established patient care protocols for the major diagnoses being admitted. Case mix coordinators capable of conducting complete and accurate MDS assessments are invaluable for facilities to sustain efficiency and maximize payment for care rendered to Medicare beneficiaries.

Greater integration and computerization of records will be mandatory requirements for providing skilled nursing care as nursing homes evolve as partners in community-wide networks, multi-health care systems, and managed care systems.

Interentity Organization

Increasingly, nursing homes are realizing the need to be a formal part of a provider network. Homes that have already begun to affiliate, or those that have been built or bought by multi-health care systems, are forerunners in the method by which nursing homes develop optimum relationships with hospitals, physicians, and other provider entities.

The challenges that typically arise tend to relate to establishing equity for long-term care within a large organization that is historically acute-care oriented (Evashwick & Holt, 2000). For example, pay scales are lower in long-term care settings. As relationships between acute care and nursing home care become more integrated, administrators must determine how to achieve parity and cooperation among respective staffs. Issues such as patient transfers (criteria for appropriate referrals, sharing of patient data, etc.) and budgeting must be resolved. Interdepartment or interequity task forces or management committees should be established to begin to develop effective ways of integrating long-term care and acute care.

In addition to acute care, the use of other services within the continuum by nursing home residents must be facilitated through organizational and managerial techniques. This may first require the nursing home staff to change their orientation to monitoring resident discharge by referring residents to rehabilitation, home care, adult day care, and other community-based services. Introducing professionals from other disciplines and other provider entities to the nursing facility staff facilitates the development of trust and collegial relationships that result in enhanced care.

OPERATIONAL ISSUES

Two of the major operational issues confronting nursing facility administrators are compliance with the extensive and ever-changing regulations imposed by state and federal governments and provision of quality care with the limited funding available from government-established payment levels. Other administrative issues include those outlined in the rest of this section.

Balancing Resident Mix

Nursing homes try to operate at full occupancy. In the 1970s and the early 1980s, homes typically ran at 97 to 98 percent occupancy. By the early 1990s, occupancy rates had begun to drop, with a national average occupancy rate of 92 percent in 1991 (Sirrocco, 1994), 88 percent in 1997 (NCHS, 2000), and 87 percent in 1999 (Jones, 2002).

One reason for the decline in occupancy is tighter state and federal regulations about who is eligible for skilled care, which has resulted in a decline in admissions. Competition has also increased. The types and availability of alternatives to community nursing homes have increased. In the past 25 years, adult day care centers have proliferated, home health has expanded, and assisted living complexes have emerged on the continuum of care as an option midway between independent senior housing and nursing facility care. Furthermore, consumer knowledge about nursing homes has changed, and families and patients are now more selective in choosing nursing facilities.

Homes are also concerned about client mix, payer mix, and level-of-care mix. A nursing home does not want to accept a large number of heavy-care, low-pay (i.e., Medicaid) residents, even if it has empty beds. A home also may not want to accept residents with special care needs if it cannot accommodate them appropriately, such as admitting more late-stage Alzheimer's patients than its Alzheimer's unit has beds. A nursing home may elect to become Medicare certified because it receives higher payment for Medicare residents. However, the home must be certain that the number of Medicare residents will offset the additional costs.

Administrators face the task of maintaining good relationships with referral sources and engaging in ongoing marketing so that their homes secure the number and types of clients they desire. In today's era of managed care, nursing home administrators also must evaluate the advantages and disadvantages of contracting with managed care providers and payers, to assure that their nursing homes remain financially viable.

Internally, the administrator must develop a discharge capability and mentality within the nursing and social work staff to move residents to the next most appropriate level of care. This gives potential residents, families, staff, and providers the confidence that, for those who may regain the ability to function independently, the home will support and facilitate their independence and a return to the community.

To maximize the resident mix, the administrator must understand the changing demand for nursing home care, be knowledgeable about the competition, develop relationships with collaborators, market services aggressively, and develop new programs or services to fill unmet demand or maximize underutilized programming capacity.

Ensuring Quality

Nursing homes have been struggling to improve quality since the 1970s. The challenge for administrators is to balance the desire to meet resident and staff needs with the funding limits imposed by low Medicaid reimbursement and stringent federal and state regulation. Moreover, the field has not yet developed consensus regarding quality outcomes for long-term care.

As the federal administrative agency for Medicare and Medicaid, the Centers for Medicare and Medicaid Services has been a leader in improving oversight and ensuring the quality of nursing home care. In 1995, the agency, then known as HCFA, issued new nursing home regulations designed to address concerns about the conditions found in nursing homes throughout the nation. These new regulations were followed in 1998 by further initiatives to improve state inspections and enforcement, and address problem nursing care providers by identifying the facilities with the worst compliance records in each state, staggering the inspection of facilities so that facilities could no longer predict inspection times and dates, requiring states to investigate consumer complaints within 10 days, allowing states

to impose financial sanctions for violations, and requiring state inspectors to revisit facilities in person to assure that violations have been corrected.

In addition to the inspection and enforcement regulations, HCFA developed best practice guidelines for long-term care. Issues addressed within guideline materials include meeting the needs of residents at risk for weight loss and dehydration and preventing complications such as bedsores. Best practice principles have inspired the adoption of innovative models of care in nursing homes nationally. Programs such as restorative care emphasize resident rehabilitation through the collaboration of a multidisciplinary professional team.

Furthermore, nursing facilities have joined other health care organizations in implementing formal quality improvement programs. Industry initiatives include the Eden Alternative, the American Association of Homes and Services for the Aged, and the Pioneer Network. Many homes also attempt to meet the standards (if not obtain formal accreditation) of JCAHO.

Beyond formal efforts, administrators strive to involve patients, families, and staff in an ongoing effort to assure quality of care and enhance patient and staff satisfaction. Creative volunteer programs, fundraising initiatives, regular surveys of residents and families, and training programs to motivate staff are all options that contribute significantly to quality.

ADMINISTRATIVE CHALLENGES

The major challenges confronting nursing home administrators include:

- The complexity of providing care to match the changing needs of resident populations
- Assuring quality of care while addressing issues related to staff recruitment, training, retention, and budget limitations
- Utilizing emerging technologies as a catalyst to address the complex needs of residents

- Providing an environment that emphasizes a homelike setting and meets the health, social, and restorative needs of residents
- Developing a strategic plan that promotes the implementation of a coordinated continuum of skilled nursing care services
- Balancing resident mix with the requirements of various federal and state payment streams
- Staying current with federal and state regulations associated with licensure, certification, and accreditation
- Introducing integrating mechanisms such as case management, information systems, telemonitoring, and interentity affiliations, which maximize the spectrum of services and quality of care
- Understanding the important role that nursing homes play in the continuum of care

CONCLUSION

Contemporary nursing homes have changed dramatically since the 1980s. Independent family operations that offered primarily a supportive environment and nursing care have evolved into sophisticated institutions that boast computers and high technology biomedical equipment. The local community convalescent center has now become part of a multi-health care system or a member of a larger multifacility nursing home organization. Administrators are highly trained and broker both internal and external community resources. Government regulations have mushroomed in an attempt to control costs yet ensure high-quality care. As the number of seniors and disabled persons grows, the number of families paying for long-term care is increasing, as are Medicaid expenditures for nursing homes.

The nursing homes of the twenty-first century will be much more sophisticated in resident care technologies, information systems, financial arrangements, and organizational structure. Their physical configurations and environment will build on the concept of small households, which focus on residents. Services such as dining will be decentralized to each household, and the physical environments will be designed with more homelike characteristics. Integration with other older adult and health care related services can be expected to increase, from greater interaction with acute care to more aggressive use of community-based services.

Nursing facilities will become more diverse and the services they offer more specialized. Homes will broker and/or provide adult day care, home care, and alternative living options such as assisted and congregate living; specialized services will be developed to care for those with Alzheimer's disease, brain injuries, and needs for orthopedic rehabilitation, ventilator care, and IV therapy. Future priorities for specific facilities will depend on the needs in the community, the skill levels of staff available for employment, the knowledge base of management, the cost to reconfigure both programming and the facility for particular services, the nursing home's role in an integrated delivery system, and the competitive marketplace. All these factors will contribute significantly to the success of the home in addressing the needs of its residents, remaining fiscally viable, and contributing to the well-being of the broader community. In this context, facilities will continue the original mission of all nursing homes: to provide a supportive and caring environment for those who require both services and a supportive living environment.

CLIENT EXAMPLES

Nursing facilities and their residents can be quite varied, as illustrated by the following examples.

Nursing Homes

Peterson's Home is a 30-bed private facility in the rural midwest. Originally utilized as a single-family dwelling, it was converted first to accommodate the needs of the family's aging parents and gradually expanded to include care for others from nearby farms. Strictly private-pay, the home is not certified for Medicare or Medicaid, and Life Safety Code requirements have been waived due to the shortage of beds in the area. Most residents require light nursing care and supervision and have come there as their final home.

The Alzheimer's Nursing Center is a 100-bed facility located in a commercial/residential area of a midsize city. The facility specializes in caring for those suffering from Alzheimer's disease. Payment is primarily private pay by individuals and families. The facility was started with a significant endowment and a large fundraising campaign from wealthy donors. Residents typically enter when their disease is sufficiently advanced that the family can no longer care for them, because of symptoms associated with the disease such as mental disorientation and behavioral problems. Residents typically remain through the final stages of the disease, and require complete care because of extreme physical dependence.

Community Care is a 99-bed facility that is part of a large regional for-profit multifacility health care organization. Approximately 70 percent of the residents are covered by Medicaid, while the remaining 30 percent are private pay. The emphasis is on light to moderate care, and most residents are expected to stay for an indefinite period of time.

The Health Center is a 16-bed unit that is part of a continuing care retirement community. Residents of the community may stay at the Health Center while recuperating from recent hospitalizations or during episodes of chronic illness when they require observation or regulation of medication. Fees are paid partially through the residents' initial entry fee account and partially through an additional daily assessment. The beds are not certified by Medicare or Medicaid. Although a few residents are permanent, the majority stay for two weeks or less.

The Elizabeth Center is a 320-bed multilevel facility in a suburban area. It provides seven distinct levels of care, including high-technology skilled care, rehabilitation services, personal care, and Alzheimer's care. It also operates its own home health agency and day care program. The center was freestanding for its first 50 years, then joined a large Catholic system. It has its own board of directors, but is closely affiliated with one of the Catholic hospitals in town that is part of the same system. The home accepts all sources of payment, depending on the level of care the resident is receiving.

The Subacute Unit is a 20-bed step-down unit of a 300-bed acute care hospital that has been licensed as a nursing facility. Patients are transferred to the subacute unit after an initial stay in one of the hospital's med-surg units. Average length of stay is 21 days. The beds are certified by Medicare, and most of those admitted are covered by Medicare or one of the HMOs with which the hospital contracts. Medicaid patients are not admitted.

Nursing Home Residents

Mrs. Taylor is a 62-year-old woman who fell and broke her hip. After three days in the acute hospital, she is transferred to the hospital's subacute unit. Mrs. Taylor spends 14 days regaining her strength while undergoing physical therapy before she is discharged to her home with home health services. Mrs. Taylor's private insurance pays for 80 percent of the cost of care in the nursing home; Mrs. Taylor pays the remainder.

Mrs. Jones is an 84-year-old woman with severe dementia. She is diagnosed with a mild heart condition and hearing loss, but otherwise is quite able to get around. She has come to live in the nursing home because she is too forgetful to live alone in her own home. Her daughter would care for her, but works during the day. Mrs. Jones's increasing loss of memory makes it too stressful for the family to provide supportive care. Mrs. Jones's estate pays her bill. However, if her estate no longer has resources, she will need to depend on Medicaid to cover her costs.

Mr. Elerby is a 72-year-old widower who has severe diabetes and congestive heart disease. Mentally, he is sharp, but his diminished vision and hearing loss make it difficult for him to read the paper, watch television, or otherwise get the mental stimulation he desires. He has had two leg amputations and finds it very difficult to care for himself, let alone maintain his home. Mr. Elerby does not have any children or other family members with whom he can live. He finally moves to the nursing home, where he receives assistance with personal care, constant monitoring of his medications, and opportunities for social and intellectual stimulation. Mr. Elerby pays for his care himself.

Mr. Frederickson is a 35-year-old man who suffered a major fall while at work as a telephone wire repairman. He has multiple fractures and is in a full body cast. Mr. Frederickson is transferred to a nursing home from Community Hospital and stays there for six months. When the full body cast is removed after four months, he begins rehabilitation with the physical and occupational therapists of the nursing facility. After another two months, he recovers enough strength and mobility to return home and continue rehabilitation on an outpatient basis. Mr. Frederickson's care is paid for by Worker's Compensation.

WHERE TO GO FOR FURTHER INFORMATION

American Association of Homes & Services for the Aging (AAHSA)
2519 Connecticut Avenue, NW
Washington, DC 20009
(202) 508-9442
http://www.aahsa.org

American College of Health Care Administrators (ACHCA)
325 South Patrick Street
Alexandria, VA 22314
(888) 882-2242
http://www.achca.org

American Health Care Association (AHCA)
1201 L Street NW
Washington, DC 20005
(202) 842-4444
http://www.ahca.org

Centers for Medicare and Medicaid Services (CMS)
7500 Security Boulevard
Baltimore, MD 21244-1850
(877) 267-2323

(410) 786-3000
http://www.cms.gov

Health Insurance Association of America (HIAA)
1201 F Street NW, Suite 500
Washington, DC 20004-1204
(202) 824-1600
http://www.hiaa.org

National Center for Health Statistics (NCHS)
6525 Belcrest Road
Hyattsville, MD 20782-2003
(301) 458-4636
http://www.cdc.gov/nchs

FACTS REVIEW

1. What types of services do nursing facilities offer?
2. How have acuity levels and functional dependencies of nursing home residents changed over the past decade?
3. What kinds of health care professionals work with nursing homes and what are their roles?
4. What is the role of nursing homes in the continuum of care services?
5. How are nursing homes paid for the services they provide?
6. How are nursing homes regulated? Accredited? Certified?
7. How have nursing homes evolved over the past 30 years? What will be the characteristics of homes of the future?

REFERENCES

American Health Care Association. (2003, February 12). *Results of the 2002 AHCA survey of nursing staff vacancy and turnover in nursing homes.* Washington, DC: Author.
Centers for Medicare and Medicaid Services. (2003). *Your Medicare benefits* (Publication No. CMS-10116 (revised April 2003), pp. 38–39). Baltimore, MD: Author.

Centers for Medicare and Medicaid Services, Office of the Actuary. (2003). *2003 CMS statistics* (Table 2, National Health Expenditure Amounts, and Average Annual Percent Change by Type of Expenditure: Selected Calendar Years 1980–2012). Baltimore, MD: Author.

Coleman, B. (1991). *The Nursing Home Reform Act of 1987: Provisions, policy, prospects.* Boston: University of Massachusetts.

Evashwick, C., & Holt, T. (2000). *Integrating acute care, long term care and housing.* St. Louis, MO: Catholic Health Association.

Gaugler, J. E., Kane, R. L., Kane, R. A., Clay, T., & Newcomer, R. (2003). Caregiving and institutionalization of cognitively impaired older people: Utilizing dynamic predictors of change. *The Gerontologist, 43,* 219–229.

Health Insurance Association of America (2003). Long term care insurance in 2000–2001. Washington, DC: Author.

Hing, E., Sekscenski, E., & Strahan, G. (1989). *The national nursing home survey: 1985 summary for the United States* (National Center for Health Statistics, DHHS Publication No. 89-1758). Washington, DC: Public Health Service. Also published in *Vital Health Statistics, 13*(97).

Jones, A. (2002). *The national nursing home survey: 1999 summary* (National Center for Health Statistics). *Vital Health Statistics, 13*(152).

Marion Merrell Dow. (1993). *Marion Merrell Dow managed care digest. Long term care edition.* Kansas City, MO: Marion Merrell Dow.

Murtaugh, C. M., Kemper, D., Spillman, B. C., & Carlson, B. (1997). The amount, distribution, and timing of lifetime nursing home use. *Medical Care, 35*(3), 204–218.

Murtaugh, C. M., Kemper, D., & Spillman, B. C. (1990). The risk of nursing home use later in life. *Medical Care, 28*(10), 952–962.

National Center for Health Statistics. (1997). *Advance data no. 289.* Hyattsville, MD: Public Health Services.

Sirrocco, A. (1994, February 23). Nursing homes and board and care homes (advance data). *Vital Health Statistics, 244.*

CHAPTER 6

Home Health

Susan L. Hughes and Megan Renehan

The U.S. home health care industry grew rapidly during the latter part of the twentieth century. At the end of the 1990s, reimbursement changes mandated by the Balanced Budget Act of 1997 (BBA '97) caused substantial industry consolidation. Nonetheless, because of underlying irreversible demographic trends, technological advances that facilitate complex care in the home, and consumer demand, home health care can be expected to continue to grow considerably in the foreseeable future. This chapter examines the development of home care in the United States, describes the payment and regulatory policies that have fostered our current complex array of home care services, details various sectors of the industry, and discusses challenges that must be met to maximize the impact of home care in the twenty-first century.

BACKGROUND

Home care policy in the United States has developed in an incremental and disjointed way. The first formal home care programs began in the 1880s. Home health care programs began to emerge in significant numbers during the Progressive Era (1905–1915). At the time, knowledge about the role of bacteria, concerns about contagious disease and poor hygiene in crowded slums, and high infant and maternal mortality rates stimulated the development of the public health nursing departments and voluntary Visiting Nurse Agencies that still exist in many communities across the United States. For the most part, these agencies focused on maternal and child health and communicable disease.

Between 1915 and 1960, a number of hospitals began to provide postdischarge care at home, and occasionally a visionary advocated the expansion of care at home for the chronically ill. At the same time, social services agencies began providing homemaker services to families with young children whose mothers were incapacitated by illness. Finally, during the 1940s, the Joint Commission on Chronic Disease was established; it produced a prestigious report in 1956.

Based on members' site visits to outstanding

SERVICE SNAPSHOT: Home Health

	Medicare-Certified Agencies, 1999	Private Agencies, 1999
Number	7,747	12,250
Clients served	2.7 million	5.1 million (est.)
Total visits	112,748	NA
Average charge	$93/visit (RN)	$90/hour (RN)
Major payers	Medicare Medicaid Out-of-pocket	Out-of-pocket Government programs Private insurance
Certification	Medicare Medicaid	May have Medicaid Other Public Programs

Accreditation	JCAHO
	CHAP (Community
	  Health Accreditation
	  Program)
		National Homecaring Council
		National League of Nursing
		Accreditation Commission
		  for Home Care

SOURCE: National Association for Home Care (2002). *Home care statistics*, 1999.

programs, the Commission Report emphasized the importance of physician involvement in home care and advocated an expanded role for homemakers (Benjamin, 1993). The commission also called for the development of organized, full-service home care programs marked by centralized responsibility, coordinated care planning, and a team approach to care. However, when the Commission Report was released in 1956, after 10 years of deliberations, little attention was paid to it because of concern over costs of hospital care for older Americans. Although Social Security Administration policy analysts were favorably impressed by Blue Cross reports of savings achieved by hospital-based home care programs, analysts were more concerned about potential excess demand for care, especially if the benefit were broadly defined to include homemaker care (Benjamin, 1993).

Therefore, when Medicare was passed in 1965,

the Part A Medicare home care benefit purposely was configured as an adjunct to acute hospital care. Eligibility criteria were so stringent that they limited use of this benefit. A similar Part B benefit was also created that did not require a prior hospitalization; however, a 20 percent co-payment deterred its use.

When first established, Medicaid identified home health care as an optional service that states could provide to poor and medically indigent persons of all ages, using a combination of state and federal funding. One year later, in 1967, home health care was moved from the optional to the mandatory category of Medicaid benefits. The benefit included skilled care, as well as select support services.

In the early 1970s, Medicare coverage was extended to persons with end-stage renal disease and adults with permanent disabilities. Social services funding for home care also increased in 1974 with passage of the Social Services Block Grant Amendments (Title XX). This encouraged states to consolidate social services and expand homemaker coverage to chronically ill adults. Meanwhile, Title III of the Older Americans Act established a network of Area Agencies on Aging to provide information and referral and chore/housekeeping services to those age 60 and older. Title VII of the same Act provided funding for home-delivered and congregate meals.

Two other developments of the 1970s also contributed to the complex composition of home care. First, appalled at the increased technological intensity, invasiveness, and emotional sterility of acute care for the terminally ill, advocates of hospice care succeeded in mandating a national hospice demonstration, and then enacting a Medicare hospice benefit for palliative care in 1982 (see Chapter 7). This promoted care at home for the terminally ill. Second, aided by space-age technology, infusion pumps made possible the "high-tech" care at home of persons requiring enteral and parenteral nutrition and intravenous antibiotics and chemotherapies.

Meanwhile, the passage of the Medicare Tax Equity and Financial Responsibility Act (TEFRA) in 1983 attempted to rein in rapid increases in hospital costs by mandating the prospective payment of Medicare hospital charges. The hospital Prospective Payment System (PPS) enabled hospitals to retain any savings achieved by shortening patients' length of stay. This provided strong incentives for hospitals to enter the home care business themselves or to transfer patients as soon as possible to home care or nursing home care.

Thus, within 20 years (1966–1986), fueled by four very basic trends—growth in the older and disabled populations, increased technological capacity, popular demand, and federal funding—home care had unintentionally become differentiated into four different models of care with multiple funding sources and differing eligibility criteria. Hospice is the subject of Chapter 7. The three models discussed in this chapter are:

- Medicare-certified home health agencies
- Non-Medicare home health agencies
- High-tech home therapy

First, an overview of aggregate home care use is presented.

NATIONAL PROFILE: ALL TYPES

In 2000, 1.5 million Americans, or about 1 percent of the U.S. population, were actively using some form of home care at any given time, and 7.8 million people had been discharged from one of the approximately 11,400 home care and hospice agencies then reported in the United States (National Center for Health Statistics [NCHS], 2000).

Clients

Table 6.1 shows the characteristics of home health users. Twice as many women as men use home health services, and use increases with age: people age 65 and older constitute 69 percent of all users; 17 percent of users are 85 years and older. People under age 65 who qualify for health care due to disabilities tended to receive a larger number of visits per person (81) than Medicare beneficiaries age 65 and older (73) (U.S. Department of Health and Human Services, 1998). Of the four geographic regions in the United States, 15.3 percent of users were from the Western states, compared to 16 percent and 26 percent from the Northeast and Midwest, respectively, and 43 percent from the South. In general, home care is widely used, without bounds of age, race, marital status, income level, geographic area, or any other characteristic.

Agencies

The number of agencies has grown markedly. In 1963, there were 1,100 home care agencies of record in the nation. The U.S. Department of the Census estimated that 19,690 home health care agencies existed in 1997. However, the Census Bureau defined *home care agencies* as "firms that provide skilled nursing services exclusively or in

Table 6.1 Characteristics of Home Health Users at Discharge in 2000

Characteristic	Percent	Characteristic	Percent	Characteristic	Percent
Age		**Gender**		**Marital Status at Discharge**	
Under 45 years	14.5	Male	36.2	Married	40.3
45–54 years	6.3	Female	63.8	Widowed	29.6
55–64 years	10			Divorced or separated	5.2
65–69 years	9.4	**Race**		Single or never married	15.3
70–74 years	10.8	White	79.1	Unknown	9.5
75–79 years	15.8	Black and other	12.4		
80–84 years	16.2	Black	10		
85 years +	17	Unknown	8.5		

SOURCE: Data from the 2000 National Center for Health Statistics Home & Hospice Care Survey. Hyattsville, MD: NCHS. Available at ftp://ftp.cdc.gov/pub/Health_Statistics/NCHS/Datasets/NHHCS/TABLE4HHC2000.XLS

combination with other services" (National Association for Home Care [NAHC], 2001). Because many private agencies do not provide skilled services, and provide homemaker/home health aide services only, this number substantially underestimates the total number of home care providers in the United States.

Services

Home care has evolved into four distinct models. The characteristics of each model differ. Figure 6.1 shows the services provided by the different home care models, which span the severity continuum. Although some home care agencies provide the full continuum of services shown, these generally are the exception, as multiple billing and regulatory mechanisms now in place discourage agencies from being full-service home care providers.

Most people with chronic disabilities need flexible combinations of, and timely access to, the 20 services shown in Figure 6.1, especially as conditions change over time. However, the organization and funding of these services in the United States has been fragmented, with no accountability across providers for the coordination and efficient management of care.

Funding

Home health care, very narrowly defined as free-standing programs (excluding hospital-based programs), was the fastest growing component of national health care expenditures during the last 40 years of the twentieth century, increasing from $0.2 billion in 1970 to $34.5 billion in 1997 and then dropping to $32.4 billion in 2000, following passage of the BBA '97 (Levit et al., 2002). Home care expenditures accounted for 0.3 percent of total health expenditures in 1970 but grew to account for 3.2 percent of expenditures in 1997 (Levit et al., 2002).

The absolute magnitude of home care expenditures ranks far behind other types of expenditures for hospital, physician, and nursing home care, which account for 40 percent, 22 percent, and 9 percent of personal health care expenditures, respectively (NAHC, 1999). However, adjusted for inflation, between 1960 and 1996, home health expenditures increased by a factor of 8.2, compared to factors of 3.1 and 2.2 for hospital and physician services respectively. (See Chapter 14 for more detail about financing.)

The major sources of payment for home care are shown in Table 6.2. Government, primarily Medicare and Medicaid, paid for roughly half of all formal

TECHNOLOGIES INTENSITY	SERVICE	SKILLED (MEDICARE-CERTIFIED)	SKILLED AND PERSONAL CARE (NOT MEDICARE-CERTIFIED)	HIGH-TECH	HOSPICE
High	Enteral/parenteral nutrition			X	X
	Ventilation/respirator therapy			X	
	Antibiotic therapy			X	X
	Chemotherapy			X	X
	Renal dialysis			X	
	Pharmaceuticals				X
	Skilled nursing	X	X		
	Physical therapy	X	X		
	Occupational therapy	X	X		
	Speech therapy	X	X		
	Medical social services	X	X		X
	Case management	X	X		X
	Nutrition service		X		X
	Full-time (24-hour) personal care		X		X
	Pastoral care				X
	Home health aide/personal care	X	X		
	Homemaker		X		
	Chore/housekeeping		X		
	Respite care		X		X
	Home-delivered meals		X		
LOW	Durable medical equipment	X		X	X

Figure 6.1 Homes Services by Degree of Skill Intensity

SOURCE: Hughes, S. L. (1991). Home care: Where we are and where we need to go. In M. G. Ory & A. P. Duncker (Eds.), *In-home care for older people.* Newbury Park, CA: Sage.

home care services in 2000. Other public programs paying for home care include the Older Americans Act, Title XX Social Services block grants, the Department of Veterans Affairs, and the Civilian Health and Medical Program of the Uniformed Services (CHAMPUS). Twenty-eight percent of home care services is paid for out of pocket by care recipients and their families, and another 24 percent is reimbursed by private insurance.

A more detailed description follows of agencies, users, and reimbursements associated with Medicare-certified skilled home care, non-Medicare certified home care, and high-tech home care. Hospice is described in more detail in Chapter 7.

NATIONAL PROFILE: MEDICARE-CERTIFIED HOME HEALTH AGENCIES

Medicare has been a driving force in the development of home health care. The 1965 legislation that

Table 6.2 Sources of Payment for Home Care, 2000

Source of Payment	Percent
Medicare	28.4
Medicaid	18.5
Other public insurance	5.2
Private insurance	23.5
Out-of-pocket	19.8
Other and private	4.6
Total	100

SOURCE: Health Care Financing Review. (2003). *Medicare and Medicaid statistical supplement, 2001.* Baltimore, MD: U.S. Department of Health and Human Services.

established Medicare (Title XVIII of the Social Security Act) created two sources of payment for home care, one under Medicare Part A and another under Medicare Part B. Both were designed to provide skilled care for those recovering from an acute episode of illness. Medicare does *not* pay for home care on an indefinite basis or for those whose major problem is chronic illness or functional disability.

The Medicare legislation also set up the criteria that a home care agency must comply with to be "certified" to receive Medicare payment. These "Conditions of Participation" specify staffing, reporting requirements, quality assurance obligations, and structural characteristics, among other conditions. Compliance is expensive and requires strict adherence by all staff to Medicare policies and processes. Thus, not all home care agencies choose to participate—and the companion "non-Medicare-certified" home care agencies have emerged. (The latter are described in the following section.)

Data on Medicare-certified agencies are relatively good because they are maintained by the federal government, and the agencies must submit information to be certified and be paid.

Traditionally, use of the Medicare home health care benefit was constrained by the review of claims done by designated fiscal intermediaries. These intermediaries were instructed to interpret the Medi-

care regulations regarding eligibility and benefits strictly so as to control use and cost. In 1989, a class action lawsuit protesting this practice (*Duggan v. Bowen*) was brought on behalf of beneficiaries, arguing that the practice violated the original intent of the Medicare legislation. The court found for the plaintiffs and mandated a broader interpretation of the definition of *homebound* and a broader limit on the number of covered visits. As a result, use of the Medicare home care benefit exploded and the number of visits and reimbursements began increasing at an annual rate of 30 percent. In an effort to staunch this fiscal hemorrhage, Congress passed the Balanced Budget Act of 1997. The BBA '97 mandated the development of a case-mix-based prospective payment system, with implementation scheduled for October 2000, and an interim payment system for use while the prospective system was in development. The interim payment system (IPS) contained new per-beneficiary reimbursement limits that had a major negative effect on the number of agencies participating in the Medicare program and on home health care payments, as will be demonstrated in sections to follow.

Clients

To be eligible for Medicare payment for home care, a person must meet the criteria delineated in the accompanying box. Although the criteria have been modified somewhat over the years, they remain focused on recovery from acute illness, not long-term maintenance or assistance with functional disability.

As shown in Figure 6.2, between 1974 and 1997, the number of clients served per year grew from less than 500,000 to 3.5 million in 1997, although it declined to 2.7 million in 2000, following the passage of BBA '97 (NAHC, 2001). The latter figure represents 7 percent of the 38.5 million aged and people with disabilities enrolled in the Medicare program. The great majority of users in 1999 (91 percent) were aged beneficiaries; 8.6 percent were younger people with disabilities. The rate of use rose from 51 users per 1,000 Medicare enrollees in 1989 to 107 users per 1,000 Medi-

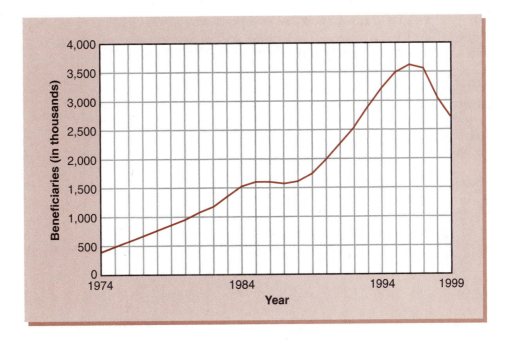

Figure 6.2   Medicare Home Care Beneficiaries, 1974–1999

SOURCE: National Association of Home Care. *Basic statistics about home care.* Available at *http://www.nahc.org/*

care enrollees in 1996, and then dropped to 85 users per 1000 in 1999, after passage of BBA '97 (NAHC, 2001).

Medicaid also pays for home health care. States establish their own criteria for acceptance as a Medicaid provider. However, states typically accept home health agencies certified to participate in Medicare as providers for Medicaid as well. In 1998, 1.2 million Medicaid recipients received home health care visits, representing 3.1 percent of the total Medicaid enrolled population. This was an increase from 1.6 percent of the Medicaid population receiving home health care in 1975. The number of people receiving Medicaid-reimbursed home care increased on average 8 percent per year, constituting the largest proportional increase in users across all types of reimbursed services (U.S. Department of Health and Human Services, 1998).

The top three principal diagnoses among Medicare home health care users in 1999 (Table 6.3)

ELIGIBILITY CRITERIA FOR MEDICARE HOME HEALTH

- Enrolled in Medicare
- Homebound, i.e., unable to leave the house, certified by a physician
- Requires skilled nursing care or physical therapy
- Needs only intermittent care, not continuous

were diseases of the circulatory system (about 31 percent), injury and poisoning (almost 16 percent), and diseases of the musculoskeletal system (more than 14 percent) (Health Care Financing Review, 2001).

The early Medicare home care reimbursement regulations attempted to ensure that the benefit

Table 6.3   Top Primary Diagnoses among Medicare Home Health Users, 1999

Admissions Diagnosis	All Discharges	Percent
Diseases of the circulatory system	855,000	31.4
Injury and poisoning	432,000	15.9
Diseases of the musculoskeletal system/connective tissue	383,000	14.1
Diseases of the respiratory system	315,000	11.6
Symptoms, signs, and ill-defined conditions	282,000	10.4
Endocrine, nutritional, and metabolic diseases, and immunity disorders	232,000	8.5
Heart failure	226,000	8.3
Diseases of the skin and subcutaneous tissue	200,000	7.4
Neoplasms	190,000	7.0
Diabetes mellitus	172,000	6.3

SOURCE: Health Care Financing Review (2001). *Medicare & Medicaid statistical supplement, 2001.* Baltimore, MD: U.S. Department of Health and Human Services.

would be used only by persons recovering from an acute bout of illness who required skilled care. Thus, beneficiaries were required to undergo a three-day hospitalization prior to referral to home care. Although this requirement was discontinued, the majority of users of Medicare-certified home health services are people who are discharged from the hospital. In 1996, about 16 percent of hospitalized Medicare patients used home care services within 30 days of discharge.

Agencies

The number of Medicare-certified home health agencies grew from 1,753 in 1967, one year after the implementation of Medicare, to an all-time high of 10,444 in 1997 (NAHC, 1999). The BBA '97 resulted in the closing of roughly one-third of all Medicare-certified agencies, with the number declining to 7,152 in 2000, a reduction of 31.5 percent (NAHC, 2001) (see Figure 6.3).

In addition to their numbers, the organizational auspice of home care agencies has changed markedly. Figure 6.4 contrasts the prevalence of organizational arrangements over time. In 1966, the Visiting Nurse Association (VNA) and Public

Health Departments accounted for 90 percent of all certified home health agencies. The Omnibus Reconciliation Act of 1980 changed the Medicare Conditions of Participation to permit proprietary providers in states without home care licensure requirements to provide Medicare reimbursed care (Silverman, 1990). Then, in 1983, Medicare prospective payment for hospital care encouraged hospitals to develop their own hospital-based or linked programs in order to streamline discharge planning and maximize patient care revenues. As a result, by 2000, VNA and public health providers dropped to 19.2 percent of total home care providers, while proprietaries increased from zero to 40 percent, and hospital-based providers rose from 6 percent to 30 percent of all Medicare-certified providers (NAHC, 2001).

Services

Services provided by skilled home health agencies include skilled nursing, skilled therapies (physical, occupational, and speech), medical social work, and home health aide. Three services constituted 97 percent of the total reimbursable visits in 1996: skilled nursing (41 percent), home health aide (49 percent),

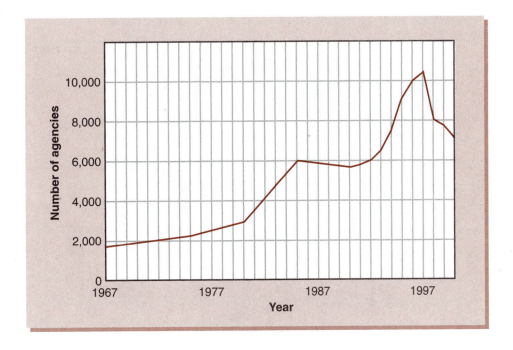

Figure 6.3   Medicare-Certified Home Care Agencies, 1967–2000

SOURCE: National Association of Home Care. *Basic statistics about home care.* Available at *http://www.nahc.org/*

and physical therapy (7 percent) (U.S. Department of Health and Human Services, 1998).

To be eligible for Medicare reimbursement, Medicare clients must be certified by a physician as needing skilled nursing or physical therapy. Other skilled services and home health aide care are then also allowable. Because of federal regulations, Medicare-certified agencies tend to offer only those services paid for by Medicare. Noncertified private agencies may offer skilled as well as support services.

Skilled personnel coordinate with staff of other organizations providing care to the client. The nurse, for example, may act as a case manager and contact the company providing durable medical equipment and the community agency providing Meals on Wheels. Coordination is usually informal rather than through any type of formal arrangement.

The total number of visits provided by Medicare-certified home health agencies by year are shown in

Figure 6.5. Annual visits rose precipitously, especially among those receiving 100 or more visits, reflecting a significant expansion in eligibility and coverage of persons with chronic care needs.

The sudden growth in visits occurred after the 1989 class action lawsuit *(Duggan v. Bowen)* that forced the Health Care Financing Administration (HCFA) to interpret the part-time/intermittent Medicare eligibility criterion more generously and to allow eligibility for enrollees who required skilled nursing *judgment,* not only skilled nursing *care.* Between 1989 and 1996, the average number of visits per user per year tripled, from 27 to 76. Following passage of the BBA '97, under the new interim payment system, the number of visits dropped dramatically. Between 1996 and 1998, the median length of stay on Medicare home health care decreased by 16 days; the decrease was especially pronounced among the proprietary providers

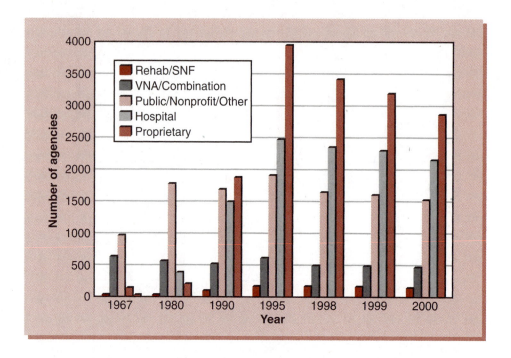

Figure 6.4   Number of Medicare-Certified Home Care Agencies, by Auspice, by Selected Years, 1967–2000
SOURCE: National Association of Home Care. *Basic statistics about home care.* Available at *http://www.nahc.org/*

(Murkofsky, Phillips, McCarthy, Davis, & Hamel, 2003). Because Medicare home health care had previously been reimbursed on a retrospective cost-per-visit basis, participating agencies had incentives to provide the maximum number of visits possible. The new PPS that was implemented in October 2000 attempted to remove this incentive by reimbursing prospectively for a case-mix-based episode of care; however, the impact of PPS on length of stay and outcomes has not been evaluated.

To constrain rapidly increasing Medicare home health care costs, the BBA '97 mandated that, as of January 1, 1998, home health coverage under Medicare Part A would be limited to a maximum of 100 visits during an illness, after a hospitalization, or after receiving covered services in a skilled nursing facility. All other home health coverage would be rendered under Part B. This shift was phased in gradually over time, at the rate of one-sixth of beneficiaries per year through January 1, 2002.

Staffing

Registered nurses (37 percent) and home health aides (28 percent) accounted for the majority (65 percent) of all full-time equivalent (FTE) staff in Medicare-certified home health agencies in 2000 (NAHC, 2001). The proportions of FTE physical therapists and licensed practical nurses (LPNs) were low, at 5 percent and 9 percent, respectively (NAHC, 2001). Social workers, occupational and speech therapists, and homemakers also may be on staff. By Medicare regulation, the majority of staff are salaried employees, although some professional staff may be on contract for a specified number of hours per month.

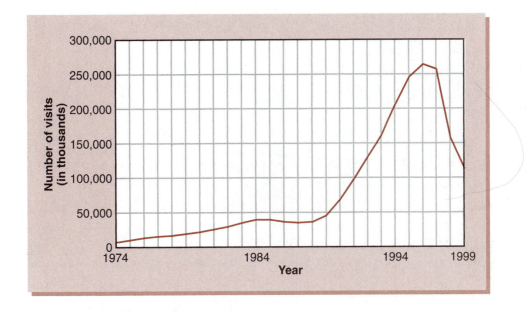

Figure 6.5   Medicare Home Care Visits, 1974–1999

SOURCE: National Association of Home Care. *Basic statistics about home care.* Available at *http://www.nahc.org/*

Home health agencies depend heavily on the availability of registered nurses and, to a growing degree, LPNs, in addition to home health aides (HHAs). At present, the industry is highly regulated. Thus, opportunities for experiments involving the substitution of less skilled personnel for more skilled personnel are limited.

Despite the fact that the acuity level of Medicare home care clients is increasing, the physician's role in home health care has been limited, with the notable exception of the Veterans Affairs (VA) Home Based Primary Care (HBPC) Program, in which physicians work closely with the home care team as primary care managers. Until the early 1990s, Medicare reimbursement rates for physician home visits were lower than those for HHAs. A randomized study of the VA home care model found that home health teams that include active physician participation reduced hospital readmission costs by 29 percent (Cummings et al., 1990). The whole issue of physician involvement in home care is being

reconsidered at present. An American Academy of Home Care Physicians has been established and the American Medical Association (AMA) has developed physician home care practice guidelines. In 1995, the HCFA increased the reimbursement for physician home visits and allowed physicians to bill for case management functions on behalf of clients. However, a national survey of 600 physicians who signed Medicare home health care plans of care in 2000 found that less than 3 percent of total home health claims were submitted for this service. Physicians reported that the reimbursement provided was too low to offset the costs of completing the paperwork required for billing (Office of the Inspector General, 2001). Thus, except for specific physician providers who specialize in providing care to homebound clients, and when the volume of clients served can offset the administrative costs of recordkeeping and billing, it is reasonable to expect that the role of the physician will not increase in importance in the future.

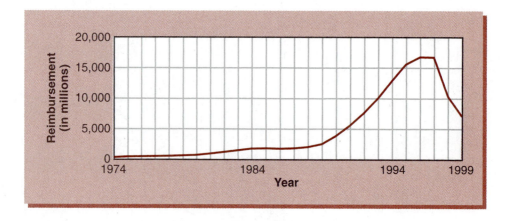

Figure 6.6   *Medicare Home Care Reimbursement, 1974–1999*

SOURCE: National Association of Home Care. *Basic statistics about home care.* Available at *http://www.nahc.org/*

Funding

Total reimbursements for Medicare-certified home health agencies expanded gradually between 1974 and 1989. As regulatory restraints on the number of visits were relaxed after the *Duggan v. Bowen* lawsuit, number of visits and concomitant reimbursements expanded dramatically, before peaking in 1997 and substantially declining following the passage of BBA '97 (Figure 6.6).

In dollar terms, expenditures for Medicare-certified home care increased from $2.5 billion in 1989 to $16.7 billion in 1997 (an annual rate of increase of 33 percent). The BBA '97 attempted to mitigate this rate of increase by mandating a change from fee-for-service/retrospective reimbursement based on cost to prospective payment based on per-beneficiary episodes of care. While the new PPS was being developed, agencies were reimbursed under an IPS that precipitously reduced expenditures to $14 billion in 1998, $9.4 billion in 1999, and $8.2 billion in 2000—a decrease of 48 percent between 1997 and 2000.

The goal of the PPS is to reward efficient providers and prod inefficient providers to change their behavior. Although the impact of IPS has been studied and reported to have decreased incidence of use among beneficiaries age 85 and older (McCall, Petersons, Moore, & Korb, 2003), the impact of PPS reimbursement is not yet known. The system relies on an 80-category case mix adjuster to set payment rates based on patient characteristics, including clinical severity, functional status, and use of rehabilitative services; it includes payment for unexpectedly high-use cases through an outlier adjustment, as well as adjustment for area wage indices. A review of PPS by the General Accounting Office (GAO) identified several areas of concern, including the 60-day episode for payment, which may be too long for many clients; the impact of payment on different types of providers in different geographic locations; and the adequacy of the case mix adjustment method with respect to accurate assessment of resource needs. As a result of these concerns, the authors urged that the impact of the new system be carefully studied by the Centers for Medicare and Medicaid Services (CMS) (GAO, 2000a).

Medicaid also reimburses for skilled home health care. In 1975, hospital and nursing home payments combined to account for 62 percent of national Medicaid expenditures. By 1998, these payments had dropped to 40 percent of total expenditures, while home health payments increased from 0.6 percent of Medicaid to 12.5 percent ($17.6 billion), reflecting the same trends toward shortened hospital length of stay, reduction of hospital admissions, and increased capacity to provide technologically complex care in the home.

Commercial insurance companies and managed care health plans typically have a benefit for skilled home care in conjunction with an acute episode of illness. Private insurance paid for 18.9 percent ($6.9 billion) of home care provided in 2000 (NAHC, 2001). Although these payers can establish their own policies, they tend to mirror federal Medicare policies. Thus, the services covered and the rates allowed are usually quite similar to those of Medicare.

Since 1994, Medicare payments to managed care plans do not distinguish home care. As a result, CMS utilization and expenditures data do not reflect home care used by managed care enrollees.

Licensure, Certification, and Accreditation

Licensing, certification, and accreditation are different for Medicare-certified home health agencies than for other forms of home care.

Licensure

Most states license a Medicare-certified home health agency as a health provider. This is typically done under the jurisdiction of the state's health department.

Certification

Home health care agencies must be certified if they are to obtain Medicare reimbursement. Similarly, most states certify agencies as eligible to participate in Medicaid based on certification by Medicare. Certification for Medicare is based on compliance with the federally mandated Conditions of Participation (COPs), which, until the late 1990s, relied mainly on compliance with structure and process standards.

The Omnibus Reconciliation Act of 1989 mandated the development and testing of client outcomes for home health care and the inclusion of client home visits in the quality assurance surveys conducted by state licensing agencies. Beginning in January 1999, CMS (formerly the HCFA) required all Medicare-certified providers to implement the OASIS system. The Outcome Assessment and Information Set, developed by the University of Colorado, is a uniform set of indicators of client outcomes. OASIS data are collected at multiple points in time during the course of each patient's treatment, including admission, follow-up, or recertification; when a patient is admitted to a hospital for any reason; when a patient returns to an agency following a hospitalization; upon discharge; or if the patient dies at home. Different pieces of data are collected at these various points in time by either a staff nurse or a therapist. CMS requires that data be gathered and submitted electronically on all Medicare, Medicaid, managed care, private-pay, and personal care-only patients. The data are then forwarded at regular intervals to an agreed-on state agency, where they are further processed, forwarded to the state home care regulatory agency, and sent to CMS.

Accreditation

Home health agencies can seek accreditation from either the Joint Commission on Accreditation of Healthcare Organizations (JCAHO) or the Community Health Accreditation Program (CHAP). JCAHO and CHAP have also developed voluntary quality assurance programs for home health care providers that incorporate the OASIS data set. Participation in JCAHO's ORYX program is mandatory for home care programs that are hospital-based or -owned and have an average monthly census of 10 or more patients. Participating agencies select measures from listed performance measurement systems, apply the measures, and submit the data regularly to JCAHO, which uses controls and comparison charts to identify performance trends and patterns that are then discussed during on-site surveys (*http://www.jcaho.org*). Currently, JCAHO certifies 4,906 home care organizations and CHAP certifies 850; thus, about 5,000 home care providers are certified. Although participation in these voluntary programs can be expensive, if providers meet the certification requirements of either of these programs, they are "deemed" to comply with the Medicare COPs and are exempt from state-sponsored regulatory surveys.

NATIONAL PROFILE: PRIVATE HOME CARE AGENCIES

Private home care agencies offer a broad range of home care services, from the skilled services available through Medicare-certified agencies to personal support provided by paraprofessionals, including personal care and homemaker/chore services. Services can be provided separately or in conjunction with any of the other models of home care. Home care is provided to persons with chronic functional disabilities who wish to remain in their homes, rather than enter an institution, as well as to those recovering from an acute illness.

Agencies

Skilled nursing and therapies can be provided by home care agencies that are licensed by the state but not certified to receive reimbursement from Medicare or Medicaid. Because providers are not required to be certified, no complete listing is currently available. According to the Bureau of the Census, there were about 20,000 home health care agencies in the United States in 2000 (NAHC, 2001). Of these, 36 percent were Medicare-certified and 64 percent were not. Therefore, it is assumed that roughly 12,000 noncertified agencies existed at that time. However, this number also may substantially underestimate the true supply, because not all providers are known.

Clients

Clients receiving care from noncertified agencies have a wider range of needs than those who are eligible for Medicare reimbursement. Clients' needs may range from around-the-clock skilled nursing to a weekly "bathe and shave" service. Those using homemaker and chore services tend to be people with functional disabilities who need assistance with ADLs and IADLs rather than skilled nursing care or therapies. The Medicaid Section 2176 Community Care Waiver and Medicaid Section 1915 (c) waivers can be applied to older adults, to younger persons with physical disabilities, to persons with AIDS, and to persons with developmental disabilities who have impairment levels that would render them eligible for nursing home care if community-based care were not available.

Services

Services provided vary, but may include case management, homemaker/chore services, and personal care, as well as the full range of skilled home care services provided by nurses and therapists.

Capital funding, start-up, and operating costs for noncertified home care providers are even less than for Medicare-certified agencies because these agencies do not need to meet Medicare requirements for personnel or financial solvency. However, because of the low rates paid by the Medicaid waiver programs in many states, many noncertified programs have found that the best way to survive in this segment of the home care field is by building volume, which entails the development of a multiunit, if not multistate, chain capacity. Private home care agencies may also exist in parallel with a Medicare-certified agency, with an exchange of appropriate referrals. However, under Medicare regulations, the two agencies must be operated entirely separately, even if owned by the same corporation or health care delivery system.

Staffing

In contrast to Medicare-certified agencies, noncertified agencies typically do not employ staff on a full-time basis. Rather, they maintain a registry of people who are willing to work on an on-call basis for an hourly fee. Skilled personnel, such as registered nurses and therapists, work on an hourly, rather than salaried, basis as they do for Medicare-certified agencies. Functional support services are primarily provided by paraprofessional workers: nurses aides (NAs), home health aides, and licensed vocational or practical nurses (LVNs, LPNs). Many of these workers are paid less than workers in the fast-food industry, have less than full-time employment, and have minimal, if any, benefits.

Bureau of Labor Statistics (BLS) data indicate that about 746,000 home health and personal care aide jobs existed in the United States in 1998 (Bureau of Labor Statistics, 2000). The overwhelming majority of these workers are women, and most have low levels of educational attainment and are economically disadvantaged (Stone & Wiener, 2001). As a result of the aging of the U.S. population, the BLS has projected that personal and home care assistance will be the fourth-fastest growing occupation by 2006, with an increase in growth of 75 percent among home health aides, specifically.

Home care workers value autonomy in their jobs and enjoy their caregiving roles. However, they want to have more input into client care plans. They need opportunities for further training and career advancement, as well as better pay and benefits.

Thus, the main challenge facing noncertified home care providers is the recruitment and retention of trained personnel. At present, noncompetitive wages, low benefits, and the challenging nature of the work are believed to cause high staff turnover rates in this sector of the home care industry. Ensuring quality is difficult when staff are part-time and on the registry of several agencies.

One possible solution to this urgent manpower issue is consumer-directed home care, a new model of care that has been tested by the Assistant Secretary's Office for Planning and Evaluation, Department of Health and Human Services (DHHS), and by researchers at Mathematica Policy Research, Inc. As its name implies, consumer-directed care enables home care consumers to recruit and manage their personal care helpers, who may be paid family members (Benjamin, 2001). This model of care has been the standard for younger persons with disabilities who are accustomed to directing their own care. However, it has only recently been tested with an elderly population. Early returns from a multisite randomized test of the model indicate that older adults who participated in the model have high levels of satisfaction with it, and several states are currently considering allowing it as an option in their waiver programs (Coleman, 2001).

Funding

Charges for home care services are roughly equivalent to those for Medicare services. However, charges are typically per hour rather than per visit. Some services may establish a minimum or a flat rate.

Although private home care agencies cannot receive payment from Medicare, they may be authorized providers for other public programs, particularly those offered by states and counties. Hence, private home care services are reimbursed by a variety of sources, including Medicaid 2176 Community Care Waivers, state block grants (Title XX), Older Americans Act Title III funds, state and local revenues, and private out-of-pocket payment. Although Title XX and OAA funding remained relatively constant during the 1990s, substantial growth has occurred in Medicaid and state funding of home care services.

Commercial insurance and managed care plans also pay for home care services. Although some may require home care agencies to be Medicare-certified, others do not, and are willing to cover care on an individual basis or to contract with an agency for coverage of eligible patients.

The Medicaid Section 2176 Home and Community-Based Care Waiver (HCBCW) was created by the Omnibus Budget Reconciliation Act (OBRA) in 1981 in an attempt to decrease the use of nursing homes by Medicaid-eligible and low-income aged, persons with disabilities, and mentally retarded persons. A modification of Social Security Act Title XIX, section 2176, allows states to apply for and receive a waiver from the federal government to modify the benefits required for Medicaid. States may expand the services covered, the eligibility criteria, or the geographic area of eligibility for increased benefits. In 1982, six states participated in the waiver, with expenditures of $3.8 million. The program has since grown to encompass all but two states, with expenditures of $8.1 billion in 1997 (Miller, Ramsland, & Harrington, 1999).

Medicaid waiver spending for individuals with mental retardation has grown the most over time, accounting for about 75 percent of total waiver expenditures in 2001, mainly because many people with mental retardation/developmental disabilities receive 24-hour support (Coleman, Fox, & Granger, 2002). The Medicaid waiver benefit increased from $10.6 billion in 1999 to $14 billion in 2001—a 32 percent increase that substantially exceeds the rate of growth in Medicaid nursing home dollars over the same time period. However, the magnitude of the waiver varies greatly from state to state.

In addition to Medicaid waivers, noncertified home care is also reimbursed in many states through programs funded by general revenue. Massachusetts, Wisconsin, California, and Pennsylvania all have relatively large state-only funded programs serving older adults (Murtaugh, Stevenson, Feldman, & Oberlink, 2000). Illinois, for example, spent $293 million of its Medicaid expenditures on home care in 2001, but also committed an additional $200 million in general revenues to its Community Care Program for older adults (Coleman, Fox-Grage, & Folkemer, 2002).

Licensure, Certification, and Accreditation

Licensing, certification, and accreditation are less stringent for private home care agencies than for Medicare agencies.

Licensure

Very few states license noncertified providers, except for business licenses. However, most states have developed mandatory quality assurance/improvement programs for providers who participate in waiver and state-revenue-funded community care programs. In most cases, structure standards are used to assess quality, and process and outcome measures are conspicuously absent.

Certification

Private home care agencies may be certified by public programs other than Medicare to be authorized providers. Certification criteria are determined by the specific program. Examples include state or county mental health departments, Veterans Affairs medical centers, and Older American Act providers selected by the local Area Agency on Aging. An agency that meets certification requirements is entitled to bill for the care provided, but must also comply with the operating regulations of the funder.

Accreditation

The Accreditation Commission for Health Care, Inc., currently accredits about 450 different home care providers, including high-tech and private home care providers. In addition, many national home care chains have developed their own internal quality assurance systems, including the initiation of continuous quality improvement programs. However, in large part, participation in quality assurance programs across providers is voluntary and hence variable. Moreover, findings are not made available to consumers.

NATIONAL PROFILE: HIGH-TECH HOME CARE

High-tech home therapy combines skilled home care professionals, advanced technology medical equipment, and pharmaceuticals. In 1968, patients without functioning digestive organs were sustained for the first time through total parenteral nutrition provided intravenously. Initially, these treatments required 24-hour-a-day hospital care. The invention of pumps in the early 1970s permitted more rapid infusion of solutions, freeing patients from tubes and bottles for up to 16 hours a day. As a result of this technology, it became possible to move this care outside the hospital to home. High-tech therapy provided at home now enables people to maintain normal lives, including resumption of work or school.

In 1983, approximately 2,500 patients received parenteral nutrition therapy at home at a cost of $150 to $250 a day, or about $200 million a year (Donlan, 1983). Since that time, high-tech home care has expanded to include respirator/ventilation therapy, intravenous (IV) antibiotics, chemotherapy treatments, and home-based renal dialysis, in addition to enteral and parenteral nutrition.

Original projections of growth in high-tech home care were glowing. The American Society for Parenteral and Enteral Nutrition estimated in 1983 that 150,000 to 200,000 home parenteral patients alone would be treated in 1990, at expenditures of up to $1.6 billion per year (Donlan, 1983). Current data indicate that these projections for growth in numbers of users and expenditures were not too far from the mark. For example:

- In 1997, an estimated 250,000 Americans used outpatient intravenous antibiotics, and this number is expected to increase annually by 15 to 20 percent. New technology has enabled the dosage of antibiotics to be timed for maximum effect with home infusion systems.
- The development of plastic-polymer catheters as replacements for steel has enabled catheters to remain in place for up to a year, an important feature for patients with long-term chronic conditions like AIDS, cancer, cystic fibrosis, or Lyme disease.
- Electric left ventricular assist devices (LVADS) and other advances enable patients with end-stage heart disease to be sustained at home on battery-operated pumps while awaiting a heart transplant.

- Advances in respiratory therapy technology have enabled chronic obstructive pulmonary disease and asthma patients to be maintained at home with oxygen concentrators and portable ultrasonic nebulizers.
- Developments in telemedicine have enabled nurses to use a two-way video hook-up to measure patient's blood pressure and pulse; listen to heart, lung, or bowel sounds through a stethoscope worn by the patients; take electrocardiograms; and remind patients to take their medicine. These systems work well with patients with diabetes, wounds, hemophilia, serious skin disorders, and anxiety attacks (McDaniel, 1997).

Although the Medicare-certified and private home health care agencies previously described account for 75 percent of the total home care industry, and are estimated to generate approximately $30 billion in health care spending, high-tech home care accounts for the remaining 25 percent of the home health care industry market. Altogether this segment of the industry, which includes respiratory therapy, infusion therapy, and durable medical equipment, accounts for another $10 billion in home care expenditures (CMS, 2002).

Clients

High-tech home care is used in the treatment of a wide variety of disease conditions that require enteral or parenteral nutrition, ventilator therapy, IV antibiotics, chemotherapy, or renal dialysis. Users also span all age groups, including "technology dependent" children, many of whom have been able to receive care at home rather than in a hospital as a result of this technology. A study of high-tech home care users at 150 home health care agencies across the United States found that one in 10 home care patients uses high-tech care, with hospices serving the largest proportion of patients (Kaye & Davitt, 1995). Complex regimens using equipment and pharmaceuticals often require that a caregiver be involved to help clients manage their care.

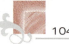

MOST FREQUENT HIGH-TECH HOME CARE THERAPIES

- IV antibiotic therapy
- Chemotherapy
- Pain medication
- Total parenteral nutrition
- Enteral nutrition
- Renal dialysis
- Respirator/ventilation therapy

Services

High-tech home care combines skilled home care professionals, medical equipment, and pharmaceuticals. The patient's physician must initially authorize care at home. A registered nurse is often involved to educate the patient and family about all aspects of care, as well as to monitor care. A specially trained technician may be involved to establish the initial set-up of equipment and supplies. Pharmacists, off-site, organize and monitor drug use. Equipment may be simple or quite complex. Initial education and ongoing commitment of the patient and family are essential to successful use of high-tech therapy in the home. In addition to high-tech therapy, the patient may have multiple conditions that require monitoring or treatment beyond the high-tech therapy, for which other home care providers and the patient's regular physician continue to be involved. The most frequent high-tech therapies are listed in the accompanying box.

Structure

Approximately 3,000 infusion companies exist nationally. These include pharmacies, hospital-affiliated organizations, regional infusion providers, and home infusion organizations. At present this segment of the home care industry is extremely fragmented and comprised for the most part of small local and regional operators. Because of increased billing complexity, limited access to capital, and payment cuts included in the BBA '97, industry analysts predict that substantial consolidation will take place in the near future (CMS, 2002).

Home care providers who wish to provide high-tech care can pursue several different options. They can start their own in-house pharmacy; however, start-up costs for this option are hefty (Brown, 1990). They can also contract with local retail pharmacies, local home care pharmacies, or local hospital pharmacies, or they can form joint ventures with a national home care chain that has expertise in this area.

A primary consideration in high-tech home care is the status of clients' homes and the capacity of clients or informal caregivers to be involved in care. Clients must have adequate space to store medical supplies, the capacity to refrigerate solutions, and the capacity to learn and adhere to a detailed care regimen.

Staffing

High-tech home care requires close collaboration of the physician, the pharmacist, the registered nurse, and, depending on the type of therapy, possibly the medical supply company. Skilled home health agencies may also participate in the client's care. However, the high-tech home care patient places a greater demand on traditional home care agencies in terms of staff and technology. Patients may require both more time and a greater level of skilled care. Both the patient and family need to be trained in care techniques, and family concerns must be accommodated by staff. The provision of high-tech home care also may demand greater physician involvement than traditional home care services. In addition, if the home care agency contracts with a separate equipment provider, services must be coordinated with emergency back-up plans and plans for equipment maintenance. Pharmacists may be involved in cases where drugs must be specially mixed and carefully monitored.

Funding

At present, some or all components of high-tech home care are reimbursed by Medicare, Medicaid, Medicaid waivers for technologically dependent children, and most private insurance. The BBA '97 also negatively affected the home respiratory and infusion therapy services market, but this segment of the home care industry experienced a quicker recovery. Home oxygen use was particularly affected, but has stabilized since 2000 (CMS, 2002).

Nursing visits to provide skilled care, patient education, supplies, and durable medical equipment (DME) are covered by Medicare; however, drugs are not covered.

Because of its perceived cost-effectiveness, the use of high-tech home care is increasing among both private insurance carriers and large employer-administered benefit plans. Such insurance can be more flexible than Medicare in covering the total cost of care. However, awareness is growing among these groups that the benefit must be very carefully managed to produce cost savings. This management may include negotiated contracts based on discounted charges with home health care agencies and medical equipment suppliers.

The billing for a high-tech client can be complex, involving up to four separate bills: one each for the home health agency skilled nurse, the pharmaceuticals, the initial equipment set-up, and the ongoing equipment monitoring.

Licensure, Certification, and Accreditation

High-tech home care providers are regulated in a complex way.

Licensure

Each service provider must meet its state's requirements for licensure as a distinct service. For example, home care agencies seeking Medicare certification must be licensed by the state department of health. Pharmacies must be licensed as pharmacies, and DME companies must have a business license. There is no single encompassing license to be a "high-tech" provider.

Certification

High-tech home care agencies that wish to seek reimbursement from Medicare must meet Medicare Conditions of Participation. Agencies can also be certified by Medicaid and select other government programs. Medical supply companies can bill Medicare Part B, which has no required COPs.

Accreditation

Participation in accreditation programs is voluntary but is viewed as advisable if a provider seeks to contract with managed care plans. About half of the 3,000 home care providers that are accredited by JCAHO provide high-tech home care, for which JCAHO has formulated specific standards of care (JCAHO, 2000). Other organizations that accredit high-tech home care providers are the Community Health Accreditation Program and the Accreditation Commission for Health Care (ACHC).

INTEGRATING MECHANISMS

Home care is an essential component of the continuum of care. However, it often functions quite separately from other services.

Structure

The diversity of home care programs is reflected in the wide variation of organizational arrangements. Many agencies provide only one model of home care, are freestanding, and relate to other providers of all types through informal relationships. At the other extreme is the large multiorganization health care system that owns all types of home care services. Under the latter, services may be well coordinated or operate as independently as if they were separate community-based agencies.

Because financing and regulations have fragmented home care delivery in a way that is not consistent with client care needs, all home care providers are faced with trying to coordinate their care with that rendered by other providers. Primarily because of stringent federal regulations, the home care providers must structure their operations in specified ways. Even within publicly funded home care, Medicare home health programs have no jurisdiction over Medicaid waiver- or Older Americans Act-funded home care services, and vice versa. Thus, the synergies, enhancements to quality, and efficiencies that could be gained by close collaboration are seldom realized. Nonetheless, for the good of patient care, cooperation across providers is important and happens on an informal basis.

Care Coordination

Home care agencies are the one provider (other than assisted living providers) who are in a client's home on a regular basis and can observe the environment and the social dynamics. Home care workers have the opportunity to assist the family in accessing the full range of health and social services needed to maximize independence at home.

However, home care may exemplify lack of clinical coordination because the several people helping a client at home may be from different agencies having no formal relationship. At present, if a person requires more than one type of home care at a time, no single individual or agency is officially in charge of that care. Home care personnel each set their own schedule, so all may arrive on the same day at the same time or too far apart. A strong and involved family may assume an active role in coordinating the care providers, but an ill individual living alone may be unable to do so.

Physician involvement in home care is minimal. Although skilled services must continue to seek physician certification, nonskilled service providers, or those paid privately, have no obligation to inform the client's physician of routine care or noted problems.

Hospital admissions and nursing home placements usually result from decisions made jointly by patients and physicians. To date, physicians have been actively discouraged from assuming a leadership role in home care, with physician home visits reimbursed at a level below that for a home health aide until 1992.

Information Systems

The information systems for home care have evolved totally separate from those of hospitals, nursing homes, or any other providers. Home care systems tend to be stand-alone and do not interface with other public or private systems. This has been exacerbated by Medicare's requirements that Medicare-certified agencies establish direct electronic billing and complete the OASIS clinical reporting. As home care enters the twenty-first century, it is well entrenched in management mechanisms that set it apart rather than allow it to function as an integrated service of the continuum.

Managed Care and Home Care

Managed care is a logical source to assume both coordination and reimbursement; however, experience with managed home care is quite limited at present.

Just as BBA '97 caused substantial retrenchment among home care providers, it also caused a significant drop in the number of managed care plans that contract with Medicare. The BBA attempted to even out reimbursement for managed care between providers in urban areas, which customarily had high Medicare reimbursement rates, and providers in rural areas, who historically received low payments. In the end, the reform drove substantial numbers of managed care plans from participation in Medicare, affecting 1.6 million Medicare beneficiaries who were forced to enroll in other plans or return to fee-for-service care (Gold, 2001; GAO, 2000b; GAO, 2001). Although Medicare reforms may help to restore the participation of managed care plans, the likelihood of their being able to assume major responsibility for coordination of services is not high at present.

Managed care plans are paid by Medicare on a capitated rate that encompasses the full spectrum of required services. Medicare does not require the plans to report the details of service actually provided. Thus, the number of people using home care, the number and type of visits, and other data about home care that are available for fee-for-service Medicare enrollees are not reported for managed care enrollees. This results in an underreporting of the use of Medicare-certified home health services by older adults and makes analysis for policy or management purposes challenging.

POLICY ISSUES

At present, the home care industry is divided into four home care models. The past 30 years have seen dramatic increases in the number of home care providers and clients, and the current political environment suggests that this trend will continue for the foreseeable future. Most analysts agree that home care is here to stay and believe that the major policy questions concern *how to manage home care* to *improve its effectiveness.* One of the major questions that remains unanswered is, "How can we streamline the delivery and management of care to maximize its efficiency and effectiveness?" Thus, methods of integrating home care services within or across providers, and methods of integrating home care services with those of acute care and other long-term care providers, are badly needed, as are methods of reimbursing care that promote efficiency across home care types.

However, despite these serious challenges, several very important advances in policy have been made in the last few years. With respect to Medicare home health, significant progress has been made in implementing both a case-mix-based prospective payment system and a case-mix-adjusted set of outcome measures. The payment system should bring some stability to the field, which was quite traumatized by BBA '97. However, it will be very important to examine the impact of PPS for home care on issues such as access and outcomes of care.

With respect to outcomes, major strides are occurring with respect to capacity to measure home care outcomes. A team at the University of Colorado tested Outcome-Based Quality Improvement (OBQI)—a continuous quality improvement methodology for home health care—in New York and 27 other states. They found significant reductions in risk-adjusted hospitalization rates and significant improvements in risk-adjusted measures of health status in treatment versus comparison-group patients (Shaughnessy et al., 2002). On the basis of these promising findings, CMS is working collaboratively with Medicare-certified providers to identify a set of outcomes that will be tested across the universe of providers.

In a landmark decision (*Olmstead v. L.C.,* 1999), the Supreme Court ruled that individuals with disabilities must be enabled by states to live in the most integrated setting appropriate to their needs and that "unjustified isolation . . . is properly regarded as discrimination based on disability" (DHHS, 2001; Rosenbaum, 2000). This ruling has very important policy implications for community care. It sent a clear message to the states that care should begin at home and that institutionalization is an option of last resort. Currently, all states are developing plans in response to this ruling.

Two other related policy developments complement this new thrust toward home care. First, CMS and the Administration on Aging are testing a single-entry community-based assessment, referral, and care system that would streamline access to care in the community for vulnerable populations. This "one-stop shopping" demonstration replicates a program that the state of Wisconsin has used for a number of years. The second policy-related program pertains to the National Family Caregiver Support Program ("HHS Releases," 2001). Many states will be using grant funds to train family caregivers of persons with long-term care needs. This legislation has been criticized by some for providing only modest relief to caregivers. However, the legislation for the first time sets the legal precedent that the government should be a partner with families caring for a member with long-term care needs.

These policy developments of the early 2000s,

coupled with the new emphasis on consumer direction previously discussed and the major epidemiologic and demographic trends described in the introduction, clearly set the stage for continued growth in home and community-based services in the future.

ADMINISTRATIVE CHALLENGES

All sectors of the home care field have undergone nearly constant change during the past 25 to 30 years. Such a demanding environment brings numerous daily challenges to administrators. The most significant issues faced by managers during the middle of the decade include:

- *Nursing shortage.* The current shortage of nurses across the nation makes it difficult for administrators to identify qualified nurses and retain them in the home care field.
- *Payment lag times.* Both Medicare and Medicaid payments are frequently delayed, requiring all agencies dealing with the government as payers to have sufficient cash flow to meet payroll and other needs despite these slow payments.
- *Mergers and acquisitions.* Although the closure of Medicare-certified agencies that was rampant immediately after BBA '97 has slowed down, mergers are still occurring. Mergers are challenging for both the agency that is being acquired and for the agency that is doing the acquiring, with respect to staffing, billing, name recognition, maintenance of referral and patient bases, and recordkeeping. They are also challenging for clients, and potentially affect client and family loyalty and satisfaction.
- *Outcomes.* Home Care Compare is a "report card" for Medicare home care agencies being made available to the public by CMS. Its purpose is to offer a suitable set of stable and relevant outcome indicators by which to compare Medicare-certified home care agencies. Other

home care providers will be challenged to develop or respond to the demand for consumer-oriented performance measures.
- *Regulatory issues.* Directors of all types of home care agencies spend a great deal of time dealing with regulatory requirements imposed by federal, state, and local governments, as well as by consumer and accreditation organizations. Compliance with new patient privacy regulations is a recent example. In an evolving field, there is always some new external pressure that requires adjustment of the home care agency's internal operations.

CONCLUSION

To conclude, a number of questions persist regarding home care in the nation. Home care has grown prodigiously in terms of providers, users, and costs. The relationships between use of home care and the use of other health care services remain unclear. Basic issues such as geographic variation in supply, utilization, and cost, determinants of scope of services provided, and organizational/management practices that maximize outcomes for specific patient groups remain to be explored. Home care has arrived and is here to stay. It is a prevalent and essential component of the continuum of care. The challenges of the future are to achieve integration and to demonstrate cost-effective outcomes.

CLIENT EXAMPLE

Fred Turner is a 35-year-old construction worker who is not married and lives alone. He falls from a third-story construction site and suffers a concussion and multiple compound fractures, including a fractured pelvis and femur. He is rushed to the emergency room of the closest hospital, and spends several days in the hospital. He is then transferred to a subacute unit for further recuperation and to begin rehabilitation. After three months, he is able to go home.

Skilled home care, rehabilitation therapies, and

home health aide services are ordered by his physician. A nurse visits three times a week for the first four weeks, and then twice a week, to check on his skin status and general medical condition. A physical therapist visits twice a week to continue the rehabilitation therapies begun in the hospital to increase mobility of his left arm, which had a minor fracture, and to maintain and increase mobility of the lower extremities. After the cast on his lower leg is removed, the physical therapist increases visits to three times a week until Fred is well enough to attend the outpatient rehabilitation clinic to continue his recovery. An occupational therapist visits immediately upon his return home to do a home assessment and recommend modifications to ensure his safety while at home. A homemaker comes twice a week to help him bathe, as the cast prevents him from getting into a bathtub or using a shower. All of these people are from a Medicare-certified skilled home health agency. Services are paid for by worker's compensation.

Durable medical equipment is ordered by the home health agency from a dealer authorized by worker's compensation. This includes a hospital bed for the first couple of weeks at home, then a walker. Worker's compensation also covers the rental costs for the equipment.

The nurse calls a private home care agency to arrange for a homemaker to come twice a week to help Fred manage household tasks, such as shopping and housecleaning. Fred pays for this service out-of-pocket. Fred's mother, who lives too far away to help on a regular basis, seeks out information about Meals on Wheels. Although many programs are only for older adults, she finds a church-based program that brings Fred a lunch Monday through Friday for the first three weeks that he is home, until he is able to manage with crutches or a walker. Fred pays the requested donation of $2 per meal.

Fred buys a lifeline signaling device at the recommendation of the home health nurse, so that, in the event of emergency, he can call for help quickly.

Services are modified as Fred recovers and gains more independence. As he transitions to use of outpatient therapy, home care services are eventually phased out. Although worker's compensation paid for the majority of home care, Fred had to pay a considerable amount out of pocket for the additional assistance that he required because he lived alone without family members to provide basic support. Each of the home care staff came according to their own schedule, and the same person was not always guaranteed. He often felt that no one was really coordinating his overall care plan. However, due to the friendliness of most of the home care providers, he felt good about his experience, and eventually made a full recovery.

WHERE TO GO FOR FURTHER INFORMATION

Centers for Medicare and Medicaid Services (CMS)
7500 Security Boulevard
Baltimore, MD 21244-1850
http://www.cms.gov

CMS OASIS Website
http://www.cms.hhs.gov/oasis

Community Health Accreditation Program, Inc.
39 Broadway, Suite 710
New York, NY 10006
(800) 656-9656
http://www.chapinc.org

Joint Commission on Accreditation of Healthcare Organizations
One Renaissance Boulevard
Oakbrook Terrace, IL 60181
(630) 792-5000
http://www.jcaho.org

National Alliance for Infusion Therapy
1001 Pennsylvania Avenue, NW
Washington, DC 20004
(202) 624-7225

National Association for Home Care and Hospice
228 Seventh Street, SE
Washington, DC 20003
(202) 547-7424
http://www.nahc.org

National Center for Health Statistics
National Home and Hospice Care Survey
Division of Data Services
Hyattsville, MD 20782
(301) 458-4636
http://www.cdc.gov/nchs/about/major/nhhcsd/nhhc sd.html

National Home Infusion Association
205 Daingerfield Road
Alexandria, VA 22314
(703) 549-3740
http://www.nhianet.org

FACTS REVIEW

1. Name four types of home care and describe their similarities and differences.
2. Who are the primary users of home health care?
3. Who are the primary payers for home health care?
4. What external factors have significantly influenced the evolution of the home health care industry?

REFERENCES

Benjamin, A. E. (2001). Consumer-directed services at home. *Health Affairs, 20*(6), 80–95.

Benjamin, A. E. (1993). An historical perspective on home care. *Milbank Quarterly, 71*(1), 129–166.

Brown, J. M. (1990, May). Home care models for infusion therapy. *Caring, 9,* 24–27.

Bureau of Labor Statistics. (2003). *National compensation survey.* Retrieved on October 20, 2004 from *http://www.bls.gov/ncs/home.htm*

Centers for Medicare and Medicaid Services (CMS). (2002). *Health care industry market update, home health.* Retrieved October 19, 2004 from *http://www.cms.hhs.gov/marketplace*

Coleman, B. (2001). Consumer directed services for older people. *Public Policy Institute Issue Brief,* 1B53, 1–16. Retrieved October 19, 2004 from *http://www.research.aarp.org/ppi*

Coleman, B., Fox-Grage, W., & Folkemer, D. (2003). *2003 state long-term care: Recent developments and policy directions.* Retrieved October 19, 2004 from *http://www.hcbs.org/files/21/1015/LTC2003.pdf*

Cummings, J., Hughes, S. L., Weaver, F., Manheim, L. M., Conrad, K., Nash, K., Braun, B., & Adelman, J. (1990). Cost-effectiveness of V.A. hospital-based home care: A randomized clinical trial. *Archives of Internal Medicine, 150,* 1274–1280.

Department of Health and Human Services (DHHS). (2001). *Letter to state Medicaid directors [Olmstead decision].* Retrieved on October 19, 2004 from *http://www.hhs.gov/ocr/olms0114.htm*

Donlan, T. (1983). No place like home. *Barron's, 6,* 21.

General Accounting Office (GAO). (2000a). *Medicare home health care: Prospective Payment System will need refinement as data become available* (GAO/HEHS-00-9). Washington, DC: U.S. General Accounting Office.

General Accounting Office. (2000b). *Medicare+Choice: Plan withdrawals indicate difficulty of providing choice while achieving savings* (GAO/HEHS-00-183). Washington, DC: U.S. General Accounting Office.

Gold, M. (2001). Medicare + Choice: An interim report card. *Health Affairs, 20 (4),* 120–138.

Health Care Financing Review. (2001). *Medicare and Medicaid statistical supplement, 2001.* Baltimore, MD: U.S. Department of Health and Human Services.

HHS releases $113 million for Family Caregiver Program. (2001). *Gerontology News, 28(3),* 6.

Hughes, S. L. (1991). Home care: Where we are and where we need to go. In M. G. Ory & A. P. Duncker (Eds.), *In-home care for older people.* Newbury Park, CA: Sage.

Joint Commission on Accreditation of Healthcare Organizations. (2000). *Standards for home care accreditation.* Retrieved October 19, 2004 from *http://www.jcaho.org*

Kaye, L. W., & Davitt, J. K. (1995). Provider and consumer profiles of traditional and high-tech home health care: The issue of differential access. *Health and Social Work, 20*(4), 262–271.

Levit, K., Smith, C., Cowan, C., & Martin, A. (2002). Inflation spurs health spending in 2000. *Health Affairs, 21*(1): 172–181.

McCall, N., Petersons, A., Moore, S., & Korb, J. (2003). Utilization of home health services before and after the Balanced Budget Act of 1997: What were the

initial effects? *HSR: Health Services Research,*
38(1):85–106.

McDaniel, C. G. (1997, July–August). High-tech home
medical care. *Consumers Digest.*

Miller, N. A., Ramsland, S., & Harrington, C. (1999).
Trends and issues in the Medicaid 1915(c) Waiver
Program. *Health Care Financing Review, 20*(4),
139–160.

Murkofsky, R. L., Phillips, R. S., McCarthy, E. B., Davis,
R. B., & Hamel, M. B. (2003). Length of stay in
home care before and after the Balanced Budget
Act. *Journal of the American Medical Association,*
289(21), 2284–2848.

Murtaugh, Stevenson, Feldman, & Oberlink. (2000).
Home care research initiative, fact sheet, fall/winter
2000. State expenditures on home and community-
based care for disabled elders. Retrieved October 19,
2004 from *http://www.vnsny.org/brief5.pdf*

National Association for Home Care (NAHC). (2002).
Home care statistics, 1999. Retrieved October 1,
2004 from *http://www.nahc.org*

National Association for Home Care. (2001). *Basic*
statistics about home care, 2001. Available at
http://www.nahc.org/consumer.hestats.html

National Association for Home Care. (1999). *Basic*
statistics about home care, 1999. Retrieved on
October 19, 2004 from *http://www.ahc.org*

National Center for Health Statistics (NCHS). (2000).
National Center for Health Statistics home and

hospice care survey. Hyattsville, MD: NCHS.
Retrieved from *http://www.ftp.cdc.gov/pub/*
Health_Statistics/NCHS/Datasets/NHHCS/
TABLE4HHC2000.XLS

Office of the Inspector General, DHHS. (2001). *The*
physician's role in Medicare home health 2001
(OEI-02-00-00620). Washington, DC: U.S. Office
of the Inspector General.

Rosenbaum, S. (2000). *Olmstead v. L.C.: Implications*
for older persons with mental and physical
disabilities (AARP Public Policy Institute, INB#30
and #2000-21). Washington, D.C.: AARP.

Shaughnessy, P. W., Hittle, D. F., Crisler, K. S., Powell,
M. C., Richard, A. A., Kramer, A. M., Schlenker, R.,
Steiner, J., Donelan,-McCall, N., Beaudry, J., Lawlor,
K. M, & Engle, K. (2002). Improving patient
outcomes of home health care: Findings from two
demonstration trials of outcome-based quality
improvement. *Journal of the American Geriatrics*
Society, 50, 1354–1364.

Stone, R. I., & Wiener, J. M. (2001). *Who will care for*
us? Addressing the long term care workforce crisis.
Washington, D.C.: The Urban Institute.

U.S. Department of Health and Human Services,
Health Care Financing Administration Office of
Strategic Planning. (1998). *Health care financing*
review, Medicare and Medicaid statistical
supplement.

CHAPTER 7

Hospice

Stephen R. Connor and Galen Miller

Most people do not want to die alone in sterile, impersonal surroundings, hooked up to machines by tubes and cut off from their family and friends and everything that is familiar. Nor do they want to die in pain. They would prefer, if possible, to spend their last days at home, alert and free of pain, among people and things they love. Hospice is dedicated to making this possible.

Hospice is a philosophy and program of care that addresses the needs of patients and families during the last phase of a terminal illness (if the disease follows its normal course, death will occur during the next six months).

A hospice program includes the patient and family, specifically trained volunteers, caregivers from the community, and an interdisciplinary team of professionals from medicine, nursing, social work, clergy, and other disciplines as appropriate to the individual case. This interdisciplinary team approach to care focuses on the patient's physical symptoms and the emotional, social, and spiritual concerns of the patient and family. No specific therapy is excluded. Decisions regarding palliative treatment lie in the agreement among the patient, the physician, the primary caregiver, and the hospice team.

The team works together to develop a plan of care and to provide services that will maximize the patient's comfort, enhance quality of life, and support the patient, family, and significant others during the terminal illness and bereavement period.

DEFINITION

Hospice programs provide a special kind of care for dying people and their families. **Hospice** in the United States is defined as care that:

- treats the physical needs of the patient as well as the emotional and spiritual needs
- uses an interdisciplinary team
- takes place in the patient's home, or in a home-like setting
- concentrates on making the patient free of pain and as comfortable as possible so the patient can make the most of the time that remains

- helps family members before and after the patient's death as an essential part of its mission
- believes the quality of life to be as important as the length of life

Receiving hospice care is always a choice for patients and families who have decided to alleviate aggressive curative or life-extending treatment for their terminal illnesses and who want to concentrate on quality of life, pain and symptom management, and psychosocial and spiritual support services for themselves and their families. As noted by Cassel, "As sickness progresses toward death, measures to minimize suffering should be intensified. Dying patients require palliative care of an intensity that rivals even that of curative efforts . . . even though aggressive curative techniques are no longer indicated, professionals and families are still called on to use intensive measures—extreme responsibility, extraordinary sensitivity, and heroic compassion" (Cassel, 1986).

Hospice recognizes dying as part of the normal process of living and focuses on maintaining the quality of life. Hospice affirms life and neither hastens nor postpones death. Hospice exists in the hope and belief that through appropriate care, and the promotion of a caring community sensitive to their needs, patients and their families may be free to attain a degree of mental and spiritual preparation for death that is satisfactory to them.

Hospice offers palliative care to terminally ill people and their families without regard to age, gender, nationality, race, creed, sexual orientation, disability, diagnosis, availability of primary caregiver, or ability to pay. Hospice cares for the patient and family as the unit of care, with all services being patient- and family-centered.

BACKGROUND

In our great-grandparents' time, birth and death in the family home were commonplace and accepted as natural events. With time and the advances of medicine, birth and death were transplanted to a new and often strange and intimidating environment: the modern hospital, where family members were merely guests and control rested with unknown health professionals.

Dr. Cicely Saunders is generally credited with establishing the modern hospice movement in Great Britain in the 1960s. Hospice derives its name from the Latin word *hospes,* which means "to be both host and guest." The basic concept was care in a special

---

SERVICE SNAPSHOT: Hospices

Number of organizations	3,200
Capacity	Variable
Number of people served per year	885,000 (2002)
Average length of stay	51 days (median 26 days)
Major payers	Medicare, Medicaid, commercial insurance
Average cost per unit	Varies, approximately $113 a day for routine home care
Licensure	State Department of Health (where required)
Accreditation	JCAHO, CHAP, ACHC
Certification	Medicare, Medicaid

SOURCE: National Hospice and Palliative Care Organization, 2003.

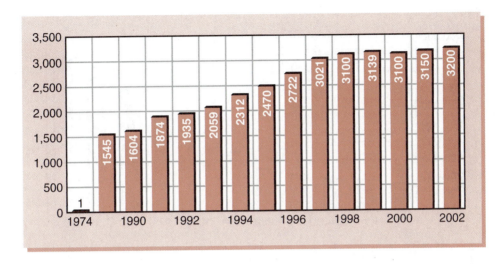

Figure 7.1   Growth in U.S. Hospice Programs 1974—2002
SOURCE: NHPCO, 2003.

facility that alleviated pain and addressed the social, emotional, and spiritual needs of the dying removed from the high-technology setting of the acute hospital. The concept was readily received and gratefully embraced by those it sought to serve.

The hospice concept spread to the United States in the 1970s. It was largely a grassroots movement that developed outside the conventional health care delivery system. These early hospices survived on shoestring budgets and depended almost entirely on charitable contributions and volunteer staff to provide the intensive and personalized care central to the hospice concept.

Hospice developed in the United States as a concept of care rather than a place for care; from the beginning the focus has been care in the patient's home. During the 1970s, hospice leaders began meeting regularly to formulate model standards for guiding development of hospice care. Creation of the National Hospice Organization (NHO) in 1978 (now the National Hospice and Palliative Care Organization [NHPCO]), provided a national forum for advocacy for the terminally ill, and discussion, education, and support of quality standards for hospices.

In 1983, Congress expanded Medicare coverage to include hospice. Many private insurers, recognizing not only the compassion associated with hospice care, but also its cost-effectiveness, began offering hospice benefits. Many states began to provide hospice benefits under Medicaid.

Hospice care continues to grow in this country as part of the mainstream health care system and social services system. Since the first hospice program provided care for patients in 1974, community-based replication of programs and services has increased to a recognized 3,200 hospice programs providing care in 2002. Figures 7.1 and 7.2 show, respectively, the growth over time in the number of hospices and hospice patients.

CLIENT PROFILE

According to NHPCO data, about 885,000 patients and families were admitted to hospice programs throughout the United States in 2002. This continues a phenomenal growth rate since the creation of the Medicare hospice benefit in 1983 (see Figure 7.2). Of these patients, approximately 665,000 died during the year, or more than 25

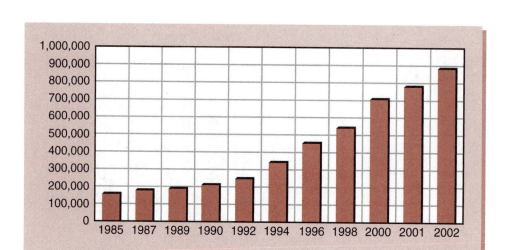

Figure 7.2   Growth in Number of Hospice Patients
SOURCE: NHPCO, 2003.

percent of the 2.4 million people who die from all causes in our country.

Slightly more women than men are served by hospice (56 percent versus 44 percent), likely due to the tendency for women to outlive men and to need care. As shown in Figure 7.3, hospices serve patients of all ages, though the great majority (81 percent) are age 65 or older. Minority patients are somewhat underrepresented in hospice care. The majority of hospice patients are white (82 percent); black patients account for 8.2 percent of patients and Hispanic/Latino patients for 3.4 percent (data from NHPCO dataset).

Figure 7.4 shows the varied diagnoses of hospice patients. The relative proportion of hospice patients with a diagnosis of cancer has continued to drop to a new low in 2001 of 53.6 percent. Heart disease is the largest non-cancer diagnosis, at 9.8 percent, followed by dementia at 6.9 percent, lung disease at 6.4 percent, stroke at 4.2 percent, kidney disease at 2.7 percent, and liver disease at 1.7 percent. Patients with HIV/AIDS now constitute less than 1 percent of the hospice population, mostly because of the success of the new protease inhibitors.

SERVICES

Hospice provides palliative care to terminally ill patients, and supportive services to patients, their families, and significant others, 24 hours a day, 7 days a week, in both home- and facility-based settings. Physical, social, spiritual, and emotional care is provided during the last stages of illness, during the dying process, and during bereavement by the medically directed interdisciplinary assessment team.

The National Hospice and Palliative Care Organization defines **palliative care** as treatment that enhances comfort and improves the quality of a patient's life. No specific therapy is excluded from consideration. The test of palliative treatment lies in the agreement by the patient, the physician, the primary caregiver, and the hospice team that the expected outcome is relief from distressing symptoms, easing of pain, and enhancement of quality of life. The decision to intervene with an active palliative treatment is based on the ability of that treatment to meet the stated goals rather than its effect on the underlying disease. Each patient's needs must continue to be addressed and all treatment options

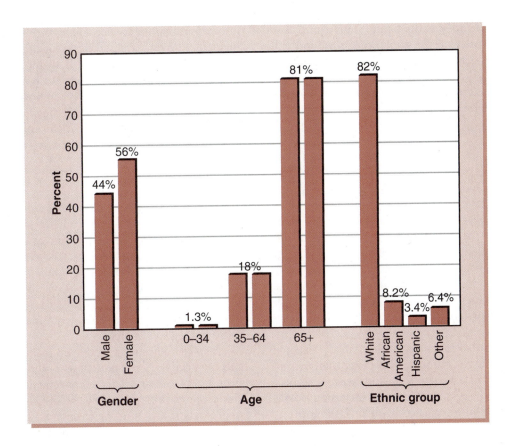

Figure 7.3 Profile of Hospice Patients
SOURCE: NHPCO, 2003.

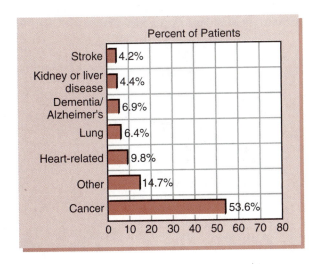

explored and evaluated in the context of the patient's values and symptoms.

Bereavement Support

Hospice bereavement services, provided by qualified staff and volunteers, begin with the initial assessment and continue through the bereavement period to help the patient and family cope with death-related grief and loss issues. Initial bereavement

Figure 7.4 Diagnosis of Hospice Patients by Percent, 2002
SOURCE: NHPCO, 2003.

assessment includes patient/family grief and loss issues; survivor(s) needs; social, religious, and cultural variables; risk factors; and the potential for complicated grief reactions.

Hospice offers a planned program of bereavement services for at least one year after the death of the patient.

Location

The focus of hospice care is to enable an individual to remain in familiar home surroundings as long as possible and appropriate. Hospice care plans reflect efforts by hospice staff and volunteers to maximize patient independence; deliver services at the convenience of the patient, family, and caregiver; arrange respite services for caregivers; bridge gaps in the patient's caregiving network; and adapt the home environment to meet the patient's physical needs.

Because individuals may reside at a residence other than their own home, a hospice program may offer services in a variety of facility settings appropriate to the patient's care needs, including hospitals, nursing homes, assisted living facilities, or freestanding hospices.

Whenever a hospice program manages or delivers care in a facility, the hospice is responsible for ensuring that an appropriate standard of care is provided in the facility, regardless of whether the hospice is responsible for the direct provision of those services. Facilities where hospice care is provided must meet appropriate licensing, regulatory, and certification requirements. Hospice policies and procedures address environmental consideration of privacy needs, including space for family gathering, 24-hour visitation and overnight stays, religious and spiritual worship, flexibility in scheduling care and accommodating individual needs, and access to services required by the patient's plan of care.

If a patient/family transfers from one hospice program to another or from home care service to inpatient service (or vice versa), the service transferring care provides a written summary that includes information about services being provided; specific medical, psychosocial, spiritual, or other problems that require intervention or follow-up; and planned follow-up by an interdisciplinary team member from the service transferring care. When hospice services are not provided directly by the hospice, there is a written agreement defining which services are provided directly by the hospice program and which are contracted out.

Staffing

A highly qualified, specially trained team of hospice professionals and volunteers work together to meet the physiological, psychological, social, spiritual, and practical needs of the hospice patient and family facing terminal illness and bereavement. The core team members required by Medicare are listed in the accompanying box. Each team member is specially trained in hospice care.

Hospice adds specialized team members to meet specific needs of each patient as outlined in the patient's plan of care. These team members may include allied therapists, art and music therapists, pharmacists, and nursing assistants. The full team works together to develop a plan of care and to provide services that will enhance the quality of life and provide support for the patient and family during the terminal illness and the bereavement period.

Hospice interdisciplinary team care represents the current standard of practice and is provided in

HOSPICE TEAM MEMBERS

- Attending physician
- Hospice physician
- Registered nurse
- Social worker
- Dietary counselors
- Clergy
- Volunteers

accordance with the code of ethics for each discipline. It is goal-directed, and promotes consistency in observations, action, interventions, and the patient's plan of care. Team care is also provided and documented in ways that ensure accountability and patient confidentiality and that meet legal and regulatory requirements.

Each member of the hospice interdisciplinary team recognizes and accepts a fiduciary relationship with the patient and family, maintains professional boundaries with the patient/family, and understands that it is the sole responsibility of each member to maintain appropriate agency and patient/family relationships.

Hospice programs provide ongoing educational experiences for staff members that include the purpose and focus of hospice care, team function and responsibility, communication skills, introduction to and review of psychosocial and spiritual assessment and symptom management, review of universal precautions, and patient/family safety issues.

Care Plan

The hospice interdisciplinary team collaborates continuously with the patient's attending physician to develop and maintain a patient-directed, individualized plan of care. Prior to providing care, a written plan of care is developed for each patient by the attending physician, the medical director or physician designee, and the interdisciplinary team. The plan of care is based on interdisciplinary team assessments that recognize the patient/family psychological, social, religious, and cultural variables and values. At minimum, the plan includes:

- patient's and family's problems, needs, and opportunities for growth
- desired goals or outcomes
- interventions directed to achieve the goals or outcomes desired by the patient, family, and interdisciplinary team
- scope, frequency, and type of services, including team interventions, pharmaceuticals, and medical equipment to be provided

- other agencies or organizations that may be involved in the care, and the role of each

Written policies and procedures concerning the development, review, and revision of the interdisciplinary team care plan address the use of advance directives in care plan development, making the plan of care available to all appropriate team members. This ensures that the care plan is followed in all care settings. The scheduling of ongoing interdisciplinary team conferences, the documentation of conference findings and conclusions, and the review or revision of the care plan by the team should occur, at a minimum, every 14 days after admission for home care and within 2 days of acute inpatient admission.

INTEGRATING MECHANISMS

Organization and Management

Hospice programs are sponsored by a variety of organizations (Figure 7.5).

Each hospice program, depending on the organizational system designed to manage the hospice, has an organized governing body that has complete and ultimate responsibility for the organization. Forty-one percent of hospice programs are community-based, not-for-profit organizations governed by a hospice board of directors. Other hospice programs are part of a hospital system, home health agency, health maintenance organization, government agency, or other health care system. The governing body determines the hospice's mission, purpose, and policies. This governing body selects, provides support to, and annually evaluates the hospice administrator.

The hospice administrator is accountable to the governing body for implementing, monitoring, and reporting on program services; for the quality of patient care; for resolution of problems; and for program improvement.

The hospice administration provides for management functions throughout the hospice program, including the delineation of staff responsibility and

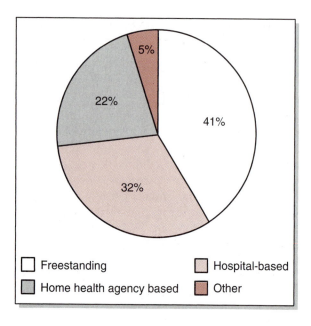

Figure 7.5 Organizational Auspices of Hospices
SOURCE: NHPCO, 2003.

accountability, and establishment of services necessary for hospice program effectiveness.

Hospices develop informal and formal collaborative agreements with other organizations to meet the full range of client needs. Mechanisms are established to coordinate administrative and clinical functions based on the characteristics of the organizations and the nature of the relationship.

Care Coordination

Providing and coordinating care involving several settings is inherent in the hospice concept, as well as a requirement for Medicare-certified hospices. The interdisciplinary team approach serves to coordinate the care provided by professionals of various disciplines. Hospice team staff interface with health professionals of other services as clients go in and out of hospital, nursing facility, home, and other settings.

Each hospice establishes its own operating policies about how to coordinate care. The hospice team may designate one individual to be the primary contact with a given client and family; alternatively, the hospice may rotate responsibilities among members of the team to accommodate a 24-hour on-call schedule.

Information Systems

At this time, no standardized management information system is required of hospices by any external authority. Just as the organizational auspices of hospices vary, so do their information systems. Hospices are likely to integrate clinical information across settings because of the encompassing nature of hospice, as well as to have accounting systems that enable management of pooled dollars because of the payment methods used by Medicare.

FINANCING

Hospices operate under various financial arrangements. Almost three-fourths (72 percent) of hospices are not-for-profit, nearly one quarter (24 percent) are for-profit, and the remainder (4 percent) are government-sponsored (NHPCO, 2003). Initial funding for a hospice may come from community support in the form of donations, fundraising events, in-kind volunteer support, grants, or other nonprofit support. Proprietary programs receive start-up funds from investors. A key issue for the hospice is whether it is willing to assume financial risk and reimbursement from Medicare, Medicaid, or insurance companies to provide and pay for the full range of hospice services. The large majority of hospice programs at present have chosen to become Medicare-/Medicaid-certified and to bill for services.

A smaller number of programs have chosen to be volunteer-based agencies that work with other government-certified providers to provide the full range of hospice services. Volunteer hospices usually provide psychosocial services such as counseling, bereavement support, volunteer services, and practical assistance.

Hospice may be a designated benefit reimbursed

as a specific service or may be paid for by its component services. Under the latter method, not all services are likely to be paid for, such as pastoral visits. Most hospices strive to receive a per diem benefit rather than for their services to be unbundled.

The Hospice Medicare Benefit established in 1983 made all Medicare beneficiaries eligible to receive hospice care as a covered Medicare benefit. Under the benefit, hospice care coverage includes:

- nursing services on an intermittent basis
- physician services
- drugs, biologicals, and infusion therapy. This includes all outpatient prescription and non-prescription medications related to the terminal illness, and parenterally administered medication or fluids needed for pain or symptom management. (A patient may be asked to pay 5 percent of the cost of outpatient drugs or $5 for each prescription, whichever is less.)
- medical social services
- counseling, including pastoral, bereavement, and nutritional
- volunteer support
- physical, occupational, and speech therapy
- home health aide and homemaker services
- medical supplies and appliances
- durable medical equipment
- short-term inpatient care for symptom management and up to five days of inpatient respite care. (A patient may be asked to pay up to 5 percent of the Medicare rate for respite.)
- bereavement follow-up services for the family for at least 12 months after the death

The per diem benefit covers all hospice services, and each day is paid at one of four levels of care, depending on patient need: (1) routine home care; (2) continuous home care; (3) general inpatient care; (4) inpatient respite care. The Centers for Medicare and Medicaid Services (CMS) updates reimbursement rates annually. Current rates can be found on the CMS website or at *http://www.nhpco.org* (from the home page, choose Technical Assistance).

The great majority of days are paid for routine home care (95 percent). Less than 1 percent of days are for continuous home care, which provides between 8 and 24 hours of nursing staffing for periods of crisis, to keep a patient at home who would otherwise be admitted to an acute care facility. General inpatient care is done through a contract with a hospital or nursing facility or hospice-dedicated facility to provide short-term inpatient care for management of severe symptoms. Inpatient respite is allowed up to five days to provide a rest for caregivers.

Anyone covered by Part A of Medicare is eligible to receive hospice care when all three of the following conditions are met: (1) the patient's physician and hospice medical director certify that the patient is terminally ill with a life expectancy of six months or less, if the illness runs its normal course; (2) the patient chooses to receive care from a hospice instead of standard Medicare benefits; and (3) care is provided by a hospice program certified by Medicare.

Medicare pays one of the per diem benefits for each day of care for two 90-day periods, followed by an unlimited number of 60-day benefit periods. At the end of each benefit period, the hospice must recertify that the patient continues to have a prognosis of six months or less. The patient may stop hospice care at any time and return to cure-oriented care. The Medicare Hospice Benefit is not required to pay for treatments or services unrelated to the terminal illness. These may be billed to Medicare separately by other providers.

Any attending physician charges can be reimbursed as usual through Part B, but all consultant physician charges must be billed through the hospice, and the hospice must have a contract with all consultant physicians seeing the patient. Although each hospice has its own policies concerning payment for care, it is a principle of hospice to offer services based on need rather than ability to pay.

Most commercial insurance companies now cover hospice and have structured their hospice benefits to mirror Medicare's model. Coverage for hospice is provided to more than 80 percent of employees in medium and large businesses (NHPCO, 2003), either through commercial insurance or through managed care companies.

Hospice care is carved out of the Medicare risk payment for HMOs. Patients can continue with their HMO and seek services from a community hospice. In this arrangement the HMO's payment is greatly reduced, along with its liability for the high costs these patients incur for their terminal illnesses. Some want to see the hospice payment carved into the HMO payments. This could encourage more use of hospice care by managed care. However, there are concerns with ensuring that these resources will be used for good hospice care rather than for other competing priorities.

Case managers sometimes try to limit services and want to unbundle hospice services and pay for only the medical components. There is also a tendency to pay only a per diem when the patient is very expensive to care for and fee-for-service when the patient is stable. When case managers understand that paying the hospice a per diem can often save them money, they are more likely to authorize the full package of hospice care.

LICENSURE, CERTIFICATION, AND ACCREDITATION

Licensure

Licensure is by state. Almost all states recognize hospice as a distinct category. In those states without licensure programs, a hospice is allowed to operate with Medicare certification and sometimes is also licensed as a home health agency, nursing home, or hospital. A number of hospices (about 200) are all volunteer programs. They are not usually Medicare-certified and often have a working relationship with another licensed health care provider.

Certification

To receive payment from Medicare or Medicaid, hospices must meet federal certification requirements. Medicare has extensive Conditions of Par-

ticipation, and Medicaid regulations mirror those of Medicare. All but a few states have the optional Medicaid Hospice Benefit. In those states that do not, a hospice that wishes to serve these patients must do so without reimbursement. Hospices certified by Medicare serve Medicare enrollees, who must meet Medicare's eligibility criteria to receive the benefit, but may also serve others, such as those whose care is paid for by commercial insurance, managed care, or out of pocket.

Accreditation

The Joint Commission on Accreditation of Healthcare Organizations (JCAHO), the Community Health Accreditation Program (CHAP), and the Accreditation Commission for Home Care all accredit hospices in the United States. JCAHO and CHAP have deemed status to grant Medicare certification along with accreditation. The JCAHO standards are part of its home care accreditation program. CHAP standards are based on the National Hospice and Palliative Care Organization's *Standards of a Hospice Program of Care*. In 2000, 74 percent of hospices were accredited, the majority by JCAHO (NHPCO, 2003).

EVALUATING OUTCOMES*

Cost-Effectiveness

Most studies of hospice to date have looked at cost-effectiveness rather than clinical outcomes. Cost-effectiveness has been a major focus in efforts to preserve funding and expand insurance and Medicare coverage for hospice care.

The National Hospice Study was funded by the Health Care Financing Administration in the mid-1980s. Results revealed that the treatment costs for

---

*This section extracted from Stephen Connor, *Hospice: practice, pitfalls, and promise* (Washington, DC: Taylor & Francis, 1998), Chapter 12: How good is hospice care?, pp. 153–170.

home-care-based hospice programs were lower than the costs of conventional care, regardless of length of stay (Mor, Greer, & Kastenbaum, 1988). The treatment costs for hospital-based programs were less than conventional care costs only for patients with lengths of stay in hospice of less than two months.

Results of the Medicare Hospice Benefit Program Evaluation have been widely reported. According to Medicare Part A data, $1.26 was saved for every dollar spent on hospice care. However, questions were raised about whether these savings are overstated as a result of patient selection effects (Birenbaum & Kidder, 1992).

In an effort to address some of these selection questions, the NHO commissioned an independent study of the Medicare data tapes (NHO, 1995). Lewin VHI analyzed data on 191,545 Medicare recipients who died between July 1 and December 31, 1992. Costs for all services were analyzed during the final 12 months of life. The study included 39,719 recipients who were hospice users. A comparison group of 123,323 patients who did not receive any hospice care was matched for age, sex, and disease.

Results of this study demonstrated that, on average, Medicare beneficiaries with cancer who enrolled in a hospice program cost Medicare $2,737 less than comparable nonusers. For every dollar spent on hospice care, Medicare saved $1.52.

Despite the size and scope of the Lewin VHI study, policymakers, payers, and industry analysts continue to challenge the cost-effectiveness of having a distinct hospice program.

Client Satisfaction

Hospices throughout the United States routinely survey the family or primary caregiver a few months after the patient's death to receive feedback on how well care was delivered. Since 1992 the NHPCO has offered a standardized family satisfaction survey for hospices to compare their results. The results submitted to NHPCO have consistently shown a very high rate of satisfaction with services. While these findings demonstrate that families and caregivers are very happy with hospice services, the results have not shown hospices where opportunities for improvement lie.

To overcome the leniency bias in such satisfaction surveys, the NHPCO worked with Brown University and the University of Massachusetts at Boston to develop a family evaluation of care to identify more effectively areas where care could be improved. This survey began to be implemented in 2003 in hospice programs throughout the country.

Measuring patients' satisfaction or perception of care is more challenging, because of the large numbers of hospice patients who are unable to communicate or who are near death around the time of admission. One standardized procedure measures whether pain was relieved within 48 hours of admission to hospice care. Patients in pain are assessed on admission and again 72 hours later and asked if "their pain was brought to a comfortable level within the first two days of care." More than 75 percent of those patients admitted in pain, and who could communicate, had their pain controlled within this time frame (NHPCO, 2003).

Quality of Life

Increasing emphasis is being placed on measuring the outcomes of hospice care. Evidence suggests that hospice provides better quality of life for both patients and caregivers (Connor, 1998). However, quality of life is an elusive construct that has been hard to measure. This is particularly the case for terminally ill patients, because of the subjective nature of care and the mental and physical effort required to complete questionnaires.

Several tools have been developed to measure quality of life. One example is the Missoula/VITAS Quality of Life Scale (MVQOL) (Byock & Merriman, 1998). This tool measures five dimensions of the patient's experience: symptoms, functional ability, interpersonal relations, well-being, and transcendence. It is a 25-question instrument that can be administered to cognitively intact patients. In answering, the patient determines the relative importance of each of the five dimensions to his or her quality of life. The remaining questions measure the patient's perception of quality of life in each area and how much it varies from a baseline. The resulting scores can help clinicians in designing and prioritizing interventions.

Evaluations

Like other health care organizations, hospices have internal quality assurance programs in place. Medicare-certified programs are required to comply with CMS regulations for quality monitoring. External accreditation by CHAP or JCAHO also provides guidelines for ensuring quality. NHPCO offers a guide called *Standards of a Hospice Program of Care: Self-Assessment Process*. The NHPCO is actively engaged in developing benchmarks for hospice practice throughout the United States.

These benchmarks will eventually lead to performance measures that are publicly reported. Such measures will have to be credible to providers, relevant to consumers, and valued by payers. They will act as a type of "report card" that will include patient measures, family evaluation of care, and other measures of program operation. As the health care system is becoming more accountable, all health care providers are being required to measure and report key information on their services.

Additional research is needed to develop useful measurement tools and benchmarks for patient satisfaction, quality of care, quality of life, and cost-effectiveness. Although these are needed for all areas of health care, they are particularly challenging for hospice because of the complexities of the physical, emotional, and social dimensions of terminal illness.

ADMINISTRATIVE CHALLENGES

The hospice industry faces a number of management challenges. In recent years, hospices have experi-

enced a shortening in length of stay, and significant changes in treatment options for the terminally ill blur the distinctions between palliative and curative care. The public's lack of awareness of hospice continues to impede use by all those who could potentially benefit from the program, and a shortage of professional staff is anticipated for the future.

- *Short length of service (LOS).* In the past decade, average length of hospice admission has declined from 70 to around 50 days. More significantly, median LOS is only 26 days, and more than one-third of hospice patients are now served for 7 days or less. These short-term patients are unable to benefit fully from hospice services, which require more time to prevent symptoms and develop a therapeutic relationship with the patient and family.
- *Palliative/curative treatment distinction.* Since the advent of the Medicare Hospice Benefit, the distinction between palliative and curative treatment has become more difficult to make. Hospices must pay for all palliative but not curative treatments. Many new treatments are not curative, but may offer life prolongation potential. Some have significant symptom burdens, whereas others relieve symptoms. Each hospice team must determine what treatments to pay for with a limited per diem payment.
- *Access to care.* For every patient who is admitted to hospice, there are nearly two others who do not receive hospice care. Only 15 percent of the general public knows that Medicare covers hospice care. Those with life-threatening illness are not being adequately informed about the availability of hospice services. Also, people of color, children, the poor, and the developmentally disabled have lower rates of hospice access.
- *Nursing and staffing shortage.* Although hospice care is appealing to nursing professionals who are motivated to provide direct patient care, the hospice community is feeling the effects of the general nursing shortage. The effects of this shortage are expected to be more acute

after 2010, as many hospice nurses are mature nurses who are more likely to leave the workforce in coming years. Similarly, projected nationwide shortages of support personnel and professional therapists may also affect the ability of hospices to bring together all the disciplines desired for a full hospice team.

CONCLUSION

The sphere of influence of hospice programs goes well beyond hospice care. Hospice organizations may provide or be involved in special care programs that provide varying levels of support to patients and families before hospice care is needed. Organizations may offer grief and loss support to patients and families living with Alzheimer's disease, long before the physical disease progresses to the final phase of the illness when hospice care is appropriate. Other examples include bereavement services provided to business and industry employees, police departments, schools, and other organizations that have been affected by traumatic loss, staff loss, or where the patient was not a hospice patient, but death occurred in another setting or in another geographic area.

A foundation of hospice recognizes death as an integral part of the life cycle and, to that end, hospice provides leadership for end-of-life dialogue among professions and the public. Hospice affirms the value intrinsic to the end of life and the psychosocial and spiritual growth possible for both patients and families during this important time. Hospice also leads the dialogue regarding the importance of the study of pain and symptom management, the value of psychosocial care, spiritual care, and family systems research related to dying and death. Hospice has provided expanded recognition that the bereavement process goes beyond what has been the traditional American response to the dying process and death.

Hospice expertise in the delivery of patient and family care by a well-trained interdisciplinary care team has led the transformation of traditional hospital and nursing care programs into patient-centered care organizations.

CLIENT EXAMPLE

Mary is a 68-year-old patient with metastatic breast cancer who was referred to hospice by her physician while in the hospital for disease recurrence. She has not responded to chemotherapy and is having pain from bone metastases. She lives with her husband of 45 years, John, who is supportive but recently had a minor heart attack. The referring physician is concerned that they are not dealing with the reality of her condition.

During hospice intake, their hopes and fears about her condition are explored. Mary is fearful that her worsening health will be hard on John's heart. John is as supportive as possible, but is still recovering from his heart condition. They have two grown children in the area who have families of their own. During the intake, it becomes apparent that both John and Mary know the seriousness of Mary's condition, but each is afraid to be honest with the other because of fear that it would cause harm.

As this conspiracy of silence is dropped, their communication improves and they are able to make plans that allow for the possibility of her death as well as her continued life. Mary's pain is controlled by medications, and she comes to understand that John's involvement in her care could help, not harm, his health.

As the next few weeks progress, Mary becomes gradually weaker. Her children and grandchildren come to visit and to help. The hospice team sets up a schedule for visitation and caregiving.

Mary and her husband get to know the various members of the hospice team. The nurses train John to administer medication to Mary. Both a social worker and a local pastor provide counseling. A dietitian works out a meal plan for Mary and one for John as well.

As her condition worsens and she is no longer

ambulatory, a wheelchair, bedside commode, and hospital bed are arranged for Mary. Aides show her husband how to help her into and out of the chair. A volunteer comes twice each week to sit with Mary while her husband goes out to handle business affairs and exercise to maintain his own health.

The social worker helps the family with arrangements for Mary's funeral. A financial counselor speaks with both John and Mary, outlining what must be done to settle Mary's estate and what measures John needs to take to prepare for life after she is gone.

With prompting from the hospice team, Mary begins to reminisce and tell her life stories into a tape recorder for the family. Her symptoms are controlled, but she begins to sleep more and interact less. Her hospice nurse tells the family about how her symptoms will change as she approaches death. As Mary becomes less responsive, all the family members begin a vigil. Mary takes her last breath on a Saturday evening when John is out of the room momentarily.

The family calls the hospice, and the hospice nurse comes to the house at 7:00 p.m. She helps everyone with the details and to say goodbye as the funeral home arrives to get Mary's body. They all stay to talk about how much Mary meant to them. John is sad that he was not with her when she died. The nurse tells him that this happens often because it is hard for someone to go in the presence of the one to whom they were closest. The hospice chaplain officiates at Mary's funeral service.

In her final six weeks of life, Mary was relatively free of pain. John was involved with her care and felt satisfied with the level of care received. Helping with her care made him feel stronger, despite his heart condition. The social worker, pastoral worker, and volunteers kept in touch with John after Mary's death to help him deal with his grief and feelings of loss. The hospice bereavement volunteer visited and invited John to a bereavement meeting where he met another widower. They became fast friends, felt comfortable reminiscing freely about their wives, and were able to help each other in the transition to living without their respective spouses. After a year, John became a volunteer with the hospice program to help give others the same support his family had experienced through hospice.

WHERE TO GO FOR FURTHER INFORMATION

Hospice programs exist in most areas throughout the country. Through the National Hospice and Palliative Care Organization Help Line, anyone can call the 800 number to locate a hospice program providing services to the terminally ill and their families in their respective location. This can also be done through the NHPCO Web site. The Help Line and Website service also provide general information on hospice care, along with referral to additional organizations and agencies providing specialized care for patients and families.

National Hospice and Palliative Care Organization
1700 Diagonal Road, Suite 625
Alexandria, VA 22314
(703) 837-1500
Help Line: 1-800-658-8898
http://www.nhpco.org

NHO Store: (for catalog or ordering of publications, video information, and hospice merchandise) 800-646-6460

FACTS REVIEW

1. What is hospice?
2. Who was the founder of the modern hospice movement?
3. List at least three characteristics found in all hospices.
4. What distinguishes hospice care from standard care of the dying?
5. Approximately how many hospices are there in the United States?
6. Approximately how many people received hospice care in the past year?

7. What are the primary payment sources for hospice?

8. Explain the Medicare hospice benefit: what is required of providers and patients?

REFERENCES

Birenbaum, H., & Kidder, D. (1992). What does hospice cost? *American Journal of Public Health, 74,* 689–697.

Byock, I. R., & Merriman, M. P. (1998, July). Measuring quality of life for patients with a terminal illness: The Missoula-VITAS quality of life index. *Palliative Care, 12,* 231–44.

Cassel, C. K. (1986). *Health care for the elderly: Meeting the challenges.* In M. B. Kapp, H. E. Pies, & A. E. Doudera (Eds.), *Legal and ethical aspects of health care for the elderly.* Ann Arbor, MI: Health Administration Press.

Connor, S. (1998) *Hospice: Practice, pitfalls, and promise.* Washington, DC: Taylor and Francis.

Mor, V., Greer, D., & Kastenbaum, R. (1988). *The hospice experiment.* Baltimore, MD: Johns Hopkins University Press.

National Hospice Organization. (1993). *Standards of a hospice program of care: Self assessment tool.* Arlington, VA: National Hospice Organization.

National Hospice Organization. (1995). *An analysis of the cost savings of the Medicare Hospice Benefit* (Item No. 712901). Arlington, VA: NHO.

National Hospice and Palliative Care Organization. (2003). *Hospice fact sheet.* Alexandria, VA: NHPCO.

CHAPTER 8

Adult Day Services

Nancy J. Cox

Adult day services (ADS) is a long-term care alternative that offers clients an opportunity to continue living at home while receiving an array of needed services in a daytime, group setting. Some people view ADS as a way to postpone or prevent the need for nursing home placement for individuals with cognitive or physical disabilities.

Increased utilization of community-based long-term care services like ADS also has positive implications for the financing of the long-term care system. In dollar terms, adult day services cost society less than other forms of long-term care. In a time of increasing health and welfare needs and shrinking resources, the economic benefits of ADS are important.

DEFINITION

Defining ADS precisely is difficult because across the country there are a variety of ADS models. Also, there is neither federal legislation regulating ADS, nor nationally mandated standards resulting in a uniform ADS model.

The National Adult Day Services Association (NADSA) has developed the following definition for adult day services. It is concise, yet broad enough to encompass the variety of program models:

Adult day services are community-based group programs designed to meet the needs of functionally and/or cognitively impaired adults through an individual plan of care. These structured, comprehensive programs provide a variety of health, social, and other related support services in protective settings during any part of a day, but less than 24-hour care. Adult day centers generally operate programs during normal business hours five days a week. Some programs offer services in the evenings and on weekends (NADSA, 2003).

BACKGROUND

The evolution of today's adult day services programs (i.e., adult day centers) was influenced by the day hospital concept, especially Great Britain's geriatric day hospitals. Predecessors to current ADS

SERVICE SNAPSHOT: Adult Day Services

Number of adult day centers	3,407 in 50 states and the District of Columbia
Population served	Adults (age 18+) in need of chronic care; average age 72
Average adult day center size	Overall enrollment of 42; average daily attendance of 25; maximum capacity of 38
Legal status	78% not-for-profit; 22% for-profit
Average cost (versus charge) per day	$56 ($46)
Major sources of revenue	Medicaid Home and Community-Based Waiver dollars, state/local funds, private pay/out-of-pocket
Average annual revenue per center	$365,208
Licensure/Certification	79% licensed or certified by the state
Accreditation	6% accredited by the Commission on Accreditation of Rehabilitation Facilities (CARF)

SOURCE: Partners in Caregiving (2003).

programs include a small number of programs originally funded in the early 1970s as Medicare demonstration projects.

The number of adult day centers in the United States has grown tremendously. Several trends have fueled the overall growth in demand for adult day services. These include the increase in the disabled older population, as well as programs now serving a younger population with chronic conditions; the growing number of baby boomers (i.e., adult children) who are more likely to be working caregivers; the expanding preference for community-based long-term care options rather than nursing homes; and a private-pay market willing to pay out of pocket for such care.

Between 1969 and 1973, fewer than 15 formal adult day centers existed in the United States (Webb, 1989). By 1978, there were 300 adult day centers, with the number increasing to 618 two years later (Webb, 1989). In 1985, a conservative estimate was 1,200 adult day centers across the country (Von Behren, 1986); in 1989, a National Adult Day Center census identified more than 2,100 adult day centers (National Institute on Adult Daycare, 1989); and in 1995, there were reported to be more than 3,000 such centers (National Adult Day Services Association, 2002). Most recently, a National Study of Adult Day Services (2001–2002), funded by The Robert Wood Johnson Foundation, was conducted by Partners in Caregiving (PIC): The Adult Day Services Program at the Wake Forest University School of Medicine. This study confirmed 3,407 adult day centers in 50 states and the District of Columbia, of which 60 percent are located east of the Mississippi River (PIC, 2003) (Figure 8.1).

The study also found that more than half of existing adult day centers are well established, having been open for 11 to 20 or more years. The vast majority are not-for-profit (78 percent), and operate under the umbrella of a large parent organization (e.g., nursing home, hospital, senior service organization). A trend noted over the years, however, is an increase in the number of for-profit adult day centers being opened, going from 16 percent of centers that are more than 10 years old to 44 percent of centers being opened from 1998 to 2002. This

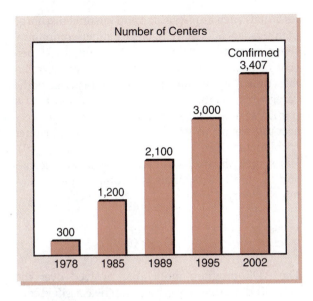

Figure 8.1   Growth in Adult Day Center Census
SOURCE: Partners in Caregiving, 2003.

entrepreneurial interest is motivated by the increase in demand, based on the trends noted here.

Although the field is in flux, with centers opening and closing on a regular basis, growth is evident, with 26 percent of all adult day centers opening between 1998 and 2002 (PIC, 2003). Growth, however, lags behind the need for the service, with 56 percent of the counties in the United States underserved (1,770 counties out of a total of 3,141). The study concluded that the current population base of the United States (based on the 2000 U.S. Census) can support a total of 8,520 adult day centers. With current need not being met in the underserved counties, 5,415 new adult day centers are needed nationwide: 1,424 in rural areas and 3,991 in urban areas.

CLIENT PROFILE

Adult day centers are designed for people who, because of physical or mental conditions, cannot remain alone during the day, but who have caregivers (typically a family member) who can take care of them when they are not at the day center. According to the PIC study, individuals being served range in age from 18 to 109, with an average age of 72. The two most prevalent groups being served (and most traditional ADS clientele) are people with dementia (52 percent) and the frail elderly (41 percent) (persons age 60 and older who are in need of supervision and/or at risk of social isolation, but do not have dementia). Target populations have, however, expanded beyond the frail elderly and those with dementia, with 24 percent of clients diagnosed with mental retardation or developmental disabilities, 23 percent physically disabled but cognitively intact (e.g., stroke, multiple sclerosis, Parkinson's disease), 14 percent with a chronic mental illness, 9 percent with HIV/AIDS, and 7 percent suffering from a traumatic brain injury (PIC, 2003). What they all have in common are disabilities that limit their ability to function independently. Selected characteristics of adult day center clients are illustrated in Table 8.1.

Adult day center clients are typically referred to as *participants*. The term emphasizes the self-

Table 8.1   Selected Characteristics of Adult Day Center Participants

Average age	72
Dementia (all forms)	52%
Frail older adults (no dementia)	41%
Medicaid-eligible or at or below the federal poverty level	60%
Need assistance with toileting	43%
Need assistance with walking	37%
Need assistance with eating	24%
White (non-Hispanic)	77%
Black (non-Hispanic)	26%
Live with adult children	35%
Live with a spouse	20%
Live in a residential setting (e.g., group home, assisted living, nursing home, foster care)	18%

SOURCE: Partners in Caregiving (2003)

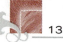

empowering philosophy of the adult day services concept. This is quite different from the terms *patient* and *client,* which may connote helplessness and need.

Most people attending an adult day center live with an adult child (35 percent) or a spouse (20 percent) (PIC, 2003). Besides providing a therapeutic environment for the person in need of care, a day center offers the family relief from the burden of caregiving. It lets caregivers who work continue to care for a loved one at home and provides a much-needed break for the nonworking caregiver. There is convincing data showing that caregiver stress is reduced by using adult day services (Zarit, Stephens, Townsend, & Greene, 1998; Jarrott, Zarit, Stephens, Townsend, & Greene, 1999).

Adult day centers help keep people in need of chronic care at home, in the community, and with family and friends for as long as possible. Adult day centers can delay or prevent institutionalization. The average length of stay at the center is two years. The number one reason for discharge is placement in a residential setting (such as a nursing home); the second reason for discharge is death (PIC, 2003).

Recruitment

Ironically, although more than 5,000 new adult day centers are needed in the United States to meet the current need, existing centers across the country are not full. As noted in the PIC study, on average, centers experience a 66 percent utilization rate (an average daily attendance of 25 divided by the average maximum capacity of 38). Adult day centers face a major challenge in maintaining census and daily attendance (PIC, 2003).

To achieve financial viability, a logical predictor of success is to keep the center full (Reifler et al., 1997). On average, one in three people who inquire will enroll (Jones, Cox, Yates, & Reifler, 1997), and a center with a capacity of 25 people per day usually needs an overall enrollment of 50 (double the average daily attendance), as everyone will not attend the program every day.

Marketing for adult day services must be ongoing. Formal referral sources, including health care pro-

fessionals such as physicians and hospital discharge planners, social service agencies, other community service providers, and employers, account for 75 percent of referrals to day centers. These formal referrals come from organizations and individuals in the caregiver's institutional and service network. Of particular note is the fact that formal referral sources account for up to two-thirds of actual day center enrollments (Henry, Cox, Reifler, & Asbury, 1999). Working with referral sources to generate referrals and to enroll participants is a complex task (Newton & Henry, 1994).

SERVICES

The ADS program model has evolved over the years. Today adult day centers can be classified into three basic models: social (adult day care), medical (adult day health care), or combination. The PIC study found that 21 percent of adult day centers are based on the medical model of care; 37 percent are based on the social model of care; and 42 percent are a combination of the two (PIC, 2003). The social and medical models are differentiated by additions to the medical model of nursing services and, in some cases, restorative and maintenance rehabilitative care. Fifty-two percent of adult day centers report having a registered nurse on site, and 33 percent have a licensed practical nurse on site (PIC, 2003).

The distinctions among the models are influenced by state licensing regulations or guidelines pertaining to payment levels. For example, California has two licensing categories: social day care and adult day health care (ADHC). In California, Medicaid (known as MediCal), reimbursement is available only for programs licensed as ADHCs. The state of Washington has identified two levels of care for state funding: Level I, referred to as adult day care, and Level II, referred to as adult day health care. In Washington, state reimbursement is based on the level of care provided, with Level II programs receiving higher payments. The main distinction between these states' two models is that skilled nursing care and rehabilitative therapy are provided by the programs licensed as ADHCs in California and as Level II programs in Washington.

The majority of adult day centers (77 percent) are open 5 days a week (Monday through Friday), 8 or more hours per day, with 11 percent open 6 days a week and 6 percent open 7 days a week (PIC, 2003). Participants may attend one or more days per week, depending on their or their caregivers' wants and needs. In most cases, the benefits of participation in the program are more apparent if participants attend at least two days (or more) per week.

Adult day centers provide a vast array of services, such as therapeutic activities, health monitoring, social services, personal care services, meals, transportation, nursing services, medication management, caregiver support services, and rehabilitation therapy. Table 8.2 lists the services commonly provided by adult day centers and the percent of centers offering each particular service. Centers that include health care services and rehabilitative therapies benefit individuals who have had strokes or are suffering from physically or neurologically degenerative diseases, such as arthritis or Parkinson's disease, as well as individuals suffering from chronic conditions such as cardiovascular and lung disease, diabetes, and similar health problems. The social model is best suited for individuals who are physically able but suffer from dementia (e.g., Alzheimer's disease) or other cognitive problems that limit their ability to function independently. These individuals need supervision and assistance with activities of daily living (ADLs), but typically do not need ongoing health care provided by a licensed nurse or rehabilitative services.

Group socialization and therapeutic activities are important parts of all models. Adult day centers provide an environment that encourages socialization through group interaction and a comprehensive activities program designed to meet the individual needs, interests, abilities, and limitations (be they physical or cognitive) of all participants. Therapeutic activities are typically planned and supervised by a qualified activity coordinator or recreational therapist. Activities offered include art therapy, group discussions (e.g., reminiscing or current events),

Table 8.2 Services Provided by Adult Day Centers

Therapeutic activities (e.g., art, music, exercise, pet therapy)	97%
Personal assistance (e.g., with meals, toileting, walking)	96%
Meals	84%
Social services	82%
Intergenerational programming	82%
Health-related services (e.g., weight/blood pressure monitoring, medication administration, glucose testing, vision/hearing screenings)	74%
Medication management	70%
Transportation	68%
Personal care services (e.g., baths/showers, hair/nail care)	64%
Caregiver support groups	60%
Nursing services (e.g., tube feeding, wound care, breathing treatments, intravenous therapy, catheter/colostomy care)	47%
Medical escort (e.g., to the doctor or dentist)	34%
Emergency respite	30%
Rehabilitation therapy (occupational, physical, speech)	28%
Medical services (dental, ophthalmology, podiatry)	12%
Overnight care	11%
Hospice	7%

SOURCE: Partners in Caregiving (2003).

games (modified physical games and word games), outings (such as shopping or visits to the zoo), music therapy, structured exercise programs, and support groups for dealing with grief or loss.

Group socialization is a major benefit for program participants. Many participants suffer from loneliness, isolation, and feelings of loss—all of which influence depression. The companionship shared among participants, as well as the warmth and caring attention provided by staff, have a positive impact on participants' mental and physical well-being. This is consistent with a *holistic* view of individuals, a philosophy that recognizes the importance of all aspects of well-being—physical, emotional, social, and environmental.

Personal care is also an essential part of all models. This is defined as help with ADLs, which may include eating, toileting, dressing, bathing, grooming, walking, and transferring. Assistance with eating may include cutting or pureeing food, cueing participants to eat, and supervising those who are at risk of choking or have other swallowing problems. Assistance with toileting includes transferring (from wheelchair to toilet) and reminding cognitively impaired participants to use the toilet to avoid accidents. Some participants are incontinent, so sometimes accidents do occur. In those instances, staff may assist participants with showering, grooming, and dressing.

STAFFING

Staffing requirements vary depending on the type of program and the state licensing regulations (if such regulations exist). Staffing levels are typically tied to daily program census. The number of full-time equivalents (FTEs) increases as average daily census increases. On average, the direct-care staff-to-participant ratio is 1:8 (i.e., one staff member for every eight participants). Recruiting and retaining qualified staff has been identified as the number two problem adult day centers face (PIC, 2003). Also, 72 percent of adult day centers have volunteers, on average, 11 volunteers per center (PIC, 2003). In some states, centers can use volunteers to meet the staffing requirements if the volunteers receive the same training as staff.

Because social-model centers do not provide health care services and are not usually funded by Medicaid, state staffing requirements are likely to be more flexible than those for programs providing health services. The only requirement for the social model may be that there are a qualified program director, activities coordinator, and program aides at the required staff-to-participant ratio. Of course, support staff providing clerical, janitorial, or financial services (accounting/payroll) are essential. These services may be provided by center staff, or a parent organization.

State regulations for programs providing health services, such as nursing and rehabilitation therapies, typically require, in addition to a program director and program aides, the following *licensed* staff:

- registered nurse(s) (on staff or consulting) or nursing staff such as licensed vocational/practical nurses
- social worker(s) (bachelor or master's degree)
- licensed recreational therapist(s)
- licensed physical and occupational therapists (if rehabilitation services are provided)

Additional staff may be mandated by state licensing regulations for adult day centers providing health services. These may include a prescribed number of hours per month of the services of a dietitian, psychiatric consultant (typically a psychiatrist, a psychologist, or master's-level psychiatric nurse), and a speech pathologist. In addition, a medical director/physician may also be required to devote a specified number of hours per month to the program.

AFFILIATION

The 2001–2002 national study conducted by PIC asked adult day centers if they are public or private and if they operate under a parent organization. Just over half (54 percent) of centers reported that they are privately owned, with 46 percent reporting that they are publicly owned (PIC, 2003). Thirty percent of all centers are freestanding facilities without a parent organization, whereas 70 percent operate under the auspices of a parent organization (PIC, 2003). When asked to identify which type of parent organization a center operates under, the most commonly reported umbrella organizations were: nursing or long-term care facility (17 percent), multiservice senior service organization (13 percent), religious organization (10 percent), and hospital (10 percent). Figure 8.2 provides a more detailed list of affiliations.

Health care organizations, such as nursing homes

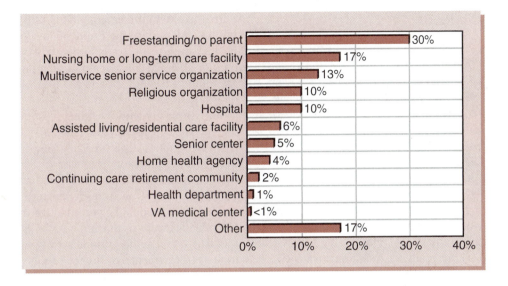

Figure 8.2   Adult Day Center Affiliations
SOURCE: Partners in Caregiving, 2003.

and hospitals, are likely to choose to establish an adult day center that includes nursing services. This medical model is more closely related to the mission of the health care organization. It might be seen as an extension of the nursing home or hospital and viewed as a continuum approach to the provision of community-based care.

LICENSURE, CERTIFICATION, AND ACCREDITATION

Licensure, certification, and accreditation for ADS are evolving as the service proliferates and matures. Adult day centers are not governed by specific regulations at the federal level. Funding or other regulatory standards usually exist at the state level, with the type of state agency overseeing adult day centers varying widely (such as a state health department/ division/bureau, state aging department/division/ bureau, or a combination of the two). The majority of centers (79 percent) report being certified or licensed by their state (PIC, 2003).

In 2001–2002, the Rutgers Center for State Health Policy conducted a 50-state survey with state government agencies, focusing strictly on adult day health programs (the medical model of care). Results show that a total of 46 states license and/or certify adult day health programs: 18 (39 percent) license only, 10 (22 percent) certify only, 8 (17 percent) both license and certify, and 10 (22 percent) neither license nor certify, but have other regulatory methods. This excludes four states (Tennessee, Idaho, Utah, and Wyoming) that designated their programs as social only (Lucas, Howell-White, & Rosado, 2003).

Only 6 percent of adult day centers are accredited (on a voluntary basis) by CARF, the national accrediting body of adult day centers (PIC, 2003). Accreditation, a joint effort of the National Adult Day Services Association and CARF, is a positive step toward quality assessment and standardization for a care model that has a great deal of variability and relatively little external regulation. Accreditation only began in 1999, so the number of centers accredited can be expected to increase over time.

FINANCING

Cost and daily fees vary by state and by adult day center, depending on the model of care and range of services offered. Surprisingly, 50 percent of centers do not know their unit cost (i.e., the cost of providing one day of care for one person) (PIC, 2003). Why? Maybe it is because most adult day centers are mission-based not-for-profits that, although they are small businesses, do not operate like businesses.

Of the 50 percent of centers that do know their unit cost, on average it is $56 per day per participant, which breaks out to $54 per day for the social model, $59 per day for the medical model, and $57 per day for the combination model (PIC, 2003). However, the average daily fee (i.e., top private-pay, undiscounted fee) is $46 per day per participant (less than cost), which breaks out to $42 per day for the social model, $56 per day for the medical model, and $45 per day for the combination model (PIC, 2003).

A predictor of success—that is, achieving financial viability—is to calculate unit cost and set fees equal to or greater than unit cost (Reifler et al., 1997). Some caregivers, however, are not able to afford the full cost of care. As a result, most centers have a sliding fee scale, offering discounts based on income. To at least break even, though, centers need to identify funds to make up for the discounts.

A variety of expenses go into the cost of operating an adult day center. As with most organizations, personnel (salaries and fringe benefits for administrative and direct care staff) is the leading expense, making up (on average) 64 percent of a center's annual budget (PIC, 1995). Nonpersonnel, direct-care expenses make up 20 percent of a budget for expenses such as dietary, program/medical supplies, and participant transportation. Nonpersonnel, fixed and administrative expenses comprise 16 percent of the budget, for expenses such as space/utilities, office operations, liability insurance, maintenance, marketing, and staff training.

Overall, the average adult day center covers 85 percent of its cash expenses with net operating revenue (i.e., fee-for-service revenue: private-pay and third-party reimbursements) (PIC, 2003). The minimum and maximum financial performances reported, were respectively, a low of 20 percent to a high of 150 percent. So, although adult day centers are financially poor, others are making a profit (or have a surplus if not-for-profit).

Forty-four percent of centers reported a deficit at the end of their fiscal years (PIC, 2003). These centers were significantly more likely (55 percent) to have been in operation for five years or less, compared with centers reporting a deficit that have been open for more than 10 years (35 percent). Overall, the combination model (49 percent) and the nonprofits (45 percent) were significantly more likely to report a deficit than medical models (39 percent), social models (42 percent), or the for-profits (39 percent).

FUNDING AND REVENUE STREAMS

Funding for adult day services is fragmented, and there is no consistency among states. Because adult day centers must piece together federal, state, and local funds, it is no surprise that the foremost problem centers face is adequate funding (PIC, 2003).

As shown in Figure 8.3, the largest source of revenue (38 percent) is third-party public reimbursements, which include federal and state funds coming into a center on a fee-for-service basis (PIC, 2003). The leading reimbursement source in this category is Medicaid Home and Community-Based Waiver dollars, reported by 60 percent of adult day centers as a source of revenue. In some states, however, this revenue stream is not available because it is a service available through waiver, not a required service (see Chapter 14). Also, in some states in which it is available, adult day centers cannot access these funds unless they use a medical model. Furthermore, there are limits on access to those participants meeting income criteria. Other sources of revenue that are third-party public reimbursements (in order of prevalence) include: state or local government, U.S. Department of Agriculture (food program), Title III of the Older Americans Act, U.S.

38%	**Third-party public reimbursements** (e.g., Medicaid Waiver dollars, state/local funds, USDA, Older Americans Act, VA)
35%	**Private pay**
14%	**Nonoperating revenue** (e.g., grants, donations)
13%	**Other operating revenue** (e.g., ancillary services, private insurance, managed care)

Figure 8.3   Adult Day Center Revenue Sources
SOURCE: Partners in Caregiving, 2003.

Department of Veterans Affairs, Medicaid Personal Care, Title XX/social services block grant, and Medicare (not for adult day services specifically, but for rehabilitation therapies such as physical or speech therapy). These additional sources of revenue may not be available in every state.

Private-pay/out-of-pocket payments constitute 35 percent of total revenue, representing the second largest source of income for adult day centers (PIC, 2003). Other operating revenue (from managed care contracts, private long-term care insurance, and ancillary services such as bathing) totals 13 percent of all revenue. Within the "other operating revenue" category, 22 percent of adult day centers report long-term care insurance as a revenue stream. Twenty-two percent of centers provide ancillary services (such as bathing, hair care, and transportation) and charge an extra fee for the service. Finally, 10 percent of centers report managed care companies as a source of revenue (PIC, 2003).

Managed care typically does not pay for adult day services as a standard benefit. However, the Social HMOs (see Chapter 14) do cover adult day services on a select basis, and some managed care companies will pay on a short-term basis if it is clear that the service substitutes for a more expensive one.

The remaining dollars coming into adult day centers, at 14 percent overall, is *nonoperating* revenue, such as United Way dollars and money from donations, contributions, fundraising events, and grants. Fifty-eight percent of centers report donations/contributions as a source of revenue, 39 percent rely on ongoing grants (such as United Way), 38 percent rely on fundraising events, and 36 percent report one-time grants as a source of revenue (PIC, 2003).

INTEGRATING MECHANISMS

People served by adult day centers often have many other needs. Those who live alone, or with families that have limited time to assist them, may need in-home care for bathing, dressing, or household chores. Participants often have health problems that necessitate the coordination of medical services. When the time comes, assistance may be needed with placement in a nursing home.

Care Coordination

Adult day centers can serve as the nexus between acute care and long-term care. They often take a holistic approach to the care needs of participants, including the provision of support services for caregivers. In this way they provide a critical care management function (Henry et al., 1999).

To help ensure that the needs and wants of both participants and caregivers are being met, adult day centers provide either a continuum of care—using a one-stop shopping approach—or create partnerships with other community service providers (Henry et al., 1999).

Information Systems

The increasing number of adult day centers has prompted the development of a variety of systems designed especially for the management of data. These include attendance, medical, billing, and payment records. Such systems are relatively inexpensive. Typically, information systems for adult day centers are freestanding and do not integrate with those for any other service.

Integrated Financing

The care model referred to as *PACE*, Program of All-Inclusive Care for the Elderly, evolved from OnLok Senior Health Services, an adult day center for frail elders; today PACE is a fully integrated, comprehensive health care program. The PACE program model is one of the few examples of a truly "seamless" continuum of care in the nation. Presently, there are 40 PACE programs nationally.

PACE is a Medicare-authorized program that serves individuals age 55 and older, who are certified by their state to need nursing home care, who are able to live safely in the community at the time of enrollment, and who live in a PACE service area. Delivering all needed medical and supportive services, the program provides the entire continuum of care and services to individuals with chronic care needs. Care and services include: adult day center services that offer nursing, physical/occupational/recreational therapies, meals, and personal care; medical care provided by a PACE physician; home health and personal care; all necessary prescription

drugs; social services; medical specialists such as audiology, dentistry, optometry, and podiatry; respite care; and, when necessary, hospital and nursing home care (National PACE Association, 2003).

PACE has all four integrating mechanisms: a multidisciplinary team-based care management system; a highly sophisticated information system; an integrated administrative structure; and capitated Medicare and Medicaid financing. The PACE model is discussed further in Chapter 14.

ADMINISTRATIVE CHALLENGES

The recent proliferation of adult day services belies the challenges faced by administrators. Among these are:

- *Financial viability.* As mentioned earlier, the average adult day center covers only 85 percent of its expenses with fees, leaving considerable fundraising and cost-shifting to be done.
- *Marketing.* Use of adult day services presents difficult choices for families, and hence most centers operate below capacity. In addition, most clients move on to an institutional setting. Constantly recruiting new clients requires energy and resources.
- *Continuum of services.* To assist participants in accessing the full spectrum of medical and social support services that they may need outside of the ADS setting, establishing and maintaining community relationships is critical.

CONCLUSION

The demand for and development of adult day centers is increasing. The following trends are influencing this growth:

- The continuing growth in the number and proportion of individuals age 65 and older—especially the very old (those 85 and older)
- The continuing efforts of public and private

health care payers/insurers to reduce costs by substituting lower-cost noninstitutional, community-based care for higher-cost nursing home and hospital care

- The aging of baby boomers, who have a preference for noninstitutional, long-term care and also have the resources to pay for such care
- The increase in the number of younger adults who have disabling chronic illnesses, and the search for cost-effective ways to maximize the well-being of this group.

Adult day centers have become a practical and appealing part of the solution to long-term care needs, offering a low-cost alternative for managing the care and promoting the well-being of chronically ill adults. Adult day centers are a viable, cost-effective community-based service option in the long-term care continuum, which help keep individuals (in need of chronic care) at home, in the community, and with family and friends for as long as possible. With widespread needs existing in the community and the profile of services and financial support becoming solidified, adult day programs continue to grow in importance and strength as part of integrated systems of care.

CLIENT EXAMPLE

Mrs. Mason is an 82-year-old widow who resides with her sister-in-law. Her husband died more than 20 years ago and her only child is a son who lives several hundred miles away in another state. One of five children, Mrs. Mason lost all her siblings in the past ten years. She was close to her siblings and often expresses how much she misses them. With the exception of her sister-in-law, she has few friends or relatives whom she sees often. Her sister-in-law is in her 80s but is highly functional both physically and mentally. The two women have always been competitive and their relationship is strained. Her son is concerned about his mother's welfare and functions as her long-distance caregiver.

Mrs. Mason's health is very frail. She has adult onset diabetes (Type II) and serious heart disease. She also has chronic obstructive pulmonary disease as a result of being a long-time smoker, who, until recently, smoked a pack a day. Her health status is further exacerbated by the fact that she was recently involved in an automobile accident and experienced hip and neck injuries. All these factors have contributed to limiting her mobility and independence at home. A retired elementary school principal, Mrs. Mason has had a great deal of difficulty accepting her decreasing ability to function independently. In addition, her increasing dependence has added to the tension in her relationship with her sister-in-law.

At the time of her accident, Mrs. Mason was hospitalized briefly and discharged home with home care. When it was time for her to be discharged from home care, the home care nurse-case manager felt she could benefit from adult day services and referred Mrs. Mason to an adult day center. The process for admission to the center began with an assessment conducted by a multidisciplinary team, including a nurse, social worker, and recreation therapist. The team assessment confirmed that Mrs. Mason could benefit from the program. A care plan was developed with the goal of controlling her diabetes, helping her adopt a healthier lifestyle, enhancing her quality of life, and reducing her risk of depression. The care plan to accomplish this included ongoing monitoring of Mrs. Mason's health status (including daily glucose testing); health education and dietary counseling; group and one-on-one counseling for depression; and encouraging socialization and participation in the activities offered by the center.

Because her income level made her ineligible for Medicaid, Mrs. Mason had to pay the private fee of $60 daily. Initially, she was reluctant to pay this fee but was persuaded by her son. Although Mrs. Mason agreed to attend the program three days a week, she initially did not adapt well. She would often refuse to come in and when she did, she would isolate herself from other participants. She told the social worker that she felt that she was not as disabled as other participants and was not sure that she wanted to continue in the program. The social worker met with other members of the team and they decided that, because of Mrs. Mason's previous experience as a teacher, she might be interested in assisting the recreation therapist in leading a group, such as a current events or book discussion group. The recreational therapist spoke with her about this and she enthusiastically agreed. Over time, her responsibilities as a "group leader" gave Mrs. Mason a sense of pride and accomplishment and had positive impact on her self-esteem. Also, participating in a depression support group and the counseling provided by the social worker helped her cope with the losses she was experiencing. Eventually, Mrs. Mason built strong relationships with other participants and staff and began to look forward to attending the program. She appeared to be less depressed and to have a more positive attitude. She also became more receptive to following her physician's orders by adopting a healthier diet. It was also apparent that attending several days a week had greatly reduced the tension between her and her sister-in-law. In sum, for about $720 per month the quality of Mrs. Mason's life greatly improved as the result of her participation in the adult day program.

WHERE TO GO FOR FURTHER INFORMATION

Commission on Accreditation of Rehabilitation Facilities (CARF)
4891 E. Grant Road
Tucson, AZ 85712
(520) 325-1044
http://www.carf.org

National Adult Day Services Association, Inc.
8201 Greensboro Drive, Suite 300
McLean, VA 22102
(866) 890-7357 or (703) 610-9035
http://www.nadsa.org

National PACE Association
801 N. Fairfax Avenue, Suite 309

Alexandria, VA 22314
(703) 535-1565
http://www.natlpaceassn.org

Partners in Caregiving
Wake Forest University School of Medicine
Medical Center Boulevard
Winston-Salem, NC 27157
(800) 795-3676

FACTS REVIEW

1. What is adult day services (ADS)?
2. What are the benefits of ADS for program participants, for family caregivers, and for society in general?
3. What are the three models of ADS and what are the key differences among them?
4. What factors are influencing the growing demand for ADS services?
5. Who are the primary payers of ADS services?
6. What does PACE stand for, and what does the model demonstrate?

REFERENCES

Henry, R. S., Cox, N. J., Reifler, B. V., & Asbury, C. (1999). Adult day centers. In S. L. Isaacs & J. R. Knickman (Eds.), *To improve health and health care 2000: The Robert Wood Johnson Foundation anthology.* San Francisco, CA: Jossey-Bass.

Jarrott, S. E., Zarit, S. H., Stephens, M. A. P., Townsend, A., & Greene, R. (1999). Caregiver satisfaction with adult day service programs. *American Journal of Alzheimer's Disease, 14*(4), 233–244.

Jones, B. N., Cox, N. J., Yates, K., & Reifler, B. V. (1997). Converting inquiries to enrollments to maintain a viable adult day center. *Pride Institute Journal of Long Term Home Health Care, 16*(4), 46–52.

Lucas, J., Howell-White, S., & Rosato, N. S. (2003). *Adult day health services across states: Preliminary results from a 50-state survey of state health policies.* Rutgers Center for State Health Policy. Available at *http://www.cshp.rutgers.edu*

National Adult Day Services Association. (2002). *Adult day services fact sheet.* McLean, VA: Author.

National Institute on Adult Daycare. (1989). *National adult day center census.* Washington, DC: National Council on the Aging.

National PACE Association. (2003). *What is PACE?* Alexandria, VA: Author. Retrieved on August 1, 2003 from *http://www.natlpaceassn.org*

Newton, G., & Henry, R. S. (1994). *Referral source marketing for adult day programs.* Winston-Salem, NC: Wake Forest University School of Medicine.

Partners in Caregiving: The Adult Day Services Program (2003). *National study of adult day services, 2001–2002.* Winston-Salem, NC: Wake Forest University School of Medicine.

Partners in Caregiving: The Dementia Services Program. (1995). *Life after diagnosis—Adult day services in America.* Winston-Salem, NC: Wake Forest University School of Medicine.

Reifler, B. V., Henry, R. S., Rushing, J., Yates, K., Cox, N. J., Bradham, D. D., & McFarlane, M. (1997). Financial performance among adult day centers: Results of a national demonstration program. *Journal of the American Geriatrics Society, 45,* 146–153.

Von Behren, R. (1986). *Adult day care in America: Summary of a national survey.* Washington, DC: National Council on the Aging/National Institute on Adult Daycare.

Webb, L. C. (Ed.). (1989). *Planning and managing adult day care: Pathways to success.* Owings Mills, MD: National Health Publishing.

Zarit, S. H., Stephens, M. A. P., Townsend, A., & Greene, R. (1998). Stress reduction for family caregivers: Effects of adult day care use. *Journal of Gerontology, 53B*(5), S267–S277.

CHAPTER 9

Housing

Jon Pynoos and Christy-Ann M. Nishita

Housing is an integral component of long-term care. The physical features of housing affect the ability of frail older persons to live safely and comfortably. Its layout and features also influence caregiver capacities to provide assistance. Service linkages with housing can enhance the ability of those with functional disabilities to age in place rather than move to more institutional settings. Housing specifically designed to incorporate services enables those who need personal assistance with physically supportive accommodations to carry out activities of daily living. Conversely, a poor housing environment can cause an at-risk person to suffer health problems that require use of health services, ranging from hospital inpatient care to durable medical equipment. Housing is an integral component in the development of a comprehensive, community-based, long-term care system.

BACKGROUND

Housing and long-term care have long been treated as separate domains, each with its own set of policies,

programs, regulations, and funding sources (Pynoos, 1992). However, early in the twentieth century, housing and services were considered together in terms of addressing social problems. For example, during the 1920s, a number of model tenements were funded by foundations and managed by social workers. Though somewhat paternalistic, this housing provided assistance in such areas as education concerning nutrition and good housekeeping.

During the Depression and after World War II, reformers hoped that their concepts would be incorporated into the policies underlying public housing. Owing to pressures to keep it from competing with the private sector, however, government-sponsored public housing had few amenities. Community facilities were limited and housing budgets pared of expenditures for social or community services. The primary role of the manager was caring for the property and collecting rent. Therefore, when adults age 65 and older with low income became eligible for public housing in the late 1950s, the pattern was well established: projects were oriented to the active well senior. Although they included some special

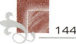

features for older people, such as emergency call buttons, few services were tied to public housing complexes. When services were provided, they had to be paid for through nonhousing sources.

In 1959, Section 202, a special housing program for older adults and those with disabilities, was created as part of the National Housing Act. Sponsors were nonprofit, and tenants initially of moderate income, just above the eligibility requirements of public housing. The designers of the program did not want Section 202 housing to function as a nursing home or even a home for the aged. Consequently, Section 202 housing projects were also built for ambulatory, independent seniors (approximately 10 percent of the units were made accessible for people under age 65 with disabilities). Several features to prevent accidents (e.g., emergency call buttons and grab bars) were included, and space for services and common activities was allowed. Services such as meals, however, were not guaranteed, and residents or sponsors were responsible for paying for them directly. The federal government's Department of Housing and Urban Development (HUD) continued to view itself as concerned only with "bricks and mortar." State programs mirrored federal ones.

Private-sector housing, composed principally of single-family houses and apartments, was also developed for independent people. Little thought was given to the eventual suitability of this housing for those who became frail (Pynoos, 1993). Private apartments, like their counterparts in the public sector, rarely included spaces for services or employed managers trained in meeting residents' service needs. In the 1950s, an increasing amount of housing was built in suburban areas in locations that were not close to services or public transportation.

During the 1970s, concern began to be raised about the suitability of the housing stock for older people who had aged in place and younger people with disabilities. Older residents who had moved into public, Section 202 housing, or even into their own homes or apartments after World War II, were now in their late 70s or 80s. Housing units that fit their needs at younger ages did not have physically

supportive environments, available services, or management trained to address their needs as they aged. When it became inefficient or too difficult to stay in their homes, frail older people, especially those with low incomes, had few residential options available. Consequently, many older people unnecessarily moved to more institutional settings, such as nursing homes or board and care homes, in sharp contradiction to their desire to age in place.

Along with the aging of the residential population, a second trend has created an additional need for supportive housing. The deinstitutionalization movement of the 1960s and 1970s placed many people with mental health problems in the community. This shift to community-based care led to the growth of special-needs housing for people with developmental disabilities, substance abuse problems, and a variety of mental health problems. However, programs and new housing alternatives expected to help those who were deinstitutionalized have been limited by funding, as well as by neighborhood opposition.

The shift toward community-based care for persons with disabilities is part of a larger trend: a recognition that the physical environment is an important determinant of the health outcomes of older adults. For example, the health care sector has looked at the home environment in its falls prevention initiatives. Falls evaluations should examine not only internal problems with vision, balance, and mobility, but also external factors, such as the presence of potential hazards in the home. The environment can also contain health hazards that can negatively affect older adults because of depressed immune system response. Older persons who take several medications or have chronic conditions are more susceptible to environmental toxins. The Environmental Protection Agency created an Aging Initiative that will study potential hazards in drinking water, indoor air, and outdoor air to create healthier homes and communities for older adults. The physical environment has a key role in preventing or lessening long-term or chronic problems, thereby creating an even greater need for supportive housing.

THE CONTINUUM OF HOUSING: CHANGING THE PARADIGMS

A long-standing assumption is that as people become frailer, they need to move along a housing continuum from one setting to another. Along this continuum are a range of housing options, such as single-family homes, apartments, congregate living, assisted living, and board and care homes, with the end point most frequently identified as a nursing home (Kendig & Pynoos, 1990).

Although the continuum of housing identifies a range of housing types (see Table 9.1), there is increasing recognition that frail older people and persons with disabilities need not necessarily move from one setting to another to obtain assistance. Semi-dependent or dependent older people can live in a variety of settings, including their own homes and apartments, if the physical setting is supportive and affordable services are accessible. The goal of maintaining older adults in the community is well-aligned with the *Olmstead* decision issued by the Supreme Court in 1999. It requires states to administer programs and services to persons with disabilities in the "most integrated setting appropriate" to their needs. A revised framework has therefore emerged that emphasizes the elasticity of the conventional housing stock in terms of its ability to accommodate a wide spectrum of frail older people and younger people with disabilities. At the same time, it stresses the importance of having a broad spectrum of housing alternatives that allow choices of settings that offer different levels of on-site services, supervision, sociability, privacy, amenities, and affordability. The following section describes the wide array of independent and supportive housing options available. The flexibility of this continuum is reflected in the fact that home modifications and services can be added to independent housing to support aging in place. The service and financial characteristics of various types of housing are shown in Table 9.2. The services available in supportive housing contrast with those available in independent housing.

Table 9.1 The Continuum of Housing

Housing Options	Level of Support: Independent	Semi-Independent	Dependent
Independent Housing			
Single-family housing*	————	——→	
Apartment dwelling*	————	——→	
Granny flat/Echo housing/Accessory unit*	——	——→	
Shared housing*	———	——→	
Supportive Housing			
Retirement community (age 55+)	————	——→	
Age-segregated apartment dwelling	———	——→	
Continuing care retirement community (CCRC)	——	————	——→
Congregate housing (20+ units)	——	————	→
Board and care home		——→	
Assisted living		————	→

* Home modifications and services can be added to independent housing to support an older adult's increasing frailty.

Table 9.2 Service and Financial Characteristics of Selective Housing Options

Type of Housing	Residents	Payment Sources	Typical Cost per Month	Services Available On-Site
Private (independent)		Tenant	Varies	Very limited
Public (independent)	Low-income	Tenant, HUD subsidies	30% of income	Service coordination, limited services
Board and care	Physically or mentally vulnerable	Tenant, SSI, long-term care insurance	$850–4,000	Physically accessible environment, meals, on-site management, services
Congregate housing (public)	Moderate ADL and IADL dependency	Tenant, HUD subsidies	30% of income	Service coordination, meals, transportation, homemaker
Assisted living	High levels of ADL dependency and cognitive impairment	Tenant, Medicaid waivers, long-term care insurance	$600–3700	Medication management, personal care, meals, housekeeping, unscheduled assistance, preventive care
Continuing care retirement communities	Middle to upper income	Private	$800–2,000	Medical services, meals, building maintenance, housekeeping, social activities

INDEPENDENT HOUSING

Most older people reside in private-sector homes or apartments. More than 8 in 10 older adults own their own homes (AARP, 2000). Although the rate of home ownership decreases with advanced old age, 78 percent of older adults over age 75 residing in the community still own their own homes (Joint Center for Housing Studies [JCHS], 2003). Certain groups, however, have lower rates of home ownership. In 2002, 80 percent of whites age 75 and older were homeowners, in comparison to 74 percent of blacks, 65 percent of Hispanics, and 59 percent of Asians (JCHS, 2003).

Apartment dwellers make up the majority of non-homeowners. Older renters differ from homeowners in that they have somewhat lower incomes, have lived in their units for relatively shorter periods of time, and occupy housing in somewhat worse condition. Older renters generally have lower incomes than homeowners. Twenty-one percent of older renters live in structures with more than 50 units, offering opportunities for economies of scale in service delivery (Naifeh, 1993).

Government-assisted housing, consisting of more than 20,000 complexes of housing for seniors, is a major potential source of service-enriched housing for low-income, frail older adults. Funded by such programs as public and Section 202 housing, USDA Rural Development, and Section 8, these complexes house more than a million seniors. Residents tend to be female, poor, live alone, and an average age of 75. Many residents are also minority older adults and increasingly at risk of institutionalization.

Visitability and Universal Design

Newly constructed homes built with accessibility features in place can support independent living. **Visitability** is a small set of basic accessibility features that enable persons with disabilities to access the main level of single-family homes, duplexes, and triplexes. The concept of visitability does not require a completely accessible house; rather, it is a narrower concept intended to assist residents, friends, and relatives who are functionally impaired, as well as future residents, to enter and get around the home. The three key visitability requirements are zero step entrance to the home, wide interior doors, and at least a half bath on the main floor.

Universal design is a concept promoting homes that are accessible, adaptable, and usable by persons of all ages and abilities (*http://www.design.ncsu.edu/cud/*). It is different from visitability because it applies to the entire home, and includes features such as variable-height counters, lever door handles, supportive bars in bathroom and shower, and bathrooms and kitchens designed to accommodate wheelchairs or walkers. Taken together, proponents of these concepts assert that it is better for housing to be accessible and supportive from the time it is built, rather than retrofitting the home when the need arises.

Aside from structural features, other design elements can be important to independent living. For example, strong color contrasts and the correct type or level of lighting can enhance visual acuity for persons with vision impairments (*http://www.lighthouse.org*). For persons with cognitive impairment, symmetrical or round configurations within the home will facilitate wayfinding and orientation. Environmental elements such as plants, murals, doors, and artwork are also important to orient these individuals to their environment (Regnier & Pynoos, 1992).

Aging in Place: Options to Remain Independent

In conventional homes without accessibility features, older adults can make changes to the home or receive services in the home to remain independent. These options support older adults in their current housing, thereby preventing or delaying a move to a more institutionalized setting.

Home Modifications

Home modifications are adaptations to existing home environments that can make it easier and safer to carry out activities such as bathing, cooking, and climbing stairs. Increasing evidence suggests that home modifications can have an important effect on the ability of chronically ill or disabled persons to live independently. Home modifications also have a role to play in multifactorial interventions to prevent falls that include risk assessment, exercise, educational materials and programming, and follow-up (Shekelle et al., 2002). Environmental factors such as privacy or sufficient space can also facilitate family and formal caregiving (Newman, 1985; Newman et al. 1990).

Only recently have there been efforts to document the prevalence of and need for home modifications. According to the 1995 American Housing Survey, 3.4 million, or 38 percent, of households with at least one member with a permanent physical activity limitation had home modifications present (see Table 9.3). However, a large number of older people who report health problems, mobility limitations, and dependency in ADLs and IADLs live in housing without adaptive features. Among older people with disabilities who express a need for home modifications, only about half of the households have the home modifications they need (JCHS, 2003).

Table 9.3 Common Home Adaptations among Households with One Member Who Has a Physical Activity Limitation

Adaptation	Number of Households
Handrails or grab bars	2,002,000
Widened doors or hallways	756,000
Ramps	736,000
Easy-access bathrooms	713,000
Easy-access kitchens	544,000

SOURCE: 1995 American Housing Survey.

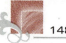

The overall low incidence of supportive features in the home is due to three major barriers. First, professionals and consumers alike lack awareness of problems in the home environment. For example, many people with disabilities, especially seniors, have a low level of awareness of the risks that the environment presents or a lack of knowledge of how home adaptations might make living safer and easier. Older people are often reported as having adapted their behavior to the environment (e.g., stopped taking baths or showers because of the danger of falling) rather than having adapted their environment to their changed capabilities (e.g., installing a hand-held shower, adding a grab bar). Among professionals such as doctors, knowledge about home adaptation is also low. Concern has been expressed that even case managers, the gatekeepers for many long-term care services, may overlook home modifications.

Second, some home modifications may be unaffordable. The majority of home adaptations are paid for out of pocket (LaPlante, Hendershot, & Moss, 1997). Costs range from less than $100 for the purchase and installation of a simple handrail or grab bar, to $100 to $800 for a portable wheelchair ramp, and $2,000 to $5,000 for a stair lift. Although some studies suggest that income does not predict unmet needs for home modification (e.g., Newman, 2003), other studies show that financial constraint is a major barrier to obtaining needed modifications (AARP, 2000).

Even though cost can be a deterrent, home modification may be cost-effective in its ability to delay institutionalization and to prevent injuries. A study by Mann (Mann, Ottenbacher, Fraas, Tomita, & Granger, 1999) compared the health care costs of a treatment group that received assistive technology and environmental interventions to those of a control group that received the "usual care services" over an 18-month period. The results indicated that the expenditures for the treatment group were significantly smaller than the control group for institutional care, nurse visits, and case manager visits. Additional evidence on cost-effectiveness may attract more third-party payers to reimburse for home

modifications, thus lessening the burden on individuals and families who must currently pay out of pocket. For example, an HMO in the Philadelphia area is providing home assessments, home safety repairs, and home modifications under its Silver Plan. The HMO contracts with the Philadelphia Corporation on Aging, a local Area Agency on Aging experienced in home modification, to provide these services.

A third barrier reported by individuals and social service agencies in obtaining home modifications has been the delivery system (Pynoos, 1993). Simple home adaptations are often made by persons with disabilities and their family members. However, many persons lack the ability to identify environmental problems and make appropriate adaptations. Decisions about such proposed changes have to take into account the resident's ability to use them, receptivity to the proposed changes, and the physical environment of the home itself. Even installing an uncomplicated grab bar on a wall requires the ability to attach the bar to a stud and position it at the correct angle and height for the person who will be using it. It is often necessary to employ a provider to assess problems and make changes. Thus, despite the modest nature of many jobs, the need for specialized skills, the low income of many persons who need adaptations, concerns about the reliability of private providers, and the difficulty of accessing occupational therapists all contribute to service delivery problems in home modification.

Innovative local and state programs have developed across the country to meet the needs of people requiring home modifications because of functional limitations. Because there is no single source of funds, many programs have pieced together resources from a variety of sources, such as Community Development Block Grants (CDBG), the Older Americans Act (OAA), the Department of Energy, Medicaid waivers, and state and local governments, in their efforts to meet the multiple needs of clients. Conventional Medicare and Medicaid remain very limited sources of funds because they pay only for medically necessary devices.

The experience of such programs illustrates both the potential and the problems that home modification and repair programs encounter:

- The need far exceeds the budgets of programs to provide services. Budget limitations highly restrict geographic areas, the types of changes programs can make, and the amount that can be spent on any individual client.
- Low-income persons often need both repairs and modifications (e.g., adding a railing to a stairway would be a solution only if the stairs themselves are in good condition and not broken, uneven, or badly lit).
- The delivery of home modification and repair services is a complex undertaking that includes assessment, estimating costs, dealing with specialized trades and unions, and managing liability and quality control.

These tasks may prove difficult for agencies more familiar with dealing with the social and health needs of clients. Nevertheless, the importance of the home environment in preventing accidents, facilitating caregiving, and forestalling institutionalization suggests that it should be included in discharge planning, preventive health programs, and community-based care. The National Resource Center on Supportive Housing and Home Modification has an information clearinghouse of home modification research, products, and innovative programs (*http://www.homemods.org*).

Clustering Services

Clustering services involves consolidating fragmented services for multiple clients. It involves bringing services to areas with a high concentration of older residents, such as in federally subsidized housing. This strategy can reduce travel time and costs, enable more efficient worker assignment, and serve more consumers. Over the last decade, there has been a growing realization that economies of scale exist in providing services to large numbers of frail seniors living in one place, as well as opportunities

for peer support. Adult day services programs, for example, have located in or adjacent to assisted living complexes. In addition to initiatives in assisted living, several demonstrations and programs have been carried out in more conventional housing settings to test models of planning, organizing, and providing clusters of services.

One of the earliest of these demonstrations, the Congregate Housing Services Program (CHSP) (Redfoot & Sloan, 1991), authorized under Title IV of the Housing and Community Development Act of 1978, provides a service-enriched setting for frail older persons. Advocates of the CHSP promoted it on the basis that it would prevent "premature" institutionalization of frail and handicapped residents of federally subsidized housing. The CHSP was carried out initially in 63 public housing and Section 202 sites, using HUD funds to pay for services such as meals, homemaking, and transportation to select groups of tenants with three ADL or IADL needs. Eligibility for and organization of the services was overseen by a service coordinator and professional assessment team. Between 1979 and 1985, approximately $28 million was spent on services to 3,500 residents of 63 public housing and Section 202 projects.

Because of controversy about whether the CHSP actually prevented institutionalization, and HUD's continued reluctance to pay for services, the program did not expand until the early 1990s (Redfoot & Sloan, 1991), with the passage of the National Affordable Housing Act of 1990. By this time, the CHSP, initially funded solely by HUD, required significant state and local funding matches that discouraged many sites from applying. Nevertheless, by 1994, the program had grown to more than 100 sites.

In another model, the New York City Visiting Nurses Association used Medicaid waivers to provide services to groups of residents living in government-assisted housing. Various personnel and health care staff are assigned to clusters of frail residents in senior housing. Staff can therefore move from one resident to another, performing various tasks rather than spending long blocks of time with individual residents. An evaluation of the VNA project found that it saved money, although residents were somewhat less satisfied because individually they received less service (Feldman, Latimer, & Davidson, 1996).

A New York City social HMO employs a model of clustering services based on group membership. The Member to Member program in New York City is a part of a nonprofit health plan for older adults called Elder Plan. Started in 1987 through a grant from the Robert Wood Johnson Foundation, program participants earn "time dollars" by providing a range of services (such as health care products or transportation vouchers) and then redeeming these credits for other needed services. Since its inception, participants have provided 115,000 hours of service to 5,000 older adults (*http://www.timedollar.org*).

Service Coordination

The concept of service coordination is an outgrowth of such initiatives as the CHSP and the Supportive Services Program in Senior Housing demonstration (Lanspery, 1992) sponsored by the Robert Wood Johnson Foundation. Through the Housing and Community Development Act of 1992, Congress authorized expenditures for a Service Coordinator Program. Service coordination is often described as the "glue" that holds a program together or the linking mechanism between residents of housing complexes and services. It is a less intensive model than the CHSP and relies more on connecting residents with services rather than providing services directly.

Services coordinated for residents include Meals on Wheels, in-home supportive services, hospice care, home health for those who meet Medicare or Medicaid eligibility criteria, transportation services, on-site adult education in areas of interest, and monthly blood pressure checks. Assistance is provided with locating other living arrangements, such as board and care, assisted living facility, or a nursing home, should it become necessary. However, the primary focus is on assisting residents to continue living in their current apartments.

The coordinators in this program do not have budgetary authority for services, but they can serve a broad group of frail older residents. According to the American Association of Service Coordinators, there were approximately 3,000 service coordinators working in Section 202, public housing, and other programs in 2003. An evaluation (Feder, Scanlon, & Howard, 1992; KRA Corporation, 1996) of the program revealed that service coordinators successfully marshal a number of new services for residents, who report high levels of satisfaction with the program.

The HOPE for Elderly Independence Demonstration (HOPE IV) program combines HUD Section 8 rental assistance with case management and supportive services for low-income seniors. It establishes a Service Coordinator position; this person makes the necessary arrangements with agencies and organizations in the community to provide these services. An evaluation of the program after two years of operation indicated that 91 percent of clients were very satisfied with the program. The receipt of services was also associated with positive outcomes such as improved social functioning, less depression, and increased vitality. Although HUD has not provided any new funding for this demonstration since fiscal year 1993, such programs would provide incentives for a range of supportive housing options if implemented on a wide scale.

Recently, HUD has taken increased responsibility for adapting its stock of housing for older adults into more supportive settings linked with services. In fiscal year 2003, the HUD budget increased funding to the Service Coordinator Program by $3 million over the previous year, to $53 million. Table 9.4 describes the different federal housing programs benefiting older adults.

SUPPORTIVE HOUSING OPTIONS

When frail older persons need a more physically supportive dwelling unit, greater supervision (e.g., with medications), more services, or more companionship than can be efficiently provided in their own

Table 9.4 Federal Housing Programs Benefiting Older Adults

Name of Program	Description	Qualifications
Public and assisted housing	Refers to rental units financed by the U.S. Department of Housing and Urban Development. Families or individuals pay no more than 30% of their income on rent.	Low-income families or individuals of all ages
Section 8 certificates/vouchers	Covers the difference in rent above 30% of the income of the family/individual to live in HUD-approved housing.	Low-income families or individuals of all ages
Section 202	Provides rental units and may include supportive services such as meals and transportation.	Very low-income persons age 62 and older
Congregate Housing Services program	Provides independent older adults living in Section 202 and public housing units with professional service coordination and services such as meals and transportation.	Very low-income persons age 62 and older with ADL limitations
Service Coordinator Program	Links older adults in Section 202 or public housing with needed services.	Very low-income persons age 62 and older
HOPE for Elderly Independence program	Combines Section 8 rental assistance with case management and support services to enable older adults to live independently.	Low-income adults age 62 and older with 3 or more problems with ADLs

homes or apartments, a move to a more supportive setting may be necessary. *Supportive housing* refers to residential living arrangements, for frail persons, that include special design features and the presence or provision of services (Pynoos & Golant, 1995). These include board and care homes, assisted living, congregate housing, and group homes. In this continually evolving field, it is difficult to categorize these housing options because their definitions blend and overlap. Moreover, regulations, when they exist, vary considerably by state. In addition, estimates of the absolute and relative size of the populations that utilize these options vary considerably because of variations in state licensing requirements, the difficulty in identifying unregulated facilities, and problems that older people themselves have answering survey questions about the type of housing they occupy.

Estimates of the number of older people living in supportive housing settings range from 1 million to 2 million (see Table 9.5). However, the stock of sup-

Table 9.5 Prevalence of Supportive Housing

Type of Supportive Housing	Number of Persons
Board and care homes	400,000
Assisted living	More than 1 million
Continuing care retirement communities	350,000–450,000

portive housing is still insufficient to meet the needs of a growing population of frail older people, much of it remains unaffordable by those with low or moderate incomes, and its quality remains difficult to judge.

Board and Care Homes

This housing type generally offers on-site management, a physically accessible environment, meals, and a range of services for physically or mentally

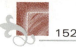

vulnerable older people and younger people with disabilities who could not continue to live independently in their previous residences. In facilities serving primarily seniors, the average age is approximately 85 (Phillips et al., 1995), about 10 years older than residents of government-assisted housing.

Studies suggest that over 30,000 board and care homes exist in the United States (Clark, Turek-Brezina, Chu, & Hawes, 1994), nearly double the number of nursing homes (Sirrocco, 1994). However, owing to their smaller size (usually between 5 and 20 dwelling units), board and care homes house only about one-fourth the number of residents (about 400,000 people) as nursing homes and include about 200,000 people under age 62. Many of the older residents in board and care homes are subsidized by state governments that add an amount to the Supplemental Security Income (SSI) that many residents use to pay for their accommodations and care. Most board and care homes are modest in nature and require that residents share rooms. Though theoretically licensed and regulated by state government, many of the smaller board and care homes remain unlicensed and enforcement is lax. These homes are often isolated from community services. Studies have suggested that board and care residents would benefit from programs brought to the homes, as well as linkages that take residents to outside activities (Goodman, Pynoos, & Stevenson, 1988).

Congregate Housing

Congregate housing refers to a wide range of multiunit living arrangements for older people in both the private and public sectors. Many Section 202 housing developments fall under this category. Older people who live in this housing generally have their own apartments that include kitchens or kitchenettes and private bathrooms. The monthly cost can range from $300 to $2,500 (*http://www.helpguide.org/*). Most of this housing has dining rooms and provides residents with at least one meal a day that is frequently included in the rent. The housing also has common spaces for social and educational activities and, in some cases, provides transportation. Sponsors of congregate housing generally do not, however, offer personal care services or health services directly. Therefore, in many states, such housing is not licensed under regulations that apply to residential care facilities or assisted living.

In line with the physical characteristics of the buildings and the limited provision of services, congregate housing attracts older people who can live independently. It especially appeals to older people who no longer want the responsibility of home maintenance or meal preparation and who positively anticipate making new friends and engaging in activities. Problems may arise, later, however, as residents age in place and need more assistance than the housing provides.

Assisted Living

Assisted living (AL) is a housing option that involves the delivery of professionally managed supportive services and, depending on state regulations, nursing services, in a group setting that is residential in character and appearance. The typical resident of an AL is female, age 83 or older, widowed, and requires help with 2.8 ADL (Assisted Living Federation of America, 2001). AL is intended to accommodate physically and mentally frail people without imposing on them a heavily regulated, institutional environment (Kane & Wilson, 1993). It has the capacity to meet unscheduled needs for assistance and is managed in ways that strive to maximize the physical and psychological independence of residents. Table 9.6 lists services typically offered in assisted living facilities.

To address the more intensive service needs of Section 202 residents, HUD has provided funding to convert certain Section 202 housing projects into assisted living facilities. HUD created an Assisted Living Conversion Program to provide private non-profit owners of eligible developments with funding

Table 9.6 Assisted Living Services

Meals
Housekeeping
Transportation
Assistance for people with functional disabilities
24-hour security
Emergency call systems in living unit
Health maintenance, wellness, exercise programs
Medication management
Personal laundry services
Social and recreational activities
Short-term respite care
Therapy and pharmacy services
Special programs for people with Alzheimer's disease or
    other forms of dementia

for the physical conversion of existing project units. The owners provide the services, either directly or through third-party sources such as Medicaid, SSI payments, or an Area Agency on Aging. HUD uses another incentive to improve the affordability of assisted living: the use of tax credits and Section 8 vouchers to pay for resident housing. Medicaid waivers are required to pay for services provided to residents.

The average monthly cost of an assisted living facility in 2002 was $2,159, but ranged from $592 in Jackson, Mississippi, to $3,696 in New York City (MetLife Mature Market Institute, 2002). Most residents pay out of pocket for their care. A long-term care insurance policy is another possible source of funding for the resident. Some states and local governments use Supplemental Security Income or Medicaid to pay for low-income residents, or the Medicaid waiver program to reimburse for services. As of 2002, 37 states provided limited Medicaid coverage of assisted living services through such sources as a home- and community-based waiver or managed care waiver.

In 2003, the Assisted Living Workgroup, made up of nearly 50 organizations, developed recom-mendations for the U.S. Senate Special Committee on Aging in many areas, including the affordability of AL (e.g., the expansion of funding for the 1915(c) Home and Community-Based waiver pro-gram and the creation of a specific SSI "living arrangement" category to cover average AL unit and board costs). Reaching consensus was difficult, but the workgroup did recommend that AL be made more affordable for Medicaid-eligible resi-dents and moderate-income residents (individuals with $25,000/year income or less) (Assisted Living Workgroup, 2003).

Varying definitions of AL around the nation have produced difficulties with regulation and accredita-tion. In the absence of federal regulation, states have established licensing criteria and regulations of their own. All 50 states and the District of Co-lumbia have some form of regulatory or licensure category for assisted living. AL facilities can attain accreditation through either of two national volun-tary accrediting organizations: the Joint Commission on the Accreditation of Healthcare Organizations (JCAHO), or the Commission for Accreditation of Rehabilitation Facilities (CARF). The standards cover a range of areas including consumer protec-tion, resident services, performance improvement, leadership, and management of the care environ-ment. In addition, the Assisted Living Workgroup recommended the creation of a National Center for Excellence in Assisted Living to develop perform-ance measures, such as measures of clinical out-comes, functional outcomes, and staff and resident satisfaction (Assisted Living Workgroup, 2003).

Assisted living facilities may also be subject to regulations governing the confidentiality of medical information. The federal Health Insurance Portabil-ity and Accountability Act (HIPAA) of 1996 sets forth "privacy" rules detailing the use and disclosure of health information. If facilities provide only so-cial services and require residents who need medical services to access those services on their own, they are not subject to HIPAA. However, if the facility employs a nurse or other licensed health profes-sional to provide medical or nursing services, any

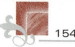

health information associated with these services will be subject to the privacy rules.

Continuing Care Retirement Communities

Continuing care retirement communities (CCRCs) are one model of the ideal continuum of care, with a range of services linked by the integrating mechanisms, including financing. CCRCs offer older people residential units, services, activities, personal care, and nursing care. Each community houses between 400 and 600 older people, often in campus-type settings. CCRCs generally require, as a condition for entry, that new residents be in reasonably good health. Once admitted, however, CCRCs are the most accommodating of all settings, because residents can remain and obtain services in the community if they experience physical or mental limitations. An insurance model is used to ensure that residents can afford services.

Most CCRCs require residents to pay entrance and monthly fees for which the community guarantees a dwelling unit, services, meals, and nursing care. Entrance fees vary widely from $20,000 to $400,000, with an average of $40,000; monthly maintenance fees range from $200 to $2,500 (Sanders, 1997). Residents generally are required to have Medicare Parts A and B. To reduce their potential liability for long-term care, some CCRCs also offer or require long-term care insurance. Generally, the CCRC option is affordable only by middle- and upper-income older people.

The typical age of entrants is 79 years. The primary reason that older adults select CCRCs is security, represented most clearly by the assurance of high-quality nursing care and personal care services. Other major considerations are the availability of medical services, meals, building maintenance, housekeeping services, and cultural and social activities. Though some communities provide most of their own services, others obtain many of them through contracts with outside organizations.

CCRCs are subject to state legislation and regulation in 38 states. The nursing and assisted living facilities in CCRCs are also subject to applicable state and federal regulations. Hence, a CCRC may hold several licenses. Voluntary accreditation is available from the Continuing Care Accreditation Commission, which has recently entered into a collaborative accreditation with CARF.

By 1997, there were approximately 1,200 CCRCs housing approximately 350,000 to 450,000 older people (Sanders, 1997). While it is predicted that the number of these facilities could double in the near future, growth may be tempered by an increase in other options, such as home care and assisted living.

INTEGRATING MECHANISMS

Housing has, for the most part, been operated quite separately from the health care system. It has not been subject to the same trends in the development of integrating mechanisms. Disjointed policies and programs have treated the residential setting in isolation, increasing service fragmentation, delivery costs, institutionalization, and consumer dissatisfaction. Moreover, the relative absence of regulations and the bias toward independent rather than dependent residents have limited the extent to which management deals with people rather than the facility. As much as housing providers may be aware of their residents' needs for services, they are reluctant to provide such services directly, because they then may be forced to become licensed as health care facilities rather than housing facilities, which would force them to comply with far more stringent regulations. Nevertheless, the models of clustering services and service coordination, mentioned earlier, are current efforts to link housing with services. The following are exemplary methods of integration.

Care Coordination

Formal on-side case management is most likely to occur in CCRCs which have a financial and a personal commitment to help residents over time and to promote their independence. Many facilities that offer board and care and some support for residents are too small to afford formal case management programs, but assist residents on an informal basis. Community-based care managers may work with residents of independent or supportive housing to help them access health care, mental health, and other services available in the community.

Integrated Information Systems

Most housing complexes maintain little information about their residents. Integrated information systems of the sophistication being developed by health care organizations are well beyond the needs of most housing entities. Moreover, the information they do keep is primarily for billing and financial purposes. Little, if any, data pertinent to health status or service utilization are maintained. Even multilevel housing complexes that may include assisted living and nursing units are likely to keep only the information required by payers and licensing authorities, and they are not likely to maintain extensive databases on the residents of other units. Small facilities may not even have their records computerized. Nevertheless, increased information concerning clients is on the horizon, as multilevel housing complexes and AL facilities become owned by large chains and vertically integrated corporations.

Capitated Financing

CCRCs were early leaders in capitated financing to the extent that they promised housing, nursing, and support services for an initial buy-in fee. However, the early CCRCs discovered that the actuarial projections underestimated longevity and the accompanying high costs of care. Regulators at the state level also became concerned about the long-term financial viability of CCRCs and passed laws related to reserves limiting CCRC commitments. Thus, most CCRCs have now modified their financial arrangements and separated or limited the

amount of health care services they commit to provide to residents without additional payments. Some CCRCs now require residents to purchase long-term care insurance to ensure that funding will be available to pay for extra services that may be needed.

The Program of All-Inclusive Care for the Elderly

The Program of All-Inclusive Care for the Elderly (PACE) is a comprehensive service program that incorporates residential services with health care and social services to enable frail, nursing-home-eligible seniors to remain in their homes. PACE became a formal Medicare benefit under the Balanced Budget Act of 1997. PACE attempts to replicate the OnLok Senior Health Services program in San Francisco that integrates Medicare and Medicaid financing and provides medical and long-term care services to nursing-home-eligible frail people in a day services setting. PACE is expected to include approximately 50 sites and 10,000 participants by 2005. Many PACE sites have added housing because a number of their participants live in deficient settings or need more supervision and help with unscheduled needs than can be provided in individual home settings. Participants in the program are assigned to an interdisciplinary team for regular needs assessment and care management. PACE's purpose is to address the needs of long-term care clients, providers, and payers. For clients, the comprehensive service package allows them to continue living independently in the community while receiving services rather than moving to institutional settings. The PACE model further demonstrates the essential link between housing and services.

The challenges to incorporating housing into an integrated continuum of care are evident. Much must be done to develop housing as an environment that supports health, particularly as people age or become disabled. Conversely, health care providers and payers must recognize the impact that housing situations can have on health. Then, efforts can be made to integrate housing and health services, and housing settings can begin to develop informal affiliations and strategies that enable services to be coordinated on a client-specific, as well as a building-wide, basis, taking advantage of the economies of scale inherent in delivering or clustering services for groups of frail people living together. The few organizations that have integrated housing with health care should be examined as models of how such integration works at present and what the potential might be to increase integration in the future.

POLICY ISSUES

Housing is increasingly recognized as an important component in the long-term health of the population. Affordable, decent, and suitable housing linked with services can help delay institutionalization, prevent accidents, increase independence, and make caregiving easier. Housing, however, has traditionally been designed for independent people; it has not been well suited to meeting the changing needs of frail older people or those with disabilities.

Faced with increasing numbers of frail older people and people with disabilities, new strategies and approaches have been developed to increase housing options, including home modifications, linkage of housing and services, and various forms of supportive housing. However, aging in place for many Americans still means living in substandard housing with inadequate supportive features or moving to more institutional settings such as nursing homes. Few affordable residential options exist other than remaining at home or living in a nursing home. Service provision to residents of government housing is still patchy, in part because of the indeterminate funding for the services and service coordination. Options such as assisted living seem to be meeting an emerging need, but a comprehensive approach that makes housing an integral part of long-term care policy is still lacking. Meeting the needs of frail older people and people with physical or mental disabilities for residential care requires a broad-based, comprehensive strategy.

Continuing the Development of Supportive Housing

The 20,000 federally assisted housing complexes for older adults remain one of the best resources for meeting the needs of low-income frail older people in residential settings. Over the past decade several national demonstrations and hundreds of state and local initiatives have experimented with adding services to such complexes. In fiscal year 2003, HUD authorized $683 million to Section 202 housing production, an increase of $4 million over the previous year. Further progress would be accelerated by physically retrofitting complexes, developing new strategies to deliver health and mental health services to residents (e.g., using HMOs, SHMOs, or PACE), and extending the concept to private multiunit apartment complexes and even neighborhoods, referred to as naturally occurring retirement communities (NORCs), that were never planned for seniors but have evolved into large concentrations of older people.

Expanding Assisted Living Options for Low-Income Frail Older People

Assisted living facilities are needed for people who require more supervision, services, and supportive environments than can efficiently be provided in government-assisted housing or in their own homes. This type of housing is capable of serving people with early to middle stages of Alzheimer's disease who may otherwise be relegated to nursing homes (Kane & Wilson, 1993). Because of its health component, AL provides opportunities for hospitals and other health/long-term care providers both to develop such housing and to play a role in service delivery.

To achieve its potential as an alternative to traditional nursing homes, AL will require new methods of financing buildings and services in ways that ensure its availability and affordability to low-income people. There are developments indicating that this goal is attainable. The state of Oregon, an innovator in this area, has made AL affordable by obtaining a Medicaid waiver that authorizes AL as an allowable service. Some long-term care insurance policies also cover AL. HUD's budget for fiscal year 2000 authorized the use of Section 8 vouchers to pay for the housing portion of AL costs, making AL an option for more low-income seniors. Thus, financing models are being tried.

Nevertheless, challenges still remain. HUD's fiscal-year 2003 budget had a $20 million decrease in the amount of funding from the previous year to fund the conversion of existing Section 202 facilities to assisted living. In addition, a continuing debate concerns how to ensure that AL remains a residential rather than medical model while at the same time protecting the safety and well-being of its residents. State licensing requirements vary. Some, in an effort to protect residents, make it illegal for the housing facility to provide the very support services required for residents to remain independent.

Promoting Visitability and Universal Design

Concepts of visitability and universal design support a school of thought that newly constructed homes should contain supportive features that benefit not only older adults, but also persons with disabilities of all ages. Many local ordinances and state laws exist that mandate visitability in housing financed with public funds, as well as nonsubsidized housing. Victories for advocates have also taken the form of voluntary programs and incentives. The voluntary approach involves consumer awareness and education on visitability. Certain localities have created builder incentives in the form of subsidies or the waiving of municipal fees.

The visitability movement is gaining momentum. As of 2003, at least 30 cities, counties, and states are promoting visitability through voluntary programs, incentives, or mandates. At the national level, a federal visitability bill, the National Inclusive Home Design Act, was introduced in October 2002. The bill would require all newly constructed single-family homes built with federal funds to meet three require-

ments: a zero-step entrance into the home, wide interior doors on the main level, and a wheelchair-accessible bathroom. Advocates view visitability as a "foot in the door" to more fully accessible, universally designed homes in the future.

Unbundling Services from Housing

Strategies such as developing supportive housing and assisted living are based on providing assistance to people with disabilities living in particular settings. However, a bona fide community-based approach to long-term care would unbundle housing and services (Pynoos, 1994; Pynoos & Liebig, 1995). Portable services would provide a broader set of choices of where to live. Though limits might still exist concerning the extent to which services could be efficiently delivered to all settings, the choice of residence would be based more on preferences for sociability, activities, and other lifestyle considerations rather than simply the need for care. For the unbundling concept to move from theory to reality, personal care, adult day services, chore, homemaker services, and transportation must be widely available. In addition, the housing must be accessible, contain supportive features, and be affordable.

Some countries, such as Denmark and Sweden, have moved relatively far in developing such a system based on entitlements to both long-term care services and housing (Gottschalk, 1995). Long-term care reform that provides more extensive service in the community would go a long way toward providing residential choices for older people and those with disabilities. Its effectiveness would also require housing assistance so that low-income people could afford to live in appropriate settings. HUD's recent efforts to allow and fund on-site service coordinators are a step in this direction.

Integrating Housing and Health

Interentity management exists in most multilevel facilities. However, most housing facilities remain separate from health care or other community-based services. Even in large health care corporations that own housing units, housing is typically in its own corporation, with little integration with other external services.

Paying Greater Attention to Environmental Context

Understanding the needs of an older person requires the examination of more than just the individual; attention must be paid to the wider environmental settings in which the person lives. Supportive features and services in the home can reduce the demand of the environment and support aging in place. The Americans with Disabilities Act of 1990 brought attention to accessibility in the broader community. Stemming from this legislation, the creation of elder-friendly communities has received increasing attention across the nation. Such communities consider matters such as the location of stores, churches, or parks; the adequacy of sidewalks; and the legibility of signage as important determinants to maintaining independence. The goal is to help older adults remain mobile and connected to the community. Future planning and policy initiatives must recognize environmental context as key to healthy aging communities.

ADMINISTRATIVE CHALLENGES

Administrators of residential settings face a host of management challenges, some of which are common across settings and some of which vary according to the type of housing. Common themes requiring managers' attention include:

- *Marketing.* All types of supportive housing and support provided in independent housing require intense marketing. Changing an existing residence or moving to a new residence is hard for anyone, and particularly for those who have problems with functioning. Moreover, the population of supportive housing tends to roll over due to the frailty of the residents, so finding new residents is an ongoing process. Housing managers must constantly work at advertising and promoting their facilities and coaching individuals and their families in making decisions.

- *Matching services with need.* Aligning the support services and physical design of a residence with a person's needs requires careful orchestration. Services must be matched with the individual's need, moderated by the desire to promote independence; financial ability is yet another factor. Initial assessment and ongoing monitoring are essential to ensure that the services continue to be appropriate for residents.

- *Funding services.* As with other services of the continuum, housing and related services may be funded by multiple streams, both private and public. In many instances, the housing manager does not even have direct access to or authority over these funds. The manager must keep current with the funding streams available and know how and when to access them.

- *Balancing housing with health care.* For many residential complexes, the balance between being a provider of housing and a provider of health care must be maintained. Residential settings that provide too much health care run the risk of being regulated and licensed as health care providers; settings that do not provide enough support face the operational dilemmas of resident dissatisfaction and rapid turnover.

CONCLUSION

Housing plays a disproportionately vital role in the lives of older adults and those with disabilities, because of the amount of time they spend in their homes and their desire to age in place. As the needs and capabilities of an older adult or someone with a disability change, a supportive home environment becomes increasingly important. A range of housing options is important to allow these people and their families to exercise choice as to their living arrangements. The old paradigm of senior housing suggested that as abilities declined, a person would move along a continuum toward increasingly supportive housing options, ending ultimately in institutionalization. A paradigm shift emphasizes the flexibility of conventional housing. Residential settings can be modified and services arranged to facilitate aging in place.

In the future, increasing the supply of affordable housing options will provide a greater range of options for low-income persons. Innovative approaches such as the unbundling of housing and services, visitability, universal design, and elder-friendly communities will stimulate new thinking about housing for older adults and those with disabilities. These housing models emphasize independence and choice. Ideally, the future should bring a wide range of housing options to enable persons to choose an appropriate setting that supports and maximizes their functioning and well-being.

CLIENT EXAMPLE

Golden Health is a multilevel senior housing complex owned and operated by a religious order that also owns a large health care system. Each service is a separate legal entity with its own board, administrators, and staff. The housing includes a privately owned townhouse, a congregate living complex, an assisted living unit, and a skilled nursing unit. An on-site clinic is run by the medical group affiliated with the hospital. All residents are automatically enrolled in the hospital's senior membership program. This gives residents preadmission enrollment to the hospital, access to the physical referral service, and other benefits.

The system's Medicare-certified home health agency attends residents of Golden Health. A private home health agency, also owned by the health care system, has a branch office in the Golden Health complex. When residents need durable medical equipment (DME), they can obtain it from the health care system's DME company at a discount. The skilled nursing unit of the housing complex is Medicare-certified. It accepts overflow from the hos-

pital. An active outpatient rehabilitation program is operated at the housing complex by the physical therapy department of the hospital and serves both residents and the community. An adult day services center operates on the ground floor of the assisted living unit.

The housing complex is also tied in with other community providers. Catholic Charities draws on residents to volunteer for its programs, as does the local Retired Senior Volunteers Program. The dietary department of the housing unit has a contract with the local Area Agency on Aging to prepare meals daily for Meals on Wheels. Residents work with nonresident volunteers to package the meals. The housing complex also obtains an allocation of taxi vouchers each month to have available for its residents who need transportation to medical appointments, stores, and other places.

The only formal arrangements the housing complex has with the hospital or other agencies are contracts. However, the staff actively participate in the local aging network, serve on committees with staff from the health care system and the community, and collaborate on specific projects. As a result of extensive informal involvement, the staff of the housing complex are generally able to help residents get assistance and advice from experts in the community that the residents might not access on their own.

WHERE TO GO FOR FURTHER INFORMATION

Administration on Aging (AoA)
Office of State and Community Programs
Wilbur J. Cohen Federal Building
330 Independence Avenue, SW
Washington, DC 20201
(202) 619-0724
Fax: (202) 357-3560
http://www.aoa.dhhs.gov

American Association of Homes and Services for the Aging (AAHSA)
2519 Connecticut Avenue, NW
Washington, DC 20008

(202) 783-2242
Fax: (202) 783-2255
http://www.aahsa.org

American Association of Service Coordinators
919 Old Henderson Road
Columbus, OH 43220
(614) 324-5958
Fax: (614) 324-5954
http://www.servicecoordinator.org

Assisted Living Federation of America (ALFA)
11200 Waples Mill Road, Suite 150
Fairfax, VA 22030
(703) 691-8100
Fax: (703) 691-8106
http://www.alfa.org

The Center for Universal Design
North Carolina State University
School of Design
P.O. Box 8613
Raleigh, NC 27695-8613
(919) 515-3082
Fax: (919) 515-7330
http://www.design.ncsu.edu/cud

National Association of Housing and
Redevelopment Officials (NAHRO)
630 Eye Street, NW
Washington, DC 20001
(202) 289-3500
Fax: (202) 289-8181
http://www.nahro.org

National Association of State Units on Aging
(NASUA)
1225 I Street, NW, Suite 725
Washington, DC 20005
(202) 898-2578
Fax: (202) 898-2583
http://www.nasua.org

National Resource Center on Supportive Housing
and Home Modification
Andrus Gerontology Center
University of Southern California
Los Angeles, CA 90089-0191

(213) 740-1364
Fax: (213) 740-7069
http://www.homemods.org

United States Department of Housing and Urban
Development (HUD)
451 Seventh Street, SW, Room 6116
Washington, DC 20410
(202) 708-1112
http://www.hud.gov

FACTS REVIEW

1. Why is housing an important component of the continuum of care?
2. Define the "continuum of housing." How has this definition changed?
3. List three supportive housing options. Specify how they are similar and different.
4. What role does HUD play in providing housing and services to older adults and those with disabilities?
5. What are sources of financing for supportive housing and home modification?

REFERENCES

AARP (2000). *Fixing to stay: A national survey of housing and home modification issues.* Washington, DC: AARP.

Assisted Living Federation of America (2001). *The assisted living industry, 2001: An overview.* Fairfax, VA: Author.

Assisted Living Workgroup (2003). *Assuring quality in assisted living: Guidelines for federal and state policy, state regulation, and operations.* Washington, DC: Assisted Living Workgroup.

Clark, R. F., Turek-Brezina, J., Chu, C. W., & Hawes, C. (1994). *Licensed board and care homes: Preliminary findings from the 1991 National Health Provider Inventory.* Washington, DC: U.S. Department of Health and Human Services.

Feder, J., Scanlon, W., & Howard, J. (1992). Supportive services in senior housing: Preliminary evidence of feasibility and impact. *Generations, 16*(2), 61–63.

Feldman, P. H., Latimer, E., & Davidson, H. (1996).

Medicaid-funded home care for the frail elderly and disabled: Evaluating the cost savings and outcomes of a service delivery reform. *Health Services Research, 31*(4), 489–508.

Goodman, C. C., Pynoos, J., & Stevenson, L. M. (1988). Board and care castaways: Older adults outside the long term care continuum. *Social Work in Health Care, 13,* 65–79.

Gottschalk, G. (1995). Housing and supportive services for frail elders in Denmark. In J. Pynoos & P. Liebig (Eds.), *Housing frail elders: International policies, perspectives and prospects.* Baltimore, MD: Johns Hopkins University Press.

Joint Center for Housing Studies. (2003). *The state of the nation's housing.* Cambridge, MA: Joint Center for Housing Studies of Harvard University.

Kane, R. A., & Wilson, K. B. (1993). *Assisted living in the United States: A new paradigm for residential care for frail older persons?* Washington, DC: American Association of Retired Persons.

Kendig, H., & Pynoos, J. (1996). Housing. In James Birren (Ed.), *The Encyclopedia of Gerontology* (pp. 703–713). San Diego, CA: Academic Press.

KRA Corporation. (1996). *Evaluation of the service coordinator program.* Washington, DC: U.S. Department of Housing and Urban Development.

LaPlante, M. P., Hendershot, G. E., & Moss, A. J. (1997). The prevalence of need for assistive technology devices and home accessibility features. *Technology and Disability 6,* 17–28.

Lanspery, S. (1992). Supportive services in senior housing: New partnerships between housing sponsors and residents. *Generations, 16*(2), 57–60.

MetLife Mature Market Institute (2002). *MetLife survey of assisted living costs 2002.* Westport, CT: Author.

Mann, W., Ottenbacher, K., Fraas, L., Tomita, M., & Granger, C. (1999). Effectiveness of assistive technology and environmental interventions in maintaining independence and reducing home care costs for the frail elderly. *Archives of Family Medicine, 8,* 210–217.

Naifeh, M. L. (1993). *Housing of the elderly: 1991* (Current Housing Reports, Series H123/93-1). Washington, DC: U.S. Government Printing Office.

Newman, S. J. (2003). Living conditions of elderly Americans. *The Gerontologist, 43*(1), 99–109.

Newman, S. J. (1985). Housing and long-term care: The suitability of the elderly's housing to the provision of in-home services. *The Gerontologist, 25*(1), 35–40.

Newman, S. J., Rice, M., & Struyk, R. (1990). Overwhelming odds: Caregiving and the risk of institutionalization. *Journal of Gerontology: Social Sciences, 45*(5), S173–S183.

Phillips, C., Lux, L., Wildfire, J., Greene, A., Hawes, C., Dunteman, G., Iannacchione, V., Mor, V., Green, R., & Spore, D. (1995). *Report on the effects of regulation on quality of care: Analysis of the effect of regulation on the quality of care in board and care homes.* Washington, DC: U.S. Department of Health and Human Services.

Pynoos, J. (1994). Housing policy for the elderly: Problems, problems and politics. In P. Kim (Ed.), *Service to the aging and aged: Public policies and programs* (pp. 93–115). New York: Garland.

Pynoos, J. (1993). Towards a national policy on home modification. *Technology and Disability, 2*(4), 1–8.

Pynoos, J. (1992). Linking federally assisted housing with services for frail older people. *Journal of Aging and Social Policy, 4*(3&4), 157–177.

Pynoos, J., & Golant, S. (1995). Housing and living arrangements for the elderly. In R. H. Binstock & L. K. George (Eds.), *Handbook of aging and the social sciences* (pp. 303–324). San Diego, CA: Academic Press.

Pynoos, J., & Liebig, P. (1995). Housing policy for frail elders: Trends and implications for long term care. In J. Pynoos & P. Liebig (Eds.), *Housing frail elders: International policies, perspectives, and prospects* (pp. 3–16). Baltimore, MD: The Johns Hopkins University Press.

Redfoot, D. L., & Sloan, K. S. (1991). Realities of political decision-making on congregate housing. In L. W. Kaye & A. Monk (Eds.), *Congregate housing for the elderly: Theoretical, policy, and programmatic perspectives* (pp. 99–110). Binghamton, NY: The Haworth Press.

Regnier, V., & Pynoos, J. (1992). Environmental interventions for cognitively impaired older persons. In J. E. Birren, R. B. Sloane, & E. Cohen (Eds.), *Handbook of mental health and aging* (pp. 763–792). New York: Academic Press.

Sanders, J. (1997). *Continuing care retirement communities: A background and summary of current issues.* Washington, DC: U.S. Department of Health and Human Services, Office of Disability, Aging and Long-Term Care Policy.

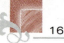
Shekelle, P., Maglione, M., Chang, J., Mojica, W., Morton, S. C., Wu, S. Y., & Rubenstein, L. Z. (2002). *Falls prevention interventions in the Medicare population.* Baltimore, MD: RAND-HCFA Evidence Report Monograph, HCFA Publication #HCFA-500-98-0281.

Sirrocco, A. (1994). *Nursing homes and board and care homes* (Advance Data Number 244). Hyattsville, MD: National Center for Health Statistics.

CHAPTER 10

Wellness

Marcia Ory, Amber Schickedanz, and Roberta M. Suber

Health promotion, disease prevention, and chronic care management are critical aspects of the continuum of care for people of all ages. Recent findings debunking myths of inevitable sickness and disability in later life highlight the importance of these concepts across the full life-course. Whether referred to as *health promotion, disease prevention, chronic care, disability management,* or *total health management,* or in lay terms, such as *self-care* or *self-management,* these concepts have the common goal of maximizing the health and functioning of the individual, and all reflect a wellness or prevention orientation and perspective (Haber, 2003).

Disease and disability are not requisite consequences of aging. Problems can be postponed or prevented through a variety of preventive services, including screening tests, counseling, immunizations, and chemoprevention, as well as broader behavioral, community, and environmental interventions. Prevention activities are the essence of formal wellness programs, but are also relevant to all the service categories delineated in the continuum

of care construct (as well as the underlying health and illness continuum).

Wellness programs may operate in home, community, business, and medical care settings. Whereas prevention activities were once seen as outside of narrowly focused, disease-oriented health services, there is now greater appreciation of the integration of prevention activities into mainstream health and social services. There is also awareness that such activities may be initiated by either clients or professionals, or represent a collaborative effort. Moreover, multiple influences on health and health behavior are now recognized, with greater attention to the influence of underlying social structures and environments on individual's health, and the need for different intervention approaches.

The management of chronic care is taking on new importance in the increasingly cost-conscious health care delivery system. After more than 30 years of nascent public efforts to link prevention with health and health care outcomes, there is finally increased consciousness of the role of prevention

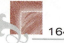

in minimizing diseases, disabilities, and injuries. Concepts such as disease management and chronic care models are attracting attention from all sectors of the continuum of care: providers, payers, regulators, and accreditation agencies (Bodenheimer, 1999; U.S. Subcommittee on Health, 2003). Coordination of care across the services and providers of the continuum is an essential link in the continuum of care. Increasingly collaborating with health care professionals or social service practitioners, individuals assume the major responsibility for coordinating their own care, while the formal system establishes a structure to enable them to do so.

This chapter highlights the salience of chronic disease and disability in older adults' lives, identifies major public initiatives for health promotion, and evaluates the success of the Healthy People 2000/2010 campaign; defines different levels of prevention and illustrates activities appropriate at each level; and outlines the potentials of prevention and challenges of chronic disease care. Practical suggestions for identifying and assessing chronic illnesses are offered. Key elements of intervention strategies, such as clinical protocols, disease management, self-management, and chronic care models, are discussed. The chapter ends with a case presentation of a chronically ill person as an illustration of how the health care system might handle a person with complex medical and social needs.

CHRONIC DISEASE, DISABILITY, AND AGING

Wellness perspectives include goals used to prevent chronic disease and disability, to delay functional decline, and to avoid adverse medical events and their associated costs (Suber, 1999). There is renewed emphasis on health promotion, preventive medicine and healthy lifestyles, screening and monitoring to ensure that individuals needing health care are identified and receive appropriate services, and proactive management of acute and chronic care across the multiple providers and sites of the continuum of care. Despite the blurring of chronic

Table 10.1 Profile of Chronic Disease and Disability

- People are living longer with more chronic diseases and disabilities than ever before
- Almost 100 million Americans live with chronic illness
- 40 million Americans are limited in their daily activities by chronic conditions, with 25 million Americans being severely disabled
- The cost for people with chronic diseases accounts for more than 75 percent of the nation's medical care costs
- The burden of chronic diseases is higher in minority populations
- Most of the available chronic care is fragmented, inappropriate, and difficult to obtain
- Chronic conditions do not always get worse; the health status of a person with a chronic condition can improve, deteriorate, or shift in either direction
- The goal of chronic care is not to cure; rather, it should be to help individuals maintain independence and a high level of functioning

SOURCE: Institute for Health and Aging, 1996; NCCDPHP, 2003a.

and acute diseases with chronic diseases having acute flare-up phases, *chronic disease* is defined as "illnesses that are prolonged, do not resolve spontaneously, and are rarely cured completely" (National Center for Chronic Disease Prevention and Health Promotion [NCCDPHP], 1999). As indicated in Table 10.1, the public health burdens of chronic diseases are well documented, with chronic diseases accounting for approximately 70 percent of all U.S. deaths and approximately 75 percent of health care costs annually.

Chronic diseases encompass a wide array of conditions, affect people of all ages, and are especially prevalent in old age, as shown by Figure 10.1. While approximately 80 percent of older adults are estimated to have at least one chronic disease, recent studies emphasize that co-morbidities, or multiple diseases, are increasingly common in old age, with certain diseases clustering, such as heart disease

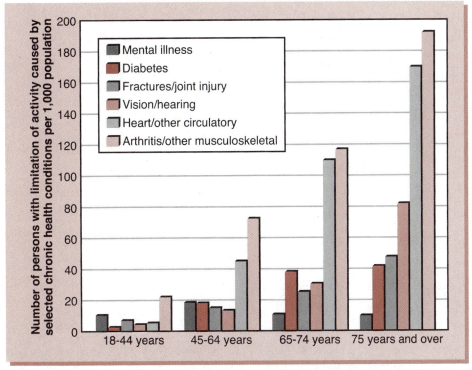

NOTES: Data are for the civilian noninstitutionalized population. Persons may report more than one chronic health condition as the cause of their activity limitation. Selected chronic health conditions include the three leading causes of activity limitation among adults in each age category.

Figure 10.1 Selected Chronic Health Conditions Causing Limitation of Activity among Adults by Age: United States, 1998–2000

SOURCE: National Center for Health Statistics [NCHS], 2002.

and diabetes (CCDPHP, 2003a; Wolff, Starfield, & Anderson, 2002). Although there is wide variability in the severity of chronic conditions, the presence of chronic disabling conditions is a major cause of severe limitation in daily activity for more than one of every 10 Americans, or 25 million people (CCDPHP, 1999).

In turn, functional limitations and disabilities are major drivers for health care and personal services. As historically defined by Nagi (1965), *disability* is a gap between an individual's capability and the demands of the social and physical environment. In recent years, investigators have refined this view by

developing a disablement model that delineates the processes involved in the movement from disease pathophysiology to impairment to functional limitation to disability (see Figure 10.2) (Verbrugge & Jette, 1994; Hazuda, Gerety, Lee, Mulrow, & Lichtenstein, 2002; Jette & Badley, 2000).

This model describes an unfolding of the disablement processes over time, illustrating the social and behavioral influences on the disablement process. It also provides a guide to points for intervention. Prevention activities at any point in the process can delay or reverse the forward movement. For example, the movement from functional limitation

EXTRAINDIVIDUAL FACTORS

Medical Care and Rehabilitation
(surgery, physical therapy, speech therapy, counseling, health education, job retraining, etc.)

Medications and Other Therapeutic Regimens
(drugs, recreational therapy/aquatic exercise, biofeedback/meditation, rest/energy conservation, etc.)

External Supports
(personal assistance, special equipment and devices, standby assistance/supervision, day care, respite care, meals-on-wheels, etc.)

Built, Physical, and Social Environments
(structural modifications at job/home, access to buildings and to public transportation, improvement of air quality, reduction of noise and glare, health insurance and access to medical care, laws and regulations, employment discrimination, etc.)

THE MAIN PATHWAY

Pathology ⟶ **Impairments** ⟶ **Functional Limitations** ⟶ **Disability**

Pathology
(diagnoses of disease, injury, congenital/developmental condition)

Impairments
(dysfunction and structural abnormalities in specific body systems: musculoskeletal, cardiovascular, neurological, etc.)

Functional Limitations
(restrictions in basic physical and mental actions: ambulate, reach, stoop, climb stairs, produce intelligible speech, standard print, etc.)

Disability
(difficulty doing activities of daily life: job, household management, personal care, hobbies, active recreation, clubs, socializing with friends and kin, child care, errands, sleep, trips, etc.)

RISK FACTORS
(predisposing characteristics: demographic, social, lifestyle, behavioral, psychological, environmental, biological)

INTRAINDIVIDUAL FACTORS

Lifestyle and Behavior Changes
(overt changes to alter disease activity and impact)

Psychosocial Attributes and Coping
(positive affect, emotional vigor, prayer, locus of control, cognitive adaptation to one's situation, confidant, peer support groups, etc.)

Activity Accommodations
(changes in kinds of activities, procedures for doing them, frequency or length of time doing them)

Figure 10.2　The Disablement Process

SOURCE: Verbrugge & Jette, 1994. Reprinted from Jette & Badley, 2000, with permission from Elsevier.

(e.g., limitations in walking) to disability (e.g., not being able to perform social roles because of impairments) can be slowed by a rehabilitation program emphasizing strength training. Chapter 17 describes disability issues in more detail.

PUBLIC HEALTH INITIATIVES PROMOTING WELLNESS

Several national initiatives begun in the 1980s provide excellent examples of public and private partnerships that have set the stage for renewed attention and resources devoted to promoting preventive health practices. These initiatives include the Healthy People 2000/2010 campaign (U.S. Department of Health and Human Services, 1990; 1999); the U.S. Preventive Services Task Force (U.S. Preventive Services Task Force, 1996) and the related Task Force on Community Preventive Services (Kahn et al., 2002); and the recent HealthierUS Initiative (Bush, 2002).

Healthy People 2000/2010

The Healthy People initiative has been called the "prevention agenda for the nation" (U.S. Department of Health and Human Services, 1990). Healthy People is a national cooperative effort by government, voluntary, and professional organizations to "improve the health of all Americans by establishing health objectives and measuring progress toward those objectives." Its purpose is to promote health and prevent disease through changes in lifestyle and other factors. Building on more than two decades of Healthy People prevention activity at the federal level, Healthy People 2010 set two broad goals: (1) increase quality and years of healthy life, and (2) eliminate health disparities among different segments of the population.

The format was streamlined to make tracking of Healthy People 2010 goals easier. Healthy People 2010 now features 467 science-based objectives, 28 priority focus areas, and 10 Leading Health Indicators, which provide a snapshot of major influ-

Table 10.2   Healthy People 2010—10 Leading Health Indicators

Physical activity
Overweight and obesity
Tobacco use
Substance abuse
Responsible sexual behavior
Mental health
Injury and violence
Environmental quality
Immunization
Access to health care

SOURCE: U.S. Department of Health and Human Services, 2002.

ences on individual, family, and community health (see Table 10.2).

U.S. Preventive Services Task Force

In 1996, the U.S. Preventive Services Task Force, which was first established by the U.S. Public Health Service in 1984, issued the first revision of its widely used guide to effective disease prevention and health promotion. The Task Force rigorously evaluated more than 6,000 studies of some 200 different interventions for more than 70 diseases and conditions. These included 53 screening tests and 11 counseling topics, ranging from preventing tobacco use to the use of aspirin and postmenopausal hormones to prevent disease (U.S. Preventive Services Task Force, 1996).

Using an evidence-based methodology, the Task Force recommended only those preventive services that demonstrate effectiveness in preventing disease, disability, or death (U.S. Preventive Services Task Force, 1996). The Task Force paved the way for the recommended standards to become the accepted standards for clinical practice. The guidelines are promoted by the U.S. Public Health Service's "Put Prevention Into Practice" (PPIP) campaign, which disseminates basic tools and materials to physicians for use in implementing the Task Force recommendations. The recommendations are also the basis for other quality initiatives, such as the Health Plan Employer Data and Information Set (HEDIS) indicators adopted by the National Committee on Quality Assurance and the managed care industry's "report cards" (National Committee on Quality Assurance, 2000).

Under the Center for Practice and Technology Assessment (CPTA), the Agency for Healthcare Research and Quality (AHRQ) is updating assessments and recommendations and addressing new topics, particularly those regarding effectiveness of behavioral counseling in primary care settings for major lifestyle behaviors such as physical activity and nutrition (*http://www.ahrq.gov/clinic/uspstfix.htm*).

Task Force on Community Preventive Services

The Centers for Disease Control and Prevention (CDC) is sponsoring a parallel Task Force (*http://www.thecommunityguide.org*) to conduct systematic reviews of evidence-based practices for population-based interventions appropriate for health care systems and community settings (Kahn et al., 2002). The Guide to Community Preventive Services targets three major areas: (1) changing risk behaviors; (2) reducing diseases, injuries, and impairments; and (3) addressing environmental and ecosystem challenges. Evidence is reviewed and recommendations for community action are offered, if evidence is warranted. For example, in-depth reviews have been conducted on interventions designed to increase physical activity; prevent tobacco use exposure and increase tobacco cessation; increase access to and use of appropriate health care services; and increase effective self-management of chronic diseases and associated risk factors.

HealthierUS

Growing recognition of the importance of personal and social responsibility for health to reduce the staggering health care problems and costs caused by preventable chronic diseases has spurred the President's HealthierUS Initiative. Sponsored by the U.S. Department of Health and Human Services (DHHS) and the Executive Office of the President, this new prevention initiative was established in 2002. Designed to help Americans live longer, better, and healthier lives by focusing on health care rather than disease care, HealthierUS is envisioned as a source of credible, accurate information to help Americans choose to live healthier lives. HealthierUS is the focal point for many governmental preventive efforts and is being implemented through Steps to a HealthierUS. The focus is on reducing the major health burden created by obesity, asthma, diabetes, heart disease, stroke, and cancer. Activities include a national health summit called "Putting Prevention First," evidence-based publications that can help guide community leaders in making prevention a top priority, and "healthy community" grants to support local communities' prevention efforts.

TRACKING PROGRESS OF HEALTH GOALS

To determine the specific priorities and measurement criteria to achieve its goals, the Healthy People 2000 Project enlisted the participation and support of representatives from national, state, and local agencies; academia; research institutions; health organizations; and citizens. In the initiative's midcourse status report, the priority areas showing the greatest progress toward meeting the objectives were heart disease, stroke, cancer, and unintentional injuries. The Healthy People 2000 objectives with the least progress were those related to diabetes and other chronic conditions, physical activity, mental health, and mental disorders. In fact, in more than a quarter of the objectives for these areas, the results were worse than the baseline data.

By the end of the decade, 21 percent of the objectives met the year 2000 targets, with an additional

Table 10.3   Achievements and Challenges in Meeting Healthy People 2010 Objectives

Areas Showing Improvements	Areas Still Needing Improvements
• Receipt of preventive services such as mammograms and Pap tests • Diabetes education • Blood glucose self-monitoring	• Influenza and pneumococcal vaccination of high-risk elders • Physician visits that include diet/nutritional counseling for medical conditions • Obesity in adults • Cigarette smoking • Leisure time activity

SOURCE: NCHS, 2003.

41 percent showing movement toward the targets. Despite positive trends, 15 percent of the objectives showed movement away from the targets; 11 percent showed inconsistent results; and 2 percent revealed no change from the baseline. Final status could not be assessed for 10 percent of the objectives (National Center for Health Statistics [NCHS], 1994).

The final reviews for Healthy People 2000 do show progress in achieving preventive services goals for older adults, especially as related to mammograms, Pap smears, flu shots, and cholesterol screening. There has been less progress in reducing financial barriers to receipt of clinical preventive services. Additionally, the nation has not done well in meeting the goal of integrating health promotion activities into existing senior services, although there has been progress in establishing patient education programs in hospital settings. Although moving in the right direction, substantial disparity by minority status persists, as does a lack of specific and culturally relevant educational materials.

Preliminary reviews from Healthy People 2010 (NCHS, 2003) highlight some achievements and some continuing challenges, especially regarding critical lifestyle behaviors associated with high disease burdens. As indicated in Table 10.3, the success areas reflect, in part, concentrated efforts to improve services and education, as well as the availability of public funding streams.

Table 10.4   Levels of Prevention and Illustrative Activities

Level of Prevention	Example
Primary	Lifestyle behaviors
Secondary	Screenings
Tertiary	Frequent monitoring to prevent complications

THREE LEVELS OF PREVENTION

As indicated in Table 10.4, preventive services are usually divided into three levels: primary prevention, secondary prevention, and tertiary prevention. These may be conceptualized along a continuum ranging from primary prevention for the well population to tertiary prevention for those with diagnosed chronic diseases and impairments or unstable status. All levels of prevention require that health services and health information be accessible to everyone. The three levels have been defined as follows (Schmidt, 1994):

- **Primary prevention** involves those activities undertaken to prevent the occurrence of disease or illness.

- **Secondary prevention** involves the detection of disease while it is asymptomatic (before symptoms appear) for that particular disease or is in an early phase, followed by appropriate intervention.
- **Tertiary prevention** involves activities undertaken to prevent the progression of symptomatic disease in individuals already diagnosed with a disease or illness and to facilitate rehabilitation, if possible.

The implications of successful prevention are profound. The degree to which many diseases and resultant functional impairments can be postponed and even prevented depends on removing the risk factors associated with the accelerated disease process. James Fries predicted that as "more research reports support the value of preventive practices in geriatrics, in areas ranging from nutrition to weight-bearing exercise programs, we may eventually see disability from chronic diseases compressed into the very last years of life" (Fries, Koop, Sokolov, Beadle, & Wright, 1998). In fact, Manton and colleagues have shown that disability rates have actually declined over the past decade, resulting in far fewer disabled adults than initially predicted with the aging of the population (Manton & XiLiang, 2001).

Fries and others have reviewed the outcomes of health programs designed to reduce health risks, and report that "age-adjusted health status has been improving, while life expectancy from advanced ages has been constant" (Fries et al., 1998). This increased "health expectancy" is as important to older adults and persons with chronic conditions as life expectancy, and "depends to a great extent on . . . physical activity, nutritional intake, social support network, access to good medical care, health education, and health services" (Haber, 1994).

Primary Prevention

Primary prevention seeks to prevent health problems from occurring. Strategies range from consumer education campaigns to access to immunizations and physician counseling. The development of vaccinations against potentially disabling conditions or possible death is one of the major medical accomplishments of the twentieth century. The CDC and other public health organizations post immunization schedules for children and adults, and host a National Immunization Awareness Month to raise public consciousness.

Healthy lifestyle habits, such as activity, good nutrition, nonsmoking, and moderate drinking, are basic to primary prevention and require no professional intervention. However, healthy lifestyle habits may have to be reinforced by special programs that encourage and support behavioral change, such as smoking cessation, nutritional or activity counseling, weight reduction, and stress reduction. Early identification and intervention to reduce or eliminate at-risk health behaviors are essential components of prevention activities across the continuum of care.

Secondary Prevention

Secondary prevention strives to identify health problems early and enable those afflicted to undergo curative treatment or to minimize the severity of the illness. The guidelines provided by the U.S. Preventive Services Task Force provide the baseline for clinical screenings today. They outline the type and frequency of clinical screening for 60 potentially preventable diseases and conditions (U.S. Preventive Services Task Force, 1996). Standard health screenings that can detect chronic conditions, such as cardiac disease or diabetes, before other symptoms are apparent include tests for high blood pressure, high cholesterol, and high blood glucose.

Routine health screenings may be an integral part of an individual's annual physical examination or may be conducted for large groups at community health fairs or health centers. Service providers who are tied formally or informally into an organized continuum of care are well positioned to conduct regular health screenings and to provide appropriate follow-up for individuals with adverse test results.

Tertiary Prevention

Tertiary prevention addresses lifestyle behaviors and therapy to keep an illness under control and ameliorate major problems. Tertiary prevention employs many of the same strategies as primary and secondary prevention, but with more specific interventions. For example, guidelines for the management of many chronic conditions require adherence to special diets, weight reduction, and regular monitoring. Complications from influenza for those with chronic conditions can lead to hospitalization or even death. Thus, annual vaccination for influenza is recommended each fall for all adults age 65 and older and for all those with chronic medical conditions, such as cardiovascular or pulmonary disorders, immunodeficiency disorders, and diabetes.

Despite the documented benefit of select preventive measures, substantial disparities exist by socioeconomic status and demographic characteristics, although the gap is narrowing across major ethnic groups for prevention activities such as self-blood glucose monitoring (CHS, 2003). Additionally, providers show significant disparity in implementation. Preventive guidelines for diabetes include recommendations for the frequency of diabetic blood glucose monitoring, annual eye exams for diabetic retinopathy, and regular foot exams to identify potential wound infections. A review of the 1995–1996 Medicare claims data found that blood glucose monitoring varied greatly by geographic region, ranging from a high of 70 percent in Idaho Falls, Idaho, to less than 9 percent in York, Pennsylvania; the rates for annual eye exams for diabetics were as low as 25 percent in some areas of the country (see Table 10.5) (Center for Evaluative Clinical Sciences, 1999).

Variance in compliance with diabetic screening guidelines is also demonstrated when traditional fee-for-service Medicare practice is compared to managed care plans, with Kaiser's Southern California Permanente Medical Group performing best in many areas. Service providers with an organized continuum of care are more apt to have information systems that trigger reminder postcards and ongoing

Table 10.5 Variations in Diabetic Screening

Screen	Percent of Individuals in Compliance at Select Sites	
	High	Low
Blood glucose	70.2%	8.9%
Blood lipid	68.9%	6.8%
Eye exam	66.1%	25.0%

SOURCE: Center for Evaluative Clinical Sciences, 1999.

education of physicians regarding screening requirements. Managed care plans and their contracted medical groups are also under closer scrutiny by government and accreditation organizations, which do not closely scrutinize the care of fee-for-service Medicare providers (Center for Evaluative Clinical Sciences, 1999).

Table 10.6 provides an example of how primary, secondary, and tertiary prevention strategies might be applied in the treatment of an individual at risk for heart disease.

BENEFITS AND CHALLENGES

Steps to a Healthier US documents the power of prevention. A DHHS report (U.S. DHHS, 2003) indicates that improvements in access to quality health care services, emphasis on health behaviors, and public prevention-oriented policies could increase American's healthy lifespan by 5 to 7 additional years and reduce costs associated with chronic diseases and disabilities. For example, 33 percent of all U.S. deaths can be attributed to three modifiable health-damaging behaviors: tobacco use, sedentary behaviors, and poor eating habits. Growing evidence from national studies by health organizations and government agencies demonstrates that the investment in proven preventive services is highly effective in saving both dollars and lives. Examples

Table 10.6   Prevention of Chronic Heart Disease

Prevention Strategies	Primary Prevention	Secondary Prevention	Tertiary Prevention
Screening	Health risk appraisal reveals lifestyle behavior risks: smoking, overweight, physically inactive	Community blood pressure screening shows high blood pressure reading	Call to Nurse Triage Phone Response with symptoms of chest pain. Sent by nurse to hospital emergency room, diagnosed with an acute myocardial infarction (MI)
Assessment	Follow-up medical evaluation: • Family history of heart disease and diabetes • Blood pressure high • Lab reports high cholesterol	Medical evaluation confirms diagnosis of hypertension; sedentary, smokes 2 packs/day, and overweight	High-risk health behaviors: smoking, sedentary, overweight Cardiologist performs full diagnostic workup, following accepted protocol for acute myocardial infarction

Interventions	• Provided education materials regarding health risks
	• Assessed to determine readiness to change health behavior
	• Counseled regarding dietary modifications
	• Advised to begin a moderate exercise program, walk 1 mile 3 times/week, gradually increasing distance and frequency
	• Advised to stop smoking
	• Administered annual flu vaccine
		• Antihypertensive drug prescribed
		• Provided education and counseling regarding dangers of uncontrolled blood pressure
		• Provided with blood pressure monitoring equipment, instructed in use
		• Enrolled in educational series on hypertension; includes dietary management and prescription drug treatment issues
		• Prescribed nicotine patch and enrolled in smoking cessation program
		• Advised to join local YMCA exercise program for older adults
		• Administered annual flu vaccine
			• Medical treatment prescribed for acute myocardial infarction following protocol, including beta blocker prescribed
			• Counseling and education for low-fat diet
			• Prescribed nicotine patch and enrolled in smoking cessation program
			• Cardiac rehabilitation program includes
			  –monitored exercises
			  –relaxation program for stress management
			  –support group to encourage adherence to healthy lifestyle
			• Administered annual flu vaccine

Goals	• Reduce health risk behaviors • Prevent or delay heart disease, stroke, or diabetes	• Reduce health risk behaviors • Prevent or delay heart attack or stroke	• Prevent another heart attack

from the CDC National Center for Chronic Disease Prevention and Health Promotion and Healthy People 2010 (CCDPHP, 2003a,c,d; U.S. DHHS, 2002) include:

- Proven clinical smoking cessation interventions cost from $1,108 to $4,542 for each quality-adjusted year of life saved.
- Cervical cancer screening among low-income elderly women is estimated to save 3.7 years of life and $5,907 for every 100 Pap tests performed.
- Each dollar spent on diabetes outpatient education saves $2 to $3 in hospitalization costs and $8.67 in total health cost (NCCDPHP, 2003).
- Intensified blood pressure control can cut health care costs by $900 (in 2000 U.S. dollars) over the lifetime of a person with Type 2 diabetes. It can also extend life by 6 months.
- In just 5 years, a foot care program can save $900 (in 2000 U.S. dollars) in health care costs for a person with diabetes who has had foot ulcers. Such care prevents amputations.
- For every dollar spent on the Arthritis Self-Help Program, $3.42 was saved in physician visits and hospital costs. Implementing an evidence-based arthritis self-help course among just 10,000 people with arthritis can result in a net savings of more than $2.5 million over 4 years. Every dollar spent on physical activity programs for older adults with hip fractures results in a $4.50 return.
- If 10 percent of adults began a regular walking program, $5.6 billion in heart disease costs could be saved.
- A 10 percent weight loss will reduce an overweight person's lifetime medical costs by $2,200 to $5,300.

Compliance with preventive standards by professionals and clients is steadily improving in many areas. However, there is still a widely held belief that it is "too late" to make a difference in the health status and functioning of older adults (Ory, Hoff-

man, Hawkins, Sanner, & Mockenhaupt, 2003). Many barriers exist to widespread implementation and use of preventive services, not the least of which has been the failure of many insurers to cover primary prevention and "maintenance" therapies. In addition to the professional skepticism and insurance coverage issues, personal and social barriers remain, such as consumers' contrary belief systems, ignorance, lack of transportation, frequent turnover in membership enrollment, and, most frequently, psychological denial. Table 10.7 gives examples of chronic disease management challenges.

Many chronic diseases, if not well managed, result in secondary conditions, which are other diseases or disabilities caused by a preexisting condition (Pope & Tarlow, 1991). Diabetes is a good example of a chronic disease for which preventive measures can greatly reduce the occurrence of complications such as blindness, amputations, and kidney disease. According to the National Center on Chronic Disease Prevention and Health Promotion at the CDC (2003b):

- Annually 12,000 to 24,000 people in this country become blind because of diabetic eye disease. Up to 90 percent of diabetes-related blindness could be prevented with regular eye exams and timely treatment, yet only 60 percent of people with diabetes receive annual dilated eye exams.
- Annually, more than 80,000 people have diabetes-related leg, foot, or toe amputations. Up to 85 percent of these amputations could be prevented with foot care programs that include regular examinations and patient education.
- Annually, approximately 38,000 people with diabetes develop kidney failure. A 50 percent reduction could be achieved through treatment to better control blood pressure and blood glucose levels.

Screening and treatment for mental illness is even more problematic than for physical conditions, and yet early intervention can be highly effective in reducing future costs and human suffering (Kessler

TABLE 10.7   Chronic Disease Management Challenges

- About 61 million Americans (almost one-fourth of the population) live with cardiovascular disease. About 90 percent of middle-aged Americans will develop high blood pressure in their lifetime, and nearly 70 percent of those who have it now do not have it under control. Despite recent advances, Americans, and especially minorities, still experience unacceptably high rates of death and disability from heart disease and stroke. The health care costs of cardiovascular disease will continue to grow as the population ages, with the cost of heart disease and stroke in the United States projected to be $351 billion in 2003, including health care expenditures and lost productivity from death and disability.
- About half of Americans age 65 and older have arthritis or another rheumatic condition. Affecting more than 40 million Americans, arthritis is the leading cause of disability in the United States, limiting some daily activities for more than 7 million people. By 2020, an estimated 60 million Americans, or almost 20 percent of the population, will be affected by arthritis, and nearly 12 million will experience activity limitations.
- More than 17 million Americans have diabetes, and about one-third of them do not know that they have the disease. Diabetes is now the sixth leading cause of death. More than 200,000 people die each year of diabetes-related complications. There has been a dramatic increase in diagnosed diabetes in the last decade, with a 49 percent increase from 1990 to 2000. With obesity on the rise, these dramatic increases are expected to continue.
- Obesity has reached epidemic proportions in America. In the last 10 years, obesity rates have increased by more than 60 percent among adults. Nearly 59 million adults are now obese, with more than 60 percent of adults reported as overweight or obese. This epidemic is not restricted to adults. In the past 20 years, obesity rates have doubled among children and tripled among adolescents. Of children and adolescents aged 6 to 19 years, 15 percent (about 9 million young people) are considered overweight.
- Approximately 4.5 million Americans have Alzheimer's disease. Prevalence increases with age. Ten percent of those age 65 and older have Alzheimer's; 40 to 50 percent of those age 85 and older have the disease. A new prevalence study forecasts a dramatic rise in the numbers of persons who will have Alzheimer's, concomitant with rapid population aging. Approximately 13.2 million older Americans will have Alzheimer's disease by 2050 unless new ways are found to prevent or treat the disease.

SOURCE: Herbert, Scherr, Bienias, Bennett, & Evans, 2003; NCCDPHP, 2003a,b,c,d.

et al., 2001; U.S. Public Health Service Office of the Surgeon General, 1999). Although at least one in five Americans experiences mental illness in a given year, there are many reasons why only a minority seek treatment, such as stigma associated with mental illness, a fragmented mental health care system, and lack of reimbursed care (Bush, 2001). Because mental health is a primary key to overall physical health, closer coordination is needed between mental health care and primary health care. As an example, depression is often present along with other medical disorders such as coronary heart disease and diabetes. The failure to detect and treat depression is critical, because depression can impair self-care and adherence to recommended medical treatments.

IDENTIFYING AND ASSESSING CHRONIC CONDITIONS

To identify and assess individuals with chronic conditions, a variety of techniques are used, ranging from self-reported response on mailed health status or "high-risk" surveys to comprehensive, interdisciplinary clinical evaluation. Health surveys may address general health status or condition-specific issues; they may be as brief as 8 or 10 questions or have more than 100 items. Health dimensions that may be assessed include physical health, functional health status, mental health, social well-being, health beliefs, and lifestyle behaviors. Health surveys may be completed by individuals or a family member, done by mail or in a doctor's office, done by interview over the phone or in person, or completed by a professional as part of a client's exam.

Many health plans and employer groups use the responses to mailed health surveys as an opportunity to promote healthier lifestyles, to identify individuals requiring more immediate medical or case management intervention, and to modify quality improvement processes. Hospitals and medical groups may use high-risk surveys to identify clients appropriate for a more comprehensive geriatric assessment process and for more intensive discharge planning services. Health systems that provide a continuum of care follow these high-risk clients when they return to the community. In total health management, all methods may be used to support primary, secondary, and tertiary prevention strategies. To the greatest extent possible, many health care providers engage the individual in the preventive process.

High-Risk Screening

High-risk screening is used to identify individuals whose health status puts them "at risk" of adverse medical events and high medical costs. High-risk screening methodology may rely on self-reported information from mailed surveys, such as the individuals' perceptions of their own health status, the presence of chronic conditions, use of medical services, functional impairments, age, and gender—all of which are considered risk factors, or predictors, of future health care needs and service utilization (HMO Workgroup on Care Management, 1996). Screening may also be conducted by professional review of information in the client's medical record, or by computerized analysis, using similar high-risk criteria and formulas for predicting possible hospitalization, functional decline, or high medical costs. The identified high-risk individuals require professional follow-up to determine if immediate medical attention or other services are needed, including interdisciplinary team assessment, integrated health management programs, or other tertiary prevention strategies. Table 10.8 delineates characteristics of clients of high-risk screening systems.

TABLE 10.8 High-Risk Screening Systems

- Target individuals with combinations of characteristics found to be associated with physical decline and medical costs, such as:
  – Age 85 or over
  – Lives alone
  – Number of chronic diseases/conditions
  – Needs assistance with activities of daily living (ADLs), such as mobility, bathing, feeding self, toileting
  – Needs assistance with instrumental activities of daily living (IADLs), such as cooking, shopping, cleaning, driving
  – Self-perception of health status
  – Recent changes in health status
  – Utilization of medical services in past year (inpatient admissions, doctor or emergency room visits)
- Provide integrated care management of individuals found to be at-risk:
  – Assessment
  – Care planning and implementation
  – Monitoring and follow-up

Health Risk Appraisals

Health risk appraisal (HRA) tools are used to identify individuals whose life health behaviors are predictive of future disease and death. Based on epidemiologic studies, life insurance tables, and similar sources, lifestyle behaviors such as smoking, exercise, and eating habits can predict the risk of dying within a specified period, such as 10 years (Breslow et al., 1997). Early primary and secondary prevention interventions can be implemented to educate and modify lifestyle behaviors and prevent or delay the onset of a chronic disease.

The Healthy Aging Initiative of the Centers for Medicare and Medicaid Services (CMS) evaluated the potential effectiveness of HRAs and programs using HRAs as a health promotion tool. The Evidence Report (CMS, 2003) concludes that health risk appraisals can have demonstrated benefits on behavior, physiological variables, and general health status. However, to maximize effectiveness,

HRAs should be part of a broader health promotion program that identifies risk factors, offers individualized feedback, and is coupled with at least one health promotion intervention providing information, support, and referrals. The report emphasizes that an HRA questionnaire alone or with one-time feedback is not an effective health promotion strategy.

Interdisciplinary Team Assessment

The interdisciplinary team assessment is a comprehensive evaluation performed by a team of professionals to clarify the complex problems of an at-risk client and to develop a realistic plan for clinical care management. Interdisciplinary assessment teams are integral components of geriatric assessment programs for frail older adults with cognitive and behavioral problems and in physical rehabilitation programs for patients with new or progressing disabilities.

The core team usually consists of a physician, nurse, and social worker who are specially trained in the specific disease or disability area, with other professionals involved as needed, such as a psychiatrist, psychologist, dietitian, pharmacist, physical therapist, occupational therapist, and speech therapist. Assessments may last from a few hours to a full day, when mental status, laboratory, and radiology testing are included. Some programs include a home assessment for clients who are unable to come to an office or who would benefit from a home environmental assessment.

A critical component of the comprehensive assessment is the family-team conference, in which the core team members meet with the client's family to review the assessment results and make their recommendations. A written report of the findings is also sent to the client's primary care physician. A follow-up study of comprehensive geriatric assessment programs found that improvement in the client's health status depended on the team's recommendations being followed later by the client's primary care physician or a clinic specializing in geriatric care and case management (Boult, Boult, Morishita, Smith, & Kane, 1998).

CLINICAL PROTOCOLS AND EXTENDED CARE PATHWAYS

Protocols, guidelines, care maps, and *critical pathways* are various names for similar tools that have been developed for guiding and monitoring the progression of care in acute and ambulatory care settings. Variations in the treatment process alert professionals to review the care for possible problems in the client's response to treatment or process of care. While it is essential that providers maintain the flexibility to exercise professional judgment for individual cases, the protocols nonetheless contribute to efficiencies in chronic care delivery. They also provide valuable data for outcomes evaluation.

The Agency for Healthcare Research and Quality (AHRQ), formerly the Agency for Health Care Policy and Research (AHRQ, 1999), maintains the National Guidelines Clearinghouse, a joint effort of AHRQ, the American Association of Health Plans (AAHP), and the American Medical Association (AMA). This can be accessed on the Web site (*http://www.guideline.gov*). The Clearinghouse contains several hundred guidelines, written and submitted by medical specialty societies, health plans, professional societies and government agencies.

Protocols began with a goal to standardize, optimize, and measure care for acute episodes, particularly hospital stays. Thus, although health screening and education, especially medication management, are an integral part of most protocols, the guidelines seldom address the broader psychosocial and community resource needs that are included in the "extended care pathway." Extended care pathways, with guidelines for continuity of care and smooth transitions between levels of care and treatment settings, improve provider communication and collaboration across provider sites and over time (see Table 10.9) (National Chronic Care Consortium, 1994). Extended care pathways are important tools *for managing care across the client's*

TABLE 10.9   Extended Care Pathways Elements

In addition to the standard clinical assessment and treatment recommendations included in a critical pathway, the extended care pathway for chronic diseases includes additional items, such as:

- Continuing care needs
- Information that is needed when client is transferred to another setting or level of care
- Psychosocial assessment
- Caregiver assessment
- Physical environment
- Psychosocial treatment
- Community support needs
- Prevention and health education

SOURCE: National Chronic Care Consortium, 1994.

lifetime or timespan of the disease itself, and are not limited to short-term episodes of care for specific symptoms.

"Disease management" programs are another approach to care that have the potential to coordinate resources "across the entire health care delivery system and throughout the *life cycle* of a disease rather than discrete medical episodes" (The Boston Consulting Group, 1995, emphasis added). The Disease Management Association of America (*http://www.dmaa.org/*) defines a full-service disease management program as having all of the following six disease management components: (1) population identification processes; (2) evidence-based practice guidelines; (3) collaborative practice models that include physicians and support-service providers; (4) patient self-management education (may include primary prevention, behavior modification programs, and compliance/surveillance); (5) process and outcomes measurement, evaluation, and management; and (6) routine reporting/feedback loop (may include communication with patient, physician, health plan and ancillary providers, and practice profiling). The programs may focus on high-volume diagnostic groups such as asthma, heart disease, low back pain, diabetes, arthritis, and depression; or low-volume, high-cost diagnoses such as HIV, multiple sclerosis, and end-stage renal disease (Faulkner & Gray's Healthcare Information Center, 1999). The best disease management programs identify those having, or who are prone to having, specific chronic diseases and provide education and coordination services to reduce deterioration.

Disease management strategies include patient education regarding early warning signs and symptoms, telemedicine devices to measure clinical indicators, and regular monitoring of data according to programmed algorithms and clinical guidelines. The patient and health care provider collaborate on a structured program of prevention, monitoring, and care. A significant contribution of the more innovative disease management companies has been the use of sophisticated information systems and data warehouses for identifying clients with early signs of chronic disease and for tracking program outcomes. As a result, disease management programs are demonstrating significant cost savings and improvement in health status. The concern is that most disease management programs focus on only one of the client's multiple chronic conditions.

Cost savings from disease management programs and the implementation of protocols have been documented in the acute care settings, with evidence of shorter lengths of stays and reduced readmissions. Disease management programs that follow clients in the community claim that avoidance of hospital admissions and emergency room visits more than justify the costs of the programs themselves (Jungkind & Corish, 1999; "Teams Slash Diabetic Admissions," 1996).

CONSUMER EDUCATION, DEMAND MANAGEMENT AND SELF-MANAGEMENT

Self-care is now seen as an essential part of health care (Ory & DeFriese, 1998). Instead of feeling threatened by patient activism, current trends are to educate and empower individuals to take an active part in maintaining their own health and function. Health education strategies to promote and maintain health and functional status span the continuum of care. For example, primary prevention programs address lifestyle behaviors such as diet and fitness; secondary prevention adds recognition of risk factors and symptoms; tertiary prevention includes treatment and teaching techniques to prevent deterioration, reduce pain, and maximize independence.

A plethora of information for consumers is available from health providers, health plans, health care organizations, libraries, bookstores, health magazines, newspapers, television, and the Internet. The self-management books distributed by health plans and providers are designed to answer basic health care questions that could avoid unnecessary emergency room or physician visits. The popularity of self-help and self-care publications and Internet health sites attests to the enormous magnitude of consumer demand for information and reassurance.

Well-informed consumers use medical services more appropriately and hence save costs (Fries et al., 1998). This evidence has led to a growing number of "demand management" strategies that provide information and services to support client decision-making and self-care. By managing the consumer's demand for medical services, demand management programs claim to reduce inappropriate health care utilization and save costs. The most popular products to come out of this movement are self-management books and the nurse "triage" or nurse advisor telephone services.

The nurse advisor call centers feature specially trained nurses available 24 hours a day to determine the need for self-care or professional care. These services are sponsored by employers, health plans, hospitals, or medical groups. The nurses handle a wide range of medical questions and possible emergencies, with the aid of computerized protocols and decision-directing algorithms.

Because certain conditions require strict adherence to diet, medication, and self-monitoring, sophisticated client education and support services have become common. The introduction of more

> ## INDIVIDUAL EMPOWERMENT TOOLS
>
> **Education/Information**
> Books
> Television
> Internet
> Counselors (peer)
> Hot lines
> Nurse advisor
> Public Health Department
>
> **Support Groups**
> In person
> On-line
>
> **Self-Monitoring Devices**
> Stand-alone
> Monitored by computer protocols
> Connected to health system

effective methods for supporting client acceptance of responsibility for health are the most recent contributions to medical self-management (Kemper, Lorig, & Mettler, 1993). These include the health education and demand management strategies, in combination with the application of research regarding helping people change health behaviors.

Self-management programs go beyond traditional information and recommendations (HRQ, 2002). To be effective, "self-management programs allow participants to make informed choices, to adopt new perspectives and generic skills that can be applied to new problems as they arise, to practice new health behaviors, and to maintain or regain emotional stability" (Lorig, 1996).

Such programs are increasingly evidence-based and draw heavily on the principles of behavior change being tested in multisite intervention studies (Ory, Jordan, & Bazzare, 2002). Concepts gaining more prominence include the importance of tailoring to client preferences, readiness to seek care, and ethnic backgrounds; the need for concrete goal setting, opportunities to develop and practice new skills, and continual monitoring and feedback; support for linkages between self-care, family care, and formal care responses; and attention to the interacting influence of the greater social and physical environment on individual behaviors. For example, the Chronic Disease Self-Management Program, developed and tested by the Stanford University Patient Education Research Center, is based on the finding that increased "self-efficacy" produces positive changes in clients. Self-efficacy is defined by Lorig and others as a person's belief or confidence in his or her ability to accomplish specific behavioral changes. The Chronic Disease Self-Management groups focus on "efficacy-enhancing strategies of skills mastery, modeling, reinterpretation of symptoms, and persuasion" (Lorig, 1996). The groups are not disease-specific and are led by trained lay persons who themselves have a chronic condition. The groups, sponsored by providers, health plans, and public agencies, help participants learn new ways of coping with universal issues of chronic disease, such as pain, fatigue, depression, managing medications, exercise, and diet.

Chronic disease support groups exist for almost every imaginable condition. Often the outgrowth of professionally sponsored group education programs, these groups meet an important need for individuals and their caregivers struggling to cope with physical, mental, and emotional stresses. Traditional support groups may meet regularly in hospitals, churches, and other community setting as well as in individuals' homes.

Self-help or support groups are also prevalent. With the popularity of the Internet, "chat groups" have emerged as yet another form of support and access to information. Although there is concern among professionals that these face-to-face and electronic groups may provide questionable and even erroneous information and "advice," the self-help phenomenon supports a more patient-centered health care delivery model in which the participants become true partners in the management of their disease. Such well-informed and motivated groups have the power to transform the health care delivery system by demanding increased access, choice, and accountability.

SYNTHESIZING CRITICAL ELEMENTS IN CHRONIC CARE MANAGEMENT

Established in 1991, the National Chronic Care Consortium (NCCC) is committed to delivering quality care for persons with chronic conditions. The NCCC identifies four critical elements for meeting this goal: integrated care management, integrated systems management, integrated information systems, and integrated financial systems (NCCC, 1995). The key elements of integrated care management reinforce many critical quality care themes discussed in this chapter: (1) provide person-centered care over the course of the chronic condition; (2) emphasize ongoing disability prevention in multiple settings; (3) integrate a comprehensive but flexible array of services across a variety of settings; (4) target those at high risk for progression, complication, and high costs; and (5) use interdisciplinary care teams and techniques such as extended care pathways to coordinate care over time and across settings.

Our current health care system does not typically provide the kind of integrated preventive care that efficiently and effectively addresses the chronic care needs of an aging society. Too often, as with disease management programs, the focus is narrow rather than comprehensive. One exception is the collaborative approach to quality improvement in chronic illness care spearheaded by Edward Wagner at Group Health Cooperative of Puget Sound as part of a Robert Wood Johnson Initiative Improving Chronic Illness Care (Wagner et al., 2001). Researchers, clinicians, health care program administrators, and policy makers are coming together to document current practices and test new models of care. Extensive clinical research and practice has led this team to visualize a chronic care model that articulates the interaction among six critical areas empirically shown to enhance health care and patient outcomes (see Figure 10.3).

The essence of this model is that it advocates collaborative interaction between an informed, activated patient and a prepared, proactive health care

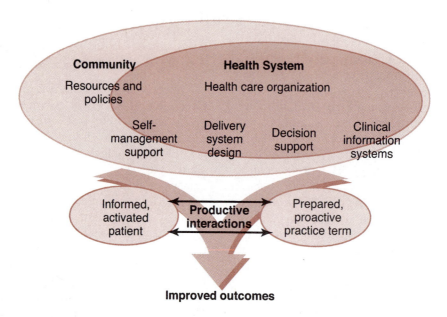

Figure 10.3 Chronic Care Model

SOURCE: Glasgow, Orleans, Wagner, Curry, & Solberg, 2001 (reprinted as Improving chronic illness care, 2003). Available at *http://www.improvingchroniccare.org*

team, and that the interactions occur within a particular health care organization that is influenced by broader social and community factors. The doctor-patient interactions are enhanced by system changes recommended by the chronic care model. Critical elements include a health care organization supportive of quality improvement processes and approaches; systematic assessments and follow-ups through enhanced clinical information systems, ready access to evidence-based treatment guidelines, and other professional information for decision supports; delivery system design that encourages team approaches and other innovative practices to meet the needs of chronically ill patients; self-management supports that aid the patient in goal setting, skill development, and long-term maintenance of recommended actions; and active referral to community resources through enhanced awareness of community linkages and partnerships.

The broad applicability of the chronic care model to prevention activities such as mammogram screening and smoking cessation has also been demonstrated (Glasgow et al., 2001). Some aspects such as linkage to community resources seem especially relevant for practices that must be supported in community settings.

CONCLUSION

The complex needs of individuals with chronic disease require the expertise of a variety of health care professionals, the availability of integrated care delivery systems, and the empowerment of individuals and their families. The system must identify individuals at risk of future disease or deterioration; provide a range of assessment, care management, education, and counseling services; and facilitate communication of essential medical and health behavior information among providers and clients. Clients and their families must be encouraged and empowered to assume responsibility for coordinating and enacting preventive measures at all three levels, to the extent they are capable of doing so.

The present system of fragmented care delivery and failures in information sharing has major health consequences for all persons, but especially for those with complex chronic conditions. Even with rapid advances in information technology, the communication network will remain dependent on the professionals' willingness to prioritize collaborative practice and shared decision making. Health promotion, disease prevention, and chronic care management require new partnerships among providers and between providers and clients to promote health and enhance personal accountability across settings and over time. Similarly, there must be a parallel recognition of the broader determinants of health and context of care. The health care and public sector must play a stronger role in providing a supportive infrastructure and coordinated structures conducive to quality chronic care management.

CLIENT EXAMPLE

Mrs. Gomez is a 55-year-old mother of 4 who immigrated to the United States from Mexico 35 years ago. She has four grown children and three grandchildren. She works full-time. Her husband, who was 10 years older, died recently. The cleaner that Mrs. Gomez works for recently got insurance in a new initiative for small business employers. Mrs. Gomez has signed up for a low-cost managed care plan.

She is sent a questionnaire to fill out and return. It asks about her lifestyle and health status. Mrs. Gomez returns the survey, and two weeks later is contacted by a nurse case manager from the health plan. Mrs. Gomez was identified as being high-risk because she is 20 pounds overweight, is recently widowed, lives alone, and reports experiencing occasional irregular heartbeats. Mrs. Gomez is asked to visit the primary care doctor she selected from the health plan's panel.

Mrs. Gomez's physician confirms that she has mild hypertension. He schedules a mammogram (her first) and Pap smear (she has not had one in five years). He recommends that she lose the 20 pounds and discusses hormone replacement therapy with her. Mrs. Gomez meets with a nurse educator and registered dietitian before she leaves. The dietitian reviews her diet, gives her information in Spanish (which she is more proficient in reading), and invites her to a weight loss support group "dinner" the following week.

The nurse educator talks with Mrs. Gomez about exercise opportunities, makes sure that she plans to fill the prescription for her heart medicine and knows how much to take, and schedules a followup appointment to monitor her progress. The nurse also arranges for a Spanish-speaking group leader to call Mrs. Gomez and invite her to a support group for recent widows.

Mrs. Gomez leaves somewhat overwhelmed with all the new information, but also with a checklist provided by the nurse to help her follow directions. She realizes that she has not been feeling well, particularly since her husband died, and believes that the help offered may renew her physical and mental well-being.

The health plan categorizes Mrs. Gomez as a high-risk enrollee who was clearly lacking preventive measures. The up-front investment of screening and counseling time may save a high-cost hospital admission. The physician, nurse, and dietitian knew they had provided basic, but essential, care to someone in need. They hoped they could encourage Mrs. Gomez to stay motivated to take her medications, participate in the support group, watch her diet, and start exercising. The care team recognizes the importance of continual feedback and monitoring at subsequent visits to provide Mrs. Gomez the long-term support she will need to make lifelong changes in her health behaviors and interactions with the health care setting.

WHERE TO GO FOR FURTHER INFORMATION

Agency for Healthcare Research and Quality (AHRQ)

540 Gaither Road
Rockville, MD 20850
Phone: (301) 427-1364
Fax: (301) 594-2283
http://www.ahrq.gov

American Public Health Association (APHA)
800 I Street, NW
Washington, DC 20001-3710
Phone: (202) 777-2743
Fax: (202) 777-2534
http://www.apha.org

Centers for Disease Control and Prevention
(CDC)
U.S. Department of Health and Human Services
(DHHS)
1600 Clifton Road
Atlanta, GA 30333
(404) 639-3534
http://www.cdc.gov

Healthy People 2010
U.S. Department of Health and Human Services
(DHHS)
200 Independence Avenue, SW
Washington, DC 20201
http://www.healthypeople.gov

National Institute on Aging
Building 31, Room 5C27
31 Center Drive
Bethesda, MD 20892
(301) 496-1752
http://www.nia.nih.gov

Partnership for Prevention
1015 18th Street NW, Suite 200
Washington, DC 20036
(202) 833-0009
http://www.prevent.org

Steps to a HealthierUS
U.S. Department of Health and Human Services
(DHHS)
200 Independence Avenue, SW
Washington, DC 20201
http://www.healthierus.gov/steps

FACTS REVIEW

1. Explain the relationship between aging and chronic diseases and disabilities.
2. Describe at least two governmental initiatives that have set the prevention agenda for the nation.
3. Delineate the three levels of prevention and give examples of prevention interventions for each level.
4. Recommend three primary prevention interventions that should be universally practiced.
5. Describe a method for early identification of individuals at risk of future chronic disease.
6. Describe a disease management program.
7. Identify the six elements in the chronic care model.

REFERENCES

Agency for Health Care Policy and Research. (1999). *National Guideline Clearing House.* Retrieved September 15, 2003 from *http://www.guideline.gov*

Agency for Healthcare Research and Quality. (2002). Retrieved September 18, 2003 from *http://www.ahcpr.gov/*

Bodenheimer, T. (1999). Disease management—Promises and pitfalls. *New England Journal of Medicine, 340*(15), 1202–1205.

The Boston Consulting Group. (1995). *The promise of disease management.* Boston: BCG.

Boult, C., Boult, L., Morishita, L., Smith, S. L., & Kane, R. L. (1998). Outpatient geriatric evaluation and management. *Journal of the American Geriatrics Society, 46*(1), 296–302.

Breslow, L., Beck, J. C., Morgenstern, H., Fielding, J. E., Moore, A. A., Carmel, M., & Higa, J. (1997). Development of a health risk appraisal for the elderly (HRA-E). *American Journal of Health Promotion, 11*(5), 337–343.

Bush, G. W. (2002). *HealthierUS: The President's health and fitness initiative.* Executive Summary retrieved September 3, 2003 from *http://www.whitehouse.gov/infocus/fitness/execsummary.html*

Bush, G.W. (2001). *President's new freedom: Commission on mental health.* Executive Summary retrieved September 3, 2003 from *http:// www.mentalhealthcommission.gov/reports/ FinalReport/FullReport.htm*

Winslow, R. (1999). Medical claims data, 1995–96. *Wall Street Journal,* April 19, 1999, B.1.

Centers for Medicare and Medicaid Studies. (2003). *Evidence report and evidence-based recommendations: Health risk appraisals and Medicare.* Retrieved September 18, 2003 from *http:// cms.hhs.gov/healthyaging/preface2c1.pdf*

Faulkner & Gray's Healthcare Information Center. (1999). *Disease management sourcebook 2000.* New York: Faulkner & Gray's Healthcare Information Center.

Fries, J., Koop, C. E., Sokolov, J., Beadle, C. E., & Wright, D. (1998). Beyond health promotion: Reducing need and demand for medical care. *Health Affairs, 17*(2), 70–84.

Glasgow, R. E., Orleans, C. T., Wagner, E. H., Curry, S. J., & Solberg, L. I. (2001). Does the chronic care model serve also as a template for improving prevention? *The Milbank Quarterly, 79*(4), 579–612.

Haber, D. (2003). *Health promotion and aging.* New York: Springer.

Haber, D. (1994). *Health promotion and aging.* New York: Springer.

Hazuda, H. P., Gerety, M. B., Lee, S., Mulrow, C. D., & Lichtenstein, M. J. (2002). Measuring subclinical disability in older Mexican Americans. *Psychosomatic Medicine, 64,* 520–530.

Herbert, L. E., Scherr, P. A., Bienias, J. L., Bennett, D. A., & Evans, D. A. (2003). Alzheimer disease in the US population. *Archives of Neurology, 60*(8), 1119–1122.

HMO Workgroup on Care Management. (1996). *Identifying high-risk Medicare HMO members: A report from the HMO Workgroup on Care Management.* Washington, D.C.: AAHP Foundation.

Improving Chronic Illness Care. (2003). *Chronic care model.* Retrieved September 18, 2003 from *http://www.improvingchroniccare.org* by selecting "The Chronic Care Model."

Institute for Health and Aging at the University of California, San Francisco. (1996). *Chronic care in America: A 21st century challenge.* Princeton, NJ: The Robert Wood Johnson Foundation.

Jette, A. M., & Badley, E. (2000). Conceptual issues

in the measurement of work disability. In N. Mathiowetz & G. S. Wunderlich (Eds.), *Survey measurement of work disability—Institute of Medicine & National Research Council* (pp. 4–27). Washington, DC: National Academy Press.

Jungkind, K., & Corish, C. (1999). Pilot acute ischemic stoke program saves $9,756 per case. *Hospital Case Management, 7*(5), 87–90.

Kahn, E. B., Ramsey, L. T., Brownson, R. C., Heath, G. W., Howze, E. H., Powell, K. E., Stone, E. J., Rajab, M. W., & Corso, P. (2002). The effectiveness of interventions to increase physical activity: A systematic review. *American Journal of Preventive Medicine, 22*(4S), 73–107.

Kemper, D., Lorig, K., & Mettler, M. (1993). The effectiveness of medical self-care first interventions: A focus on self-initiated responses to symptoms. *Patient Education and Counseling, 21,* 29–39.

Kessler, R. C., Berglund, P. A., Bruce, M. L., Koch, J. R., Laska, E. M., Leaf, P. J., Manderscheid, R.W., Roseheck, R. A., Walters, E. E., & Wang, P. S. (2001). The prevalence and correlates of untreated serious mental illness. *Health Services Research, 36,* 987–1007.

Lorig, K. (1996). Chronic disease self-management: A model for tertiary prevention. *American Behavioral Scientist, 39*(6), 676–683.

Manton, K. G., & XiLiang, G. (2001). Changes in the prevalence of chronic disability in the United States black and nonblack population above age 65 from 1982 to 1999. *Proceedings of the National Academy of Sciences USA, 98,* 6354–6359.

Nagi, S. (1976). An epidemiology of disability among adults in the United States. *Millbank Memorial Fund Quarterly, 54,* 439–467.

National Center for Chronic Disease Prevention and Health Promotion, Centers for Disease Control and Prevention. (2003a). *Chronic disease overview.* Retrieved September 15, 2003 from *http:// www.cdc.gov/nccdphp/overview.htm*

National Center for Chronic Disease Prevention and Health Promotion, Centers for Disease Control and Prevention. (2003b). *Diabetes: A serious public health problem.* Retrieved August 20, 2003 from *http://www.cdc.gov/nccdphp/bb_diabetes/index.htm*

National Center for Chronic Disease Prevention and Health Promotion, Centers for Disease Control and Prevention. (2003c). *Healthy aging: Preventing disease and improving quality of life among older*

Americans. Retrieved September 3, 2003 from *http://www.cdc.gov/nccdphp/aag/aag_aging.htm#3*

National Center for Chronic Disease Prevention and Health Promotion, Centers for Disease Control and Prevention. (2003d). *Preventing obesity and chronic diseases through good nutrition and physical activity*. Retrieved September 15, 2003 from *http://www.cdc.gov/nccdphp/pe_factsheets/pe_pa.htm*

National Center for Chronic Disease Prevention and Health Promotion, Centers for Disease Control and Prevention. (1999). *About chronic disease*. Retrieved September 15, 2003 from *http://www.cdc.gov*

National Center for Health Statistics. (2003). The Healthy People 2010 database. Retrieved September 15, 2003 from *http://wonder.cdc.gov/data2010/ABOUT.HTM*

National Center for Health Statistics. (2002). *National Health Interview Survey: Chartbook on trends in the health of Americans*. Retrieved September 15, 2003 from *http://www.cdc.gov/nchs/data/hus/hus02cht.pdf*

National Center for Health Statistics. (1994, December). Current estimates from the National Health Interview Survey, 1993. *Vital and Health Statistics*, Series 10 (no. 190), Table 62.

Issue brief: The elements of integrated care management. (1995). Bloomington, MN: National Chronic Care Consortium.

Conceptualizing, implementing and evaluating extended care pathways. (1994). Bloomington, MN: National Chronic Care Consortium.

National Committee for Quality Assurance. (2000). Health plan and employee data and information set. Washington, D.C.: NCQA.

Ory, M. G., & DeFriese, G. H. (Eds). (1998). *Self-care in later life*. New York: Springer.

Ory, M. G., Hoffman, M. K., Hawkins, M., Sanner, B., & Mockenhaupt, R. (2003). Challenging aging stereotypes: Strategies for creating a more active society. *American Journal of Preventive Medicine*, *25*(3S2), 164–171.

Ory, M. G., Jordan, P. J., & Bazzarre, T. (2002). The Behavior Change Consortium: Setting the stage for a new century of health behavior-change research. *Health Education Research*, *17*(5), 500–511.

Pope, A. M., & Tarlow, A. R. (1991). *Disability in America: Toward a national agenda for prevention*. Washington, DC: National Academy Press.

Schmidt, R. M. (1994). Preventive healthcare for older adults: Societal and individual services. *Generations*, *18*(1), 3–38.

Suber, R. (1999). Innovative information technology improves care management. *Managed Care & Aging*, *6*(1), 3, 6.

Teams Slash Diabetic Admissions, Emergency Department Visits. (1996). *Disease State Management*, *2*(12), 133–135.

U.S. Department of Health and Human Services. (2003). *Steps to a HealthierUS: A program and policy perspective: The power of prevention*. Retrieved September 20, 2003 from *http://www.healthierus.gov/steps/summit/prevportfolio/Power_Of_Prevention.pdfU.S.*

U.S. Department of Health and Human Services. (2002). *Healthy People 2010*. Retrieved September 20, 2003 from *http://www.healthypeople.gov/LHI/lhiwhat.htm*

U.S. Department of Health and Human Services. (1999). *Healthy People 2010: Fact sheet: Healthy people in healthy communities*. Retrieved September 20, 2003 from *http://www.healthypeople.gov/Publications/HealthCommunities2001/default.htm*

U.S. Department of Health and Human Services. (1990). *Healthy People 2000: National health promotion and disease prevention objectives*. DHHS Publication No. (PHS) 91-50213. Washington, DC: U.S. Department of Health and Human Services.

U.S. Preventive Services Task Force. (1996). *Guide to clinical preventive services* (2d ed.). Baltimore, MD: Williams & Wilkins.

U.S. Public Health Service Office of the Surgeon General. (1999). *Mental health: A report of the Surgeon General*. Rockville, MD: Author.

U.S. Subcommittee on Health. (2003). *Eliminating barriers to chronic care management in medicine* (Serial No. 108-6). Washington, DC: U.S. Government Printing Office.

Verbrugge, L. M., & Jette, A. M. (1994). The disablement process. *Social Science & Medicine*, *38*, 1–14.

Wagner, E. H., Glasgow, R. E., Davis, C., Bonomi, A. E., Provost, L., McCulloch, D., Carver, P., & Sixta, C. (2001). Quality improvement in chronic illness care: A collaborative approach. *The Joint Commission's Journal on Quality Improvement*, *27*(2), 63–80.

Wolff, J. L., Starfield, B., & Anderson, G. (2002). Prevalence, expenditures, and complications of multiple chronic conditions in the elderly. *Archives of Internal Medicine*, *162*, 2269–2276.

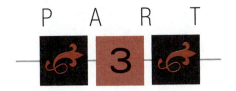

P A R T

3

Integrating Mechanisms

A continuum of care is more than a set of services alone. To function as an efficient *system* of care, the services must be pulled together in daily operations. Four basic integrating mechanisms are essential: interentity management, care coordination/case management, integrated information systems, and financing. Dramatic changes have occurred in each of the integrating mechanisms since the 1990s. Moreover, the integrating mechanisms have emerged as the leading challenge of creating the continuum of care for the twenty-first century. The chapters in this part describe each of the integrating mechanisms and their current stage of development, as well as public policy and ethics—issues that cut across services.

CHAPTER 11

Organization and Management

Thomas G. Rundall and Connie J. Evashwick

The continuum of care, as defined in Chapter 1, is more than a collection of fragmented services; it is an integrated system of care. Organizational integration of long-term care is achieved when multiple services across the continuum of long-term care are linked together through formal relationships. There are four integrating mechanisms that are key to the success of integrated continuum of care delivery systems. As presented in Chapter 1, these integrating mechanisms are

- Interentity organization and management
- Care coordination
- Integrated information systems
- Integrated financing

This chapter discusses the first of these integrating mechanisms: interentity management and organization and structure for the continuum of care. Appropriate structure is a prerequisite for the other three integrating mechanisms to occur. Organizational structure puts in place the processes and management systems that enable care coordination, information systems, and financing systems to operate effectively.

Integration of services offers considerable benefit to an organization (see box). However, integration also requires deliberate management actions and appropriate allocation of resources.

ORGANIZATIONAL ARRANGEMENTS TO ACHIEVE SERVICE INTEGRATION

Integration of long-term care services into a continuum can be achieved through different types of organizational arrangements and led by any of several types of organizations, including health care provider organizations (e.g., health care delivery systems), purchasers (e.g., Medicare or Medicaid), or government agencies (e.g., state departments of health or human services).

BENEFITS TO ORGANIZATIONS OF INTEGRATING SERVICES

- Increased efficiency
- Economies of scale
- Wider distribution of risk
- Greater bargaining power
- Expanded market:
  - Automatic referrals
  - Product appeal to customers
- Improved customer satisfaction
- Enhanced quality and outcomes

Integration at the Health Care Provider Level

Services integration by health care providers can be achieved through a variety of arrangements. The two extremes are informal networks or formal arrangements, with the latter ranging from affiliation agreements and contracts to corporate ownership of a continuum of services.

Networks

Organizational networks are clusters of legally separate organizations that are formed to pursue goals that could not be attained by an individual organization acting alone, such as community-based social and health-related support services that are linked together for clients by a case management program. Organizational networks take numerous forms, ranging from informal to formal, from dyads to networks including dozens of organizations, and from networks in which the member organizations are loosely coupled to vertically integrated networks with centralized policy and operational management structures.

Many transorganizational goals encourage organizations to participate in network arrangements. Valued space, equipment, specialized personnel, or other resources may be shared so that each organization in a service delivery system need not pay the cost of acquiring these resources. Organizations may pool their purchasing of goods and services in order to obtain discounts from suppliers. In some networks, organizations may collaboratively produce a product or service, or they may decide to work together toward some common and mutually agreed-on goal, such as improved coordination, integration, or quality of services provided to clients.

Interorganizational relationships among organizations in a network can be structured by formal instruments, such as contracts or memoranda of understanding, and in some cases the network may be formally organized as a corporation. Alternatively, networks can be based on informal personal ties or the implicit personal commitments made by organizational leaders (Bardach, 1998). In health care markets with substantial managed care penetration, reducing the cost of service delivery and improving organizational financial performance will be important motivations for forming a service network, and such networks will be more likely to have formal contracts and memoranda.

For many years, organizational networks have been created to coordinate services among organizations serving many different client groups, including the mentally ill (Broskowski, 1981; Turner & Tenoor, 1978), the terminally ill (Alter, 1988b), seniors (Alter 1988a), HIV-positive patients (Mor, Fleishman, Allen, & Piette, 1994), and people with physical disabilities (Minnesota Department of Human Services, 2003). Indeed, in most communities there are numerous health and social networks operating simultaneously.

The following example illustrates the types of arrangements and operating procedures found in an organizational network designed to offer comprehensive care to hospice clients.

Long-Term Care Network Example: The Home-Based Hospice Care Network

The Home-Based Hospice Care Services exemplifies the long-term care network. Hospice services are delivered in two counties by a small network of seven medical and social service organizations.

- Hospice Care, a freestanding private organization, does not provide direct medical or nursing care, but rather coordinates the care being delivered by other agencies.
- Visiting Nurse Association (VNA), a nonprofit, public health organization that has a specialized hospice nursing program, provides in-home health care.
- Family Social Services, a private agency, provides social casework services directed at the social needs of the patient and his or her family.
- Voluntary Action Center sends volunteers to the home to provide respite for the family and friendly visiting for the patient.
- Hospital Pastoral Care provides spiritual support and bereavement counseling with the family for up to one year after death.
- National Cancer Society, the local chapter, provides essential medical equipment and supplies on a sliding fee scale.
- Community Hospital provides inpatient medical treatment, when needed, in a specialized hospice unit.

The hospice network is loosely coupled: the financing and delivery of services remain within the purview of each individual organization. The board of directors of Hospice Care consists of representatives of the member organizations and prominent members of the community. They set policy, plan program direction, and work on fundraising activities to maintain the core hospice agency that provides the coordination and integration. Client services provided by agencies in the network are financed through different funding channels: Medicaid, private insurance, governmental subsidies, private contributions, and others. In general, money flows to the agency providing the service and not through the central hospice coordinating agency.

Terminally ill patients typically require periods of intense care in which multiple services of short duration are provided. The hospice network approach matches this service need. Hospice patients are cared for by an interagency team comprised of staff from the seven participating agencies. They meet with the family every week to plan and coordinate services. The urgent nature of hospice care creates a climate in the community that permits the medical and social service providers to come together voluntarily and act in a unified way. Administrators of the seven organizations meet regularly to assess and solve systemic problems, and workers perceive themselves as members of a team.

As suggested by the hospice network example, the structure of any given network depends on the nature of the client's problems, the types of organizations involved, the nature of client flow through the system, the resources available, and the level of trust that organizations have in one another.

Creating a freestanding organization, such as Hospice Care, to provide centralized patient care coordination is not always necessary or desirable. Often, a natural lead agency, such as a regional hospital or nursing home, may play this key role. However, as pressures increase on the network from regulators, payers, or consumers to document quality of care and client outcomes, the creation of formal relationships may become essential. For example, many hospices began as network models, like the one described here. By 2003, 80 percent of hospices were Medicare-certified, implying formal structure and a consolidated organization.

Ownership

An alternative way in which services are integrated over time and across organizations is through ownership by a single "umbrella" organization. More than 60 services have been identified as integral to a complete continuum of care (see Chapter 1) (Evashwick, 1987). In a pluralistic society such as the United States, it is unlikely that any single organization will own all these services. However, as a result of the organizational diversification trend of the 1980s and the integrated delivery systems trend of the 1990s, some large regional health care systems do indeed own many of the major services of the

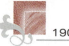

continuum of care through sole ownership, partnership, joint ventures, and other multi-institutional arrangements.

When many services are linked together through ownership, it is easier to instill a common culture supporting important features of long-term care, including disability prevention, maintenance of at-risk individuals in community settings, effective case management, and client self-management of chronic conditions. Management strategies and structures to support the integration of cross-site, multispecialty care programs may be implemented. Moreover, a common information system is feasible (if not yet always in place). This allows providers in all settings to share meaningful information about a client's condition, effectiveness of services provided, and overall cost of care. Case management is common in "owner" services delivery systems, both because the system is likely to benefit from efforts to manage client referrals, and because the system has control over referrals and the client's care experience at the point of service delivery. The use of case management to achieve client and system goals is widely perceived as indicative of a quality long-term care system, and research verifies that small caseloads, specific targeting criteria, and case manager training, authority, and intensity of effort contribute to successful outcomes (see Chapter 12 and Scharlach, Giunta, & Mills-Dick, 2001). These attributes of the ownership strategy create tremendous potential for effective use of the continuum of care.

Most of the services identified in the accompanying box are owned by Sutter Health, but in some communities, the services are provided through a joint venture with another organization, such as the VNA, or by contractual arrangements with local agencies. This system of care makes it possible for Sutter Health to implement care management successfully in support of the philosophy and goals of long-term care. Indeed, the Continuous Care Management Department of the Sutter Sacramento Sierra Region was the inaugural (2003) winner of the Franklin Award of Distinction by the American Case Management Association and the Joint Commission on Accreditation of Healthcare Organi-

SUTTER HEALTH

Sutter Health is a regional system located in Northern California, extending from the San Francisco Bay Area to the foothills of the Sierra Mountains. In 2003, the continuum of care at Sutter Health consisted of more than two dozen acute care hospitals, numerous medical groups and aligned independent practitioner associations, and many outpatient services that support integrated long-term care. Continuum services included:

Adult day services
Advance respiratory care
AIDS center
Allergy clinics
Alzheimer's disease programs
Alzheimer's residential care center
Arthritis and rehabilitation center
Asthma center
Diabetes program
Dialysis centers
Family home companions
Health resource and wellness center
Hearing and speech centers
Home care
Pain management
Physical therapy clinics
Pulmonary rehabilitation program
Rehabilitation centers
Skilled nursing facilities
Transitional living center

zations (American Case Management Association, 2003).

The award recognizes Sutter Health's commitment to a collaborative philosophy and an interdisciplinary process for case management. Sutter Health was judged to excel in providing a case management service that is functionally comprehensive and outcome oriented. The key to Sutter Health's

SELF-ASSESSMENT FOR SYSTEMS INTEGRATION PARAMETERS

1. Governance structures support goal development and improve the ability of individual care providers to work together as a single system.
2. Management strategies and structures support cross-site, interdisciplinary integration efforts.
3. Information technology systems allow providers in all settings to share meaningful information about clients, costs, and operations.
4. Financing systems promote a system-wide management of cumulative costs, tied to care outcomes.
5. The needs of high-risk populations are identified.
6. A full array of effective and efficient services is provided.
7. Care management is focused on disability prevention and organized around defined populations.
8. Seamless care is provided across settings and over time.
9. Clients are involved in care management and self-care activities.

SOURCE: NCCC, 1995.

was a nationwide collaborative of hospitals, large nursing facilities, and health care systems that sought to develop the tools and recognition required to coordinate and fund the continuum of care. Created in 1990, NCCC promoted integrated care until it closed its operation in 2003. NCCC members came to consensus on the organizational elements fundamental to integration of care. The Self-Assessment for Systems Integration (SASI) identifies nine parameters by which organizations can measure their "readiness" to integrate. These parameters, which expand on the four integrating mechanisms, are shown in the accompanying box.

TECHNIQUES FOR ORGANIZATIONAL INTEGRATION

Whether a continuum of care is a network or an ownership model, effort must be dedicated to achieving service delivery in an efficient, cost-effective, high-quality manner. Organizations that have achieved successful integration have developed integrating mechanisms that foster and support coordination of care across the continuum of disease prevention, acute care, and long-term care services. Common management techniques that increase the likelihood

PROVIDERS' MANAGEMENT TECHNIQUES FOR INTEGRATION USED BY PROVIDERS

• Share a vision
• Create management team
• Educate board
• Identify leaders
• Unify marketing
• Centralize purchasing
• Align human resource functions
• Coordinate clinical care
• Establish disease management

success is to link patients with the right care at the right time and place of services, regardless of the payer. The case managers do not make decisions for Sutter patients, but rather give patients the information they need to make informed choices from the array of services available within the Sutter Health system as well as the community (American Case Management Association, 2003).

The National Chronic Care Consortium (NCCC)

of coordination across the continuum of care are outlined in the accompanying box.

Share a Vision

Organizations that have similar visions or that can arrive at consensus on a single, shared vision find that this common ground greatly facilitates collaboration. A shared vision of the ultimate goal of client care keeps many organizations working together in concert despite daily challenges and episodic problems. An initial shared visioning session and a statement of joint purpose is one technique used by organizations that strive to coordinate their services.

Create Management Team

For the continuum to function optimally, administrative support is essential. Establishing an interentity executive management team (and other interentity management teams as appropriate) consisting of the senior managers of the services involved is one way to do this. Within the executive team, the authority of the participants should be comparable. Such a management team might consist of the administrator of the nursing home, the head of the home health agency, the director of patient care services of the hospital, the manager of the senior housing complex, the head of case management for a preferred medical group, and the vice president of community relations of the integrated delivery system. A similar management team might comprise the managers of each of the organizations that have specific responsibilities, such as the person responsible for human relations at each of the organizations involved. The key to such committees is that the members must have official responsibility to make decisions regarding the allocation of resources, including staff.

Educate Board

Board support is also critical. When creating a continuum, boards frequently merge or create overlapping governance structures to ensure broad-based decision making and support for the integrated system. Educating the board(s) about organizational relationships, whether collaborative or ownership, may require special sessions. Boards must also understand and accept new per-formance expectations that reflect collaboration across services.

Unify Marketing

One of the advantages of a continuum is its ability to attract clients and thus capture market share, yet many organizations fail to promote their continuum as a comprehensive, integrated set of services available to clients as highly desirable one-stop shopping. Each service may already have its own promotional material, own logo, own colors, and the like. Giving up a separate identity entirely is difficult for any service or organization and is probably not necessary. Nonetheless, joint marketing of the services constituting the continuum is possible and desirable. Overall, consumers are looking for simplicity in the maze of the health care delivery system. Any organization that promises this (and can deliver) will be well received by consumers, as well as by payers. Thus, those services engaged in the continuum of care should collaborate on joint marketing materials and approaches.

Centralize Purchasing

Each component of the continuum will generate a certain volume of commerce, such as purchases of durable medical equipment, clinical and laboratory supplies, office supplies, and information technology. By centralizing purchasing, the integrated continuum ensures that certain types of purchases, such as computers, communication systems, and the software that run them, are compatible across all component services. Also, bulk purchasing enables the system to purchase supplies at lower prices, thus reducing costs across the entire system. Finally, centralized purchasing enables the system to have flexibility in supplying individual services and to implement management techniques such as "just in time" inventory control, again increasing the efficiency with which services are provided.

Align Human Resource Functions

When organizations work closely, regardless of the organization arrangements, staff will come to expect similar treatment, pay, and benefits. An organization that owns several clinical services may find that industry standards vary across services. For example, job titles may be similar in different services, but the job functions may be quite varied. Similarly, pay scales are much lower for nurses who work in nursing facilities and home care than for those who work in hospitals. Particularly when the units are all owned by the same organization, these differences conflict with employees' expectations of a single set of organizational policies.

The human resources staff can help ensure staff commitment to integration by reviewing and revising job descriptions and titles, examining pay scale and fringe benefit compatibility, and conducting educational programs for all employees about the implications of integrated care for performance evaluations, pay parity, career ladders, and other human resources issues. Differences that cannot be resolved in the short term may be dealt with by a clear explanation of the issues to employees and a plan for long-term resolution.

Coordinate Clinical Care Coordination of clinical care is not likely to happen on an extended basis unless the continuum formally builds it into the structure and operating processes. It is not enough to offer a continuum of care; the care delivered to clients must be coordinated such that the client sees the right provider for the right problem at the right time. Case management is the most common form of coordination. It refers to a method of linking, managing, and coordinating services to meet the varied and changing health needs of clients.

In the context of the continuum of care, case management involves periodically assessing clients' needs; planning a program of further diagnostic services, treatment, and support services; referring clients to appropriate providers; assisting clients in making appointments; following up to ensure that services were provided as planned; and communicating regularly to providers and clients as necessary to ensure that all have current and accurate information regarding the clients' status and service plan. With the growth of managed care, case management of clients with complex long-term care needs has become important not only to coordinate

services but also to control costs. Clearly, coordination of clinical care is at the heart of integrated care systems and is vitally important to the success of the system. Case management is discussed in Chapter 12 in greater detail. Integration of patient information is another critical element that facilitates coordination of care across providers. This is discussed in Chapter 13.

Establish Disease Management The majority of expenditures for acute and long-term care services are for the treatment of individuals with chronic diseases. Management of individuals with chronic disease—often called disease management—is essential to fulfilling the vision of a coordinated continuum of care. Protocols for disease management are being developed and implemented in many health care delivery systems. Disease-management techniques have been developed for people with asthma, diabetes, heart disease, stroke, and depression, among other conditions. Chapter 10 describes disease management in detail.

By carefully tracking the treatment provided to these people, providing disease prevention services information, improving prescription drug compliance and management, developing community-based care and self-care programs, and regularly monitoring the person's health status, improvements can be achieved in clients' health at reduced cost to the system. Sophisticated disease management programs span service settings and thus involve awareness and cooperation of multiple providers, all working together to help the client prevent and/or control illness.

Integration at the Payer Level

Although few private and public models exist in which services are integrated through payer organizations, three are discussed here: the continuing care retirement community (CCRC), the Social Health Maintenance Organization (S/HMO), and the Program for All-Inclusive Care for the Elderly (PACE). Each of these approaches to organizing the continuum of long-term care services is discussed in detail elsewhere in this book (Chapter 9 for CCRCs, Chapters 8 and 14 for PACE, Chapter 14 for S/HMO). This chapter briefly describes these approaches with regard to organizing the continuum.

CCRCs are models of care integrated through private payers. CCRCs offer older people housing, meals, social services, activities, personal care, and nursing care (Medicare, 2003a). CCRCs provide different levels of care based on the residents' needs. Care levels range from independent living apartments to skilled nursing in an affiliated nursing home, with on-campus units often referred to as the "health center." Residents move from one setting to another based on needs, but continue to remain part of the CCRC community. A CCRC typically houses between 400 and 6,500 older residents. Most CCRCs require residents to pay a large entry fee and also a monthly fee. Residents may be required to have Medicare Parts A and B, and some CCRCs also offer or require long-term care insurance. CCRCs may be regulated by the state department of insurance for their fiscal solvency, as their financing structure is based on insurance principles.

Although the range of services offered by CCRCs is limited, the great advantage of these organizations is that they allow residents to obtain services on their residential "campus." Furthermore, the CCRC arranges services and, to some extent, payment for service delivery. CCRCs are a relatively expensive model of integrated long-term care for older people, but those who can afford the entrance and monthly fees are assured access to nursing care, personal care services, meals, building maintenance, housekeeping, and cultural and social activities. Some CCRCs own the necessary space and equipment and hire staff to provide these services directly, whereas others contract for at least some services through outside organizations.

A *S/HMO* is a health plan that provides a comprehensive array of health, medical, and support services for Medicare beneficiaries who voluntarily enroll and pay a premium for the services (Medicare, 2003b). S/HMOs provide the full range of Medicare benefits offered by a standard Medicare HMO, plus additional services, including care coordination, prescription drug benefits, chronic care benefits (covering short-term nursing home care), a full range of home and community-based services, adult day care, respite care, and medical transportation. Although each model operates somewhat differently, medical care is typically available through preferred provider arrangements with physicians and hospitals, and case managers arrange and coordinate the care for those needing long-term care services.

The premiums paid by enrollees supplement capitation payments to the S/HMO from Medicare and Medicaid. These funds are pooled to provide the source of funds with which the S/HMO either delivers or purchases service. S/HMOs require co-payments for certain services. In brief, the S/HMO is an innovative approach to integrating medical and long-term care services, financed through capitation payments, enrollee premiums, and co-payments, with the S/HMO bearing the financial risk for all covered services. Currently, four S/HMOs are participating in Medicare: the S/HMOs associated with Kaiser Permanente, Portland, Oregon; SCAN, Long Beach, California; Elderplan, Brooklyn, New York; and Health Plan of Nevada, Las Vegas, Nevada.

The *Program of All-Inclusive Care for the Elderly (PACE)* is a model of organizing long-term care services that replicates the OnLok Senior Health Services Program in San Francisco (Medicare, 2003c). The distinguishing characteristic of PACE programs is that they serve frail seniors, all of whom must have been approved for nursing home admission. PACE enrollees must be at least 55 years of age, live in the PACE service area, be screened by a team of medical professionals, and sign and agree to the terms of the enrollment agreement. An enrollee's service needs are determined by PACE's interdisciplinary team of care providers.

PACE offers and manages medical, social, and rehabilitative services. The PACE service package must include all Medicare and Medicaid services provided by the respective state's Medicaid program. At a minimum, a PACE organization must provide 16 additional services, including primary medical care, social services, restorative therapies, personal care and supportive services, nutritional counseling, recreational therapy, social work, pharmaceuticals, and nursing facility care. When an enrollee is receiving adult day care services, these services also include meals and transportation. Services are available 24 hours a day, 7 days a week, 365 days a year. Generally, these services are provided in an adult day health center setting, but may also be provided in the client's home and via referral to other providers, such as medical specialists, laboratory and other diagnostic services, and hospital and nursing home care.

PACE provides services using either a consolidated or brokered model of service provision. Each requires different organizational arrangements. In the consolidated model, a multidisciplinary team plans and delivers primary care and most other services, and controls the resulting costs. In the brokered model, case managers purchase services and carefully manage patients' access to and use of services. Care that is delivered by other organizations, such as nursing homes and hospitals, is closely monitored and managed, but PACE has somewhat less control over care and expenditures than under the consolidated model.

PACE assumes financial risk for acute and long-term care services. Hence, the financial viability of PACE depends on its ability to support frail participants in noninstitutional settings. PACE receives a fixed monthly payment per enrollee from Medicare

MANAGEMENT TECHNIQUES FOR INTEGRATION USED BY PAYERS TO SUPPORT THE CONTINUUM OF CARE

- A single intake form
- A single patient identification number
- Case management
- Pooled categorical funding
- Single contracting of services to all clients regardless of source of coverage

and Medicaid. Persons enrolled in PACE also may have to pay a monthly premium, depending on their eligibility for Medicare and Medicaid. Currently, 25 sites are fully operational PACE programs, located in 14 states, and each site has about 200 enrollees.

Payers use a variety of integrating mechanisms to support the continuum of long-term care services. Examples are delineated in the accompanying box. With these integrating mechanisms, clients' access to multiple-provider organizations is enhanced, coordination of care is strengthened, and financial constraints on the use of services are reduced.

Integration at the Government Level

State governments have taken the lead in formulating long-term care policy and developing integrated models of care. In many states, state government controls or influences financing, organization, and delivery of long-term care services. For example, states have administrative authority over home and community-based services authorized under Medicare and the Older Americans Act. They also are responsible for enforcing federal standards governing nursing homes and home health agencies receiving reimbursement from Medicare and Medicaid. States have used their legislative authority to foster long-term care services, including payment to home and community-based long-term care services and have developed case management systems to authorize and control use of community-based services. States have demonstrated the ability to cut the red tape of categorical funding to facilitate movement across service provider lines.

One example of a state-initiated effort to integrate long-term care services is Minnesota Senior Health Options (MSHO), a health care program begun in 1997 for Minnesota seniors, age 65 and older, who are eligible for Medical Assistance and Medicare (Minnesota Department of Human Services, 2003). Enrollment in MSHO is voluntary. A Medicare waiver allows MSHO to be paid a capitated amount for each enrollee. Funds from the state's medical assistance program are also committed to

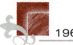

this program, enabling MSHO to contract with health plans to provide services to enrolled members. MSHO combines the health care and support services that normally are offered by separate programs into one seamless package to make it easier for people to obtain these services. MSHO is administered by the Minnesota Department of Human Services, in partnership with three health plans: Medica, Metropolitan Health Plan, and UCare Minnesota. Upon enrollment, the member must choose one of these health plans. The health plan assigns a care coordinator to each enrollee to help with paperwork and gaining access to needed health care and support services.

MSHO provides a wide array of services, including doctor visits, emergency room care, hospitalization, dental care, lab and X-rays, durable medical equipment, prescription drugs, personal care attendant services, home health services, community-based services, nursing home care, transportation, and interpreter services. As of August 2003, MSHO had nearly 5,000 enrollees.

State governments use a variety of integrating mechanisms to support the continuum of long-term care. Examples are shown in the accompanying box. These integrating mechanisms enable clients to access multiple-provider organizations more easily;

increase the coordination of services across the continuum; and reduce financial barriers to the use of services poorly reimbursed, or not reimbursed, by some categorical funding streams.

BARRIERS TO INTEGRATION

Formal policies and internal management mechanisms are required to ensure that continuity of care occurs. Even so, clients' prior experiences, geographic location, physician preferences, and informal relationships all affect what services are used. Even ownership in and of itself does not guarantee coordination of services. Examples are rampant of organizations that acquired or initiated services within their own organization or network, only to find that referrals for these very types of services went outside their system (Evashwick, 1987).

The accompanying box lists typical barriers that must be overcome if integration is to be achieved. These may inhibit integration across different service organizations or across different service units within the same organization. Knowing the challenges, an organization can initiate the appropriate management techniques, as described in the previous section, to overcome barriers and create seamless care from the client's perspective.

Even managed-care systems, such as HMOs and preferred provider organizations, have difficulty integrating diverse services. Although managed care imposes financial incentives to use services within the given preferred provider network, some services may not be included in the networks, and in many instances clients can go outside the preferred provider network if they choose to pay additional charges. Moreover, managed care covers primarily acute and episodic care, and more recently, disease management. Long-term care support services may be paid for by the individual or by an array of government programs. Financing thus remains fragmented.

The geographic location and organizational structure of the systems may also deter coordinated delivery of the continuum of services. Because services may have been added for different reasons and at

---

MANAGEMENT TECHNIQUES FOR INTEGRATION USED BY STATE GOVERNMENTS TO SUPPORT THE CONTINUUM OF CARE

- A common intake form
- Case managers with responsibility to the state program, not to the collaborating agencies
- Team management (program managed by a team of managers from multiple collaborating agencies)
- Pooled categorical funding

BARRIERS TO ORGANIZATIONAL INTEGRATION

- Different service eligibility criteria
- Separate financing streams
- Conflicting regulations
- Differing organizational cultures
- Client and staff loyalties
- Geographic boundaries
- Professional cultures and preferences
- Poor communication patterns
- Inadequate information systems
- Lack of board support
- Absence of leadership
- Incompatible missions and goals
- Imbalance of organizational resources to commit

different times, they may be housed organizationally in separate divisions and at different levels, and reporting relationships may change as the organization restructures—a seemingly endless process engaged in by most large corporations delivering health and medical services.

Often when related businesses are consolidated into one organization, economies of scope are achieved—efficiencies in the management and operations of the separate, but related, units. Economies of scope have been difficult to achieve in health care continuums. For example, many continuums of care have been created by hospitals acquiring physician practices, nursing homes, home health care agencies, assisted living facilities, and other service organizations. The cultures of these organizations vary, as do the societal expectations for their performance. A great deal of detailed knowledge is required to understand the market for each of these services and their respective payment schemes. Each service has different regulations, different payment

systems, different accreditation requirements, and different performance expectations. Managing these different types of health services in a comprehensive continuum of care has proven more difficult than many believed at first.

TRENDS

A complex environment and recent trends have added further barriers to integration.

The Balanced Budget Act of 1997 (BBA) substantially reduced Medicare reimbursements to providers and instituted major changes in how long-term care providers are paid, installing prospective payment systems (PPS) for skilled nursing facilities, Medicare-certified home care agencies, long-term care hospitals, rehabilitation hospitals, and psychiatric hospitals. Each PPS has a different patient assessment instrument and case mix metric for provider payment. The drastic changes caused by the BBA caused a backlash of disintegration, particularly in stimulating major health care delivery systems to divest long-term care services. The combination of reduced Medicare payments and the time and energy required to implement new payment systems caused providers to focus on their core businesses and refrain or withdraw from activities involving other services. For example, nearly one-fourth of Medicare-certified home health agencies were closed, including many owned by hospitals and health systems. Similarly, many hospitals closed subacute units rather than deal with implementing the PPS for skilled nursing facilities.

The Health Insurance Portability and Accountability Act of 1996 (HIPAA) also caused concern about integration. HIPAA, which began to be phased in for providers in 2003, required internal security precautions to protect patient information, placed constraints on the sharing of information among health care providers and health plans, and regulated contractual relationships, all of which have potentially negative effects on integrating services. The regulations and rules established by the Centers for Medicare and Medicaid Services (CMS) attempt to balance the goal of maintaining the privacy of patient information with the need of health care provider organizations to share patient information among clinical providers caring for a patient, other employees, and health plans paying for the care provided. Health care organizations functioning in a formal network of providers—what HIPAA regulations refer to as an *organized health care arrangement (OHCA)*—are explicitly recognized, and sharing of protected medical information among providers in such networks is permitted (CMS, 2003). The health care field has had little time to test the appropriateness and flexibility of HIPAA requirements across many patient circumstances, provider networks, and care settings. However, at this point it does not appear that HIPAA presents any insurmountable barriers to integrating care across providers. Nonetheless, for a period of several years, it inhibited serious attention to integration among some provider and payer organizations.

The backlash to managed care has had both direct and indirect effects on integration. To the extent that managed care plans have championed case management, disease management, and prevention, all funneled through a single payment system, the closure or withdrawal of managed care plans has narrowed access for some consumers to one means of integrating care. The indirect effect of stalled managed-care expansion on integration begs the question of whether managed-care plans, which presumably integrate many services, offer higher quality and/or lower cost than fee-for-service systems.

Measuring quality has become a foremost priority for all components of the health care delivery system. Thus, one of the most important questions to be asked about continuums of care is: Do they produce better client outcomes than the traditional fragmented health care system? This also is the hardest question to answer. Client outcomes are difficult to measure. The state of the art for measuring outcomes or quality is nascent. Even for well-studied services, such as hospital care, or conditions, such as heart problems, for which extensive research has been done, expert consensus on benchmarks and quality measures is weak or lacking. Long-term care is far behind acute care in measuring outcomes.

Outcome measures are altogether lacking for comparisons across systems of care encompassing several services.

A few pilot programs, such as PACE, do have aggregate data on outcomes of integrated systems, but irrefutable data differentiating the contribution of each component of integration (e.g., case management, information systems, pooled financing, managed-care structure) for each subgroup of the population (aged, well versus healthy, functionally disabled, etc.) are not available. Moreover, the challenge of examining and differentiating both long-term and short-term outcomes makes this type of research exceedingly difficult.

In tight financial times, organizations find it difficult to allocate resources to concepts that are not supported by concrete data that project likely results. Thus, the absence of data inhibits the development of integration efforts; yet, without the implementation of integration, it is not possible to accrue the data needed to measure and document outcomes.

CONCLUSION

Models of continuum of care take on a wide range of forms, from loosely affiliated networks to highly centralized ownership. The organizational form of a continuum of care may evolve as the continuum gains experience with its partners and the community and as it confronts new environmental challenges. Adapting to change, and managing the consequences of a turbulent environment, will be central to the future success of continuums of care. Much remains to be learned about creating and maintaining a successful continuum. The organizational arrangements of the ideal continuum of care are still being developed. Management techniques, from sample contracts to managed care pricing to extended patient care protocols, are also being developed and tested.

What is certain, however, is that successful continuums of care, no matter what model, target population, or services are included, require changes in management structures and techniques that override individual service goals and emphasize the effectiveness of the continuum as a whole. The first step is changing the orientation of the managers and clinicians. Each management function and client care activity should be thought of not from the perspective of *my* organization, but from the perspective of the full continuum of care, and also from the clients' perspective—because they will be part of the continuum not only on the first day of their illness, but on an ongoing basis through periods of both wellness and illness.

The promise of integrated systems offering a continuum of care is great. The long-term success of America's health care system depends on achieving the improvements in system performance described in this chapter. In the coming decade, the movement to develop continuums of care will grow to the extent that these systems can be shown to have delivered on their promise.

FACTS REVIEW

1. List five benefits to an organization of creating an integrated continuum of care.
2. Name five internal barriers that must be overcome to create a continuum of care.
3. Describe four management techniques that can be used to facilitate integration at each of the following levels: provider organization, payer, state government.
4. Discuss external challenges that impede the integration of services.
5. Articulate why deliberate management techniques are necessary to achieve integration of clinical services.
6. Describe two alternate ways that continuums of care can be structured, and discuss the strengths and weaknesses of each model.

REFERENCES

Alter, C. (1988a). The changing structure of elderly service delivery systems. *The Gerontologist, 28,* 91–98.

Alter, C. (1988b). Integration in interorganizational hospice care systems. *The Hospice Journal, 3,* 11–32.

American Case Management Association. (2003). Franklin Award. Retrieved November 12, 2003 from *www.acamaweb.org* (click on "Franklin Award").

Bardach, E. (1998). *Getting agencies to work together: The practice and theory of managerial craftsmanship.* Washington, DC: Brookings Institution Press.

Broskowski, A. (1981). *Linking health and mental health.* Newbury Park, CA: Sage.

Centers for Medicare and Medicaid Services. (2003). Health Insurance Portability and Accountability Act of 1996. Retrieved November 8, 2003 from *http://cms.hhs.gov/hipaa*

Evashwick, C. J. (1987). Definition of the continuum of care. In C. Evashwick & L. Weiss (Eds.), *Managing the continuum of care: A practical guide to organization and operations,* 23. Rockville, MD: Aspen.

Medicare. (2003a). CCRC. Retrieved November 12, 2003 from *http://www.medicare.gov/nursing/alternatives/other.asp*

Medicare. (2003b). S/HMO. Available at *http://www.medicare.gov/nursing/alternatives/SMHO.asp*

Medicare. (2003c). PACE. Available at *http://www.medicare.gov/nursing/alternatives/Pace.asp*

Minnesota Department of Health Services. (2003a). Minnesota disability health options. Available at *http://www.dhs.state.mn.us/health care/msho-mndho/MNDHO/htm*

Minnesota Department of Human Resource. (2003b). Minnesota senior health options (MSHO). Retrieved October 28, 2003 from *http://www.dhs.state.mn.us/healthcare/msho-mndho/msho.htm*

Mor, V., Fleishman, J. A., Allen, S. M., & Piette, J. D. (1994). *Networking AIDS services.* Ann Arbor, MI: Health Administration Press.

National Chronic Care Consortium. (1995). *Self-assessment for systems integration tool.* Bloomington, MN: NCCC.

Sharlach, A. E., Giunta, N., and Mills-Dick, K. (2001). *Case management in long-term care integration: An overview of current programs and evaluations.* Berkeley, CA: University of California, Berkeley Center for the Advanced Study of Aging Services.

Turner, J. C., & Tenoor, W. J. (1978). NIMH community support program: Pilot approach to a needed social reform. *Schizophrenia Bulletin, 4*(3), 319–334.

CHAPTER 12

Case Management

Monika White

Case management is a leading technique for efficient and effective coordination of care. In the conceptual framework of an integrated continuum of care (Chapter 1), it is identified as one of the four essential integrating mechanisms.

Case management developed in response to the increased complexity of health care. It is a way to meet the multiple objectives of various players and have everyone win. Clients and their providers benefit from case management through the focus on the full range of client and family needs. The case manager's knowledge of resources and service quality and a commitment to finding alternatives and options to costly services and institutionalization have resulted in generally well-satisfied clients and families.

Case management also serves the goals of providers. Case management focuses on facilitating access to information and services for individuals with designated risk factors. In recent years many health care systems have implemented this process to help stem runaway costs, reduce service fragmen-

tation, and simplify multiple provider and payer interactions while striving to improve the quality of care.

Case management is well suited for use across the full continuum of care. For example, with older adults case managers tend to work with the more vulnerable, at-risk populations, often to prevent lengthy or inappropriate institutionalization by coordinating care from a range of long-term care services. These services span health, mental health, and a variety of community and in-home services that enable the client to maintain independent living to the extent possible. The process of identifying clients; conducting an assessment or evaluation to understand problems and needs; developing a plan of care; and locating, arranging, coordinating, or otherwise obtaining services through purchase or referral is the work of case management.

Case management can link systems and settings and facilitate client movement through coordination and collaboration. It enhances communication among varied parties who may have roles in a

SERVICE SNAPSHOT: Case Management

Name:	Case manager, also called care manager, service coordinator, care coordinator
Functions:	Assessment, client identification, case planning, service coordination, and follow-up
Number:	Unknown—likely thousands
Number of clients served:	20 to 80 active at any time per case manager
Cost (@private pay):	$150–$400 per assessment; $50–$150 per hour of service
Payment sources:	Private, Medicaid, Medicare (under select circumstances), Older Americans Act, other publicly funded programs, long-term care insurance, health plans
Discipline:	Social work, nursing, other
Certification:	Currently offered by multiple organizations for individual professionals

comprehensive plan of care—physicians who need to be kept informed of outcomes, assisted living facility managers who desire to keep residents in place, or payers who require documentation. The emphasis on crisis prevention and education fits well with the principles of managed care. As more managed-care systems integrate acute and long-term care and services shift to outpatient areas, case management can ease transitions with the end result of improving care and keeping clients well.

BACKGROUND

Every discipline can claim its part in the origination of case management. Case management existed in the early 1900s in settlement houses and charity organizations. It continued to be used by social workers and nurses in public welfare, health, and mental health programs. In the 1970s and 1980s the federal government funded community-based research and demonstration projects to test long-term care coordination approaches and financing. Most of the programs served dependent populations and

were financed under Medicare and Medicaid waivers. Through these projects, the clinical and coordination activities conducted in many human services programs began to take shape and systematize the case management function.

The demonstrated success of case management in these projects led states to include the process in programs to control costs of home and community-based care. Case management was also incorporated in hospital-based demonstration projects funded by a major private foundation to improve health care for older adults. During this time, community-based case management continued to evolve outside the acute care setting. Simultaneously, health care professionals were developing case management systems to improve patient care within the hospital.

Case management has now expanded to many types of health and social service settings, as well as private practice. As further indication of growth and acceptance, in recent years private insurance companies, managed care programs, employers, and private family members have been willing to pay for case management services.

DEFINITION

Case management can be defined as a process of identifying issues and problems experienced by individuals and families and developing, implementing, and monitoring solutions to address them. Regardless of the educational background, discipline, or professional practice arena of the case manager, the job requires interpersonal and clinical skills; knowledge of eligibility criteria for programs and benefits, community resources, and costs of care; understanding of service delivery systems; and ability to establish and maintain relationships with service providers.

Descriptions of case management use varying terms and have multiple meanings. The flexibility of the concept has both contributed to a lack of consensus about its definition and led to widespread usage in diverse contexts. The term has been used interchangeably with others, including *care management, care coordination, service coordination,* and *managed care,* although some make distinctions. Examples of definitions found in the literature often highlight specific characteristics that describe case management.

COMPONENTS

Although many variables combine to give case management its definition in specific situations, there is general agreement on its components. The accompanying box lists the major components of case management.

Case Identification

Case management begins with efforts to define and target the desired population. It includes outreach activities that publicize the services and identify referral sources. Determination of eligibility and appropriateness for case management are achieved through established intake procedures. Acceptance for service may be based on such criteria as age, income, diagnosis, acuity, high risk, or high cost. Eligibility may be mandated by a payer or be set by

CORE COMPONENTS OF CASE MANAGEMENT

- Case identification
- Assessment/evaluation
- Care plan development
- Implementation/coordination
- Follow-up
  - Monitoring
  - Reassessment

the case management program. Referrals for case management may be made in writing, by telephone, or through in-person screenings. Not everyone requires case management, nor is this service ever free. Therefore, identifying and serving only appropriate cases is essential to the program's long-term financial viability.

Assessment

An assessment determines the needs and provides information from which to develop an individualized care plan. An individual case manager, such as a social worker or a nurse, or a multidisciplinary team may conduct the assessment. Multiple instruments, some standardized, are used to evaluate the individual. Often broader in scope than a medical or psychiatric examination, questions regarding physical and mental health, functional ability, family and social supports, the home environment, and financial resources are included to determine the full range of capabilities and needs. Others connected with the individual may be interviewed for further information; these may include family members, physicians, friends, service providers, and attorneys. This type of assessment may be conducted in various settings for different purposes, including in the hospital to provide information for discharge or in the home to determine level of care needed to maintain independence. The goal of this comprehensive process is a complete view of the individual and her or his circumstances.

Care Plan

A care plan is developed to address the needs and problems identified in the assessment. It includes agreement with the individual and involved family members on goals and priorities. Some of the factors that affect solutions are cost restraints, availability and accessibility of services, and the extent of family involvement. The plan outlines the problems, type and level of assistance needed, roles of client and family, who will provide the services, and desired outcomes. Knowledge of service options, local resources, delivery systems, quality providers, financial alternatives, available benefits, and eligibility requirements for assistance are critical to the plan.

Service Coordination

The case manager implements the care plan by arranging and coordinating services delivery. This includes coordinating informal assistance, such as that provided by family members, and facilitating transitions between services or settings. A case manager's authority to arrange services specified in the care plan depends on the program and the payer. Some can only make referrals to service providers and are limited to the role of broker. Others can negotiate and even purchase services. Previously arranged formal contracts may establish costs and referral procedures for some services. The case manager's knowledge of the service system, expertise in establishing relationships with providers, and ability to work with the client and family to make decisions and accept services are key to successful implementation of the care plan.

Follow-Up

Follow-up activities are conducted to ensure continuity, respond to changes in the individual's condition, and address any problems in care delivery. The setting again determines the nature and duration of the task. In an acute care facility, the care manager monitors the patients throughout their stay. In community and in-home settings, ongoing monitoring contacts are specifically planned weekly or monthly. Monitoring helps determine the continued effectiveness and appropriateness of services. Monitoring is also an important cost-containment measure. Periodic contact with the individual, the family, and service agencies provides a communication channel that can reduce problems and avert crises. In addition, a formal reassessment is scheduled at regular intervals or can be triggered by changing circumstances. This helps ensure that the care plan remains relevant to the current situation.

Other Functions

Additional activities that may be associated with the core components of case management include education and training of the client and caregivers, advocacy with agencies and providers for services or benefits, counseling, and solving problems. Often utilization review, quality improvement activities, and professional consultation are combined with the case management function.

THE CASE MANAGER

Who performs (or should perform) the case management function remains controversial. Case management is not a discipline, but a locus of responsibility. Many different people can carry this responsibility: professionals, paraprofessionals, volunteers, family members, and sometimes clients themselves.

Case management may be seen as the province of a particular discipline in relationship to the needs of the individual client. For example, nurses are likely to do case management when the need is for acute care; social workers are likely to be involved when the concerns are for long-term care; and physicians are the managers when the need is for primary care. However, there is much overlap and ongoing change.

The practice of case management focuses on a set of tasks and activities that demand considerable knowledge and skills requiring professional intervention. The case manager always serves as a partner or team member, working with the client; involving many members of natural support systems such as family, friends, and neighbors; and engaging professionals, such as physicians, attorneys, and home care providers. Case managers often work in multidisciplinary teams, bringing health and psychosocial expertise and perspectives together.

Case managers perform many roles. The type of program usually determines the range and level of responsibility. Case managers in managed care, for example, may have a significant gatekeeper role to minimize the use of inappropriate or specialized services. Case managers in publicly funded community programs often have a strong role as advocates who work to obtain the full range of services needed by their clients. In programs that emphasize more face-to-face contact with the individual and family members, case managers play important roles as counselors and mediators.

The organizational locus determines lines of authority. The actual location of case management services within an organization is an important design decision. Many organizations develop a separate program, unit, division, or department to maximize flexibility, assure equality with other departments, and facilitate program funding. In hospitals, it is most often located in nursing or social work departments. Others position case management as a marketing program or attach it to a specific target population such as seniors, AIDS, or Alzheimer's victims. The location or position of case management is a crucial design decision and will affect its authority, utilization, and acceptance by internal as well as external entities.

Accountability

Case management almost always deals with multiple "clients." Regardless of the setting, case managers are accountable to the recipient of the care, family members, the service providers, and the organizations that employ them. Often funding for case management is received from outside the organization or program, adding yet another layer of accountability. The case management function requires significant autonomy and independent judgment and, therefore, trust. To whom and how case management is accountable is an important administrative consideration. The balance between autonomy and accountability requires administrative sanction and support.

Provider versus Independent

A key concept in case management has been its objective and impartial perspective. Therefore, it has long been considered a potential conflict of interest for the case manager, as the coordinator of services, also to be part of the provider of care. The controversy is focused on the premise that case managers will coordinate what they or their agencies provide and may not consider more cost-effective or appropriate resources. Others argue that coordinating provider-based services enhances continuity and offers greater opportunities to control costs and quality. There has been strong opposition to reimbursement for provider-based case management and current legislative debate about the issue.

Recent mergers and the development of new companies point toward combining case management with direct services such as home care. This is particularly true in the private practice sector, where a number of ventures are capitalized to capture the fee-for-service case management market. Many of the most experienced and best-known case management programs are part of organizations that also provide health, mental health, and home care services. The most common model, however, remains separate.

CASE MANAGEMENT PROGRAM DESIGN

The designs of case management programs vary significantly. Programs tend to fall into medical or nonmedical models although a third category is a combined or consolidated model. Within these broad models are subsets of case management. Table 12.1 summarizes the types and their key characteristics which define the population served, the setting in which the case manager works with the client, the major focus of the case management activity, and how service is reimbursed.

Key Characteristics

Populations and settings. Case management is being used to manage the care of individuals who are high risk and have high-cost, complex problems. Increasingly, it is also being used for those with chronic disabilities and problems. The trend is to institute case management in all settings where these

Table 12.1   Summary of Case Management Types and Key Characteristics

Type Medical	Population	Setting	Focus	Financing
Primary care	Patients	Doctor's office; clinics	Prevent, diagnose, treat, monitor	Private pay; insurance; Medicare; Medicaid
Acute care	Patients	Hospital; acute, subacute facilities	Facilitate flow of care; discharge; prevent readmission	Private pay; insurance; Medicare; Medicaid
Other medical (including home health)	Medically dependent, complex or problems	Skilled nursing facility; home, special facility	Treat, monitor, supervise, prevent, rehabilitate	Private pay; insurance; Medicare; Medicaid
Managed care	Enrollees; high-risk high-cost	Primary/acute settings	Authorize, verify services and utilization; manage benefits/costs	Private pay; employer; Medicare; Medicaid
Long-term care insurance	Enrollees	Home; assisted living; skilled nursing facility	Authorize, verify services and utilization; manage benefits/costs	Private pay Reimbursement per LTCI plan
Non-Medical				
Community/ in-home	Community functional/ cognitive disability	Noninstitutional	Coordinate wide range of nonmedical care; keep independent	Private pay; waiver funds; grants/contracts
Nursing facility	Ongoing need for skilled care, supervision; chronic problems	In-home, community, or facility	Monitor, prevent decline; link to needed resources	Private pay; some insurance; waiver funds; grants/ contracts
Mental health	Complex, chronic psychiatric problems	In-home community-based group home	Education; life skills, adaptation; compliance monitoring	Private pay; some insurance; some Medicare, Medicaid; grants, contracts
Other	Usually well; need advice, counseling	Community	Resource/service information, referrals	Private pay; grants, contracts

individuals receive care. This calls for a broad definition that applies to primary, acute, and long-term care; to medical and nonmedical psychosocial arenas; to community and institutional settings; and to many subgroups of people with disabilities and chronic illnesses. Case management may involve service arrangement only, or, with varying degrees of authority, purchase of services. Additionally, the setting may determine if the case manager serves primarily a client advocacy or a gatekeeper function or must achieve some combination of the two.

Purpose. Case management is instituted by an organization for any of several primary reasons. When minimizing the length of stay is important, case management is used primarily to facilitate and smooth the transition of care. For individuals at home, the focus shifts to coordination of multiple community-based services. In long-term care management, monitoring over time to prevent decline takes on added emphasis. In contrast, the purpose of case management programs that serve generally well populations with short-term information or counseling is to provide resource and service referrals. Cost containment is often the underlying reason for implementing case management. Overall, case management is an appropriate response to the complexity of the health and social services systems, not only for individuals needing help for themselves or their families, but also for professionals who cross settings to get their clients served.

Funding. A key characteristic is funding. Financing most commonly defines the population, the level of staffing, and a myriad of other design elements. Funding for case management depends largely on its relationship to health or medical care or social supports. The medical types are reimbursed through private pay, private health insurances, Medicare, Medicaid, and HMOs. The nonmedical, social support models are funded through special Medicaid waivers, both public- and private-sector contracts (such as a county or corporate program), public and private grants, and private pay. Nonprofit organizations such as community services agencies and churches often finance these programs through fundraising events and private donations.

Duration. Another variation is the duration of time that case management is actually provided. Applebaum and Austin (1990) distinguish between the short-term case management offered in conjunction with direct services, such as that provided by hospital discharge planners and home health agencies, and comprehensive long-term care case management. The latter is characterized by greater intensity of involvement with patients/clients (allowed by smaller caseloads), a broader range of provided services, and a longer duration of involvement based on client functional capability. The length of time a client receives case management depends on a combination of factors, including program purpose, target population, funding, and individual need.

Caseload size. A program that emphasizes resource information and referral may have large caseloads that involve only one or two brief contacts. Individuals with complex needs may be case management clients for a year or more and be part of smaller caseloads. Publicly funded programs often have specific guidelines regarding caseload size that are related to the frailty level of the target population.

Types of Case Management

As shown in Table 12.1, there are both medical and nonmedical types of case management, each with some key characteristics.

Primary care. Primary care case management is usually planned by the primary care physician or a physician-led team that includes a nurse and social worker, rehabilitation therapist, or other specialist, depending on the needs of the client. Physician-led case management teams often operate out of specialty clinics, such as geriatric assessment programs, and serve designated populations, such as HIV/AIDS or Alzheimer's victims or rehabilitation patients.

Contact with the client's primary care physician is an important aspect of case management practice, regardless of the setting. The physician is key not only in providing or verifying important information, but also in supporting and assisting with implementation of the care plan in difficult situations. Primary care physicians may employ or contract with individual or agency case managers to provide linkages to health and community services to augment care and continuity (see White, Gundrum, Shearer, & Simmons, 1994).

Acute care. Case management in inpatient and outpatient acute settings has become a normal part of hospital care. Hospital case managers are usually nurses and tend to be assigned to specific units such as cardiac or oncology. They follow high-risk patients throughout the hospitalization to facilitate services, treatment, and paperwork such as insurance authorizations. A patient with a history of multiple hospitalizations, high utilization of the emergency room, or noncompliance may be followed by the hospital case manager through other settings as well, including home, to assure continuity of care and address medically related issues. Where clinical guidelines or protocols are used by a hospital, the nurse case manager may be responsible for ensuring that all tasks specified by the protocol are accomplished and performed according to the designated schedule.

Other medical care. A variety of complex medical problems can be monitored through case management. Whether clients are in a facility or living independently, the involvement of a case manager will expedite appropriate care and provide the individual with an advocate if difficulties arise.

Until recently, case management was often terminated as soon as a client was admitted to a congregate setting or skilled nursing facility. Now follow-up is often continued whenever it is deemed necessary and to the extent that reimbursement allows. Because reimbursement is most commonly tied to an acute episode or medical problems, insurance or private pay is the major source; however, some hospitals are providing case managers to follow patients into the community to assure compliance with and appropriateness of treatment and care.

Home health care. As patients leave hospitals earlier, an increasing array of treatments (such as hospice care, ventilator care, and general infusion therapy) that were formerly done only in hospitals are now part of home care, and lend themselves to a case management approach. Some businesses are developing case management programs for their fee-for-service clinical plans that stress the use of home care when appropriate. Some home care agencies are partners with managed care home programs that use case management teams consisting of a home health case manager, a doctor, ancillary services, and the payer. Their focus is patient and family education and an increased level of independence for the patient.

Long-term care insurance. A number of long-term care insurance (LTCI) products now cover in-home and community-based services, such as day services, transportation, and meals. Case managers who are either employed by the insurance company or are contracted for these purposes perform underwriting and benefits determination, assessment, care planning, and monitoring tasks. Whether and to what extent the insured population utilizes case management depends on the policy design. Some policies require enrollees to use case management and make it a part of the benefits received; others recommend it and may deduct the cost of the case management from the available benefits if used. Still others combine a requirement for planning the care with an option for implementation and monitoring.

Managed care. Managed-care organizations integrate financing and service delivery and utilize case managers to achieve good quality care while controlling utilization and costs. Many managed-care organizations are expanding to incorporate a broad array of services for members. This model is a good example of a combined medical and nonmedical model in which the case manager can coordinate acute, primary, community, and in-home services to implement the most appropriate level of care and services possible at the best cost. Through its monitoring activities, case management contributes greatly to prevention and compliance, areas that can represent significant savings.

Case management in insurance and managed care arenas is to be distinguished from utilization review. The verification of eligibility or membership, the authorization of services, and benefits management are, in fact, a large part of the activities conducted by case managers, but one of their most important tasks is the identification of high-risk and high-cost clients. These clients then have more opportunities to receive appropriate care and assistance in maintaining and managing their health status.

Community/In-home care. Case management in the community focuses on the coordination of nonmedical, nonskilled services for individuals with functional or cognitive disabilities. A primary goal for this type of case management is to keep people living as independently as possible in noninstitutional settings. Referrals for case management are received from a wide variety of sources and settings, including health, social services, mental health, other home care providers, physicians, attorneys, and families. The case manager, in turn, refers or purchases services from these same types of sources and others, including home health, nursing homes, and assisted living or other residential facilities. The community-based case manager will have broad knowledge of the available resources and how to access them. He or she also works closely with informal supports such as families, friends, neighbors, and church groups to assist in serving the client.

Funding for community-based case management comes primarily from public sources such as Medicaid, the Older Americans Act (OAA), or other waiver programs established to prevent institutionalization. These focus on specific populations, such as persons with AIDS or those age 60 and older who are eligible for OAA services. Private foundations also provide funding for community-based case management, usually to test innovative methods for short periods of time. Private, fee-for-service case management is mostly used by families with the means to purchase consultation and monitoring services.

Mental health. Case management has long been an approach to working with the mentally ill. It continues to be an effective approach to keeping individuals with complex mental health problems in the community. The primary function of the case manager is to provide the client with life skills and

to coordinate services that support independent living. Monitoring tasks assure regular contact and the ability to intervene if problems arise. An important addition to using case management in mental health is integrating behavior change theory and motivational interviewing to assist clients to take more personal responsibility for change and goal attainment in the case management process. (Hackstaff, Davis, & Katz, 2004). In some areas, special funding is available through state and county programs for extended periods of case management services.

Triage and referral. Case management is generally considered to be most appropriate for individuals or families with complex, multiple, or long-term problems. Though this is still true, there are many situations in which one-time or short-term assistance is needed, such as consultation about coping with an ill family member or information about housing options. Agencies such as senior centers, family service, and community social, medical, or mental health centers often provide such services by telephone or in person. When funding allows, community agencies prefer to employ professionals with case management experience to provide assessment, consultation, information, and referral services, because of their expertise in problem identification, care planning, and resource acquisition. These types of programs often identify the need for case management and provide access to appropriate case management services.

Integration. Integration of acute and long-term care or medical and nonmedical services is a goal of many organizations and funders. The need for and interest in integration is evident in the health care systems development pursued extensively during the 1990s. Acquisitions, mergers, affiliations, and network development bring hospitals, physicians, clinics, home health care agencies, and home and community-based services together into vertically integrated systems. Other efforts are based on agreements to collaborate rather than to formally integrate, but the ability to provide easier access, less fragmentation and duplication, better tracking of information, and an opportunity to control costs and quality is enhanced. Case management is one of the most effective integrative mechanisms available today. As integrated systems emerge, the role of the case manager must evolve to span service boundaries.

Network development. Several case management networks have been established to link community-based programs and services together at national, state, regional, and local levels. Network organizations, such as Family Caring Network in Massachusetts, contract with insurance companies to conduct underwriting and benefits determination assessments and have several hundred care management members that provide these and other related services. State and local networks have been developed for easy access and referrals. In addition, a number of telephone networks exist, including the Work Family Directions (also based in Waltham, Massachusetts), that contract with large businesses to provide information and referral services at the local level for employed caregivers and retirees.

Overall, network development slowed in the late 1990s and early 2000s. On the rise is the acquisition of for-profit, private care management practices by home care agencies or other practices for development of regional and national companies. Two examples of successful companies in 2003 were LivHome, based in Los Angeles, and Senior Bridge, headquartered in New York.

Other case management networks are developing direct partnerships with corporate employee assistance programs. One example is RBA's Independent Practice Association in Fort Lauderdale, Florida. RBA is a private care management company with regional and national corporate contracts. Individual professionals joining this network receive referrals as well as enhancements for their practices and benefits for their clients. Another is a new, innovative relationship between a national professional association and a private corporation. One example is the National Association of Professional Geriatric Care Managers (NAPGCM) and LifeCare, Inc., a large, privately owned employee benefits organization, which have formed "The GCM Guild." Full members of NAPGCM are eligible to join the Guild and are given priority referral status by LifeCare for its clientele throughout the country. LifeCare is assured of access to professional care managers who meet their association's practice standards and are specialists in working with older adults and their families; Guild members get expanded referral and visibility opportunities and access to LifeCare's informational resources.

What is clear is that case management is provided at the local level—but family needs are national. Thus, it is important for professionals to be linked through some mechanism with those who need them. Though not all prior networks have been successful, efforts to improve these relationships continue.

OUTCOMES

With its potential to reduce fragmentation and make efficient use of resources, case management can be a welcome cost-containment strategy both in terms of time saved and actual dollars spent.

Quality Measures

Measuring outcome is difficult for several reasons: case management is a process rather than an outcome, the role and function of case management are not always clear, and case management is often enmeshed with many other services. Most efforts to date have focused on timeliness, responsiveness, completion of forms and reports, and client satisfaction surveys.

The most consistent outcomes associated with case management are based on "costs, service utilization, functional capacity, family functioning and quality of life" (Scharlach, Guinta, & Mills-Dick, 2001, p. 64). Facilitating and managing acute and primary care have resulted in savings of millions of dollars. Community-based programs are still struggling to prove their impact with hard data. This is due in part to a lack of funding for both quantitative evaluation and adequate information systems.

Increasingly, funders are requiring development

of outcome measures. Woodside and McClam suggest that case managers can begin to relate what they do with the benefits their clients receive by "linking their activities to the objectives of the organization . . . and to the cost of services delivered" (2003, p. 257). Better data are anticipated as client tracking software becomes more affordable and systems become more compatible across organizations.

Information Systems

Information systems to facilitate case management have been available for years for both inpatient and community-based models. However, no system has been universally adopted. Keeping resource information current is a challenge. Moreover, interface with client records maintained by clinical providers has not been achieved.

In spite of technological readiness and a few attempts, tracking of information about case management services has not yet been achieved on a widespread basis. Client information is compiled within controlled environments such as hospitals and insurance companies, but data on the actual time, expense, and outcomes of the case management itself are not collected. This is an important task for the future, especially as case managers increasingly follow clients longer and across settings and funding sources. Measuring both process and outcomes will be easier when standardized information systems are adopted by a broad spectrum of programs.

Standards

At the present time, case management as a function is not licensed. Care managers may have licenses in their clinical disciplines, such as social work or nursing.

Standards for any client services are important to ensure ethical, moral, and professional behavior and practice. Because case managers are trained in many disciplines, standards tend to be drawn from those professional backgrounds. For example, the American Nurses Association has developed standards for nursing case management; the National Association for Social Workers has social work case management standards; and both the National Council on Aging and the National Association of Professional Geriatric Care Managers have established standards for case management with seniors. Cross-disciplinary standards have yet to be developed. Leadership toward this effort is emerging through the formulation of a variety of case management credentials.

Case Management Education and Credentialing

Case managers have primarily learned their practice on the job. Seminars, workshops, and training through conferences and short courses by professional associations and universities have been offered for some time. Education for a specific degree in case management is controversial, but curriculums are being developed at a number of universities. Although there is agreement about the core components and function of case management, consensus has not yet been reached about standards, curriculum, or the need for a separate degree or credential.

There are several reasons to promote certification of case managers. Proponents of certification argue that it is important not only to professionalize case management, but also to be acceptable to payers and funders who look to credentials as a standard of quality. Moreover, certification allows consumers, funders, and employers to identify case managers who have proven their knowledge by passing an examination and who have met education and experience criteria to sit for the test.

The late 1990s saw a proliferation of efforts to credential case managers through development of certification examinations. To date, there are nearly 20 national groups offering case management certification; the majority of them focus on nursing and rehabilitation professionals. Table 12.2 lists selected credentialing organizations and the certification given. Certification is of individual practitioners rather than agencies, although accreditation

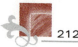

Table 12.2 Selected Case Management Credentialing Organizations

Organization	Credential
• American Institute of Outcome Case Management	Case Manager Certified (CMC)
• Certification of Disability Management Specialists Commission	Certified Disability Management Specialist (CDMC)
• Commission for Case Management Certification	Certified Case Manager (CCM)
• Commission for Rehabilitation Counselor Certification	Certified Rehabilitation Counselor (CRC)
• Healthcare Quality Certification Board of the National Association for Healthcare Quality	Certified Professional in Healthcare Quality (CPHQ)
• National Association of Certified Care Managers	Care Manager, Certified (CMC)
• National Association of Social Workers	Certified Social Work Case Manager (C-SWCM)
• National Board for Certification in Continuity of Care	Continuity of Care Certification, Advanced (A-CCC)
• Rehabilitation Nursing Certification Board	Certified Rehabilitation Nurse (CRRN)
• URAC (formerly Utilization Review Accreditation Commission)	Case management program accreditation

for case management organizations and companies has been implemented by URAC.

Estimates are that there may be as many as 30,000 to 40,000 certified case managers in the country (mostly nurses). Nevertheless, many professionals do not seek this specific credential. One reason is that there is currently little demand for credentialed case managers. Second, case managers tend to identify with their own disciplines (e.g., social work, nursing, psychology) and therefore must continue to meet education, continuing education, and employment requirements of the state in which they are licensed. Still, interest in certification programs is growing, and it is anticipated that the numbers of and demand for credentialed case managers will continue to increase despite reservations from many leaders and practitioners.

CONCLUSION

As long as complex financing and regulations, fragmentation, duplication, and gaps in the health care system remain, case management will continue to be an essential component of service delivery. It is becoming increasingly important as the growth in continuum of care systems develops and clients must transition through hospital, physician, home care, and long-term care services. In spite of the fact that many issues regarding case management have not been put to rest, its ranks are expanding daily.

CLIENT EXAMPLE

To illustrate the role of case management in different settings, brief summaries of three cases are presented.

Acute Care

A 66-year-old man with a history of coronary artery disease was scheduled for aneurysm repair surgery at a hospital that used case management with vascular patients. At each step of his transfer from the vascular unit to the operating room and to the surgical intensive care unit, a primary nurse was designated for his care. The vascular unit nurse was assigned the case manager role of coordinating the patient's overall care throughout his stay and involving the family.

The nurse case manager made sure that all diagnostic tests ordered by the physician were performed on a timely basis, that results were reported promptly to the physician and recorded in the patient's record, and that postsurgery treatment protocols were followed by all shifts. When serious complications necessitated a return to surgery, the case manager smoothed the transition, and the patient stayed only a few days beyond the allotted DRG for major vascular surgery. As part of the discharge plan, a referral was made to the hospital's community case management program for in-home help and follow-up.

Physician Office

During a routine examination a physician noticed that his 50-year-old patient seemed especially distressed. The physician learned that the patient's wife had just been hospitalized with a stroke after learning that she had cancer. The physician contacted a community-based case manager who was able to go to the home to visit the husband. The case manager called the hospital social services department and alerted the wife's social worker to the situation to aid in discharge planning. The case manager discussed local cancer counseling and support resources with the husband and gave him referral information. A follow-up call indicated that the client had contacted a cancer support organization and arranged respite care and participation in a caregiver's support group.

Community-Based Program

A 79-year-old widow lived alone in her own home with no nearby relatives, but kept in contact with her daughter, who lived out of state. Alarmed on her last visit by her mother's weight loss and confusion and the unkempt state of the house, the daughter contacted her mother's physician, who referred her to a care coordination program. An in-home evaluation by the case manager indicated that the mother had impaired memory and judgment, poor personal hygiene, and difficulty with regular meal preparation and performance of household tasks.

The case manager helped the daughter to arrange and coordinate services that included a homemaker to help with bathing, meal preparation, and housekeeping, and a senior center with adult day services that provided transportation. After a checkup by her physician, it appeared that the mother's health problems were due to poor nutrition. An appointment with a nutrition specialist was made to improve her diet, and a follow-up visit with her physician was scheduled. The daughter was able to stay with her mother to work with the case manager to get the services in place. The mother's condition improved and the daughter returned home, knowing that the case manager would continue to monitor her mother's situation.

WHERE TO GO FOR FURTHER INFORMATION

The widespread interest in case management has stimulated a diverse body of regularly published literature.

American Case Management Association
10310 West Markham Street, Suite 209
Little Rock, AK 72205
(501) 907-2262
http://www.acmaweb.org

Case Management Society of America (CMSA)
8201 Cantrell Road, Suite 230
Little Rock, AR 72227
Phone (501) 225-2229 Fax (501) 221-9068
http://www.cmsa.org

Commission for Case Management Certification
http://www.ccmcertification.org

National Academy of Certified Care Managers
244 Upton Road
Colchester, CT 06414-0669
(800) 962-2260
http://www.naccm.net

National Association of Professional Geriatric Care Managers (NAPGCM)
1604 N. Country Club Road
Tucson, AZ 85716-3102
(520) 881-8008
http://www.caremanager.org

FACTS REVIEW

1. What is case management?
2. What are the components of case management?
3. How is case management financed?
4. Explain how a case manager's authorities and activities vary according to organizational base.
5. What benefits can be expected from case management? For the client? For the provider?

REFERENCES

Applebaum, R., & Austin, C. D. (1990). *Long-term care case management: Design and evaluation.* New York: Springer.

Hackstaff, L., Davis, C., & Katz, L. (2004). The case for integrating behavior change, client-centered practice and other evidence-based models into geriatric care management. *Social Work and Health Care, 38*(3), 1–19.

Scharlach, A. E., Guinta, N., & Mills-Dick, K. (2001). *Case management in long-term care integration: An overview of current programs and evaluations* (Report for the California Center for Long-Term Care Integration). Berkeley, CA: Center for the Advanced Study of Aging Services, University of California–Berkeley.

White, M., Gundrum, G., Shearer, S., & Simmons, W. J. (1994, Summer). A role for case managers in the physician office. *Journal of Case Management, 3*(2), 62–68.

Woodside, M., & McClam, T. (2003). *Generalist case management: A method of human service delivery.* Pacific Grove, CA: Brooks/Cole-Thomson Learning.

CHAPTER 13

Integrated Information Systems

Lisa R. Shugarman and Rick Zawadski

This chapter addresses integrated information systems by describing a model for an information system integrating medical and social services information across providers and payers. It discusses some of the benefits of such a system, as well as barriers to implementation.

BACKGROUND

The effective clinician uses information from the client, and knowledge of similar clients and problems in the past, to determine a plan of care. Likewise, information drives policy making about health and human services. In recent years, the volume and complexity of information have increased exponentially. Tools and systems have been developed and are still being developed to help capture, organize, and coordinate a variety of data sources into an **integrated information system.**

Health and human services are the most information-intensive service industries. Early information systems focused on accounting and external

reporting, but it soon became clear that information also would be needed to support care-related decisionmaking at the client, provider, and payer levels. The delivery of a single service requires identifying information on the patient or client, assessing service need, tracking and describing services provided, and billing multiple funders. Often, even within a single provider agency, for example, the clinicians, the accounting department, and the managers will collect their own overlapping information. In a network of multiple providers or programs, this information is often gathered repeatedly by each service provider. Multiple sets of overlapping information are not only duplicative and inefficient, but also limit the usefulness of the information gathered. Knowledge of other service use would be helpful to the clinician and total participant cost information would help manage and develop more cost-effective services.

Policymakers rely heavily on information about the programs for which they are responsible to make next year's funding decisions, to document outcomes or even justify the very existence of the program. The payers of many services provided to those who need long-term care (i.e., Medicare, Medicaid, etc.) rely on others to provide the service and feed information back to the source agency for reimbursement and oversight. Because large portions of state and federal budgets are appropriated for these programs, the public agencies responsible for Medicare and Medicaid have specific and substantial reporting requirements.

DEFINITION

An **integrated information system (IIS)** is an array of multiple information sets linked together in an organized way. **Information sets** are groups of similar items often collected together. Examples include client characteristics, health and functional assessments, service use, and service billing information. The multiple information sets may be collected at different times by different members of the service agency. Instead of collecting information separately for each need, an information system links or connects information collected by different units in the agency and makes it available to everyone who needs it. *Organized* means that there is a well-defined plan for collecting and linking information sets to meet multiple information needs in the most efficient and effective manner. An IIS is more efficient because it eliminates the need for duplicate data collection; one entry serves all. More importantly, an IIS makes more information available to all users, allowing new and expanded use of information to improve service quality and increase efficiency.

Integration of information can occur at many levels. Within the agency providing a single service, information can be linked across departments; for example, between clinical staff and accounting. Integrating fiscal and client data allows the measurement and tracking of service cost and the assessment of cost/benefit and cost-effectiveness. In the multiservice agency, an IIS would link information across different services and would integrate information across agencies for a given participant.

Chronically ill persons are not conveniently divided into acute and long-term care segments; their problems and needs are interrelated. Integrating information across services and provider systems provides a comprehensive picture of participants, a description of their health needs and conditions, the services they receive, the cost of their care, and the outcomes of treatment. Altogether, this information allows provider-based managers of care to make decisions that improve the quality and limit the total cost of chronic care (and aids policymakers in making resource allocation decisions and planning for the needs of the population).

CLIENT EXAMPLE

A single individual could receive services for which there are several payers and providers. Currently, there is no system-wide method for linking data across programs and providers about an individual. Take for example, the case of Mrs. C. Mrs. C., a recent widow whose husband provided much of her care, was diagnosed a year ago with uncontrolled diabetes and congestive heart failure. Since the death of her husband, Mrs. C. has been unable to pay her bills, keep her apartment clean, or adequately prepare food. She has not paid the rent and the landlord is trying to evict her. She appears to have few assets, but insists that she is related to the King of England and is an heiress. Mrs. C. does not have a working telephone, her refrigerator has been disconnected, there is no food in her house, and she remembers eating little in recent days. She lives with two uncaged birds and a small dog. She is eligible for Medicare and Medicaid.

What services does Mrs. C. need? Clearly, she requires some level of both medical and social service intervention. Medical services include physician care to assess and treat her diabetes and heart failure, and possibly hospital care and pharmacy services to stabilize her conditions, as well as mental health, dental, and vision services. She may also need other medical services. The social services Mrs. C. might need include personal assistance, housing, homemaker services, transportation, protective supervision, and companionship. These services might be provided in the community or, quite possibly, in an institutional setting.

How will Mrs. C. get the services she needs? She is eligible for Medicare and Medicaid services and may very well be eligible for other services provided by state and local governments. The challenge for Mrs. C. will be in navigating through the system. Considering her fragile state, she will need assistance.

The challenge in the current system is that programs operate in "unintegrated payer silos of care." The typical long-term care client will require services funded by several different agencies or programs

(such as Medicare and Medicaid), and these programs currently do not share information about the persons they serve. As shown in Figure 13.1, an individual might access medical services from Medicare, Medicaid, or private-pay sources (both out of pocket and commercial insurance) and receive social services from federal, state, and locally funded public programs or through private pay. There is considerable overlap in the set of services these payers provide. The lack of information sharing may result in duplicated services and may result in little or no coordination of care for the client. Lack of integration creates problems in payment to providers and stymies efforts to plan and allocate scarce resources at a societal level because we cannot

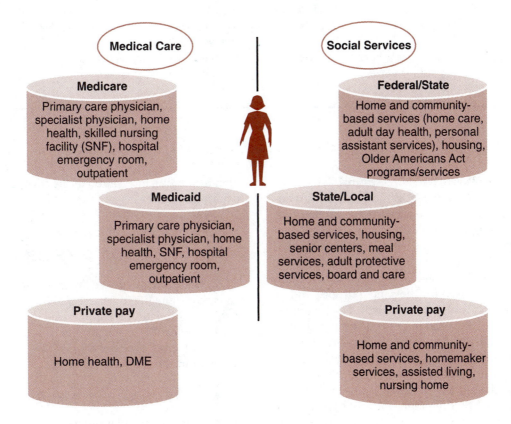

Figure 13.1   Unintegrated Payer "Silos of Care"
SOURCE: Wilber, 2000.

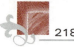

 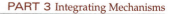

Table 13.1   Fragmentation in Clinical and Fiscal/Management Information Systems

Information Source	Purpose
Minimum Data Set (nursing home)	• Resource Utilization Groups (RUGs)—used for case mix payment of Medicare-funded skilled nursing care under a prospective payment system and, in some states, for Medicaid nursing home reimbursement • Care planning
Outcome and Assessment Information Set (OASIS)	• Home Health Resource Groups (HRGs)—case mix payment of home health services under a prospective payment system • Outcomes assessment • Quality assurance
Inpatient Rehabilitation Facility Patient Assessment Instrument (IRF PAI)	• Case Mix Groups (CMGs)—payment for inpatient rehabilitation under a prospective payment system
Hospital discharge data	Diagnosis Related Groups (DRGs)—case mix reimbursement of inpatient services under a prospective payment system
Outpatient claims data	Ambulatory Payment Classification Groups (APCGs)—case mix reimbursement of hospital-based outpatient services under a prospective payment system
Current Procedure Technology (CPT) codes	Used by multiple providers (inpatient, outpatient, physician, SNF, home health, etc.) to classify patient visits
International Statistical Classification of Diseases and Related Health Problems, 10th revision (ICD-10)	Used by multiple providers (inpatient, outpatient, physician, SNF, home health, etc.) to classify patient diagnoses and conditions

integrate services across funding streams. Table 13.1 shows examples of different clinical and fiscal/management information systems used for different purposes. The fragmentation illustrates the challenge to integrating information when there are discrete systems and each system uses its own metric for assessing client need and care—in some cases, the metrics may be used for the same purpose and in others for very different purposes. For example, functional status is used both for determining clinical care and as the basis for reimbursement (as in the Minimum Data Set for nursing homes).

This table provides examples of information sources and their varied uses. Many information sources are used for reimbursement of specific services and some may serve other purposes as well. Additionally, some information sources that are commonly used across provider types could be help-ful in facilitating integration at the client and fiscal/management levels.

A MODEL INTEGRATED INFORMATION SYSTEM

A model for an integrated information system to manage an integrated service program for a long-term care population is summarized in Figure 13.2. The boxes identify different sets of information or files. Lines show the connections or links between information sets.

Components of the System

Many pieces of information are needed to manage and deliver high-quality services to a long-term care population in a cost-effective way. These data ele-

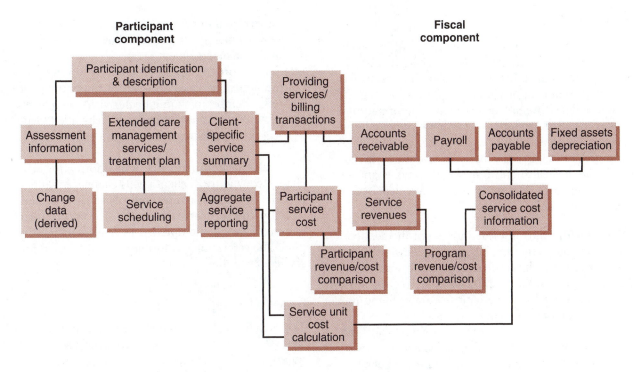

Figure 13.2   Model Integrated System for a Chronic Care Organization

ments can be grouped in different ways. In multi-service agencies, there may be several information sets covering the same area; for example, the service recording forms for the day care center may duplicate those of the hospital.

The conceptual model information system is divided into two major areas: the participant (clinical) component and the fiscal/management component. Major information sets in each area are identified and described. Examples of items included in each set are presented and data collection source and frequency are discussed.

Participant (Client) Information

Identification and Description

Central to an IIS is the basic information identifying and describing the participant. This information

is collected at the time of application or enrollment and is used by everyone within the system. The master participant record would include:

1. Identifying information: name, address, telephone, family contact, Medicare, Medicaid, and insurance numbers.
2. Demographic information: gender, ethnicity, date of birth, marital status, and living arrangements.
3. Program status information: eligibility/membership status, application date, referral source, reason for referral, enrollment, and closing date.

Data collection frequency. This information is relatively stable. Information is recorded at the time of enrollment and updated as changes occur (for example, change of address or change in program status).

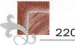

Assessment

Before determining the service needs of a chronic care participant, the older person's health and functional status must first be assessed. The assessment should include information on all areas influencing service decision making. Assessment information is used to define major health conditions for condition-based demonstrations. Assessments should be repeated at regular intervals to monitor change. Change in health and functional status is an outcome measure. The participant assessment record would include:

1. Health status information: major medical conditions, active medications, review of major health systems, and general health status.
2. Functional status information: level of assistance needed in activities of daily living and instrumental activities.
3. Cognitive status information: short- and long-term memory, reasoning skills, and the ability to make decisions on his or her own behalf.
4. Environmental information: assessment of living environment for barriers to independence and safety (e.g., stairs and bathroom facilities).
5. Informal support information: assessment of the informal support (family, friends, and neighbors) available and the assistance they can and do provide.

Data collection frequency. This information changes over time and must be assessed at regular intervals, such as quarterly or semiannually. Changes in assessed status will be an outcome measure derived from the comparison of assessments at different times.

Service/Treatment Plan

A service or treatment plan is developed by the care management team based on assessment information. The plan is integrated and cuts across all service areas. The participant and/or family is involved in the development of the plan. The service/treatment plan record would include:

1. Service goal information: list of prioritized care management goals developed by the participant and care management team.
2. Service orders: specification of the type and amount of services ordered for the participant (e.g., number of home health visits, frequency of adult day center attendance, scheduled medical procedures, and active medications).

Data collection frequency. This information will change constantly as client needs change. An initial plan is developed at the time of assessment and stored with the assessment record. The service plan record is continually updated to reflect changes in plan. The service plan information will be used for service scheduling.

Service Use

The benefit of the system is the services provided to the chronically ill person. The service use record tracks all the health and human services provided to a participant by all service departments or agencies. This information is collected and organized by service type and amount and is summarized for a given time period. The participant's service record would include:

1. Delivered services information: date, provider, type, and amount of health and health-related services provided to the participant by all providers. Services include number of admissions and days of hospitalization, nursing home days, inpatient and outpatient physician visits and procedures, home health and in-home supportive services, durable medical equipment, prescriptions, adult day services, therapy, and medical transportation.
2. Service coordination: date, type, and amount of care management and coordination service provided to the participant by the provider or its affiliated agencies.

Data collection frequency. This information is collected as individual service records, on an ongoing basis. Service information is summarized and reported for specified time periods, such as on a monthly or a quarterly basis. Service patterns can be compared across participants and providers and tracked over time. Service use also can be compared to service plan to assess compliance—one measure of service quality.

Fiscal/Management Information

Service Revenue

Services are paid in many ways: physicians may be reimbursed per visit or procedure; hospital stays by DRGs; adult day centers by day of attendance and monthly capitation. One important data set, then, is the amount billed and received for health and health-related services. The service revenue record would include:

1. Service charge information: the date and amount charged for each health and health-related service provided to participants.
2. Payment information: the amount of payment received for each service from each funding source and the basis for payment.
3. For those who participate in prepaid health plans, capitation amounts per enrollee.

Data collection frequency. This information is collected, along with individual service records, on an ongoing basis. Total service charge information by participant is computed on a monthly basis. Revenues for all chronic care services are reported by funding source.

Service Costs

Charges do not necessarily reflect costs. Whenever possible, an attempt should be made to capture costs of services. Cost information can be ascertained through the agency's fiscal system or independently gathered from estimates of time, facilities, and materials needed to provide the service. A chart of accounts is established and expenses collected. An expense reporting system is used to integrate different types of expenses and group them by service area. The program cost record would include:

1. Personnel cost information: salaries and benefits for staff involved in the delivery of services by service area.
2. Materials and supplies information: cost of materials and supplies used in the delivery of services. Costs are grouped by service area.
3. Facility cost information: cost of facilities, use of equipment, and general overhead used in the delivery of services. These costs are also grouped by service area.

Data collection frequency. Ideally, this information is derived from the agency's general ledger system and reported on a regular (i.e., monthly) basis. Otherwise, cost information could be estimated on a periodic basis from multiple sources, such as time analysis, or prorations of facility use. Total expenditures by cost centers are compared to service counts for the same time period to measure cost per unit of service. Cost information is compared to revenue received by service and overall by participant.

Integration across Funding Streams

The model described in the preceding section is a general model for the integration of participant and fiscal data within a single provider organization. The system becomes more complex when one attempts to integrate multiple funding streams. The same service may be paid for by more than one payer or program (i.e., both Medicare and Medicaid pay for home health services). Figure 13.3 depicts the challenge of integrating across funding streams. The most effective way to reduce duplication of service provision, improve coordination of care across providers and payers, and quite possibly reduce the cost of care is not only to integrate information across different components within a single organization or for a single client, but also to integrate information across providers and different funding streams.

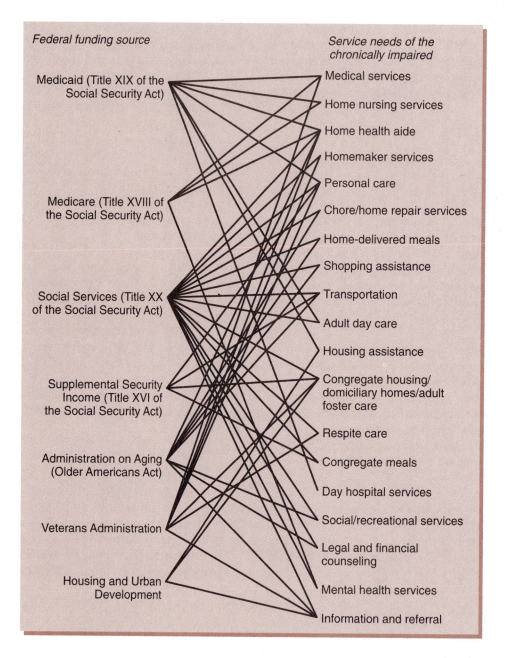

Figure 13.3   Major Federal Funding Sources for Long-Term Care Services
SOURCE: General Accounting Office, 1979.

INTEGRATED INFORMATION SYSTEMS: STATE OF THE ART

Many good information management applications and tools are available today. Other industries, however, have been more aggressive in the development and use of information systems than health and human services. Banking has adopted common standards and developed a worldwide financial network. The aerospace industry has organized large bodies of information and has developed expert systems to assist decision making. Police departments are using pen-based computers and wireless connections that allow them to access national databases and automatically record traffic tickets with a few marks of a pen on an electronic pad. Most industries now use *open architecture*—information systems built around core sets of data connected together that can be used by multiple applications and can work on many different kinds of computer equipment. Although these applications have little to do with health services, they demonstrate innovative technologies that could be applied.

Hospital Information Systems

Numerous applications have been developed for hospitals. Every major hospital and medical center has a computerized accounting system and a DRG billing system to help collect, organize, and document medical information to ensure appropriate reimbursement. Most hospitals also have other specialized information management applications; for example, for medical, laboratory, pharmacy, and facility management records. Most of these specialized applications are subsystems—highly developed information systems that address a specific area and need. Unfortunately, many of these subsystems do not share information, resulting in duplication of information and effort.

Recent trends in hospital information management have led to the integration of these subsystems into multifunction acute care information systems. Using a modern database management system, mul-

tiple applications can share information from different areas, producing powerful and efficient systems. Many of these excellent systems use the latest technology. This move toward integrated systems in hospitals is one that is both laudable and oriented to the future. Unfortunately, to date, these systems have focused on the short-term acute care encounter, and do not incorporate community-based chronic care services such as day care and in-home services, nor do they collect health and functional assessment information, or track information over time.

Health Plans and Managed Care

Health plans have developed large, sophisticated information systems to track information on their members over time. As with hospitals, most use multiple subsystems. The good systems are more integrated and maintain membership information, coordinate service scheduling, collect services provided by multiple providers, and track and monitor costs. These systems are designed for managing traditional health care services for a generally healthy population. Many of the principles and techniques of IIS would be applicable to chronic care management, but existing systems do not include long-term care services and are not designed to manage the more intensive and ongoing needs of a chronic care population. More promising is the IIS work of the social health maintenance organizations (S/HMOs), which includes case management and select long-term care services for a portion of their participants.

Long-Term Care Information Systems

Computer applications have been developed for specific long-term care providers. There are information systems for nursing homes, home health agencies, and adult day care centers. As with the other health services, many of the available applications focus on specific functions of these agencies, such as billing and external reporting. Multifunction integrated systems are also beginning to emerge in these industries, but these systems focus on only one service industry; few integrate information across even two services. Some innovative community service organizations, however, have developed common intake and assessment forms, and an IIS to link different community agencies serving the same client base.

One example of an IIS for long-term care is that of San Mateo County, California, located in the Bay area (near San Francisco). San Mateo's Department of Aging and Adult Services (DAAS) runs several case management programs, including the Medicaid waiver for home and community-based services, an AIDS case management program, the In-Home Supportive Services program (a state-funded, consumer-directed personal care program), and Linkages (a case management program for elders and disabled adults at risk of institutionalization who are not eligible for other case management programs). In addition to the case management programs, the county department runs Adult Protective Services and a guardianship program.

The DAAS is currently working to integrate information across all of these programs. It is adopting a single assessment instrument, the Minimum Data Set for Home Care (MDS-HC, the community-based analogue to the Minimum Data Set used in all Medicare/Medicaid-certified nursing homes), to collect information on functional, clinical, and social support needs of its clients. This assessment instrument will be the basis for care planning. The information system the county is implementing will incorporate information gathered with the assessment into routine reporting activities. The most important aspect of the new system will be its capability to share information across the various providers in DAAS through the Internet. An added feature of this new system is its ready capability to consolidate all reporting activities for which the county is responsible, at the local, state, and federal levels.

The state of Michigan also adopted the MDS-HC for care planning and reporting of the various home and community-based services programs the state runs. Unlike the San Mateo County system, which only links community-based services, Michigan's information system links the MDS-HC assessment information from multiple home and community-based programs with the nursing home MDS, enabling state planners and policymakers to understand the broader long-term care needs of Michigan residents, as well as their costs. The developers of the state's information system are currently working on an Internet-based application that will allow the sharing of information in real time.

Chronic Care Information Systems

Today, although some very good information systems have been developed for different segments of the health care industry, none of these systems by itself fully meets the needs of chronic care management. Chronic care management integrates all health care services—acute care and long-term care, medical and social services, institutional and community-based services—into a coordinated chronic care program. Chronic care management requires more information than is typically used by health plans because the managers' involvement lasts for years, not days, as is usually the case with hospitals. A comparable set of information requirements are found in the capitated long-term care demonstrations. These demonstrations have developed integrated systems for chronic care management, but all of their services are delivered through or controlled by a single provider. Much can be borrowed and learned from the information systems developed in these other health areas to build an effective IIS for chronic care groups.

In California, legislation was passed (A.B. 1040) to promote the integration of chronic and long-term care in demonstration projects at the county level. This legislation allowed the implementation of a pilot project aimed at integrating the financing and administration of chronic care services, to create a network of providers in up to six counties in the state.

Goals for this legislation include delivering services in the least restrictive environment appropriate for a particular consumer; providing alternatives to unnecessary use of acute care hospitals; providing a continuum of social and health services that foster independence and self-reliance for the consumer; achieving greater efficiencies through consolidated screening and reporting requirements; and identifying ways to expand funding options for the pilot program to include Medicare and other funding sources. This innovative program from California will serve as an example for other states of the integration of chronic care services, making accessibility and continuity of services optimal for the consumer.

Electronic Medical Records

An **electronic medical record (EMR)** offers the technical ability to integrate information across providers and settings. **Vertical integration** refers to the integration of all sources of information for a single individual across providers (e.g., primary care, hospital care, postacute or rehabilitative care, and long-term care). **Horizontal integration** refers to the integration of information across similar types of providers (e.g., across primary care providers or across nursing homes).

Several initiatives have already started working toward the development of a comprehensive EMR, as well as on strategies for overcoming many of the barriers that EMR adoption faces (Lieber, 2004). The Continuing Care Record initiative has been working to develop a common data set that can be passed electronically from one clinician to another when a patient is transferred between care settings. Having a common "vocabulary" is a cornerstone of the development of any IIS.

Another initiative has focused on creating systems that allow providers on different technical platforms to "talk" with each other. The Integrating the Healthcare Enterprise initative has developed technical frameworks that allow providers to transfer radiology images across systems developed by different vendors. Rather than require providers to purchase new software, so that it is common across locations, these frameworks provide a method by which systems on different technical platforms may exchange information.

While national initiatives seek to define a model EMR, individual organizations are pursuing their own. Internal EMRs are being implemented in a variety of health care settings across the country. The Veterans Health Administration was the first to implement a nationwide, system-wide EMR for all covered individuals, integrating acute and long-term care, community-based (e.g., outpatient physician office, home health care) and institutional care (e.g., hospital, SNF, hospice, rehabilitation), laboratory, and radiology. More limited examples of EMRs are seen in managed-care organizations, such as Kaiser Permanente, and in other covered populations; however, they do not necessarily cover the broadest range of health care, integrating both acute and long-term care.

A variation of the EMR that would facilitate integration of long-term care with acute care is an EMR that a person could take with him in the form of an electronic card that could be "read" by any health care provider with whom the person comes in contact. Currently, privacy issues (discussed more fully later in this chapter) are the primary barriers to development of this model of the EMR. Even in the face of these barriers, the initiatives described earlier are paving the way for widespread use of IIS.

Methods of Integrating Information

To this point, there has been little discussion of computerization. The information collected is important, but it is only as useful as the information system in which it is housed. Effective computerization does make the process of integrating information easier, but the key ingredient is *integration*—integration of key information for clinical, management, and policy decision making. Information from different service providers and the categories discussed earlier must be integrated into a common, client-specific information base. A number of methods can be used to integrate information. These include manual compilation of data, automated (i.e., computer) systems, and the Internet.

BENEFITS OF AN INTEGRATED SYSTEM

Any health and human service organization has a number of different audiences or consumers of information. An IIS potentially benefits all those in contact with the system.

Clients and Clinicians

Most importantly, the client can benefit from IIS. An integrated system would reduce the need for different providers to gather duplicative information. Information that is easily accessed can improve the quality of service plans. Automated scheduling can increase service plan compliance. Changes in health and functional status could be used as outcome measures and used to monitor quality.

Currently, the Minimum Data Set (MDS), the assessment instrument used by all Medicare- and Medicaid-certified nursing facilities in the United States, is sent to the Centers for Medicare and Medicaid Services (CMS) in an electronic format. The computerization of the MDS has made it possible to share information with consumers about the quality of care in nursing homes. This initiative makes facility-level quality indicators available on the Internet to help consumers choose a nursing home. The OASIS data system for home health has made it possible for a similar quality indicator system to be displayed for home care consumers. Before the computerization of the MDS and OASIS, these efforts and systems would not have been possible.

In addition, better information across services over time will enable clinicians to improve quality of care, because they will be able to evaluate the effectiveness of various clinical practices.

Program Managers

Program managers can use the IIS to actively manage, rather than merely administer, the managed chronic care program. The IIS would produce regular and timely reports on the number and charac-teristics of participants served, the type and number of services provided, and the cost of care. Managers could set cost and service use goals and use the IIS to monitor performance. Service plans could be automatically compared with service use to assess service plan compliance—one measure of the quality of care. A good IIS would reduce administrative costs by eliminating duplicate entry of data and by automating internal and external reports. Finally, the IIS would provide information to help the manager track costs and outcomes across individuals and over time to continually evaluate and refine the service program.

External Funders

External funders impose many reporting requirements so that they can monitor how their funds are being spent. Often the external payers that fund health and social services for older populations and the disabled are government agencies. These agencies implement numerous regulations that stipulate which services may be reimbursed, at what level they are reimbursed, and the process by which they are reimbursed. An IIS could be an extremely efficient way to maintain regulatory compliance. By coding services and revenues by funding source, the same IIS could be used to produce separate reports for each funding agency. In addition to gathering cost data across time and place, the IIS could also meet funder requests for demographic and assessment information.

The Balanced Budget Act (BBA) of 1997 was important legislation that will influence the way health care is provided for many years into the future. The BBA moved long-term care providers one step closer to integration by requiring nursing facilities and home health agencies to electronically report assessment data, in addition to the administrative data already collected. As mentioned previously, all Medicare- and Medicaid-certified nursing facilities must report MDS data (a comprehensive assessment used as the basis for care planning and reimbursement) to CMS. Likewise, all Medicare-certified home health agencies must report (an assessment used as the basis for outcomes assessment and quality assurance) data to CMS. The collection of this data in an electronic format aids the study of outcomes by linking assessments for a single client/resident over time, allowing providers to examine changes in clinical and functional status. Additionally, data can be aggregated to study quality of care at the facility level. The MDS data is being used for this very purpose in CMS's Nursing Home Compare Initiative, as mentioned earlier.

Insurers

Today, with the involvement of multiple funding streams and service providers (as shown in Figure 13.3), little is known about the total cost of chronic care. Until we can integrate information about the needs and costs of the population across providers and payers, we will not be able to integrate and better coordinate care for those with chronic or long-term care needs. The goal should be to allocate scarce resources fairly and efficiently in an integrated system for all long-term care consumers while focusing on continuity of care. Until comprehensive information about costs is known, the price of long-term care insurance will continue to be high and risk adjustment unrefined.

Policymakers

Policymakers want to know about the relationship between acute and long-term care and the impact of alternative service delivery and financing models. By integrating information on acute and long-term care, an IIS could provide this information. Does good chronic care reduce the use of hospital days? Does it enhance independence? By tracking costs and revenue information by funding source, the financial participation of different public and private funders can be determined. The model IIS could be used to assess the impact of different funding methods on participant characteristics, client satisfaction, services, and costs. Simply tracking costs across

providers will provide information that is very important but rarely captured—*the total cost of chronic and long-term care.*

BARRIERS TO IMPLEMENTATION

If the benefits of information are so clear, why haven't more providers and payers collaborated to develop these systems? The development of an IIS is not easy; it often involves many changes in and across organizations. Moreover, many new information systems have created more problems than benefits, especially during the initial development period. In the interest of presenting a balanced view, this section discusses some of the factors that have been impediments to the development of an IIS.

Commitment

Many senior executives, providers, and policymakers pay lip service to the benefits of information, but are not willing to make it a priority. An effective IIS cannot be built without a substantial commitment of time and resources.

Resources (People, Time, and Dollars)

The development of a good IIS will take considerable time, money, and organizational energy. Lack of resources is a common reason cited for not developing an IIS. (The upfront costs for developing an IIS can be considerable. One needs to consider the costs of purchasing needed software and hardware in addition to the costs of training personnel to use the new system.) However, there are opportunity costs associated with *not* integrating and using information. Duplicate recordings, missing information, lost reimbursement, and duplicate service provision are all expensive. Though difficult to measure precisely, the cost benefit of an IIS can be estimated, and this task should be done before

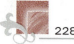

implementation. In the long run, the cost savings realized from the improvement in service coordination could be considerable.

Shared Objectives

The development of an IIS requires agreement on objectives from all the parties concerned. The clinician wants timely and complete participant information, the manager wants summary information on all areas, the fiscal manager wants to track and control costs. An IIS can meet the information needs of many audiences; however, these different objectives should be clearly stated, shared, and built into the system.

Interagency Cooperation

Perhaps the biggest barrier to integrating information is lack of cooperation by participating organizations. Most service organizations are unaccustomed to sharing information; funding silos are a major barrier to this effort. Changing the way providers do business to meet an external request is difficult. It is relatively easy for a single service to move once management has made a commitment. A collaboration is more complicated and requires the commitment of many. Cooperating agencies will have to see clear benefits before they can be expected to extend the effort required. Nationally publicized report cards, such as those produced by the National Committee for Quality Assurance (NCQA), have forced providers and payers to accept public sharing of data.

Willingness to Change

Change is difficult even when the alternative is clearly better. Most people prefer the familiar; change takes time and effort. An IIS will cause problems and the organization should be prepared for them. The best way to minimize resistance to change within an organization is to involve those who will be affected by the change in the development process.

Privacy and Security

Privacy concerns are raised by integration. Sharing of data across multiple services and providers will increase the threat to privacy of personal information. The Health Insurance Portability and Accountability Act (HIPAA)—a large and complex piece of legislation passed by Congress in 1996—included efforts to address potential problems arising from the computerization and standardization of medical records and other sources of personal health information. Among other provisions, HIPAA mandated the development of rules to protect the privacy of health information. The Department of Health and Human Services, which was tasked with fleshing out this mandate with specific rules, eventually established a privacy rule, which creates a new federal-level floor of protection for health information. The privacy rule defines health information, specifies who can access and share it, and details the conditions under which this information can be shared. The penalties for violating the privacy rule can be substantial, leaving many organizations, providers, and state policymakers nervous about developing integrated information systems.

HIPAA also details how protected health information should be kept secure and private. The security of this information (that is, the means by which information remains confidential) is the organization's responsibility. Administrative procedures and physical safeguards, such as password-controlled access to data, must be implemented in organizations that deal with protected health information. Protections (e.g., encryption for data transfer) and confidentiality agreements can be built into the IIS to safeguard privacy. However, the threat remains; increased access means greater potential abuse. Increased vigilance will be required and participants may be required to sign releases regarding their personal information. The benefits of IIS for the participant should outweigh the costs and justify these risks. The costs of improving system security are considerable, but security enhancements to information systems are required by law and should not be used as an excuse not to develop IISs.

CONCLUSION

With health care at the forefront of public concern and scrutiny, accurate records and cost containment are more important than ever. Competition among health care providers and greater oversight by public agencies now necessitates not only satisfactory service, but also a continuum of care to serve the many needs of acute and long-term care clients—all at a reasonable cost. The health and human services sector is finally joining other industries in realizing the importance of IISs in accessing data records and providing quality care. Recently enacted government regulation is aiding the move to integrated systems by requiring the computerization of client information. All of this means that health care organizations must equip themselves with IISs to maximize quality, manage costs, and meet external reporting demands from both payers and consumers.

WHERE TO GO FOR FURTHER INFORMATION

American Health Information Management Association
(866) PRECYSE
http://www.ahima.org

American Medical Informatics Association
4915 St. Elmo Avenue, Suite 401
Bethesda, MD 20814
(301) 657-1291
http://www.amia.org

Centers for Medicare and Medicaid Services (CMS)
7500 Security Boulevard
Baltimore, MD 21244-1850
(877) 267-2323 / (410) 786-3000
http://www.cms.gov

Get Care
700 Murmansk Street, Suite 4, Bldg. 590
Oakland, CA 94607
(510) 986-6700
http://www.getcare.com

Health Insurance Portability and Accountability Act of 1996 (HIPAA)
http://www.cms.gov/hipaa

Healthcare Information and Management Systems Society (HIMSS)
230 East Ohio Street, Suite 500
Chicago, IL 60611-3269
(312) 664-4467
http://www.himss.org

Medicare/Medicaid Integration Program
http://www.hhp.umd.edu/

Nursing Home Compare
Official U.S. Government Site for People with Medicare
http://www.medicare.gov/nhcompare/home.asp

Web MD
http://www.WebMD.com

FACTS REVIEW

1. What is an IIS?
2. What are the two major components of a model information system for managing chronic care? What are their subcomponents?
3. What contribution can an electronic medical record make toward creating an IIS? Give two examples of current progress toward creating an EMR.
4. List two audiences that would benefit from an integrated system, and describe why and how they would benefit.
5. List four barriers to the implementation of an IIS.

REFERENCES

General Accounting Office. (1979). *Entering a nursing home: Costly implications for Medicaid and the elderly.* Washington, D.C.: General Accounting Office.

Lieber, S. (2004). Someday we'll all be on the same page: The long journey toward common health data record-keeping is well under way. *Modern Helath Care, 34*(8), 24.

Wilber, K. H. (2000). Managing services for older adults. In R. Path (Ed.), *Handbook of social welfare management* (pp. 521–533). Thousand Oaks, CA: Sage.

CHAPTER 14

Financing

William E. Aaronson

Long-term care, as described throughout this book, includes a range of services, from personal support to complex medical care. Thus, when it comes to understanding the financing of long-term care, it is necessary to understand that payment for services varies considerably by the service under consideration and the recipient of that service. A vast array of federal, state, and local programs contribute to meeting long-term care needs, either directly or indirectly, through the payment for or provision of goods and services, in-kind transfers, or cash assistance. Long-term care insurance had a slow start, but is now established as an increasingly important source of payment. In addition, the user of services is frequently expected to pay in full or contribute financially for use of the service. No single program, public or private, has been designed to support the full range of long-term care services on a systematic basis.

Moreover, the costs of long-term care to the individual and family are difficult to ascertain because much of the care is rendered informally, and the remainder is likely to be provided by multiple sources, with changes in both informal and formal support over time. No comprehensive data exist on the lifetime costs of long-term care, except on a condition-specific basis, and even then estimating the total lifetime cost of long-term care is problematic.

Nonetheless, to envision a future of a well-organized system of long-term care, the financial realities of the present must be understood, despite the limitations of the data. Although this chapter presents issues related to the financing of some of the key services of the continuum, of necessity it stops short of a full treatment of the financing of the continuum.

QUANTIFIABLE EXPENDITURES FOR LONG-TERM CARE

Caring for people with chronic, multifaceted health problems over an extended period of time usually involves the use of a variety of services. National data on expenditures for nursing homes and home

Table 14.1 National Health Expenditures Aggregate Amounts by Type of Expenditure: Selected Calendar Years 1980–2001

Type of Expenditure	1960	1970	1980	1990	1995	1996	1997	1998	1999	2000	2001
						Amount in $ Billions					
National health expenditures total	26.9	73.2	245.8	696.0	990.1	1,039.4	1,092.7	1,150.0	1,219.7	1,310.1	1,424.5
Hospital care	9.3	28.0	101.5	253.9	343.6	355.2	367.6	378.4	393.7	416.5	451.2
Physician and clinical services	5.3	13.6	47.1	157.5	220.5	229.4	241.0	256.8	270.2	288.8	313.6
Other professional services	0.6	1.4	3.6	18.2	28.5	30.9	33.4	35.5	36.7	38.8	42.3
Dental services	2.0	4.7	13.3	31.5	44.5	46.8	50.2	53.2	56.4	60.7	65.6
Other personal health care	n/a	n/a	3.3	9.6	22.9	25.8	27.7	30.2	33.6	36.7	40.9
Nursing home and home health	0.9	4.4	20.1	65.3	105.1	113.5	119.6	122.7	121.9	125.5	132.1
Home health care	0.1	0.2	2.4	12.6	30.5	33.6	34.5	33.6	32.3	31.7	33.2
Nursing home care	0.8	4.2	17.7	52.7	74.6	79.9	85.1	89.1	89.6	93.8	98.9
Prescription drugs	2.7	5.5	12.0	40.3	60.8	67.2	75.7	87.3	104.4	121.5	140.6
Medical products & durable medical equipment	n/a	n/a	53.1	33.1	39.7	42.4	44.0	45.4	47.7	48.9	50.1
Government admin & net cost of private health insurance	1.2	2.7	12.1	40.0	60.4	61.1	60.8	64.3	73.2	80.7	89.7
Government public health activities	0.4	1.3	6.7	20.2	31.4	32.9	35.4	38.0	40.9	44.1	46.4
Investment	n/a	n/a	12.3	26.4	32.6	34.2	37.2	38.2	41.0	47.7	52.0
Research[1]	0.7	2.0	5.5	12.7	17.1	17.8	18.7	20.5	23.5	29.1	32.8
Construction	1.0	3.4	6.8	13.7	15.5	16.4	18.5	17.7	17.6	18.6	19.2

[1] Research and development expenditures of drug companies and other manufacturers and providers of medical equipment and supplies are excluded from research expenditures. These research expenditures are implicitly included in the expenditure class in which total expenditures occurred.

NOTE: Numbers may not add to totals because of rounding.

SOURCE: Centers for Medicare & Medicaid Services, Office of the Actuary, National Health Statistics Group, 2003.

health are reasonable proxies for the cost of providing long-term care, even though these data reflect the provision of some short-term care and exclude data on provision of select long-term care services, such as adult day services. Expenditures for hospitals include dollars spent on hospital-based nursing beds and hospital-based home care programs, some of which may be for long-term care. Dollars spent on social support programs, such as nonmedical adult day services or home-delivered meals, are not counted as "personal health care expenditures" in national data. Moreover, the costs to the individual and family, ranging from the costs of housing to time lost from work for caregiving, are not measured directly and can only be estimated from survey data.

Table 14.1 compares national health expenditures for selected years from 1960 to 2001. In 1960, combined expenditures on nursing home and home health care represented only about 0.4 of 1 percent of total health care spending. By 1997, spending on long-term care specific services had risen to 11 percent of total personal health expenditures. Expenditures for nursing home care in 1997 were $85.1 billion, compared to $0.8 billion in 1960; home care spending rose from $0.1 billion to $34.5 billion during that period of time.

However, following the enactment of the Balanced Budget Act (BBA) in 1997, expenditures on home health and nursing home care leveled off and fell compared to other health expenditures. Whereas total expenditures rose by 5.2, 6.1, and 7.4 percent respectively in the years 1998, 1999, and 2000, home health expenditures declined, by –2.8, –3.7, and –1.8 percent respectively. Nursing home care expenditures rose by more modest amounts: 4.7, 0.5, and 4.7 percent respectively. Long-term care spending (home health and nursing homes) remained at approximately 11 percent in 2001, as seen in Figure 14.1. These changes were partly due to the establishment of prospective payment systems for nursing homes and home care providers—and partly to changes in market dynamics. The result was severe financial stress on nursing homes generally and on home health agencies and providers in particular.

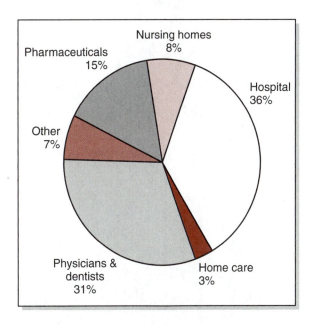

Figure 14.1   Distribution of Personal Health Expenditures, 2001

SOURCE: Centers for Medicare and Medicaid Services (CMS). *http://www.cms.gov*

Aggregate data may be misleading because they do not reflect relative use of services. For example, hospital charges are roughly $1,500 per day for a community hospital, while nursing costs range from $160 to $250 per day, and home care visits cost about $100 per visit. In addition, use varies considerably; hospital length of stay is time-limited, whereas nursing home and home health care tend to be longer in duration. Daily costs and sources of payment become relevant in determining long-term care arrangements because often more than one service configuration could be used to meet a consumer's needs.

Cost per unit of service is one consideration; payment source in a fragmented system of payment is another. Table 14.2 shows the relative payment contribution for selected services (total expenditures, hospital, nursing home, and home health) for selected years from 1965 to 2001. This enables one

Table 14.2 Personal Health Care Expenditures Aggregate and Per Capita Amounts and Percentage Distribution, by Source of Funds: Selected Calendar Years 1980–2001

Amount in Billions

Year	Total	Out-of-Pocket Payments	Third-Party Payments			Public			Medicare2	Medicaid3
			Total	Private Health Insurance	Other Private Funds	Total	Federal1	State and Local1		
Total										
1965	41.1	18.5	28.1	10.0	2.3	15.7	4.8	5.5	—	—
1980	214.6	58.2	156.4	60.6	9.2	86.6	62.8	23.8	36.3	24.7
1990	609.4	137.3	472.1	203.6	30.6	237.9	174.2	63.7	107.3	69.7
1998	1,009.4	175.2	834.2	341.3	54.8	438.2	335.0	103.2	204.3	160.0
1999	1,064.6	184.4	880.2	365.8	56.8	457.6	347.5	110.1	206.3	173.5
2000	1,137.6	194.7	942.9	397.1	56.3	489.5	371.1	118.4	216.8	188.3
2001	1,236.4	205.5	1,030.9	437.2	56.7	537.0	406.6	130.4	234.5	208.5
Hospital Care										
1965	14.0	8.8	2.8	5.7	0.3	8.4	2.2	3.1	—	—
1980	101.5	5.3	96.3	36.1	5.0	55.2	41.5	13.7	26.4	10.6
1990	253.9	11.2	242.7	97.1	10.3	135.2	102.7	32.4	67.8	27.6
1998	378.4	11.9	366.5	120.8	19.7	226.0	181.3	44.7	121.3	61.0
1999	393.7	12.5	381.2	128.7	20.6	231.8	185.3	46.6	122.0	66.0
2000	416.5	13.1	403.4	139.3	22.0	242.1	193.0	49.1	125.9	69.9
2001	451.2	13.8	437.4	152.1	22.1	263.1	209.4	53.7	135.0	77.1
Nursing Home Care										
1965	1.5	0.8	0.9	0.0	0.1	0.8	0.2	0.3	—	—
1980	17.7	7.1	10.6	0.2	0.8	9.6	5.7	3.9	0.3	8.9
1990	52.7	19.8	32.9	3.1	3.9	25.9	15.8	10.2	1.7	23.2
1998	89.1	24.9	64.2	7.4	4.6	52.3	35.0	17.2	10.2	40.1
1999	89.6	25.4	64.2	7.5	4.5	52.2	34.3	17.9	8.4	41.8
2000	93.8	26.2	67.6	7.3	4.1	56.2	37.7	18.5	9.5	44.6
2001	98.9	26.9	72.0	7.5	3.7	60.9	41.8	19.0	11.6	47.0

Home Health Care

Year										
1965	0.09	0.01	0.08	0.00	0.07	—	—	—	—	—
1980	2.4	0.4	2.0	0.3	0.4	1.3	0.8	0.5	0.6	0.3
1990	12.6	2.3	10.3	2.9	1.0	6.5	4.4	2.0	3.3	2.1
1998	33.6	6.6	26.9	8.3	1.4	17.3	13.2	4.1	10.1	5.4
1999	32.3	6.6	25.7	8.1	1.6	16.0	11.8	4.2	8.6	5.6
2000	31.7	6.3	25.4	7.8	1.3	16.3	12.0	4.3	8.6	6.1
2001	33.2	6.3	26.9	7.0	1.2	18.7	13.9	4.9	9.9	7.1

SOURCE: CMS, Office of the Actuary, National Health Statistics Group, 2003.

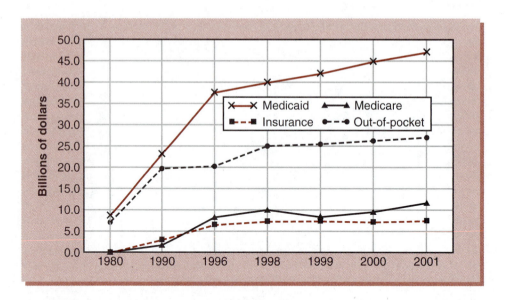

Figure 14.2   Nursing Home Sources of Payment by Selected Years
SOURCE: CMS. *http://www.cms.gov*

to compare the relative payment contributions of government versus private sources, as well as interagency differences within the federal and state governments. Figure 14.2 shows the dramatic growth in out-of-pocket payment for nursing home care in comparison to payment by Medicaid, Medicare, and health insurance (including long-term care insurance). All payers, largely due to the medical and rehabilitative aspects of care, equally support home health care spending (Figure 14.3).

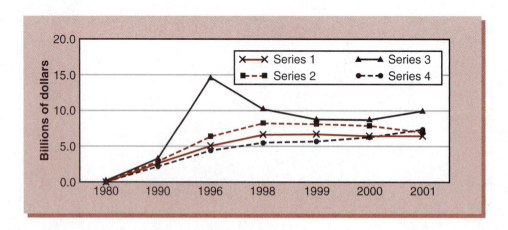

Figure 14.3   Home Health Sources of Payment by Selected Years
SOURCE: CMS. *http://www.cms.gov*

Older adults pay privately for a much higher percentage of long-term care costs than they do for acute care. In 2001, Medicare paid 11.7 percent of the bill and Medicaid, 47.6 percent. In recent years, the share paid by private health insurance, including long-term care insurance, has grown from less than 1 percent to 7.6 percent. Due to extensive Medicare and private insurance coverage of acute care services, the hospital patient's out-of-pocket share of total spending for inpatient hospital costs in 2001 was only 3 percent (for deductibles, co-insurance, and noncovered stays). However, about 27 percent of all spending for nursing home services is paid privately by the users of nursing home services and their families. For home health care, consumers pay about 19 percent of the total bill. The proportion of the nursing home bill for which patients are responsible has declined steadily since the introduction of Medicare and Medicaid. In 1970, consumers paid 53 percent of the total bill, in comparison to the government's share of 41.2 percent and private insurance at 0.3 percent.

The accelerated growth of expenditures for long-term care, coupled with the "demographic imperative" (the projected expansion of the older population, which is the heaviest user of long-term care services), portend continued future growth in spending for long-term care. Policymakers have grown increasingly concerned in recent years about the viability of the Medicare Trust Fund and the tax burden of Medicaid. In 1997, Congress enacted legislation as part of the BBA that was intended to curtail the growth in public spending on both short-term and long-term care through the Medicare and Medicaid programs without placing additional financial burdens on consumers. This legislation has had a profound influence on the way in which providers are compensated for services, and as a result, has serious long-term consequences for consumer access to the continuum of care.

RECENT LEGISLATION

The BBA of 1997 (Pub. L. No. 105-33) was signed into law by President Clinton in August 1997. This legislation created the greatest change in the Medicare and Medicaid payment programs since their inception in 1965. The payment methodologies and levels were changed for hospitals, nursing homes, home health agencies, rehabilitation hospitals, long-term care facilities, physicians, and health plans (health maintenance organizations—HMOs). Although the changes were phased in over time, in general, they seriously undermine flexibility in payment for a broad-based continuum of care. According to the HCFA summary of the legislative changes, the purposes were to:

- Extend the life of the Medicare Trust Fund and reduce Medicare spending
- Increase health care options available to America's seniors
- Improve benefits for staying healthy
- Fight Medicare fraud and abuses

The major thrust of the BBA was simple: reduce Medicare and Medicaid expenditures, and save the Medicare Trust Fund. The provisions of the legislation were directed at providers and were not intended to reduce consumer benefits. However, the ability of providers to participate fully in the continuum was constrained, and access for consumers diminished.

Some of the more important provisions included revisions in Medicare payment to skilled nursing facilities (SNFs) and Medicare HMOs: requiring prospective payment systems (PPSs) for other long-term care providers previously exempt from PPS, including long-term care hospitals, psychiatric hospitals, rehabilitation hospitals, and home care; significantly cutting in home health care; changing hospital medical education and disproportionate share payments; imposing consumer protections and access to information through CMS, and supporting managed care initiatives, such as Program of All-inclusive Care for the Elderly (PACE) and Medicare+Choice. Home health care was a special target. Congress mandated the introduction of a PPS for home care services, and in the interim ordered a 15 percent reduction in payment for home care services.

In 1999 Congress reconsidered many of the provisions of the BBA relating to the Medicare and Medicaid programs in the context of the long-term viability of the Medicare Trust Fund and the objective to manage the federal budget. *The Balanced Budget Refinement Act of 1999* ameliorated the financial impact of the initial BBA on providers.

In 2000, in an effort to prevent further erosion of Medicare+Choice plans, Congress passed the *Medicare, Medicaid, and SCHIP Benefits Improvement and Protection Act (BIPA)*. (SCHIP stands for the State Child Health Insurance Program.)

The *Balanced Budget Refinement Act of 1999* was passed at a time of optimism about the achievability of a balanced budget and a zero national deficit. Those hopes vanished with the recession of 2001 and a return to deficit spending. State budgets were particularly hard hit by a combination of reduced tax revenues and commitments made when the economy was still booming. Medicare and Medicaid will come under increasing pressure because they are big-ticket items for both federal and state legislatures.

The *Health Insurance Portability and Accountability Act of 1996 (HIPAA)*, though predating the BBA, only began to have direct impact on providers in 2002 and 2003, when regulations regarding security of patient information were fully implemented. In some ways, HIPAA may be perceived as inhibiting integration of care. However, other provisions in this act may have a further-reaching effect in terms of increasing the affordability of long-term care insurance, and thus providing future benefit to long-term care providers.

In 2003, Congress passed the *Medicare Prescription Drug Improvement and Modernization Act*. This law rivaled the BBA in the sweeping changes it brought to the Medicare program. At a projected cost of $400 billion over 10 years, this bill initiated payment by Medicare for prescription drugs for Medicare enrollees. It also promoted the role of private insurance and managed care in serving Medicare beneficiaries. As the implementation of the laws

rolls out, the impact on chronic care disease management and the continuum of services will be examined.

PAYMENT SOURCES FOR LONG-TERM CARE

More than 80 different federal programs, and an uncounted number of state and local programs, contribute to the financing of long-term care services. Only the major current and potential sources of funding are highlighted here. What each does not cover is as important as what it does cover. The principal source of public payment for medical and rehabilitative services for older Americans and those with permanent disabilities is the Medicare program. For long-term nursing and personal care services, Medicaid is the primary public purchaser of services. However, private long-term care insurance is beginning to emerge as an important source of payment for nursing homes, assisted living, and home care.

Consumers also have access to provider-sponsored integrated delivery systems that allow for pooling of public and private resources, such as Medicare managed-care plans (Medicare HMOs), social HMOs (S/HMOs), and PACEs. These programs range in degree of integration from broad health and medical coverage in the case of Medicare HMOs to complete integration of social, personal, and health services in the case of PACE. Several states have initiatives to pool long-term care service and funding programs that emanate from state government. As of 2003, Wisconsin, Minnesota, California, Florida, and Maryland have implemented major changes to facilitate coordination of long-term care services and/or payment programs.

Personal out-of-pocket expenses continue to be a major source of financing of many forms of long-term care and senior housing options. The financial condition of seniors has improved considerably since the inception of Medicare and Medicaid. As shown in Table 14.3, the percent of the older population living in poverty has declined from 28.5 percent in 1966 to 9.9 percent in 2000. Growing senior

Table 14.3   Age 65 and Older Living in Poverty

Year	Persons in Poverty (millions)	Percentage of Total
1966	5.1	28.5
1970	4.8	24.6
1980	3.9	15.7
1985	3.5	12.6
1990	3.7	12.2
1991	3.8	12.4
1992	3.9	12.9
1993	3.8	12.2
1994	3.7	11.7
2000	3.3	9.9

SOURCE: CMS, 2003; Department of Commerce, Bureau of the Census, 2003.

wealth means greater demand for asset protection. This is expected to foster a more favorable climate for growth in the private insurance market and in alternative and more efficient delivery systems.

MEDICARE

Medicare is a public entitlement program for people age 65 and older, and those who are permanently disabled due to blindness, select other disabilities, or kidney failure. It was enacted in 1965 as Title XVIII of the Social Security Act of 1935. From its inception in 1965, the primary purpose of the Medicare program has been to provide older citizens with protection from the high costs of acute medical illness, particularly costs associated with inpatient hospital care. Hence, in determining what Medicare will and will not pay for, a boundary has historically been drawn between services that are oriented toward the treatment of acute illness and services that are primarily custodial in nature. In 2003, 41.7 million Americans, or about 14 percent of the total population, qualified for Medicare. Every older American who is eligible for Medicare is eligible for retirement benefits under Social Security. Growth in Medicare enrollment slowed in the 1990s as a result of the Great Depression era decline in birth rate. However, baby boomers (born between 1945 and 1960) will turn 65 years of age beginning in 2010, which will place an increasing strain on the system. Very high birth rates following the close of World War II, combined with economic growth and growing longevity, have fueled substantial population growth among that age cohort.

The most recent estimate from the Congressional Budget Office is that the Medicare Hospital Insurance and Supplementary Medical Insurance Trust Fund will be bankrupt by 2015 without major structural changes (revenues and expenditures) in the system. Income to the Hospital Insurance Trust Fund exceeded outlays for the first time in several years in 1998. However, this was a short-lived phenomenon. Hospital expenditures rose by 8.3 percent in 2001, an increased level not seen for a decade. The BBA was a contributing factor to the decline in outlays in 1998, but the legislation in late 1999 restored many of the cuts in provider payments.

The Medicare program provides some limited long-tem care coverage as an entitlement, without means testing. However, the long-term care benefits are focused on short-term episodes, not long-term management. Nonetheless, Medicare is relevant to a discussion of long-term care financing for three reasons. First, because so many older people have chronic health problems, payers of care for older adults are inevitably payers for long-term illnesses. Second, as a result of managed care and other social trends, there is a growing emphasis on primary health care as a point of entry into a continuum of health and health-related services, and Medicare funds primary care. This trend is further supported in legislation such as the BBA, which encourages integrated delivery systems (e.g., PACE). Third, Medicare explicitly does not pay for custodial long-term care services. However, the BBA encouraged greater participation in Medicare risk contracts by nontraditional insuring entities. Medicare HMOs have typically included more short-duration long-term care than would be available via traditional Medicare. Although CMS has attempted to make coverage information readily available (see *http://cms.gov/consumer*), consumers as well as many professionals remain confused about what Medicare does and does not cover. Many older people still do not realize that Medicare does not protect them from most of the costs associated with long-term care.

Congress passed Medicare legislation in 1965 on a crest of concern about the welfare of older U.S. citizens. Its purpose was to protect older people from the high costs of acute medical illness, particularly the costs associated with inpatient hospital care. It was never intended to cover long-term care.

Table 14.4 shows the services covered by Medicare and the co-payment rates as of 2003. The benefit structure was affected by the BBA, most notably coverage for home health care. Home health care following a hospitalization will continue to be covered under Medicare Part A, hospital insurance. However, home health visits not related to a hospital stay were shifted into Part B (supplemental medical insurance—SMI) coverage over a six-year period of time. Roughly 95 percent of Part A beneficiaries are also enrolled in Part B, but enrollment is not universal.

The majority of Medicare dollars are spent on

Table 14.4   Medicare Part A Benefit Structure for the Year 2004

Services	Benefits	Medicare Pays	Patient Pays
Hospitalization			
Semiprivate room and board, general nursing and other hospital services and supplies	First 60 days 61st to 90th days > 90th day in benefit period Lifetime reserve of days	All but $876 All but $219 per day All but $438 of lifetime reserve days; nothing once lifetime reserve used	$876 $219 per day $438 per day for reserve days; all cost beyond
Skilled Nursing Facility Care			
The patient must have been in a hospital for at least three days, enter a Medicare-certified SNF, and meet other program requirements	First 20 days 21st to 100th day Beyond 100th day	100 percent coverage All but $109.50 per day Nothing	$0 Up to $109.50 per day All costs
Home Health Care			
Medically necessary skilled care, home health aide services, medical supplies, etc.; BBA excluded visits to draw blood only	First 100 visits after hospital discharge covered under Part A; other Medicare-approved visits covered under Part B (BBA change)	100 percent of approved visits covered; 80 percent of approved amount for durable medical equipment (DME)	$0 for visits; 20 percent for DME $0 if covered by Part B (SMI); if no Part B coverage, all costs

SOURCE: CMS. *http://www.cms.gov*

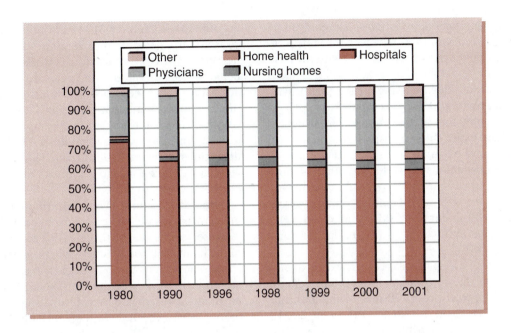

Figure 14.4   Medicare Provider Payment Distribution for Selected Years

SOURCE: CMS. *http://www.cms.gov*

hospitals and doctors (see Figure 14.4). Table 14.5 shows that of the $234.5 billion spent by Medicare in 2001 only $11.6 billion was spent on nursing homes and $9.9 billion on home health care. The amount spent on home health care and nursing home care combined amounted to 11.2 percent of the Medicare budget for 1997, representing a dou-

bling of proportion of the Medicare budget for long-term providers from 4.3 percent in 1990. However, largely due to reductions in home health, spending on nursing home and home health accounted for only 9.2 percent of total Medicare expenditures in 2001. The growth in Medicare expenditures for home care and for nursing home care was one of

Table 14.5   Medicare Provider Expenditures for Selected Years (in billions)

	Hospitals	Physicians	Home Health	Nursing Homes	Total Medicare
1970	5.4	1.7	0.1	0.1	7.7
1980	26.4	8.0	0.7	0.3	37.5
1990	68.7	29.2	3.0	1.7	111.5
1997	123.7	46.4	12.8	11.2	214.6
2001	135.0	63.9*	9.9	11.6	234.5

* Category enlarged to include clinical services.

SOURCE: CMS. *http://www.cms.gov*

the principal reasons that Congress targeted these providers for reductions in payment through prospective payment systems within the framework of the BBA.

The Medicare skilled nursing facility (SNF) benefit provides up to 100 days of coverage per spell of illness. To qualify for coverage, a Medicare beneficiary must have experienced a hospital stay of not less than 3 days and be admitted to the SNF within 30 days of the hospital discharge for the same diagnosis. The first 20 days are fully covered. The beneficiary is liable for a co-payment amount for all covered days after the 20th day. In 2003, the Medicare SNF co-payment amount was $109.50 per day for days 21 through 100.

Payment for nursing home care increased as a proportion of the Medicare budget, from 0.8 percent in 1980 to 1.6 percent in 1990 and to 5.2 percent in 1997; it remained at that level through 2001. Three factors have contributed to the increase in Medicare skilled nursing use.

First, Medicare beneficiaries must meet relatively restrictive functional criteria for Medicare SNF coverage. The Medicare SNF regulations stipulate that a beneficiary must require skilled nursing care or skilled rehabilitation services. The regulations explicitly state that individuals who require custodial care only are *not* eligible for Medicare SNF coverage. The distinction between custodial care and need for skilled care and rehabilitation is not precise.

In the mid-1980s, denial of Medicare claims for skilled nursing care, and especially for home care, reached very high levels. This led to a lawsuit against the Department of Health and Human Services (*Smith v. Bowen*). In settling that suit in 1988, the Health Care Financing Administration (now CMS) issued a directive that liberalized the definitions of who required skilled nursing and rehabilitative care.

The second factor was the passage of the Medicare Catastrophic Coverage Act (MCCA) of 1988. This eliminated the three-day hospital stay requirement. Although the MCCA was repealed in 1989, it produced a significant rise in the use of Medicare-authorized skilled nursing home use.

A third factor was the growth of subacute nursing units (see Chapter 5). As a way to use excess capacity and generate new revenue streams, many hospitals converted unused beds to skilled nursing beds. Medicare paid for one year of start-up costs and three years of cost-based reimbursement. A hospital could discharge patients from DRG capitated payment and readmit them to the hospital's skilled nursing units, for which it would be paid on a per diem basis, set according to costs. This system provided a significant incentive for hospitals to transfer eligible patients to skilled care.

These three policy events contributed to a dramatic increase in Medicare payment for skilled nursing care during the 1990s. The BBA removed many of the financial incentives for having a subacute unit. Nonetheless, the transfer patterns and clients' needs are unlikely to change quickly. The skilled nursing payments by Medicare may decline slightly but are more likely to continue to remain stable during the early part of the 2000 decade.

Table 14.6 shows the sources of payment for home health care from 1970 to 2001, projected to the year 2012. As shown in Figure 14.3, Medicare was the largest purchaser of home health services in 1996, but was on par with other purchasers after that year. In 1980, the Medicare program covered 29 percent of expenditures for Medicare-certified home care agencies. By 1996, the proportion covered by Medicare had grown to 45 percent. However, the BBA of 1997 had a devastating effect on the financing of home care. The decline was also reflected in the Medicare proportion of total expenditures, which fell to 29.8 percent in 2001 and is projected by the CMS Office of the Actuary to remain at that level through 2012. Congress was simply concerned that if home care expenditures continued to rise at the pace experienced in the 1990s, this line item alone could overwhelm the Medicare budget.

Although Medicare pays fully for medically necessary home care, home care services are covered only under the following conditions: the patient has the potential for recovery or improvement, only intermittent (not 24-hour) care is required; the patient requires skilled nursing or physical therapy; the patient is bedbound. These criteria often have been

Table 14.6 Home Health Care Expenditures Aggregate and Per Capita Amounts, Percent Distribution and Average Annual Percent Change by Source of Funds: Selected Calendar Years 1980–2012 (in billions)

Amount in Billions

Year	Total	Out-of-Pocket Payments Total	Third-Party Payments Total	Private Health Insurance	Other Private Funds	Public Total	Public Federal[2]	Public State and Local[2]	Medicare[3]	Medicaid[4]
Historical Estimates										
1980	2.4	0.4	2.0	0.3	0.4	1.3	0.8	0.5	0.6	0.3
1990	12.6	2.3	10.3	2.9	1.0	6.5	4.4	2.0	3.3	2.1
1998	33.6	6.6	26.9	8.3	1.4	17.3	13.2	4.1	10.1	5.4
1999	32.3	6.6	25.7	8.1	1.6	16.0	11.8	4.2	8.6	5.6
2000	31.7	6.3	25.4	7.8	1.3	16.3	12.0	4.3	8.6	6.1
2001	33.2	6.3	26.9	7.0	1.2	18.7	13.9	4.9	9.9	7.1
Projected[1]										
2002	36.2	6.4	29.8	7.0	1.2	21.6	15.9	5.7	11.1	8.7
2003	38.3	6.4	31.8	7.1	1.3	23.4	17.2	6.2	11.9	9.5
2004	40.9	6.7	34.2	7.4	1.4	25.4	18.8	6.7	13.0	10.3
2005	43.7	7.1	36.6	7.8	1.4	27.3	20.1	7.2	13.9	11.2
2006	46.9	7.6	39.3	8.5	1.6	29.3	21.6	7.7	14.8	12.2
2007	50.1	8.1	42.0	9.0	1.7	31.3	23.1	8.3	15.7	13.2
2008	53.3	8.5	44.9	9.6	1.8	33.5	24.6	8.9	16.7	14.3
2009	56.7	8.9	47.8	10.1	1.9	35.8	26.2	9.5	17.6	15.5
2010	60.4	9.5	50.9	10.7	2.0	38.2	28.0	10.2	18.6	16.8
2011	64.5	10.2	54.3	11.3	2.1	40.8	29.9	11.0	19.8	18.2
2012	68.9	10.9	58.1	12.1	2.3	43.7	31.9	11.8	21.0	19.8

[1] The health spending projections were based on the 2001 version of the National Health Expenditures (NHE) released in January 2003.

[2] Includes Medicaid SCHIP Expansion and SCHIP.

[3] Subset of federal funds.

[4] Subset of federal and state and local funds. Includes Medicaid SCHIP Expansion.

SOURCE: CMS. Office of the Actuary, 2003.

vague and enforcement difficult. The 1997 BBA provisions limiting payment and changing the payment system created financial problems for home health providers. Many reduced service availability, and nearly one-fourth of Medicare-certified home care agencies closed. In particular, the BBA mandated development of a prospective payment methodology for home care, reduction in the labor component of the cost basis for reimbursement (interim payment system), and overall reduction in home care expenditures. As a result of the BBA's draconian cuts in Medicare payment, Medicare home care expenditures declined after 1998.

Medicare was once again changed at the end of 2003 with the passage of the Medicare Prescription Drug, Improvement, and Modernization Act of 2003 (MMA). This act brought radical changes affecting all facets of the health care delivery system, including providers, insurers, manufacturers, and consumers alike. The bill moved Medicare beyond a program focused strictly on acute care and recognized the need to pay for prevention and chronic care as well. Payment for prescription drugs for Medicare enrollees was a major element of the law, as noted in its name. However, the law also made major changes in coverage of other benefits, such as suspending the cap on therapy services, adding coverage of select diagnostic services, and streamlining access to new technologies. Major modifications were also made to the payment systems for almost all providers. Full provisions can be found on the CMS Web site at *http://www.csm.hhs.gov/medicarereform.*

The MMA established the Chronic Care Improvement Program, "the first large-scale chronic care improvement initiative under the Medicare Fee-for-Service Program" (*http://www.cms.hhs.gov/medicarereform*). This demonstration has initially funded 10 regional organizations to offer self-care guidance and support to Medicare beneficiaries with chronic illnesses, specifically congestive heart failure, diabetes, and chronic obstructive pulmonary disease. Improving communication of clinical information across providers is an explicit provision of this program.

The MMA will be implemented over an extended period of years. The impact on chronic care for individuals and the population thus remains to be determined. Regardless of how the details evolve, the legislation is positive overall for the continuum of care in recognizing that, to achieve quality, acute care and long-term care cannot be separated.

MEDICAID

Medicaid is a major payer of long-term care services, particularly nursing home care. Medicaid was enacted in 1965 as Title XIX of the Social Security Act of 1935 for the purpose of paying for health care for low-income people. It is administered and funded jointly by the federal government and the governments of each of the states, territories, and District of Columbia. Each state operates a separate program that conforms to broad federal guidelines for participation. These guidelines set parameters within which the states determine eligibility, set the scope of benefits, and manage the system of payment for health care providers. In general, each state also determines the payment methods and rates for services provided to Medicaid recipients and the criteria under which providers are eligible to participate. Thus, Medicaid is not a single program, but a collection of 50 state programs that fall within a range of options determined by the federal government.

Medicaid is a means-tested program: only the poor qualify for Medicaid coverage. Table 14.7 shows a breakdown in Medicaid eligibility between the years 1975 and 2003. There are two levels of Medicaid eligibility. The primary eligibility for Medicaid is receipt of cash assistance, such as Supplemental Security Income (SSI), or Temporary Assistance for Needy Families (TANF) for a younger population. Medical Assistance Only (MAO) eligibility arises when people are ineligible for cash assistance, but generate extensive medical costs and become indigent in the process. States have the option to provide MAO eligibility and the discretion to set the level of allowable income and assets. The majority of U.S. residents age 65 and older are eli-

Table 14.7 Medicaid Recipient Trends for Selected Years, 1975–2003 (in millions).

	1975	1980	1985	1995	1997	2001*	2003
Total	22.1	21.6	21.8	36.2	38.7	46.1	50.7
Age 65 years +	3.6	3.4	3.1	4.2	4.6	4.8	5.0
Blind	0.1	0.1	0.1	0.1	0.1	0.1	0.1
Disabled	2.4	2.8	2.9	5.9	6.5	7.8	8.4
Dependent children	9.6	9.3	9.8	17.6	18.7	23.1	25.2
Adults with children	4.5	4.9	5.5	7.8	8.3	10.4	12.0
Other Title XIX	1.8	1.5	1.2	0.6	0.6	n/a	n/a

* The large increase in enrollment between 1997 and 2001 can be attributed in part to a change in definition.

NOTE: Eligibility categories may not add to totals as some recipients are classified in more than one category.

SOURCE: CMS, 2003. Enrollment and beneficiary projections were prepared by the Office of the Actuary for the President's fiscal year 2003 budget.

gible for Social Security and thus are less likely to have high income than younger adults who are working. Thus, older Medicaid recipients are eligible either as medically indigent or as MAO.

The medically needy are those whose income and resources are great enough to cover daily living expenses (according to income levels set by the state) but not large enough to pay for medical care. If the income and resources of a medically needy individual are above a state-prescribed level, the individual must first incur a certain amount of medical expense that lowers the income to the medically needy level. This is referred to as the "spend-down" requirement.

As a result of state variations, people with identical circumstances may be eligible to receive Medicaid benefits in one state but not in another. Even individuals in the same state with similar incomes may not be equally eligible for benefits, because of welfare rules.

The financial criteria used to determine whether an applicant qualifies for Medicaid coverage in a nursing home are complex, and vary across the 50 state Medicaid programs. Furthermore, many people who do not qualify for Medicaid prior to nursing home admission become eligible once they enter a nursing home, because their income and assets are

insufficient to pay the costs of nursing home care over an extended period of time. In addition, many people pay for their nursing home care privately for months or years, and then become eligible for Medicaid after their private resources are depleted. Such persons are considered to have spent down to Medicaid eligibility. Essentially, Medicaid acts as a safety net for those entering nursing homes in the event that their personal resources are insufficient to pay for continuing care.

As shown earlier in Table 14.7, in 2003 about 12 percent of those age 65 and older were enrolled in the Medicaid program at some point during the year—about 5.0 million people. This also represents about 10 percent of total Medicaid recipients for 2003. The proportion of Medicaid recipients age 65 and older has been declining slightly, while the proportion of older adults living in poverty has declined substantially. Table 14.8 shows the distribution of benefits according to eligibility categories. Although older persons represented only 12 percent of Medicaid recipients in 1997, they accounted for 30.4 percent of Medicaid expenditures in 1999. The percent of Medicaid dollars spent on those age 65 and older dropped to 27.7 percent by 1999, but the percent spent on the blind/disabled increased from 41 to 43 percent. Again, this is largely because

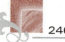
Table 14.8 Distribution of Medicaid Benefits by Eligibility, 1995 and 1999

	Fiscal Year Vendor Payments (in millions)		Percent Distribution	
	1995	1999	1995	1999
Total	120,141	152,629	100.0	100.0
Age 65 years and over	36,527	42,347	30.4	27.7
Blind/disabled	49,418	65,668	41.1	43.0
Dependent children under 21 years of age	17,976	21,018	15.0	13.8
Adults in families with dependent children	13,511	15,637	11.2	10.2
Other Title XIX	1,499	5,131	1.2	3.4

NOTE: Totals do not necessarily equal the sum of the rounded components.
SOURCE: CMS, 2003.

eligibility for Medicaid is related to long-term care use, especially nursing home care.

Unlike Medicare, state Medicaid programs have always provided coverage for both skilled care related to acute illnesses and custodial care for persons with long-term disabilities. However, the breadth of the Medicaid benefit package varies from state to state, and access to Medicaid payment for these services is limited to people who lack the financial resources to pay for their own care.

The federal government's share of medical expenses is tied to a formula based on the per capita income of the state. As a minimum, the federal government will pay 50 percent of the Medicaid expenses incurred by the state. This ranges up to 78 percent in the lower per capita income states. Although poorer states have a smaller percent liability for long-term care expenses, they have substantially smaller tax bases and thus have tended to provide service configurations closer to the minimum required for participation in the Medicaid program. Thus, wealthier states, despite lower federal contribution, have tended to be more innovative and provide richer arrays of service configurations.

Medicaid requires states to offer a specified minimum core set of services. Beyond the requisite core, states vary greatly with regard to the services they include in their plans and the groups eligible to receive these services. Major long-term care services provided under Medicaid include nursing facility care and home health care. Other long-term care services that may be covered by a state include private nursing services, clinic care, physical therapy and related services, inpatient care for patients 65 or older in institutions for mental disease, inpatient psychiatric services for individuals under age 21, personal care services at home, adult day services, and assisted living. However, not all states cover these services equally.

In addition, states may cover certain other home and community-based services under one of several waiver programs. Section 2176 of the Omnibus Budget Reconciliation Act of 1981 is also referred to as home and community-based services (HCBS) or 1915(c) waivers. This waiver program enables states to provide services to people who would otherwise be eligible for nursing home placement. However, each waiver request must be reviewed and approved by the secretary of the U.S. Department of Health and Human Services. At present, all states have waiver programs. The waivers may, however, not cover all populations or all geographic areas of the state.

Several studies have analyzed the results of 2176 waiver programs. The results are mixed at best. However, it is clear that Section 2176-waivered services are quite useful in putting together a community-based continuum of care for people who may be eligible for nursing home placement. Section 2176 also allows community dwellers to qualify for Medicaid more easily. Thus, the program is a helpful component in assembling a care continuum for frail seniors and younger people with disabilities who are poor or near-poor.

MEDICAID-COVERED SERVICES

Medicaid was designed by Congress to be a medical assistance program to the poor. As such, covered services are similar in many respects to those of the Medicare program. Table 14.9 lists the federally mandated benefits and optional services for which the federal Medicaid program will reimburse state expenditures. Medicaid covers a wide range of medical services, including physician services, hospital care, diagnostic and treatment modalities, home health care, and skilled nursing facility care. The distinction is that Medicaid will—and principally does—pay for long-term custodial care in a nursing home.

Table 14.10 shows the distribution of Medicaid provider payments between the years 1970 and 2001. Between 1990 and 2001, nursing home payments declined as a proportion of total payments,

Table 14.9 Federal Medicaid Mandated and Optional Services

Mandatory Services	Optional Services
Inpatient hospital services	Podiatrist services
Outpatient hospital services	Optometrist services
Rural health clinic and Federally Qualified Health Center (FQHC) services	Psychologist services
Laboratory and x-ray services	Medical social worker services
Nurse practitioner services	Private duty nursing
Nursing facility (NF) services and home health services for individuals age 21 and older	Clinic services
Physician services and medical and surgical services of a dentist	Physical therapy
	Occupational therapy
	Speech, hearing, and language disorder therapies
	Prescribed drugs
	Dentures
	Prosthetic devices
	Screening services
	Preventive services
	Rehabilitative services
	Intermediate care facilities/Mental retardation services (ICF/MR)
	NF services for people under age 21
	Personal care services
	Transportation services
	Case management services
	Hospice care services
	Inpatient and NF services for people age 65 and older in institutions for mental diseases (IMDs)

SOURCE: CMS, 2003.

Table 14.10 Medicaid Provider Expenditures for Selected Years (in billions)

	Hospitals	Physicians*	Home Health	Nursing Homes	Total Medicaid
1970	1.4	0.3	0.01	0.5	2.9
1980	5.6	1.4	0.2	4.9	14.5
1990	16.6	4.1	1.1	13.0	42.7
1997	36.2	9.3	2.6	22.6	91.1
2001	44.8	12.5	3.9	28.1	121.3

*Category enlarged to include clinical services.
SOURCE: CMS, 2003.

while home health care payments increased (see Figure 14.5). This is due to the increased availability of community-based services, the broader coverage provided by 1915(c) waivers, and the growing tendency for states to participate in the waiver program.

Unlike Medicare, which provides limited nursing home coverage for all Medicare beneficiaries, the Medicaid program provides relatively broad nursing home coverage to a limited population—the poor who cannot afford to pay the total costs of their own care. More than 78 percent of all public spending for nursing home care flows through the Medicaid program (U.S. Department of Health and Human Services, 1994). Medicaid also accounts for more than 40 percent of all public and private spending for nursing homes. In 1992, about 1.5 million persons over the age of 65 received some public assistance for the costs of their nursing home care through Medicaid.

As shown in Table 14.11, in 1998, state Medicaid programs spent $40.1 billion for nursing home care. Medicaid expenditures for older persons in nursing homes increased from $8.8 billion in 1980 and to a projected $91.9 billion in the year 2012. In 1998, Medicaid spending for nursing home care for seniors exceeded Medicare SNF expenditures by a ratio of approximately 4 to 1. This contrasts considerably to 1990, when the ratio was 12 to 1. During the same period of time, the proportion of

private, out-of-pocket payment declined from 43.2 percent of total to 27.9 percent. Medicaid contributions as a proportion of total payment remained around 45 percent between 1990 and 1996. Thus, public payers are picking up a larger portion of the total bill for nursing home care. While Medicaid continues to be the most important payment source, Medicare as a source of payment grew the most rapidly during that period of time.

Medicaid also pays for home health care services. The financing of home care services under the Medicaid program occurs primarily under three different coverage options in state Medicaid plans: (1) home health care services; (2) personal care services; and (3) home and community-based waiver services. Home health care services are a mandatory service, meaning that all states are required to cover home health services for certain groups of Medicaid enrollees. They are similar in scope to Medicare-covered home care, except that conditions for eligibility may be more lax. Personal care services and home and community-based waiver services, in contrast, are optional services, meaning that states may elect to provide coverage for these services, but are not required to do so.

Personal care services are semiskilled or non-skilled services provided to Medicaid beneficiaries who need assistance with basic activities of daily living (ADLs) in their own homes. Personal care providers are generally nonlicensed persons who pro-

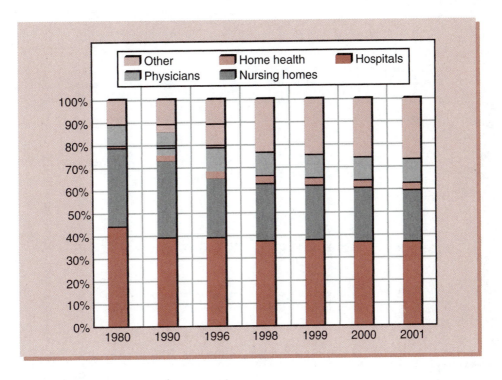

Figure 14.5   Medicare Provider Payment Distribution for Selected Years
SOURCE: CMS. *http://www.cms.gov*

vide individuals who have functional disabilities help with bathing, grooming, dressing, housekeeping, toileting, and other basic living activities. They may be employed by a community agency, or they may work under direct contract to the state Medicaid agency. Federal regulations defining reimbursable personal care services are relatively broad, and only stipulate that they be:

- Prescribed by a physician
- Provided under a written plan of treatment
- Provided by a qualified individual
- Supervised by a registered nurse
- Provided by someone who is not a member of the recipient's family

The Omnibus Budget Reconciliation Act of 1990 modified Medicaid coverage of personal care serv-

ices by expanding the definition of *personal care* to include services provided outside the recipient's home. This modification allows a personal care provider to be paid for shopping, transportation, and other services provided outside the home. This provision took effect in all states in 1995.

Home and community-based waiver services (HCBS) were first authorized under the Omnibus Budget Reconciliation Act (OBRA) of 1981. HCBS are not Medicaid state plan options, as coverage of these services requires a separate application to the CMS.

The Medicaid home and community-based waiver program allows states to cover a broad array of non-medical community-based services that otherwise cannot be covered by state Medicaid plans under federal law. These services can be covered *only if* the states demonstrate to CMS that such coverage

Table 14.11 Nursing Home Care Expenditures Aggregate and Per Capita Amounts, Percent Distribution and Average Annual Percent Change by Source of Funds: Selected Calendar Years 1980–2012 (in billions)

Amount in Billions

Year	Total.	Out-of-Pocket Payments	Total	Third-Party Payments Private Health Insurance	Other Private Funds	Total	Public Federal[2]	State and Local[2]	Medicare[3]	Medicaid[4]
Historical Estimates										
1980	$17.70	$7.10	$10.60	$0.20	$0.80	$9.60	$5.70	$3.90	$0.30	$8.90
1990	52.7	19.8	32.9	3.1	3.9	25.9	15.8	10.2	1.7	23.2
1998	89.1	24.9	64.2	7.4	4.6	52.3	35	17.2	10.2	40.1
1999	89.6	25.4	64.2	7.5	4.5	52.2	34.3	17.9	8.4	41.8
2000	93.8	26.2	67.6	7.3	4.1	56.2	37.7	18.5	9.5	44.7
2001	98.9	26.9	72	7.5	3.7	60.9	41.8	19	11.6	47
Projected[1]										
2002	103.7	27.3	76.4	7.7	3.3	65.3	44.7	20.6	12.1	50.8
2003	108.2	28.3	79.9	8.2	3.3	68.4	46.5	21.9	11.8	54
2004	113.3	29.3	83.9	8.9	3.4	71.7	48.6	23.1	12	57
2005	119.8	30.9	88.9	9.5	3.4	76	51.6	24.3	13	60
2006	126.8	32.2	94.6	10.4	3.5	80.7	55	25.7	14.1	63.5
2007	134.3	33.7	100.6	11.2	3.6	85.8	58.5	27.3	15	67.4
2008	142.1	35.1	107.1	12.1	3.6	91.3	62.3	29	16.1	71.6
2009	150.3	36.3	114	13	3.7	97.3	66.4	30.9	17.3	76.2
2010	159.1	37.7	121.4	14	3.8	103.6	70.8	32.8	18.5	81
2011	168.7	39.4	129.3	15	3.8	110.5	75.5	34.9	19.8	86.2
2012	178.8	41.1	137.6	16	3.8	117.8	80.5	37.2	21.2	91.9

[1] The health spending projections were based on the 2001 version of the National Health Expenditures (NHE) released in January 2003.
[2] Includes Medicaid SCHIP Expansion and SCHIP.
[3] Subset of federal funds.
[4] Subset of federal and state and local funds. Includes Medicaid SCHIP Expansion.

SOURCE: CMS, Office of the Actuary, 2003.

is cost-effective. States must demonstrate to CMS that spending for home and community-based waiver services will be offset by reduced expenditures for nursing home care of at least an equal amount. Persons receiving services under home and community-based care waivers must meet the same level of care criteria used by states to certify Medicaid coverage for nursing home care. Limits are also placed on the number of individuals who may receive home and community-based waiver services annually, to maintain cost-effectiveness.

Typical services provided by states under home and community-based waiver programs include case management, nonmedical day services, personal care services, nonmedical transportation, homemaker services, and respite care. Although some of these services can be offered under regular state Medicaid plans, the waiver program also allows states to provide these services under regulatory requirements other than those that are applied to regular state plan services. For example, a state may limit home health care services to two visits per week under its regular Medicaid program, but allow a higher number of visits for home and community-based waiver recipients. Or a state may provide personal care services under a waiver program without a requirement that these services be authorized by a physician, allocating that authority to professional case managers instead.

PAYING FOR HOME AND NURSING HOME CARE: UNDERSTANDING PUBLIC CONTRIBUTION

Home health care and nursing home care are integral to the continuum of care. Both provide interim care during periods of illness and convalescence, and both to some degree provide long-term supportive care. The distinction between medically necessary rehabilitative and convalescent care and long-term custodial care is essential to the roles played by Medicare and Medicaid in financing care services. In particular, anyone responsible for identifying, securing, and coordinating services for older adults must have a clear understanding of what Medicare and Medicaid will pay for.

States also vary in the amount of their own general revenue funds that they allocate to community-based service programs for seniors other than Medicaid. An extremely important feature of the public long-term care system is the lead role that state governments have in shaping the characteristics of local financing and delivery systems for long-term care services. Consequently, where older persons live can have a great impact on their access to publicly financed long-term care.

Integrated financing mechanisms are based on the coordination of several financing systems, with Medicare and Medicaid at the core.

For purposes of comparison, Tables 14.6 and 14.11 show the growth in Medicare and Medicaid spending for home health care and for nursing home care respectively from 1985 to 2001 (actual) and projected to 2012. These tables show clearly the effects of the BBA on Medicare spending after 1997. In the case of nursing homes, the sharp growth in spending levels off; for home care providers, the expenditures actually decline. Regardless of intent, reduced expenditures are bound to translate into reduced access. Lower payment at the institutional level results in fewer resources for staff; fewer staff hours means fewer clients served.

PRIVATE LONG-TERM CARE INSURANCE

A market for insurance against the high costs of long-term custodial care emerged slowly, but has strengthened in recent years. Private long-term care insurance became available in the 1980s, and accounts for about 8 percent of nursing home expenditures. The market for long-term care insurance proved difficult to establish, for several reasons.

One relates to the nature of the event insured. Half the people currently in their 50s are expected to require long-term care at some point in their lives. Thus, unlike the need for acute care, the need for long-term care is not a random, but a highly probable, although delayed, event. Because the likelihood of requiring services increases with age, insurance must be purchased well in advance or be prohibitively expensive, because actuarial risk increases with age.

However, individuals in their 50s are not inclined to view long-term care as a current priority compared with other purchasing decisions. The existence of the Medicaid program as an insurer of last resort has led some potential consumers to consider alternate strategies to provide for future long-term care needs. Individuals who choose to self-insure by setting up investment accounts for this purpose rely on Medicaid to act as a stop-loss, assuming coverage when assets are spent down to the eligibility level.

Lack of actuarial experience with long-term care provoked fears that the availability of insurance could induce demand as individuals sought more services than they otherwise would. As a deterrent, insurers designed the first wave of long-term care policies with coverage restricted to nursing home care. For these reasons, from the potential policyholder's perspective, the benefits of long-term care insurance accrue mainly to heirs, who view insurance as a means of protecting a future bequest, and to the Medicaid program, in the form of reduced costs. The perceived shortcomings of long-term care insurance led industry observers to conclude that expansion in this market would be limited until products changed to allow coverage of a variety of long-term care services, tax treatment was made commensurate with other types of insurance, and benefits were better coordinated with Medicaid so that benefits accrue to the policy holder.

Largely due to progress made in correcting these private long-term care insurance deficiencies, the market has grown substantially in recent years. Policies are now available that cover both institutional and noninstitutional long-term care services. Some offer a "pool of money" option that maximizes flexibility in how covered benefits are distributed across services. This option allows beneficiaries to trade off benefits from one type of care to another. Policies

that adjust the level of benefits for inflation, though expensive, are now also widely available. Finally, many link eligibility to functional status rather than diagnosis.

The Health Insurance Portability and Accountability Act of 1996 (HIPAA) provided a number of protections to insured individuals. Two sets of provisions affected the marketability of long-term care insurance policies. One had to do with safeguards for the consumer purchasing the insurance. The second set of provisions dealt with the tax incentives provided for purchasers of long-term care insurance and the use of said benefits. Health insurance is heavily government subsidized, through tax incentives to employers to provide health insurance to employees and tax breaks to individuals who buy and use insurance. HIPAA attempted to bring the tax incentives for long-term care insurance in line with those of standard health insurance products. Under HIPAA, premiums can be deducted as a medical expense for those who itemize tax deductions, subject to age-indexed limitations. Employers can deduct the cost of long-term care premiums as a business expense, and premiums are not treated as employee income. However, because the legislation did not allow long-term care insurance to be included as an option in a "cafeteria"-style menu of benefits, many observers felt that it did not go far enough in promoting expansion of this benefit. A study by the Health Insurance Association of America (HIAA) showed that the number of long-term care insurance policies grew tenfold between 1987 and 2001, from 815,000 to 8.3 million (see Figure 14.6). More than 1.4 million individuals purchased policies during the 2-year study period. They also found that the average annual premium was coming down in price. For example, a policy with similar daily coverage cost a 65-year-old $1,002 in 1999, but only $996 in 2001. In 2001, there were 4,700 employers offering long-term care insurance, and the employer market passed 1.3 million policies. The number of policies sold by 2001 through employers represented 25 percent of the total policies sold in that year.

Finally, some states have attempted to coordinate

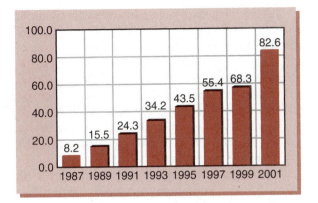

Figure 14.6 Long-Term Care Insurance Policies Sold by Year (in millions)
SOURCE: HIAA, 2003.

privately purchased long-term care insurance with Medicaid benefits, allowing individuals to protect some portion of their assets. For example, in some states, individuals can purchase special policies that guarantee to protect some or all assets from Medicaid spend-down. Sold in partnership with each state's Medicaid program, these policies pay benefits equal to the amount of assets the policyholder wants to protect.

FINANCING SOCIAL CARE NEEDS

Most social care needs of older people and younger people with disabilities are taken care of within family and social networks. Adequate availability of a social support system is essential to a continuum of care. However, not every social system is able to provide an adequate level of support for those who become frail or disabled. Social Security was the first and still one of the more important government efforts to provide economic security and social stability for older and disabled people.

The Older Americans Act (OAA) was first legislated in 1965, the same year as Medicare and Medicaid. The passage of the OAA, like the Medicare

program, was largely due to the political pressure that escalated following the 1961 White House Conference on Aging. Programs funded through the OAA are designed to improve the lives of older people in the areas of income, emotional and physical well-being, housing, employment, social services, and civic, cultural, and recreational activities.

The OAA provides grants to state Agencies on Aging, which in turn fund Area Agencies on Aging (AAAs) to plan, coordinate, and advocate for a comprehensive services system for older persons (see Chapter 18). The OAA was intended to fund the purchase of a variety of social services to meet needs identified by state and AAAs. Priority was to be given to in-home services, home-delivered meals, case management, day services, and protective services.

The primary purpose of the OAA was to enhance life for people age 60 and older, regardless of income. However, because resources are scarce, OAA programs have tended to concentrate on those with the greatest social and economic need. Thus, meeting social support needs of older people was treated separately for purposes of public funding, and resulted in further segregation of medical and social needs.

The OAA has had limited impact on the provision of long-term care services, because of the small size of the budget. However, AAAs have amassed considerable expertise in the provision of community-based services. The AAAs are frequently included in or directly manage allocation of 2176 waiver funds for purchase of community-based long-term care services. They are also often providers of the services.

Thus, although OAA-sponsored services may be limited in scope and quantity, control of 2176 waivered services, along with OAA-funded services, make AAAs important partners in developing capitated systems of care providing integrated and coordinated social, as well as medical, services. Moreover, the intent and scope of the OAA has resulted in AAAs developing specific expertise in long-term care case management; a source of funding, however small, that encouraged the development of community-based agencies; and a multilevel approach to advocacy that has increased public awareness of the need for long-term care services and financing.

FINANCING THE CONTINUUM

Historically, the major impediment to the development of a continuum of care has been the system (or nonsystem) of financing services for people with complex or long-term, chronic care needs. A continuum of care is based on adequate and accessible financing. However, the sources of financing are fragmented and not guided by a uniform national policy on long-term care. Because the financing programs are fragmented and often have contradictory regulatory and reporting requirements, providers of services have been unable to pool funds and allocate resources through an internal process to match a client's needs for the appropriate care in the appropriate sequence.

The concept of managed care for an older, chronically ill beneficiary population, based on capitated payment, is particularly appealing. It provides incentives to integrate services and provide services to clients at a point where it adds most value to the client at least cost to the health plan. The capitated payment serves as an integrated system of finance, and the needs of case management and utilization review suggest that information systems should be integrated as well. Thus, managed care plans exhibit the key elements necessary for the development of an integrated and coordinated system of care.

Ultimately, integrated financing systems will be the key to the integration of long-term and acute care services for a defined chronically ill population. The Medicare program, as discussed previously, has been entering into capitated risk contracts with HMOs since 1985. The advantage of integrated financing over fee-for-service financing is that clients of the system are more likely to receive services at the point at which they add the greatest value. In theory, this should increase quality of services, reduce duplication, and, consequently, help to control system costs.

The BBA ostensibly was intended to facilitate access to coordinated care. Although the results have been less than desirable, and may have deepened fragmentation, the conclusion is clear. Systems of care must be created organizationally, not by payers. In theory, managed care is supposed to accomplish this by providing an organizational mechanism to plan, coordinate, and evaluate care for individuals who are enrolled in managed care plans, as well as a financing mechanism.

The merger of financing and delivery systems into a broader community perspective will allow providers to focus on delivering services within the financial constraint of the price paid by the purchasers in the form of insurance. The merger of financing and delivery can occur in provider-driven or purchaser-sponsored networks. However, it appears that provider-sponsored networks may be more effective at developing an integrated service system for enrolled persons over a period of time, while purchaser-sponsored networks are more likely to overcome obstacles to system development in the short run. Congress explicitly recognized the value of provider sponsorship as part of the BBA. Medicare+Choice specifically recognizes provider service organizations (PSOs) as contracting agents for Medicare managed care.

Three models of integrated financing will be presented, all of which have been promulgated in federal legislation and reinforced within the framework of the BBA and then again in the MMA. They are Medicare managed care, S/HMO, and PACE. Each of these models takes a unique approach to the integration of social and support services into the payment and delivery model.

Medicare Managed Care

The Tax Equity and Fiscal Responsibility Act of 1982 (TEFRA) legislated the availability of Medicare risk contracts to qualified HMOs that enroll Medicare beneficiaries. Essentially, the plan was to begin moving Medicare beneficiaries into managed care plans on a voluntary basis. This approach was a radical departure from the indemnity approach taken by the Medicare program through its fiscal intermediaries. The risk-contracting program was expanded under the BBA of 1997 to include contracting with nontraditional organizations, such as PSOs. The intent of the Medicare+Choice program was to encourage the growth in provider-sponsored delivery systems.

Medicare risk contracts are a means to transfer risk of beneficiary service use from CMS to the risk contractor, usually an HMO, or a qualified managed care plan, including a PSO. The HMO enters into a contract with CMS whereby CMS pays the HMO a capitated payment per enrollee per month. The HMO is then required to provide all Medicare-covered services, with the HMO at risk for Medicare service costs that exceed the amount paid per capita by Medicare. HMOs in turn share the risk with providers by negotiating favorable pricing structures, often capitated rates, with the provider for a defined list of services to be made available to enrollees. The latter arrangement results in sharing risk directly with the provider organization.

The Medicare HMO can add benefits over and above what is required by Medicare regulations. For example, many Medicare HMOs waive the three-day hospital stay and co-payment requirements for nursing home admissions. In addition, the Medicare HMO may charge a premium over and above the Medicare Part B premium collected by CMS. These premiums vary according to the richness of benefits. The BBA required CMS to publish a comparative analysis of all Medicare managed-care plans, including benefits and premiums. This comparison can be viewed in full on the CMS Web site.

The Medicare risk-contracting program experienced an early rapid growth in the number of HMOs entering into risk contracts with CMS to provide Medicare services. The contracts became available in 1985. By 1987, there were 149 risk contracts covering 0.8 million Medicare beneficiaries. Since 1987, the number of risk contracts initially declined to 82 by 1992, but enrollment rose to 1.4 million. Although there have been a number of problems with the implementation and management of Medicare risk contracts since they were in-

troduced as part of TEFRA (Porell & Tompkins, 1993), many of the challenges have been met as the managed care organizations have become more sophisticated in managing the care of an older, chronically ill population.

HMOs with Medicare risk contracts have emphasized provision of medical services and medical components of long-term chronic care to the general exclusion of custodial care. Medicare-covered services include hospital stays, rehabilitation services, physician services, extended care in an SNF, and skilled home health services.

The BBA included substantial provisions with regard to Medicare managed care. The new program was known as Medicare+Choice. Two provisions are important to the financing of the continuum. First, Medicare+Choice expanded the scope of provider eligibility. PSOs were included along with traditional HMOs as potential contracting organizations. According to the CMS legislative summary, "PSOs are public or private entities established by or organized by health care providers or a group of affiliated providers that provide a substantial proportion of health care items and services directly through providers or affiliated groups of providers. Affiliated providers share, directly or indirectly, substantial financial risk, and have at least a majority financial interest in the PSO." While this sounds like the ideal basis on which to develop an integrated system, market response has not been very favorable.

The second change relates to payment methods. The method for calculating the capitation rate was altered, in many cases resulting in a reduction of rates for contracting HMOs. Table 14.12 shows that Medicare payment rates for managed care did decline between 1997 and 1998. The result has been that many HMOs have withdrawn from Medicare risk contracts. On January 1, 1999, roughly 407,000 persons were dropped from Medicare managed-care plans, signaling a large-scale retreat by HMOs from the Medicare market. Thus, while the BBA was intended to increase managed care participation, its short-term effect was the opposite.

The Medicare, Medicaid, and SCHIP Benefits

Table 14.12 Medicare Managed Care Payment Rates, Part A, USPCC Rates for Selected Years

Year	Retrospective	Prospective
1985	$127.42	$129.66
1990	$160.06	$171.35
1995	$255.46	$251.61
1996	$277.01	$274.84
1997	$292.23	$297.81
1998	$265.28	$271.26
1999	$274.27	$277.67
2000	—	$286.18

SOURCE: CMS. *http://www.cms.gov*

Improvement and Protection Act of 2000 (BIPA) was passed precisely to protect 5.6 million Medicare beneficiaries enrolled in Medicare+Choice plans. Inclusion in the new program required that plans apply to CMS, but the benefits included additional funding to enhance provider networks and better risk-adjustment methods to assure appropriate premium levels to the health plans. Although CMS projected continued decline in terms of access to Medicare+Choice plans, the decline in access is expected to slow, partially as a result of changes made by MMA. CMS has also engaged in a demonstration with Preferred Provider Organizations (PPO) and open-access HMOs being recognized as Medicare managed-care plans. Access to these plans is likely to grow, as is enrollment in private fee-for-service plans. Each of these alternatives will be available at higher premiums based on the degree to which the service base is enriched.

Benefits and Problems Associated with Medicare Managed Care

The most important distinguishing feature of a Medicare HMO compared to traditional Medicare financing is that the HMO manages the care of the enrollee. That is, the HMO assigns a care manager or managers to assess the care delivered by the HMO

network of providers. Each enrollee is required to select a primary care physician. Thus, the care is coordinated and managed between the primary care physician and the HMO. Under traditional fee-for-service Medicare financing, a client may go to the physician of choice—primary care or specialist physician. Older persons with multiple chronic conditions may need the care of multiple specialists (specialties vary according to organ systems affected by disease). Thus, care is often fragmented and clients may be in jeopardy if one specialist prescribes a treatment that is contraindicated in the treatment of another disease. For example, a cardiac specialist may prescribe walking to improve cardiac function, but the orthopedic specialist orders limited weight-bearing on a deteriorating hip joint. Polypharmacy is another area where problems may arise: two physicians may prescribe drugs that interact in a harmful way. In managed care, these problems are theoretically reduced because one physician is managing care and an HMO care manager is assessing all care delivered to that client.

However, there is less than universal agreement about the benefits of managed care. The primary care physician must seek approval for certain services recommended for individual consumers. The managed-care plan can and often does deny services that are ordered by a physician. Though Medicare benefits appear to be more liberal under the managed-care approach, many consumers perceive that access is more restrictive. For example, although managed-care plans generally provide more liberal coverage of short-term nursing home stays—intended to allow substitution of less expensive subacute care in a nursing home for more expensive hospital care—the plan has the prerogative to allow or deny the admission. Under traditional Medicare coverage, after a three-day hospital stay, admission to an SNF is approved provided that the patient meets the medical criteria. Many critics contend that managed-care plans use economic criteria to make care decisions as well.

Managed care enrollment has been growing among the general public at a much faster rate than among the Medicare population, largely because those covered under employer-based insurance have far less freedom of choice than do Medicare beneficiaries. Thus, concerns about access are not limited to Medicare beneficiaries. Also, some states have implemented required managed care participation for Medicaid enrollees. The BBA has several consumer protection clauses. Additional legislation has been passed at state and federal levels to protect consumer rights while promoting managed care.

With changes in payment and increased risk to HMOs, many plans have either pulled out of the Medicare market altogether, severely reduced benefits, and/or raised premiums. One of the first benefits to go was the prescription drug benefit. The current approach of Medicare HMOs that insure in local markets is to differentiate products and charge higher premiums for enriched benefits packages. However, the role of prescription drugs as a competitive feature for managed-care plans changed completely with the passage of the Medicare Prescription Drug, Improvement, and Modernization Act of 2003. A CMS report showed that the percent of the Medicare population with access to plans providing drug coverage declined from 65 to 50 percent from 1999 to 2002, but recovered to 60 percent, largely because of the introduction of the PPO demonstration and private fee-for-service plan options.

An analysis of enrollment data on the CMS Web site (*http://www.cms.gov/healthplans/statistics/mpscpt/*) shows that Medicare managed-care enrollment dropped from 5.5 million in June 2002 to 5.0 million in June 2003. Traditional HMO enrollment dropped from 4.9 million to 4.5 million. However, demonstration, PSO, PPO, and fee-for-service plan enrollments increased from 207,894 to 286,911.

A study by the Mathematica Policy Research (Achman & Gold, 2002) concluded that managed-care organizations that withdrew from Medicare+ Choice had lower enrollments, higher premiums, and less generous benefit packages, indicating that they were not very competitive in the Medicare market. The decline in HMO enrollment and the increase in alternative plan enrollments (albeit small) suggests that the Medicare managed-care market may be more similar to the general managed-care

market, in that consumers demand more open-access plans over limited-access options under traditional HMOs. Managed-care organizations that offer such plans may be more competitive in the general market and so may offer Medicare enrollees better value.

S/HMO: Health and Social Care Managed-Care Demonstrations

A number of federally sponsored demonstration projects since the late 1970s have focused on innovative ways to finance and deliver long-term care services. The Social HMO (S/HMO) project was initiated by Brandeis University in 1985. The S/HMO builds on the Medicare risk contract, but provides long-term care services in addition to the traditional Medicare-covered services. Thus, the S/HMO was an innovative approach to the integration of medical and long-term care services, financed through capitation and enrollee premiums, with the S/HMO being the risk-bearing agent.

The initial HCFA demonstration funded two different models: purchaser-sponsored and provider-sponsored (Harrington & Newcomer, 1990). There were two purchaser-sponsored S/HMOs: Kaiser-Permanente Northwest (Medicare Plus II) in Portland, Oregon, and a partnership between Group Health, Inc. and the Ebenezer Society (Seniors Plus) in Minneapolis, Minnesota. There were also two provider-sponsored S/HMOs: the Metropolitan Jewish Geriatric Center (Elderplan) in Bronx, New York, and the Senior Health Action Network (SCAN Health Plan) in Long Beach, California. Each of the S/HMOs was free to develop its own benefit structure, eligibility criteria, and service system organization. One of the four, the Ebenezer Society, dropped out, but the other three continue.

The sponsorship had more effect on the initial experience under the plan than on the actual benefit structure. Basically, each S/HMO was established as an integrated organization to provide a comprehensive array of health, medical, and custodial care services for Medicare beneficiaries who voluntarily enrolled and paid a premium for services. The enrollee premiums supplemented resources pooled from Medicare and Medicaid. That is, each plan was paid a capitated rate per enrollee by Medicare and Medicaid to provide agreed-on services. The two sources were pooled and used as the source of funds with which to either deliver or purchase services.

The project was a demonstration and in the start-up phase, HCFA bore some of the risk. The S/HMOs were to assume full financing risk at the end of a 30-month period. This aspect provided applicants with financial incentive to embark on the project. One of the aspects of this type of program is that there is considerable start-up cost and initial risk up to the point where enrollment reaches a critical mass. The S/HMO has sufficient risk-management experience to (1) control medical and chronic care costs, (2) identify a balanced benefit structure, and (3) set premiums that are marketable and fiscally responsible.

In response to a congressional mandate to continue the S/HMO demonstration and expand the number of sites, HCFA established a second generation of S/HMO projects in 1995. The goal of the second generation of sites was to determine whether Medicare HMOs that receive additional capitated fees make a concerted effort to apply geriatric principles, and that added long-term care benefits can achieve better outcomes than those achieved by traditional Medicare HMOs. Implementation of second-generation S/HMOs stalled because of constraints imposed by the revised reimbursement methodology.

The BBA allowed the continuation of the first- and second-generation S/HMO demonstrations until 2001, with an evaluation of the demonstrations occurring in 2000. However, the MMA further stipulated that the S/HMOs be blended into the Medicare Advantage program by the end of 2006. The 2000 evaluation (Sutzky et al., 2000) found merit in the S/HMO model, but agreed with Congress that the S/HMOs should be treated as other Medicare managed-care plans (Thompson, 2002).

The projects have demonstrated that S/HMOs can successfully manage risk, even when nontraditional health care services are included, such as custodial nursing home care. Thus, the evaluation of these projects may result in a better understanding of how

to provide Medicare managed care to an older population that is at risk for use of custodial as well as restorative health care services.

PACE: A System for the Frail Elderly

PACE stands for Program of All-Inclusive Care for the Elderly. It is a replication of a program initiated by OnLok Senior Services of San Francisco. OnLok has had more than 30 years of experience in providing community-based services for frail seniors, using a model of adult day health services as an organizing hub. In 1983, OnLok received its first waivers from Medicare and Medicaid to offer services designed to meet the health and health-related needs of its more than 300 frail participants. The distinguishing characteristics of OnLok and its replication projects are that they serve the frail elderly, all of whom are certified for nursing home admission; use adult day services as the hub around which services are organized; and assume risk for acute and long-term care services, both institutional and community-based. This was a conscious decision to serve this high-cost, long-term care population and to bear the financial risk of service delivery.

The BBA has further ensconced the concept of PACE by making it a Medicare benefit. The BBA defines eligibility as follows: "PACE-program-eligible individuals are 55 years of age or older; require the nursing facility level of care; reside in the service area of the PACE program; and meet other eligibility conditions imposed under the PACE program agreement."

OnLok uses a consolidated, rather than brokered, model of care. In a brokered model, case managers purchase services or control access to services (e.g., Medicare managed care or S/HMOs). In a consolidated model, a multidisciplinary team plans, organizes, and delivers most care, including primary care. Care that is delivered by other organizations, such as hospitals and nursing homes, is closely monitored and managed. The tight control of a consolidated model allows OnLok to keep costs below the capitated payment rates.

PACE is similar to S/HMOs in that it requires the pooling of funds from Medicare, Medicaid, and member fees. However, there are key distinguishing features. First, because the program is directed specifically at the nursing home eligible population (i.e., frail elderly), Medicaid plays a bigger part in financing the care. Each PACE site negotiates a Medicaid capitation rate with the state's Department of Health Services. Rates are set in accord with the costs of nursing home care. The state Medicaid program then pays PACE at the predetermined monthly rate for each Medicaid-eligible person participating. PACE sites also receive a Medicare capitation rate that is based on a variation of the standard adjusted annual per capita cost (AAPCC) method. While the AAPCC method uses standardized per capita rates of payment adjusted by four demographic cost factors (age, sex, welfare status, and institutional status), PACE's rate is determined using a single, higher Medicare cost adjuster that more accurately reflects the population's frailty and utilization experience.

Persons not eligible for Medicaid pay the portion of the total contributed by Medicaid, and participants usually quickly spend down to Medicaid limits. Once Medicaid-eligible, the Medicaid capitation rate takes effect. Less than 1 percent of participants are fully self-pay (i.e., not eligible for either Medicare or Medicaid).

The BBA provided a solid platform on which to expand the PACE replication project. In particular, the language in the BBA is based on the integrated model of financing and service delivery apparent in the OnLok model and in the other PACE demonstration models. The BBA states that "a PACE program is defined as a program of all-inclusive care for the elderly whose services are delivered by a qualified PACE provider—a provider of comprehensive health care benefits that is a public or private, nonprofit entity organized for charitable purposes under section 501(c)(3) of the Internal Revenue Code of 1986." Additionally, the legislation allows for up to 10 demonstrations per year in which for-profit entities will be allowed to operate PACE programs.

The legislation states further that individuals participating in the PACE program may be eligible for both Medicare and Medicaid, for Medicaid-only, and, in some cases, for Medicare-only. However, payment method is only specified for the Medicare portion of the integrated contribution. That is, the BBA requires that a PACE organization be treated like other managed-care entities under Medicare+ Choice options. However, the capitated rate was to be adjusted to account for the frailty of the population served through the program. Still, the rate must be set below what the actuarial cost of a comparable, non-PACE population would be. In other words, PACE programs must produce services more efficiently than other systems that provide services to frail populations. The demonstrations indicated that this is possible, but increasing system efficiency may result in increasing financial squeeze as the initial benefits of PACE are matched by other non-PACE systems of care that are likely to develop.

PACE is based on the provision of a full range of community-based services, including primary care and long-term care. Various payers, Medicare and Medicaid in particular, pay for different service elements. The BBA captured these elements in defining the scope of benefits (HCFA BBA Legislative Summary, 1999). The legislation defines the scope of services as follows:

- Regardless of the source of payment, PACE providers must make available all items and services covered under both Titles XVIII and XIX without any limitations on amount, duration, or scope; and without application of deductibles, co-payments, or other cost sharing.
- Enrollees must have access to benefits 24 hours per day, every day of the year, and services must be provided through a comprehensive, multidisciplinary system that integrates acute and long-term care services.
- Providers must arrange for the delivery of all covered items and services not provided directly by the entity itself.
- The PACE program agreement must include a written plan of quality assurance and improvement and a set of written safeguards (including

a patient bill of rights and grievance and appeals procedures).

The legislation sets a limit on growth of PACE programs, allowing for the establishment of up to 40 sites in the first year and 20 additional sites in succeeding years. However, the market has not responded with a great deal of enthusiasm. As of 2004, there were only 22 approved PACE sites operating in 17 states, each with about 200 enrollees.

PUBLIC POLICY AND FINANCING THE CONTINUUM

The high degree of complexity, fragmentation, and local variation in long-term care reflect the current financing mechanisms. Although the intent of the BBA was to increase coordination and efficiency of services, it has actually served to increase rather than to decrease the fragmentation. This has occurred as the result of two important changes. First, the changes in payment for HMOs resulted in the withdrawal of health insurers from the Medicare managed-care program, rather than increased participation as a result of the Medicare+Choice provisions. Second, the changed payment system for nursing homes and other long-term care providers has increased rivalry between hospitals and nursing homes for clients that would increase the case mix index for nursing homes (resulting in higher payment rates under prospective payment).

Federal policy is often a blunt instrument. However, it is clear that efforts to restructure long-term care into a more coherent *system* of care must inevitably involve changes in the state and federal programs that fund long-term care. Although the BBA set the tone for reform of the health care system for older persons, the provisions may actually have the short-term effect of reducing access to needed services. The longer-term effect has not yet been evaluated.

In any new or revised programs for Americans needing long-term care, several policy issues must be addressed. These include:

- What services should be covered
- What eligibility criteria should be used for determining who should receive benefits (including whether the program should be an entitlement or means-tested) and how care for beneficiaries should be managed
- What the responsibility of the family and individual should be
- What respective roles the federal and state governments should play in the organization and management of the program
- Which financing mechanisms and incentives should be used to encourage a rational, efficient, and effective integrated approach to a continuum of long-term care

Covered Services

A continuum of care consists of elements that are integrated. Identification of the services or elements to include and the payer responsible is the first step in creating the continuum. Consensus exists that the Medicare program should cover services that are clearly medical or rehabilitative in nature. Services that are generally considered to be critical services for chronically impaired people to remain in their homes include nonmedical support services, such as homemaker/home health aide services, personal care, adult day care, and services that temporarily relieve family caregivers of their responsibilities (generally referred to as *respite care*). Federal programs currently provide relatively little support for care in the home, and these are the services most people prefer.

The BBA was an attempt by Congress to encourage greater use of managed health and long-term care through the Medicare+Choice provisions and the PACE allowance under the Medicaid program. Expansion of PACE in particular will provide greater opportunities for states to facilitate the development of continuums of care for older people who may require nursing home care otherwise. The Medicare Prescription Drug, Improvement, and Modernization Act of 2003 further promotes managed-care participation to facilitate coverage of prescription drugs for Medicare enrollees.

In general, policymakers are concerned about the cost of health and long-term care programs across the spectrum, as well as expanding the base of federal support for chronic care costs beyond the very significant level at which these services are currently supported under Medicaid. Policymakers are concerned that expanded nursing home coverage for long stays may end up protecting assets for some nursing home residents who are likely never to return to the community. The effect of the expanded coverage, financed with public dollars, may be to protect assets of older people for children or other relatives to inherit. There is general agreement that preservation of wealth for individuals is not a government responsibility.

Protection of assets is the role of insurance, so part of the answer may lie in more effective long-term care insurance. Regardless, long-term care insurance is an essential ingredient of a continuum. Federal and state policymakers should continue to look for ways to promote and facilitate long-term care insurance markets, while protecting consumers.

Eligibility

There are two aspects to eligibility for benefits. First is the "objective" condition of the consumer. Most discussions about new publicly financed benefits have based eligibility for long-term care benefits on a person's inability to perform ADLs, including the functions of bathing, dressing, getting in or out of a bed or chair, and eating. Using ADLs allows long-term care benefits to be targeted to a limited number of people and also enables the new benefit to be provided without regard to certain medical criteria commonly used to establish eligibility for health benefits. Eligibility criteria for health benefits, such as prior hospitalization or need for skilled nursing care, often have little to do with the social service

needs of a chronically impaired population and can limit access to services needed by a long-term care population. Limitations in three ADLs has typically been proposed as a threshold for eligibility for new long-term care programs; the number three is intended to target services for people with severe disabilities.

The second eligibility issue relates to resources, both financial and personal. In a publicly funded program, eligibility must be based on sound stewardship of public resources. The question is how much burden individuals and families can be expected to bear in terms of the risks and consequences of the ill health to which one is exposed as a result of the aging process. In Congress, much of this debate centers on the types and levels of benefits, as well as consumer contribution, in the Medicare and Medicaid programs. These are among the more difficult public policy issues. The burden of caring for failing family members touches the lives of countless Americans, including members of Congress and state legislatures.

Role of the States and the Federal Government

Far more than the federal government, states have the lead role in formulating, financing, and implementing long-term care policy. States administer home and community-based services authorized under the Medicaid and Older Americans Act programs (through state Agencies on Aging). They also have responsibility for implementation and oversight of federal standards governing nursing homes and home health care agencies receiving reimbursement under the Medicaid and Medicare programs. Long-term care systems vary considerably across states.

Over the past 25 years, some states have made major strides in dealing with the complexities involved in coordinating the various federal home and community-based long-term care programs to overcome what they believe is a bias in federal funding for institutional care. State initiatives have included development of methods to control access to institutions through preadmission screening mechanisms; development of case management systems to authorize and control use of community-based services (sometimes through designation of local agencies to act as single entry points for long-term care services); and consolidation of state administration of the various long-term care service programs. In addition, some states have spent substantial state dollars to support home and community-based long-term care services to be responsive to the strong preference of seniors and younger people with disabilities for such care.

States will continue to play the largest role in providing for the welfare of their citizens. However, the federal government has a role in leveling differences in performance across states and in providing guidance and funding for innovations in service delivery that individual states may not have the ability to support. For example, PACE was a local movement that started in San Francisco, only the federal government can provide the support needed to expand the program through demonstration grants and through reform of the Medicare and Medicaid payment systems. The pivotal role that Medicare and Social Security play in any system will require the federal government to continue to provide leadership for system reform. The BBA was one such radical effort to overhaul the system of payment for the Medicare program. The Medicare Prescription Drug, Improvement, and Modernization Act of 2003 ensured the role of the private sector in the financing of Medicare benefits.

The federal government also influences long-term care access through tax policy. One reason that long-term care insurance did not become established earlier was the lack of tax incentives to encourage purchase of long-term care insurance by employees and individuals. Tax policy can also be directed at employers, to encourage support for employees with aging family members who may require personal and support care services.

Another critical area is consumer protection. For example, research has shown that older persons tend to buy too much insurance, especially Medigap insurance to cover services not paid for by Medi-

care. The BBA requires that CMS provide information to help consumers select the proper level of coverage. Consumers have limited ability to estimate their risks and to evaluate comparative coverage from multiple sources. HIPAA provides additional protection to consumers purchasing long-term care insurance. HIPAA also extended previous protections to Medicare managed-care enrollees. Thus, consumer protection is a critically important role at both the state and federal levels.

CONCLUSION

The development of a continuum of care depends heavily on integrated financing systems. HMOs with Medicare risk contracts, S/HMOs, and PACE sites have shown that it is possible to provide a more integrated and coordinated system of care for seniors and people with disabilities. However, many questions are left unanswered as to the proper balance between services to meet health and social needs. Emphasis on capitated risk contracts is likely to continue to expand as states, as well as the federal government, embark on health reform plans affecting Medicare and Medicaid.

Rather than consider any one model to be complete, providers interested in developing a continuum of services will need to be creative in pooling diverse streams of funding. S/HMOs and PACE programs do precisely that. The key to successful development of an integrated financing system is to tap into sources of client funding that support social as well as medical needs. Because no single source of payment covers all needs, creative providers must develop strategies in the following four areas.

First, the provider will need to assemble dynamic networks of physicians, health, long-term care, and social service agencies such that services financed by a variety of payer programs can be provided within the network. The package of services should be identified in line with what is necessary and feasible given the likely benefit limits of an integrated financing package. Institutionally based services provided by nursing homes and hospitals are essential, but may not be the ideal focus of an integrated service package for older adults and the chronically ill.

Second, the provider must be prepared to assume actuarial risk for the population. That is, the provider should have some type of health plan, HMO, or other managed-care component. However, partnership with an established managed-care plan may be preferable, especially if the managed-care plan has experience administering a Medicare or Medicaid risk contract. As shown in the S/HMO demonstration, this experience reduces start-up costs considerably.

Third, the provider must become astute at negotiating risk arrangements with such payers as Medicare, Medicaid, private insurers, HMOs, and others. The provider must meet the needs of the payers, but have sufficient leverage to deliver the required services to the target population within capitated payment levels for the bundle of services offered. In the process, the initiating provider must negotiate risk agreements with other provider members of the network. Thus, the initiating provider organization must have sufficient leverage with other provider organizations in the market area, as well as with service purchasers, in order to negotiate simultaneous agreements and fit the multiple pieces of the puzzle into one frame. Risk will be greatest during the start-up phase, so the initiating provider should seek financial backing when and wherever possible.

Finally, the market, consumers, and physicians, in particular, must be experienced in managing care and be prepared for the implications of a capitated, managed system of care for older persons, especially those who are chronically ill, and for younger people with disabilities. This includes providing services, or access to services, that meet social, personal, and medical needs. The less ready the market, the greater the marketing costs will be, and the less effective the results.

WHERE TO GO FOR FURTHER INFORMATION

American Association of Retired Persons (AARP)
601 East Street NW

Washington, DC 20049
(202) 434-2300 / (800) 424-3410
http://www.aarp.org

Centers for Medicare and Medicaid Services (CMS)
7500 Security Boulevard
Baltimore, MD 21244-1850
(877) 267-2323 / (410) 786-3000
http://www.cms.gov

Health Insurance Association of America (HIAA)
1201 F Street NW, Suite 500
Washington, DC 20004-1204
(202) 824-1600
http://www.hiaa.org

Health Insurance Portability and Accountability Act of 1996 (HIPAA)
http://www.cms.gov/hipaa

Long Term Care University
http://www.ltcuniversity.com/index.html

Medicaid
http://www.cms.gov/medicaid/

Medicare
http://www.cms.gov/medicare/ for professionals or *http://www.medicare.gov* for beneficiaries

Medicare+Choice Plan
http://www.cms.gov/healthplans/reportfilesdata/default.asp

Medicare Fee-for-Service Program
http://www.cms.hhs.gov/medicareform

National Health Care Expenditure Tables
http://www.cms.hhs.gov/statistics/nhe/projections-2001/

Programs of All-Inclusive Care for the Elderly (PACE)
http://www.cms.hhs.gov/pace/default.asp

FACTS REVIEW

1. Describe the system of financing health and long-term care services for persons age 65 and older in the United States.

2. Compare and contrast the roles that Medicare and Medicaid play in financing a continuum of services.
3. Describe the benefits and problems of the BBA and MMA as they pertain to the financing of long-term care.
4. Describe the types and levels of managed care programs that are available to older people.
   a. Medicare Advantage
   b. S/HMO
   c. PACE
5. What are the most important policy issues relating to financing services that must be faced at the federal and state levels? Explain two options for resolving each issue.

Note: For the most recent updates on MMA regulations and implementation, see *www.cms.gov/ medicarereform*

REFERENCES

Achman, L., & Gold, M. (2002). *Medicare+Choice 1999–2001: An analysis of managed care plan withdrawals and trends in benefits and premiums.* Washington, DC: The Commonwealth Fund (*http://www.mathematica-mpr.com*).

Centers for Medicare and Medicaid Services, Office of the Actuary, National Health Statistics Group. (2003). Retrieved on October 19, 2003 from *http://www.cms.hhs.gov.*

Harrington, C., & Newcomer, R. (1990). Social health maintenance organizations. *Generations, 14*(2), 49–54.

Health Insurance Association of America. (2003). *Long-term care insurance in 2000–2001.* Washington, DC: Author.

Porell, F., & Tompkins, C. (1993). Medicare risk contracting: Identifying factors associated with market exit. *Inquiry, 30,* 157–169.

Sutzky, S., Alecxih, L. M. B., Duffy, J., & Neill, C. (2000). *Review of the Medicaid 1915c Home and Community-Based Services Waiver program literature and program data—Final report prepared for: Department of Health and Human Services, Health Care Financing Administration.* Washington, DC: The Lewin Group.

Thompson, T. G. (Secretary, U.S. Department of Health and Human Services). (2002). *Evaluation results for the Social/Health Maintenance Organization II Demonstration (A report to Congress).* Washington, DC: CMS.

U.S. Department of Health and Human Services, Assistant Secretary for Planning and Evaluation. (1994, March). *Cost estimates for the long-term care provisions under the Health Services Act.* Washington, DC: Office of Disability, Aging, and Long-Term Care Policy.

CHAPTER 15

Public Policy

Richard H. Fortinsky

"Long-term care is hardly new . . . [y]et it is largely within the past few years that Americans have become aware of the emergence of long-term care as a modality different in character and scope from the kinds of acute medical care to which medicine has been primarily oriented" (Wessen, 1964). This excerpt, from an article published before the passage of Medicare, Medicaid, and most other public policies affecting long-term care today, serves as a sobering reminder of how little the public perception of long-term care has changed. In the taxonomy of this book, the article cited called for the development of a continuum of care to address the long-term care needs of people of all ages with physical and mental disabilities.

The delivery of long-term care services is heavily influenced by public policy. However, the United States has no unifying long-term care policy. Instead, public policies at federal, state, and local levels have developed in very incremental and fragmented fashion, at times focused on financing specific services in the continuum of care (discussed in Chapter 1), at other times focused specifically on one pop-ulation group needing long-term care, and at still other times focused on regulatory oversight of services financed by public funds. This chapter examines the dynamics underlying public policy formulation and implementation in relation to individuals with long-term care needs. In an effort to complement rather than duplicate the other chapters in this book, this chapter presents and elaborates on a framework for understanding who needs long-term care policy, where public policy originates, what and who influence the development of public policy in the long-term care arena, and how major public policies concerning long-term care have been shaped to date. This framework is intended to illuminate the complex interplay among policymakers, interest groups, and the political climates and sensibilities that have influenced long-term care policy development to date. Figure 15.1 outlines this framework, which includes three domains: populations needing long-term care; types of policies; and levels of policy making, all of which take place in a particular political climate, as discussed later in this chapter.

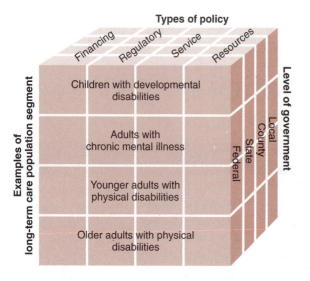

Figure 15.1   Framework Illustrating Domains of Policy Development in the Context of Long-Term Care

NOTE: Illustrative rather than exhaustive list of populations, based primarily on major groups eligible for state Medicaid waiver programs discussed in this chapter.

SOURCE: Evashwick, C. (2004). *The Continuum of Long-Term Care Slide Package.* Long Beach, CA.

POPULATIONS NEEDING LONG-TERM CARE

As discussed in Chapter 2, the total population with long-term care needs is commonly categorized according to type of functional disability. Figure 15.1 lists selected population groups categorized in this fashion: people with developmental disabilities and mental retardation; those with chronic mental illness; younger people with physical disabilities; and older adults with physical or mental disabilities, or both. Additional groups with long-term care needs include people with brain injuries, HIV/AIDS, degenerative neurological conditions, and end-stage kidney disease, to mention just a few. Public policies have been developed to provide a range of home and community-based services for individuals in each of these classified groups and, as will be shown below,

many states operate parallel programs for these different populations, due to the incremental way in which these public policies are formulated and implemented.

As illustrated by Figure 15.1, policies can be formulated to target one or more cells within the cube. For example, service financing policies developed at the state level can address one or more populations needing long-term care. Generally, the more inclusive the policy (i.e., the more cells represented), the greater the likelihood that it will favor improvement of the long-term care continuum ideal. Moreover, the prevailing political climate at the time of policy formulation (e.g., highest priority given to needs of the population; highest priority given to cost containment) will likely influence the success of the policy initiative.

Veterans of the American armed forces and older Americans represent examples of systems that have been developed because of the political clout of the sector, rather than the needs of specific individuals with conditions requiring long-term care. Indeed, because of their political importance, entire sets of public policies have been developed and implemented to finance, organize, and deliver health care and related services to these population segments. Chapter 21 in this book devotes full attention to the Department of Veterans Affairs and the health care system designed to provide for the health and long-term care needs of the veteran population; Chapter 18 describes the Older Americans Act service system for seniors.

TYPES OF PUBLIC POLICIES AFFECTING LONG-TERM CARE

Public policies in the health arena can be grouped into four major types, depending on the aspect of health care with which they are primarily concerned: financing, service organization and delivery, regulation to ensure service quality, and health resources availability. Some legislation includes more than one type of provision.

Financing Policy

Medicare and Medicaid are examples of financing policies, in that they specify funding mechanisms to pay for health-related services, specify the types of services that are eligible to receive funding, and specify the target populations eligible for funded services (Brown & Sparer, 2003). Chapter 14 provides greater detail about the characteristics and consequences of public policies concerned primarily with financing. This chapter discusses how financing policy in the health sphere has or has not contributed to the development of a continuum of care for people with long-term care needs.

Service Organization and Delivery Policy

Public policies may also authorize the development of direct health care services and mandate how these services will be organized and delivered. At the federal level, the Veterans Affairs Medical Centers and associated inpatient and outpatient health services were established pursuant to these types of public policies (see Chapter 21 for more details). At the state level, these types of policies created state mental health hospitals and group homes for people with chronic mental illnesses (see Chapter 20 for more details).

Most of these policies, however, have limited their authority regarding service organization and delivery to specific settings of care and do not focus on how care might be coordinated between these settings and settings outside their authority. For example, no policy guides how services within and outside the Department of Veterans Affairs should be coordinated for veterans who use services in both systems. Indeed, an important source of the fragmentation of long-term care discussed throughout this book is the lack of long-standing and effective public policy directives regarding how Medicare- and Medicaid-funded services might be organized and delivered to achieve greater coordination from the viewpoint of a continuum of care.

The Tax Equity and Fiscal Responsibility Act of 1982 (TEFRA) marked the first attempt to legislate an alternative method of health care delivery under Medicare. Under TEFRA, health maintenance organizations (HMOs) and other health care providers were encouraged to assume risk for Medicare beneficiaries by providing mandatory and, optionally, additional services for a capitated rate. Chapter 14 provides greater detail about Medicare risk contracts. TEFRA initiated a voluntary movement of HMOs and other health care providers into the Medicare managed-care market, a movement that peaked in the mid- to late-1990s. However, primarily because of Medicare capitation rates that are insufficient to support the relatively costly Medicare population, between 1998 and 2001 the number of managed-care plans participating in Medicare risk-sharing plans (now referred to as Medicare+Choice) dropped by nearly half, from 346 to 179 (Brown & Sparer, 2003). From the viewpoint of long-term care continuum advocates, even in its heyday the Medicare managed-care policy initiative did not legislate an expanded range of benefits that encompass long-term care services. The only significant benefit that was added to many Medicare+Choice plans to attract Medicare beneficiaries was prescription drug coverage, but this benefit did not last long before the expense became prohibitive.

The Balanced Budget Act (BBA) of 1997 included public policy more oriented toward service organization and delivery. The BBA legislated the development of integrated delivery models incorporating acute and long-term care services for persons age 55 and older eligible for long-stay nursing facility care, based on the original OnLok model and subsequent demonstration sites for the Program of All-Inclusive Care for the Elderly (PACE). The BBA also enabled Medicare and Medicaid funds to be pooled to improve service organization and delivery at PACE provider sites. Of course, as with Medicare risk contracting, providers must be willing to accept the negotiated financing terms set by Medicare (capitated rate) and state Medicaid programs if they are to participate as PACE sites. In September 2003, the nation had a total of 42 PACE sites in

23 states (*http://www.natlpaceassn.org*), including demonstration sites established before the BBA made the PACE model a permanently recognized provider type under both the Medicare and Medicaid programs. The BBA legislation related to PACE site replication represents the most progressive move to date toward health service organization and delivery on a national level, and could help set the stage for future advances in public policy that would further improve the continuum of care for people with long-term care needs.

Regulatory Policy

An important example of public policy in the area of regulation is the Omnibus Budget Reconciliation Act of 1987 (OBRA), which significantly strengthened the capacity of federal and state agencies to monitor the quality of care provided in long-stay nursing facilities. OBRA was implemented following a highly influential report from the Institute of Medicine that demonstrated the delivery of relatively poor quality of care in America's long-stay nursing facilities and proposed a comprehensive set of recommendations designed to improve nursing facility quality (Institute of Medicine, 1986). As a result of OBRA, a uniform resident assessment and care planning system was implemented nationwide, and the use of physical and chemical restraints in nursing facilities has been dramatically reduced (Capezuti, Strumpf, Evans, Grisso, & Maislin, 1998; Hawes et al, 1995).

Riding on the momentum created by OBRA, the Centers for Medicare and Medicaid Services (CMS) has engaged in vigorous efforts to initiate regulatory policy to improve quality throughout all sectors of health care (Docteur, 2001; Jencks, 1995). In 2002, CMS implemented the Nursing Home Quality Initiative as a matter of public policy. This initiative involves the publication and wide dissemination of quality-of-care "report cards" for all nursing facilities, using data from the uniform assessment form developed as a result of OBRA. For home health care, CMS introduced the Home Health Quality Initiative (HHQI) policy initiative, in which

quality report cards are based on data from the federally mandated Outcome and Assessment Information Set (OASIS). Though these initiatives are not necessarily aimed at coordinating services, they mark important advances in quality monitoring because they focus on health-related outcomes (e.g., whether the service recipient improved in level of functioning or severity of symptoms).

As described further later in this chapter, Medicaid home and community-based waiver programs have been established in an effort to provide comprehensive care to different populations with long-term care needs. The U.S. General Accounting Office (GAO) released a report in 2003 contending that greater regulation of these waiver programs is required to assure quality care (U.S. GAO, 2003). CMS is likely to formulate public policy in response to this report, and waiver programs will likely undergo increased regulatory scrutiny.

Health Resources Policy

The Public Health Service Act authorized the establishment of the Health Resources and Services Administration (HRSA), located within the U.S. Department of Health and Human Services. Just as CMS is responsible for implementing policies formulated by Congress in the realm of health financing policies, HRSA is responsible for implementing policies formulated by Congress in the realm of health resources policies. In federal fiscal year 2003, Congress appropriated nearly $7 billion to HRSA for its activities, which include expanding the availability of primary care professionals and clinics to underserved populations. HRSA includes a Bureau of Health Professions, which is responsible for helping to assure access to quality health care professionals in all geographic areas and to all segments of society through appropriate preparation, composition, and distribution of the health professions workforce. This bureau also has the responsibility to improve access to a diverse and culturally competent and sensitive health professions workforce.

Pressing health resource policy issues affecting the population with long-term care needs include the shortage of nurses, the shortage of paraprofessionals such as home health aides and personal care providers, and the shortage of health care providers with expertise in geriatrics (Kovner, Mezey, & Harrington, 2002; Sochalski, 2002; Ward & Berkowitz, 2002). In addition to initiatives implemented by the health professions themselves, HRSA has responsibility for implementing training programs to attract individuals to work in these professions. For more information, visit the HRSA Web site at *http://www .hrsa.gov.*

Health resources policy also pertains to building construction to support the delivery of health care services. For example, the Hill-Burton Act passed shortly after World War II funded the construction of acute care hospitals and nursing homes. The National Housing Act and its amendments in the 1950s created apartment-style living quarters for people with disabilities and older adults, with special design features intended to support their independent living (see Chapter 9 for more details). These policies were concerned with the "bricks and mortar" aspects of health resources, and offered little guidance about the types and organization of services to be provided within the walls of these facilities.

LEVELS OF POLICY MAKING

Public policy formulation occurs at four different levels of government: federal, state, county (in most states), and local. At the federal level, members of the Senate and House of Representatives formulate most public policy, but responsibility for policy implementation and oversight is in the hands of federal and state agencies. Table 15.1 summarizes major federal legislation formulated and implemented over the past 40 years that provides funds for health and supportive services to people with long-term care needs. This table shows how multiple pieces of legislation cover the same types of services, but often for different target populations. Moreover, jurisdictional responsibility for implementing and monitoring legislation varies consid-

erably, with federal responsibility for Medicare, state responsibility for Medicaid, and state and local responsibility for the Older Americans Act. Appendix A lists the main federal laws pertaining to various aspects of long-term care.

States pay for more types of long-term care services, through Medicaid and an array of other public programs, than the services Medicare pays for from the federal level. Thus, states are the major drivers of most long-term care policies. This results in 50 different approaches to long-term care delivery systems.

Public policy also can be formulated in the judicial branch of government. In 1999, the U.S. Supreme Court decided the *Olmstead v. L.C.* case, which held that the retention of persons with disabilities in institutional settings was discriminatory and a violation of the Americans with Disabilities Act of 1990. The Olmstead Act exemplifies a federal-level public policy that may have far-reaching effects for one segment of the population with long-term care needs. The Olmstead Act directs states to discharge from institutional settings individuals with mental disabilities determined to be candidates for residence in community-based settings, provided that the placement can be reasonably accommodated, taking into account resources available to the state and the needs of others with mental disabilities. This policy, spurred by the Supreme Court decision, has set in motion state-level initiatives across the country to "transition" eligible individuals from long-stay nursing facilities and mental health chronic care facilities into community settings, as well as to make communities more accessible to persons with disabilities. It remains to be seen whether a true continuum of care can be established in the community for individuals affected by the Olmstead Act. However, this single public policy has set the stage for meaningful change in the organization and delivery of services to persons with long-term care needs, particularly in states where movement in this direction has been incremental at best.

At the state level, legislatures can formulate policies regarding how state revenues might be used to

Table 15.1 Features of Major Federal Legislation Affecting Individuals with Long-Term Care Needs

Legislation	Year(s) Passed	Target Population	Major Covered Services	Primary Jurisdictional Responsibility
Medicare (Title XVIII of Social Security Act)	1965	• Age 65 and older • Under 65; disabled • End-stage renal disease	• Acute care hospitals • Rehabilitation hospitals • Short-stay nursing facilities • Home health • Hospice • Mental health • Physician visits	Federal
Medicaid (Title XIX of Social Security Act)	1965	• Poor	• Long-stay nursing facilities • Home health • Physician visits • Prescription drugs	State
Social Services Block Grants (Title XX of Social Security Act)	1974	• All ages and disabilities, but specifics vary by state	• Home and community-based services that vary by state	State
Medicaid Home and Community-Based Waiver programs	1981	• Poor or near poor • Medically eligible for long-stay nursing facility • Target populations vary by state	• Personal care • Case management • Homemaker • Adult day care • Respite care	State
Mental Health	1967, 1971, 1986	• Persons with mental illness • Persons with mental retardation or developmental disabilities	• Community mental health centers • Long-stay nursing facilities (ICF-MR)	State
Older Americans Act	1965	• Age 60 and older	• Home-delivered and congregate meals • Senior centers • Information and referral • Transportation • Legal	State (State Units on Aging); local (Area Agencies on Aging)
Veterans Administration	1963, 1972, 1975, 1980	• Military veterans	• Hospital • Nursing facility • Physician visits (at VA sites) • Home health • Adult day care • Prescription drugs	Federal

fund new initiatives. Over the past 20 years, a large number of state legislatures have enacted policies to expand in-home and community-based services for those with long-term care needs. In many cases, financial and medical eligibility for state-funded programs created by these policies are less stringent than eligibility criteria for Medicaid-funded home and community-based services, although the range of services available under these programs may be identical. State legislatures also can formulate policies specifying sources of revenue that could be used to pay for new programs. For example, in Pennsylvania state lottery revenues are earmarked for social and health-related services available to the older population.

Public policies at the state level also may be formulated by agency administrators to modify the ways in which Medicaid funds are used to make services available to the state's population. For example, all Medicaid waiver programs originate at the state level with agency administrators, who must gather evidence that expanded home and community-based services will be cost-effective in relation to long-stay nursing facility services for the pro-

jected population served. State applications are submitted to federal administrators at the CMS for approval, but state-level policymakers are responsible for initiating these programs.

To illustrate the extent to which state agency administrators have formulated public policy for persons with long-term care needs, Table 15.2 shows the number of states that had operational Medicaid home and community-based (HCBS) waiver programs in federal fiscal year (FY) 2002 for different populations with long-term care needs; total Medicaid expenditures for all states combined for each HCBS waiver program in FY 2002; and the growth in Medicaid expenditures from FY 1997 through FY 2002 for each of these HCBS waiver programs for all states combined. All states except Arizona and Washington, DC, had a Medicaid waiver program for people with mental retardation or developmental disabilities (MR/DD) in 2002. Most states had a Medicaid waiver program for older people and people with disability combined (A/D), and many others had a separate Medicaid waiver program for each of these two groups separately. A smaller number of states had Medicaid waiver programs in

Table 15.2   Number of States with Medicaid HCBS Waiver Programs for Different Targeted Long-Term Care Populations, Total Expenditures for Each Program, Federal FY 2002, and Percentage Increase in Expenditures for Each Program from FY 1997–FY 2002

Targeted Long-Term Care Population	Number of States with Medicaid HCBS Waiver Program, FY 2002	Total Expenditures, FY 2002	Percentage Increase in Expenditures, FY 1997–FY 2002
People with mental retardation or developmental disabilities	50*	$12,033,760,444	90%
Older people and people with disabilities	37	$3,078,938,741	139%
People with physical disabilities only	27	$395,252,762	124%
Older people only	18*	$515,826,827	164%
People with brain injuries	16	$104,730,372	187%
People with HIV/AIDS	16*	$66,174,721	−28%
People who are technology dependent or medically fragile	14	$88,821,656	54%
People with mental illness	3	$32,362,266	674%

*Includes the District of Columbia (Washington, DC).

SOURCE: Data provided by Medstat. See Eiken & Burwell, 2003.

2002 for other specialized populations with long-term care needs. In states with multiple Medicaid waiver programs, each program has its own administrative structure within state government.

Table 15.2 also shows that a large majority of Medicaid waiver program expenditures (nearly 75 percent) in 2002 were for programs for the population with MR/DD, followed by A/D waiver programs (19 percent). All of these programs experienced significant growth in expenditures between FY 1997 and FY 2002, except the program for people with HIV/AIDS, which experienced a substantial decline in expenditures. These programs stand as the most visible and pervasive examples of how persons with long-term care needs have benefited from public policy formulation and implementation at the state level.

A related area of state public policy formulation is the appropriate balance between long-stay nursing facility care and home and community-based care, because Medicaid spending on nursing facility care accounts for more than 75 percent of all Medicaid long-term care spending (Feder, Komisar, & Niefeld, 2000). Most states have attempted to redress this imbalance by crafting public policies to limit the supply of nursing facility beds and to expand home and community-based care programs for different long-term care populations, as shown in Table 15.2. A few states have taken more dramatic measures to reduce nursing facility service, especially Oregon, which has for a decade aggressively moved to discharge nursing facility residents and serve them in a variety of community-based settings, including adult foster care and assisted living facilities (Feder et al., 2000; Zimmerman et al., 2003).

At county and local levels, elected officials with legislative authority include county commissioners, city and town officials, and "district" officials. Examples of policy initiatives that can help address the needs of persons with long-term care needs are integration of Older Americans Act funds with county-level funds to help coordinate long-term care services (Fortinsky, 1991), and local referenda that propose to fund long-term care services from new local tax revenues. It is beyond the scope of this chapter to fully elaborate on county and local levels of policy making, but these efforts can be expected to increase as the baby boom cohort ages and develops health-related needs of their own and their parents begin to replace concerns related to educating their children in local schools.

WHAT AND WHO INFLUENCES PUBLIC POLICY DEVELOPMENT: INTEREST GROUPS AND POLITICAL CLIMATE

Public policy unfolds in a highly active political process, regardless of the level of policy formulation. In fact, by its very nature, the entire legislative process often begins with ideas or proposals submitted to policymakers by citizens or by leaders of interest groups representing specific constituencies. As policymakers and their staff members disseminate drafts of bills, interest groups with opposing views insert themselves into the policy-making process. Thus, public policy development is influenced first and foremost by interest-group politics, and many groups operate from a position of enlightened self-interest.

The number of interest groups influencing the public policy development process at the national level has grown dramatically over the past two decades. By the mid-1990s, there were more than 100 such national organizations focused on issues affecting the older population alone (Binstock & Day, 1996). These interest groups helped persuade Congress in the late 1980s to pass legislation to expand benefits of the Medicare program through the Medicare Catastrophic Coverage Act in 1988. Unfortunately, an interest-group backlash quickly followed, because the final legislation would have linked the cost of Medicare premiums to income and assets. Congress repealed this act just one year later. These events demonstrate the power of interest groups on the policy-making process.

There are also scores of interest groups representing other populations needing long-term care (e.g., persons with developmental disabilities or mental retardation). Many of these groups have focused their lobbying efforts primarily on maximizing independent living, assuring equal access to employment and educational opportunities, and optimizing community inclusion of people with disabilities. These interest groups' efforts were rewarded with the passage of the Americans with Disabilities Act of 1990, considered landmark federal legislation for people with disabilities (although not directly addressing long-term care needs of this population).

From the viewpoint of elected or appointed officials charged with formulating public policy at the national level, policy development would be easier if many or most interest groups supported a similar position on a policy topic. This rarely occurs in the real world. However, during 2 periods over the past 40 years, sufficient consensus was reached that major federal legislation was passed, or was seriously entertained, affecting the vast majority of individuals with long-term care needs.

The first period was in the 1960s. Three of the most influential public policies that directly affect the vast majority of individuals with long-term care needs to this day—Medicare, Medicaid, and the Older Americans Act—were born at the same time, in 1965. At that time, the national political climate was highly oriented toward addressing the needs of the population, in areas of life as wide-ranging as civil rights and health. In the health arena, federal policymakers responded to calls from a broad spectrum of interest groups, ranging from consumer advocacy organizations to physician and hospital professional associations, to craft public policy that would offer health insurance coverage (Medicare) and a wide range of community-based supportive services (Older Americans Act) based on the most important perceived needs of older Americans, as well as health insurance coverage for poor Americans of all ages (Medicaid). Under Medicare, perceived needs of older Americans were interpreted primarily as medical care and hospital care, pat-

terned after private health insurance policies available at the time (Schlesinger & Wetle, 1988). Perceived needs under the Older Americans Act were comprehensive in scope and highly consistent with needs in any population requiring long-term care, particularly social support, employment, and legal assistance (see Chapter 18). Under Medicaid, a joint federal-state program with most authority resting with states, perceived needs were primarily medical care and hospital care for poor, younger Americans, particularly children with single parents. Moreover, the costs associated with implementing these new public policies were not viewed as insurmountable barriers.

Since that time, however, cost containment has become a major feature of the political climate surrounding public policy development, even while the population requiring long-term care has grown dramatically and the range and expertise of interest groups have grown in size and political effectiveness. Medicare and Medicaid have grown rapidly, straining federal and state budgets; the Older Americans Act has not fully achieved its initial goals because of insufficient financing. Consequently, there has been a much less unified view in the past 20 years, compared to in 1965, that the needs of the population should be the overriding priority in fashioning public policy.

This change in the political climate was firmly in place in the late 1980s and early 1990s, when many of the disparate interest groups representing the different populations needing long-term care formed a coalition in an effort to influence public policy at the federal level. Known as the Long-Term Care Campaign, this coalition of interest groups officially formed in 1989, with a reported 60 million members from 140 national organizations (Binstock & Day, 1996). The philosophy of this coalition was that insurance coverage for long-term care should be based on need (i.e., level of disability) rather than on age or economic status. This philosophy was consistent with a political climate that placed priority on the needs of the population. The late Claude Pepper, then a U.S. Representative from Florida, in 1989 introduced a bill influenced by evidence provided by the Long-Term Care Campaign; it would have provided long-term home care insurance coverage to persons of any age who were dependent in two or more activities of daily living, such as dressing and bathing (Binstock & Day, 1996). In 1993, then-President Clinton proposed a similar long-term care insurance coverage plan as a component of his administration's initiative to reform health care (Binstock & Day, 1996). In part because of the political climate of cost containment, these policy formulations were not enacted into law; however, without the formation of the Long-Term Care Campaign coalition, it is unlikely that such policy formulations would have been designed at the federal level. Since then, most coalition members of the Long-Term Care Campaign have refocused their efforts on Medicare and Medicaid reform issues, some of which relate directly to long-term care services (e.g., expansion of Medicaid waiver programs) but many of which do not (e.g., a Medicare prescription drug benefit).

At the state level, interest groups representing different populations requiring long-term care influence elected officials and state agency administrators responsible for formulating public policy. Advocacy groups representing people with developmental disabilities and younger adults with physical disabilities are particularly influential in promoting policy options that lead to independent living. Medicaid HCBS waiver programs have served as important instruments of public policy in this regard, and Table 15.2 provides evidence, in terms of expenditures, about the relative success the various interest groups have had in helping to grow these programs for their constituents requiring long-term care.

From the viewpoint of the continuum of care framework (see Chapter 1), a critical lesson from this brief review of interest groups can be drawn: as long as different constituency groups act only in their own interests and influence policy development accordingly, the promise of more unified long-term care policies and a true continuum of care for the populations with long-term care needs will continue to be elusive.

MAKING POLICY DEVELOPMENT MORE FAVORABLE TO THE LONG-TERM CARE CONTINUUM

This chapter closes by presenting principles that attempt to cut across the elements of the framework depicted in Figure 15.1. If various long-term care constituency groups could agree on principles to be advocated, the nation might begin to develop consistent policies across sectors. Public policy development in the future might then be a more effective mechanism for the growing, diverse population in the United States with long-term care needs.

Independent living. For nearly three decades, independent living has been a major thrust of interest groups representing children and younger adults with physical, mental, and developmental disabilities requiring long-term care. Needs of older adults more often have been cast by interest groups as favoring home and community-based care over long-stay nursing facility care. Independent living across the lifespan may be a more effective principle to voice in the political process surrounding policy development, because it speaks directly to a public policy goal from the perspective of those whose needs are the true targets of public policy.

Maximum potential. Closely related to the principle of independent living is the principle that all individuals with long-term care needs, regardless of age, should have access to services that will help them achieve their maximum physical and mental potential. By following this principle, public policy can be formulated to reinforce the importance of habilitation and rehabilitation services and mental health services in the continuum of care for individuals with long-term care needs. The Americans with Disabilities Act of 1990 and the Olmstead Act of 1999 represent federal legislative achievements of this principle; the next generation of public policy might focus on state initiatives that attempt to improve service coordination consistent with the principle of maximum potential.

Consumer direction. Over the past decade, a number of states have introduced consumer direction into Medicaid-funded home-based services for people with disabilities (Benjamin, 2001). Younger persons with disabilities have spurred these initiatives to a much greater degree than older persons. These initiatives enable care recipients themselves to arrange and supervise personal care assistants and other in-home service workers, without the requirement of an independent care supervisor or case manager. Although numerous challenges remain in assuring that consumer direction yields high-quality care and controlled expenditures, this principle may become more popular over time as the baby boom cohort moves into advanced age (Knickman & Snell, 2002).

Flexible fund pooling. Particularly for those individuals eligible for both Medicare and Medicaid (dual eligibles), regardless of age, fund pooling can lead to creative approaches to coordinating service organization and delivery. Little is known about how many younger individuals with long-term care needs are dually eligible; most policy initiatives to date have focused solely on individuals age 55 and older (e.g., PACE legislated by the BBA in 1997). As of 2000, seven states had sought federal approval for demonstration programs that would, in the tradition of PACE sites, involve pooling Medicare- and Medicaid-funded services into a more comprehensive package for dual eligibles, nearly all of whom have long-term care needs (U.S. GAO, 2000). These initiatives have proven challenging, and at least two of these seven states eventually dropped plans to proceed, but states such as Minnesota and Wisconsin have successfully sustained fund pooling in limited ways (U.S. GAO, 2000). Other states attempting to merge program funding or authorities include California, Florida, and Massachusetts. The principle of flexible fund pooling is a critical feature of any effort to achieve a true continuum of care for people with long-term care needs. Moreover, greater flexibility may attract health care providers to the long-term care population, such as home care organizations that are starting to use innovative care

management techniques to care for people with chronic illness (Kodner & Kyriacou, 2003).

CONCLUSION

The twenty-first century dawned during a period of enormous growth in the use of information and communication technologies (Masys, 2002). This phenomenon adds an entirely new layer of complexity to the policy-making process. For example, near-instant access to information and communication have enabled greater numbers of existing and new interest groups to organize and become involved in the policy-making process. In addition, opinion polls about every topic of public interest (and many of little interest!) can be conducted, and results analyzed and prepared for public consumption in a matter of hours. As noted earlier, policy making always has been an intensely political process; information and communication technologies have enabled ever-larger numbers of individuals to enter this process. In the context of long-term care policy development, thoughtful and creative uses of these new technologies by interest groups and policymakers alike could greatly enhance efforts to achieve greater coordination across populations requiring long-term care, types of policy in long-term care, and levels of policy development.

Finally, health care administrators are advised to remain abreast of changes in public policy affecting long-term care financing, organization and delivery, regulation, and health resources, because models of care are constantly introduced, tested, and evaluated. Research results from long-term care experiments initiated by public policies are regularly published, and the health care research community has renewed its efforts to be responsive to the needs of policymakers who wish to formulate long-term care policy based on the most current scientific evidence (Kemper, 2003). Factors that will likely stimulate policy formulation affecting long-term care include the continued strengthening of interest groups, the aging of the diverse baby boom birth cohort, and the prospects of fiscal constraints on the Social Security and Medicare programs (Knickman & Snell, 2002). The process of policy formulation, program experimentation, and program evaluation will continue to evolve in the growing area of long-term care for the foreseeable future.

FACTS REVIEW

1. Name four basic types of public policies and describe the primary function of each.
2. What is the role of lobbying in creating public policy?
3. Explain how and why long-term care policy in the United States is fragmented.
4. Name three major pieces of federal legislation that pertain to long-term care, summarize what each covers, and discuss the contributions and shortcomings of the legislation in the context of the broad field of long-term care.
5. What are Medicaid waivers, and how do they relate to long-term care?
6. Describe three principles that you would favor to guide long-term care policy making, and discuss the effect that each would have on legislation; cite examples if possible.

WHERE TO GO FOR FURTHER INFORMATION

American Association of Retired Persons (AARP)
Legal Council for the Elderly
601 E Street, NW
Washington, D.C. 20049
(202) 434-2145
http://www.aarp.org

American Association of Homes and Services for the Aging (AAHSA)
2519 Connecticut Ave., NW
Washington, D.C. 20008

(202) 783-2255
http://www.aahsa.org

Centers for Medicare and Medicaid Services (CMS)
7500 Security Boulevard
Baltimore MD 21244-1850
(877) 267-2323
http://www.cms.hhs.gov

International Longevity Center (ILC)
60 E. 86th Street
NY, NY 10028
(212) 288-1468
http://www.ilcusa.org

National Association of State Units on Aging (NASUA)
1201 15th Street, NW
Suite 350
Washington, DC 20005
(202) 898-2578
http://www.nasua.org

National Institute on Disability and Rehabilitation Research (NIDRR)
400 Maryland Avenue, S.W.
Washington, DC 20202-7100
(202) 245-7316
http://www.ed.gov

National PACE Association
801 North Fairfax Street, Suite 309
Alexandria, Virginia 22314
(703) 535-1565
http://www.npaonline.org

U.S. Administration on Aging (AoA)
Washington, DC 20201
(202) 619-0724
http://www.aoa.gov

Health Resources and Services Administration
U.S. Department of Health and Human Services
Parklawn Building
5600 Fishers Lane
Rockville, Maryland 20857
http://www.hrsa.gov

REFERENCES

Benjamin, A. E. (2001). Consumer-directed services at home: A new model for persons with disabilities. *Health Affairs, 20,* 80–95.

Binstock, R. H., & Day, C. L. (1996). Aging and politics. In R. H. Binstock & L. K. George (Eds.), *Handbook of aging and the social sciences,* 4th ed. (pp. 362–387). San Diego, CA: Academic Press.

Brown, L. D., & Sparer, M. S. (2003). Poor program's progress: The unanticipated politics of Medicaid policy. *Health Affairs, 22,* 31–44.

Capezuti, E., Strumpf, N. E., Evans, L. K., Grisso, J. A., & Maislin, G. (1998). The relationship between physical restraint removal and falls and injuries among nursing home residents. *Journals of Gerontology: Medical Sciences, 53,* M47–M52.

Docteur, E. (2001). Measuring the quality of care in different settings. *Health Care Financing Review, 22,* 59–70.

Eiken, S., & Burwell, B. (2003). *Medicaid HCBS Waiver expenditures, FY 1997 through FY 2002.* Cambridge, MA: MedStat.

Feder, J., Komisar, H. L., & Niefeld, M. (2000). Long-term care in the United States: An overview. *Health Affairs, 19,* 40–56.

Fortinsky, R. H. (1991). Coordinated comprehensive community care & the Older Americans Act. *Generations, 15,* 39–42.

Hawes, C., Morris, J. N., Phillips, C. D., Mor, V., Fries, B. E., & Nonemaker, S. (1995). Reliability estimates for the Minimum Data Set for nursing home resident assessment and care screening (MDS). *The Gerontologist, 35,* 172–178.

Institute of Medicine (1986). *Improving the quality of care in nursing homes.* Washington, DC: National Academy Press.

Jencks, S. F. (1995). Measuring quality of care under Medicare and Medicaid. *Health Care Financing Review, 16,* 39–54.

Kemper, P. (2003). Long-term care research and policy. *The Gerontologist, 43,* 436–446.

Knickman, J. R., & Snell, E. K. (2002). The 2030 problem: Caring for aging baby boomers. *Health Services Research, 37,* 849–884.

Kodner, D. L., & Kyriacou, C. K. (2003). Bringing managed care home to people with chronic, disabling conditions. *Journal of Aging and Health, 15,* 189–222.

Kovner, C. T., Mezey, M., & Harrington, C. (2002). Who cares for older adults? Workforce implications of an aging society. *Health Affairs, 21,* 78–89.

Masys, D. R. (2002). Effects of current and future information technologies on the health care workforce. *Health Affairs, 21,* 33–41.

Schlesinger, M., & Wetle, T. (1988). Medicare's coverage of health services. In D. Blumenthal, M. Schlesinger, & P. B. Drumheller (Eds.), *Renewing the promise: Medicare and its reform* (pp. 58–89). New York: Oxford University Press.

Sochalski, J. (2002). Nursing shortage redux: Turning the corner on an enduring problem. *Health Affairs, 21,* 157–164.

U.S. General Accounting Office (2003). *Long-term care: Federal oversight of growing Medicaid home and community-based waivers should be strengthened* (GAO-03-576). Washington, DC: U.S. GAO.

U.S. General Accounting Office (2000). *Medicare and Medicaid: Implementing state demonstrations for dual eligibles has proven challenging* (GAO-00-94). Washington, DC: U.S. GAO.

Ward, D., & Berkowitz, B. (2002) Arching the flood: How to bridge the gap between nursing schools and hospitals. *Health Affairs, 21,* 42–52.

Wessen, A. F. (1964). Some sociological characteristics of long-term care. *The Gerontologist, 4,* 7–14.

Zimmerman, S., Gruber-Baldini, A. L., Sloane, P. D., Eckert, K., Hebel, J. R., Morgan, L. A., Stearn, S. C., Wildfire, J., Magaziner, J., Chen, C., & Konrad, T. R. (2003). Assisted living and nursing homes: Apples and oranges? *The Gerontologist, 43(suppl 2),* 107–117.

CHAPTER 16

Ethical Considerations

Leslie A. Curry and Terrie Wetle

Appreciation of the ethical dimensions of health care has grown in recent years as a result of four major trends: (1) the emergence of the patient or client as an informed health care consumer, (2) protection of individual rights to privacy of medical information, (3) continued advances in medical technology and science, and (4) the changing nature of the patient-health care provider relationship in managed care systems.

Ensuring the appropriate consideration of ethical concerns of individuals as they are cared for within and across the long-term care continuum is challenging for health care providers and administrators. Ethical care is influenced by factors that are consumer-based, provider- and family-based, and system-based. Health care consumers have individual characteristics and preferences that must be understood and respected. Providers and family members experience competing responsibilities and obligations, and may be influenced by negative stereotypes regarding disability or misguided paternalism. Finally, health care systems face challenges in terms of organization, financing, and regulation

of services across the continuum. Chronically impaired persons (especially frail older adults) are likely to have diminished opportunities for making autonomous choices in community-based care, as well as in institutional settings such as nursing homes and acute care hospitals.

Ethical concerns arise in balancing individual safety and autonomy in community-based settings, in determining the level of participation of patients in treatment and care decisions, and in developing appropriate relationships between residents and care providers in various institutional settings, such as nursing homes and assisted living. Health care administrators are charged with creating and fostering support systems that encourage all involved parties to appropriately address the many ethical issues that arise during delivery of services across the continuum.

This chapter: (1) provides an overview of key ethical concepts relevant across the continuum of care; (2) discusses their significance with regard to home and community-based services, congregate living arrangements, acute care hospitals, nursing homes, and managed-care settings, as well as the full continuum of care; (3) identifies system-wide factors that may pose ethical dilemmas in service delivery; and (4) gives examples of management techniques that administrators can employ to deal constructively with ethical considerations of care.

OVERVIEW OF ETHICAL CONSIDERATIONS

Rose Anderson is 83 years old and has lived in her own small home since the death of her husband 11 years ago. She has begun to show signs of poor judgment and memory problems, including leaving her door unlocked when she goes out, leaving the burner on after she has finished making tea, and getting lost when she took the wrong bus home. After a small fire in her kitchen, her daughter insists that she move to a congregate living facility. Rose refuses, saying she wants to stay in her own home.

An understanding of four principal ethical considerations is fundamental to a thoughtful discussion of issues that arise as individuals receive health services across the continuum of care. These principles are autonomy, beneficence, paternalism, and justice.

Autonomy

Autonomy is the right of the individual to *make decisions for herself or himself,* and is a central value in Western cultures. Autonomy is generally considered at two levels. The first is **agency** or **decisional autonomy,** the freedom to decide among options. The second is **action** or **executional autonomy,** the freedom to carry out the course of action chosen.

For older adults and younger people with disabilities, the freedom to choose among options is potentially constrained by several factors. The range of options itself may be constrained by lack of information, limited personal resources, or well-documented gaps in the current system of services. Chronically impaired people may be precluded from making choices because of assumptions (correct or not) about their ability to participate in such deci-

sions. Most important, older adults as a group are more likely to suffer limitations in their capacity to make decisions due to impaired cognitive ability. These cognitive impairments may be a result of mental illness, dementia, or other mental or physical problems that alter the individual's understanding of his or her surroundings. Symptoms such as impaired memory, disorientation, and poor judgment directly impair ability to participate in decisions; additionally, capacity to participate in care decisions may fluctuate over time.

Determining an individual's capacity to make certain decisions is an inexact science. The term *competence* is primarily a legal definition rather than a medical definition, and while some cognitively impaired clients may be formally determined to be incompetent by a probate court, many do not go through this procedure (Kapp, 2002). The formal assessment of competence or decisional capacity is itself highly complex and rich with ethical implications. Most ethicists and clinicians prefer the concept of *task-specific competence,* which recognizes that individuals may have the decisional capacity to make some decisions but not others. For example, an individual with mild cognitive impairment may be capable of expressing wishes regarding assignment of a particular home health aide, yet be incapable of understanding a full range of treatment options for mid-stage breast cancer.

Surrogate Decision Making

For those who are so impaired as to be unable to participate in treatment decisions, a hierarchy of standards should be used in the decision-making process. Most preferred are *advance directives,* formulated by individuals while competent, which declare preferences regarding future treatment. Potential benefits of advance directives include ensuring that patient wishes are clearly articulated, decreasing emotional burden on the family members who are required to make end-of-life decisions for their loved one, and minimizing the possibility that surrogate decisionmakers will make a choice that is inconsistent with the individual's values. Advance directives may be informal letters or written statements that provide an indication of patient wishes, or formal legal documents, such as a living will or durable power of attorney. For most patients, clear, written statements of preference are not available, despite federal legislation encouraging completion of advanced directives (see below). Thus, the physician or other professional must often rely on reports from family, friends, or other caregivers regarding past statements or behaviors that indicate what the patient would want in the current circumstances. The principle of substituted judgment is then used to determine the appropriate course of action.

Substituted judgment means that the decision-maker uses knowledge of the client's preferences and actions prior to incapacitation to make the decisions the person would have made in these circumstances were she or he still competent. Unfortunately, evidence indicates that there is often poor correlation between surrogate decisions and patient wishes regarding treatment decisions, including care at the end of life (Ditto et al., 2001; Smucker et al., 2001). When the decisionmaker's knowledge is not adequate to apply the principle of substituted judgment, the principle of *best interest* applies.

Best-interest decisions balance the expected burdens and benefits to the client of alternative actions. The best-interest standard is considered less desirable than substituted judgment because of its deemphasis on personal autonomy and because of potential disagreement regarding the true best interest of the client. In some cases, the appointment of a guardian to participate in treatment decisions on behalf of the incapacitated individual may be necessary. To address the special ethical concerns of the cognitively impaired, advocates and providers have begun to develop creative approaches to decision making, including durable powers of attorney, more detailed living wills, and other forms of advance care planning by proxy (Volicer et al., 2002).

Related Ethical Concepts

In addition to the ethical principles tied to individual rights and responsibilities, a number of ethical concepts guide the health care professional's actions and consequently affect individual autonomy. **Beneficence** is a primary human value; simply put, it means doing good for others. A related value is nonmaleficence, which is embodied in the direction of the Hippocratic oath to "first, do no harm." Those in the helping professions place strong importance on beneficence: it forms a basis for professional codes of ethics for medicine, nursing, and social work. Ethical dilemmas frequently involve the balancing of beneficence and the wish to protect the client's autonomy and individual right to decide for himself or herself.

Paternalism is the making of decisions for another. **Weak paternalism** refers to making decisions for another who is unable to make them independently (e.g., the cognitively impaired). **Strong paternalism** refers to making decisions for another who *is* capable of making them. Although paternalism is often used in a pejorative sense, professionals in the continuum of care are often called on to make decisions for clients whose ability to care for themselves is impaired.

An individual's right to confidentiality and privacy is among other ethical and legal issues made more complex across a continuum of care. Individual control over the nature and type of information shared with care providers is challenged by the requirements of the system in several ways. Detailed clinical and financial information is necessary in the determination of eligibility for particular services or programs, developing appropriate care plans, and processing reimbursement for expenditures. Clients may be unaware of the distribution of such personal information, even when they have signed releases or other legal documents authorizing access to medical records and financial data.

Because of increasing public concerns regarding privacy of health information and access to medical records, the federal government passed legislation intended to restrict access to records and to extend additional protections. The Health Insurance Portability and Accountability Act (HIPAA) of 1996 (Pub. L. No. 104-191) is comprehensive legislation addressing insurance portability, accountability, and

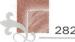
administrative simplification. The portability aspect of the legislation assures that individuals moving from one health plan to another will maintain continuity of coverage and will not be denied coverage under the preexisting condition clauses. The accountability aspect of the legislation increases the federal government's fraud enforcement authority in several areas. It directs the Department of Health and Human Services (DHHS) Secretary and Inspector General, working with the Attorney General, to coordinate federal, state, and local law enforcement programs to control fraud and abuse with respect to health care plans and to conduct investigations, audits, evaluations, and inspections relating to delivery of and payment for health care. The administrative simplification component addresses privacy and security of health information. This section of HIPAA was implemented later than the others and has caused considerable concern among health care providers as they work to comply with the regulations. In the first part of this HIPAA section, the Secretary of DHHS is directed to set standards for coding and transmitting health and billing information that is electronically exchanged.

The intent of the HIPAA privacy rules is to protect individuals from unnecessary disclosure of their personal health information, and to give each person control of how such health information is disclosed. The HIPAA statute, though critical in protecting privacy of individuals, also presents significant challenges for health care systems in terms of information sharing and provision of patient care (Gostin, 2001). Individuals may give permission for their own health information to be disclosed for research and other purposes. In most cases, use of individually identifiable health information requires informed consent, but there are circumstances in which health information may be used for research purposes without individual consent. Such use requires approval of a waiver by an institutional review board (IRB) or privacy board, with assurance that the research involves no more than minimal risk, that appropriate protections are in place to protect identifiers from improper use or disclosure,

> ## INDIVIDUALLY IDENTIFIABLE HEALTH INFORMATION
>
> "Information created or received by a health care provider, health plan, public health authority, employer, life insurer, school or university or health care clearing house that relates to past, present, or future physical or mental health or condition of an individual, the provision of health care to an individual or the past, present or future payment of health care to an individual."
>
> SOURCE: Pub. L. No. 104-191, Aug. 21, 1996, p. 91.

and that a plan exists for destruction of identifiers at the end of the research.

For additional information regarding the use of covered health information for research purposes, see *http://www.hhs.gov/ocr/hipaa/guidelines/research.pdf*. Compliance with HIPAA regulations is required if one is either (1) a "Covered Entity" (i.e., a health plan, a health care provider, or a health care clearing house), or (2) one who exchanges (sends or receives) covered information. In most cases, disclosure of health information requires consent from the individual, although some minimal necessary disclosures can be made for the purposes of treatment, payment, and health care operations. A helpful guide to understanding this aspect of HIPAA can be found at the DHHS Web site: *http://www.hhs.gov/ocr/hipaa/privacy.html*.

Health care professionals and their staff should be fully aware of the legal requirements, as well as their ethical duties, to protect confidentiality and to fully inform clients as to information-sharing requirements. As in all other areas of medical ethics, knowledgeable informed consent must be obtained prior to sharing personal information. Particular care must be taken in developing informed consent and patient's rights documents, both of which are frequently written at inappropriately high reading levels (Hochhauser, 1999).

APPLYING CONCEPTS ACROSS THE CONTINUUM

Home and Community-Based Services

Bill Smith is 76 and has somewhat limited mobility due to a long-standing respiratory problem. He lives alone and has trouble taking care of himself. He frequently skips meals, does not take medications as prescribed, and has not been doing appropriate wound care for a foot sore exacerbated by his diabetes. He was referred to the visiting nurse association by a local care management agency, but he is refusing home-based care because he does not want a stranger in the house. His only daughter, who lives and works 45 minutes away, has been trying to convince him to move into an intermediate care setting. She has expressed resistance to caring for her father at home.

KEY CONCEPTS

- **Evaluating risk and client preferences**
- **Balancing individual autonomy and safety**
- **Identifying roles and rights of family members**

Individual autonomy is perhaps most strongly asserted in the home care setting, where people live in a familiar environment that may support expression of personal authority and preferences. Home-based care provides individuals the opportunity to make decisions of both greater and lesser magnitude (such as health care treatment and meal times). Control over one's environment has long been viewed as a basic human motivation. Several studies indicate that the presence or absence of control exerts important influences on emotional and physical well-being. Many people receiving services at home express a strong interest in the choice and scheduling of home care workers and in determining the tasks they perform.

However, for most of those being cared for at home, external factors in the continuum of care influence the degree to which true autonomy may be exercised. The involvement of care management agencies, managed-care organizations, and families in arranging and delivering care in the community has very real implications for individual autonomy. It is increasingly common for acute, institutional, and home-based services to be coordinated through care management agencies, which perform screening, assessment, care planning, and monitoring functions. Care managers act as both gatekeepers and advocates for their clients, struggling with competing responsibilities of enhancing autonomy, ensuring safety, and justly allocating services. The continual weighing of safety and risk is intrinsic to the care management process. Strong preferences to remain at home, particularly when combined with client's overestimation of personal ability to function independently and underestimation of the risks associated with staying at home, complicate the care manager's responsibility to construct a safe plan of care.

Key elements of care management that can enhance individual autonomy include sharing information regarding the full continuum of appropriate services, encouraging client participation in decision making, providing processes and structures to resolve disagreements between clients and care managers, and understanding issues of control and preferences in decision making.

An important first step in autonomous decision making is the communication of relevant information, such as eligibility criteria and restrictions, availability of services, financing mechanisms, and costs of care. Provision of complete and readily understandable information is essential to enabling older persons and their agents to appropriately balance safety and autonomy concerns (Kane & Kane, 2001).

The primary assumption underlying the concept of autonomy in home and community-based services is that clients wish to be (and ought to be) involved in decisions regarding their care. Though many individuals with chronic care needs prefer to actively participate in care planning, others are comfortable with a lesser degree of involvement (Benjamin & Matthias, 2001).

Several factors may influence client preferences regarding the level and nature of control they wish to exert in the care planning and management process. Health beliefs, symptom interpretation, strategies of service utilization, and care preferences have all been shown to be influenced by cultural experience (Cornelison, 2001). Socioeconomic status, education, and work experience also influence understanding and expectations of the health system, as well as trust in authority figures and willingness to express preferences regarding control. Secular and personal life events also influence preferences regarding control in care planning. Preferences may also change over time as health or cognition deteriorates. The environment and circumstances under which preferences are elicited may also influence expressed preferences regarding control. For example, the client about to be discharged from a hospital after an acute health event may express different preferences regarding control in care planning than that same person after several weeks of recuperation at home.

Care of frail older adults or people with disabilities living in the community frequently involves family members and other informal care providers. This raises ethical concerns regarding the nature and scope of family involvement in planning for and providing needed services. Balancing of interests, rights, and responsibilities must occur among the care recipient, the family and other informal caregivers, and formal health care providers. Dilemmas arise when interests of individual family members conflict. For example, a frail widowed parent may wish to move into an assisted living facility in Florida in order to be near a friend, while the children prefer her to live close to them in the northeast.

Changing dependency relationships also challenge accustomed family dynamics. When there are no clear expectations regarding what is to be reasonably expected for one generation to provide for another, feelings of guilt or abandonment may result. Expectations about the duties and responsibilities among generations in a family vary substantially among different cultures. Some may value formal

health care providers as key partners in caring for a dependent family member; others believe that relatives should be the exclusive caregivers. Inattention to these diverse perspectives may present challenges to arranging care in the community that involves culturally appropriate integration of formal and informal supports.

CONGREGATE LIVING ARRANGEMENTS

Fredrika Wolens moves into her new senior housing apartment. Soon she has piles of papers and garbage on her balcony and all over her apartment. She refuses to allow staff in to clean up or to throw away anything. "These are my things, I need them." Her neighbors begin to complain about the smells from her apartment, and two have asked to move to other floors.

KEY CONCEPTS

- Balancing individual and communal rights and responsibilities
- Defining justice in congregate settings

By their nature, congregate living arrangements require individuals to accept some limits on autonomy in order to gain the security and benefits provided by living in a communal setting. Such limits may be imposed through what Collopy (1993) describes as **intrusive beneficence,** where the individual may be denied autonomy in the name of her own well-being as defined by others. In the exercise of intrusive beneficence, social limitations may be misconstrued as mental aberrations, physical frailty may be mistaken as indicative of cognitive frailty, and periodic lapses as proof of permanent incapacity.

The ethical concept of **justice** is especially pertinent in congregate living settings, where there is daily balancing of individual preferences with group needs and wants. More than at any other point in the continuum, the issue of personal privacy and rights in the context of community safety is central to life in a congregate setting. One definition of *justice* is the concern with the fair distribution of benefits (or cost and harms) among individuals. Rawls (1971) argues that liberty should be distributed in such a way as to maximize liberty among *all* individuals and that public goods should be distributed so that the least advantaged benefit most. Although individual residents are entitled to liberty and privacy, these rights must continually be considered in relation to responsibilities and rights of others in the community.

HOSPITALS

Selena Jones is ready to be discharged from a hospitalization related to her second stroke. She has been told that she is unable to care for herself at home alone. She insists that she will go to live with her son and his wife. The daughter-in-law privately asks the discharge planner to insist that a nursing home is the only alternative. "My husband can't say no to his mother, but it would be a nightmare to have her come live with us."

KEY CONCEPTS
- Patient self-determination
- Influence of system factors on autonomy
- Balancing rights and preferences of family members

Issues of autonomy for impaired or frail older patients are raised at many points during a typical acute care hospital stay; patients are faced with decisions of both great and lesser consequence. The Patient Self Determination Act (PSDA) was implemented in late 1991. This federal law requires health care facilities such as hospitals and nursing homes to inform patients, at the time of admission, of their rights to participate in health care decisions and to execute advance directives, such as living wills, or to designate a surrogate decisionmaker or health

care agent. The law also requires facilities to have policies that allow individuals to exercise these rights and document in the patient's medical record whether the individual has a formal advance directive. Finally, the PSDA also mandates that providers train their staff and educate the community about advance directives.

Empirical studies generally indicate that the PSDA has not had the desired impact of increasing patient involvement in end-of-life decisions (The SUPPORT Investigators, 1995). Problems persist in patient awareness of advance care planning options and processes, interinstitutional transfer of advance directives, and participation of ethnic minority groups in advance care planning (Lahn, Friedman, Bijar, Haughey, & Gallagher, 2001; Baker, 2002).

Recent research suggests that preferences for end-of-life care are highly contextual—that is, they are largely influenced by the specific circumstances surrounding the decision. Systems of care can support health care professionals by allowing time to build trust with patients and continuing advance care planning conversations over time, prior to a medical crisis (Prendergast, 2001).

Historically, much attention has focused on the ethical concerns around physician-client relationships and specific medical care decisions, such as the right to refuse treatment. Recent discussions have begun to acknowledge the critical importance of involving the client in planning continuing care arrangements after hospital discharge. Discharge planning, a function required of hospitals by JCAHO guidelines, is viewed as the main method for ensuring that clients' continuing care needs are met and that they are supported to function at the highest possible level upon returning home from a hospital stay. Comprehensive discharge planning, typically conducted by advanced practice nurses, has been shown to reduce hospital readmission rates and decrease costs of care (Naylor et al., 1999).

Several factors unique to discharge planning challenge the protection of individual autonomy in that process. Often there is great urgency to arrange needed services, especially in light of the ever-increasing demands for early discharge. Patients are often under severe emotional stress associated with an injury or impairment. Systems factors, such as availability and allocation of resources, as well as fragmentation in services and issues of access, also present difficulties for discharge planners. An individual's ability to exercise clear and considered choices is constrained by these factors, as well as by the opinions of family members and other caregivers.

Discharge planning often involves making choices about the nature and amount of care that will be delivered at home. Individuals vary in their reactions to this process, including the degree of control they wish to exert in the decisions that are made. Ethical dilemmas may arise for hospital staff (often social workers) who are responsible for this activity and who feel pressured by conflicting demands of clients, family members, and their own hospital administration. Full exploration of patient preferences, family circumstances, available data, and value systems are recommended to ameliorate these pressures.

NURSING HOMES

George Brown has been in the nursing home for seven months, during which time he had a private room. Because of a new admission that fills the last available bed, a roommate is moved in with George. Soon there are big problems. George does not like the fact that the roommate is forgetful and that he is incontinent. "He messes around with my things and he smells. I always had my own room except in the army. I can't sleep with him here. Move me or let me go home."

KEY CONCEPTS

- Risk of exclusion from health care decisions
- Balancing individual choice with institutional needs

Residents of nursing homes are at increased risk for inappropriate treatment and inadequate decision-making processes, such as being inappropriately excluded from health care decisions. The very nature of nursing homes may reinforce feelings of dependence and encourage learned helplessness. The limited involvement of physicians in most institutional care makes it unlikely that the client and physician will even know one another, let alone develop a trusting relationship. Older people are especially vulnerable to being excluded from discussions due to frailty, advanced age, prevalence of dementia, and biased practice patterns or care providers (Shawler, Rowles, & High, 2001).

Since passage of the nursing home reform laws in the late 1980s, concerted efforts have been made by policymakers, providers, and advocates to enhance the participation of nursing home residents in decisions that affect their daily lives. Though important improvements have been achieved in many institutions, resident involvement in treatment decisions remains quite constrained, particularly with regard to end-of-life care. Alternative models, such as advance proxy planning, are being evaluated, and offer promise for residents who lack decision-making capacity (Cantor & Pearlman, 2003).

Although some anecdotal evidence suggests that individuals are not interested in or comfortable with discussions about future health events or treatments, studies in both hospitals and nursing homes have demonstrated that many people appreciate the opportunity to exercise control and express preferences over future medical care.

The current emphasis on autonomy in medical care decision making in nursing homes often overlooks other important issues for residents. Additional concerns among residents include the right to choose their own roommates, timing of meals and bedtimes, menus, when to make and receive phone calls, and a myriad of other daily decisions most of us take for granted. The problems and concerns involved in balancing individual rights and preferences with the needs of the group, discussed earlier in this chapter, are clearly evident in nursing home settings.

A major challenge for administrators and staff is to identify opportunities for flexibility and choice, and to support resident preferences whenever possible. As innovative strategies for caregiving are developed, and as philosophy and practice change, resident rights and quality of life are enhanced. Current research is examining mechanisms to include residents in defining essential aspects of a good quality of life in nursing homes (Kane, 2003). One example of how philosophical and policy changes may enhance patient autonomy is the effort over the past decade to reduce the inappropriate use of physical and chemical restraints with nursing home residents. Combining a change in philosophy of care with research that demonstrated effective alternatives to restraints fueled an advocacy movement that changed practice in many institutions.

MANAGED-CARE ENVIRONMENTS

Ms. Dalia is a 79-year-old retired school teacher who suffered a stroke while gardening. After a brief hospitalization, she was discharged to a subacute unit of a nursing home for rehabilitation. Upon reaching the short-term functional goals of the rehabilitation protocol, she returned to her home with a very limited number of home health visits for continued rehabilitation. The visiting nurse believes that Ms. Dalia would benefit from more rehabilitation visits, but the HMO care manager enforces the limited number, citing company guidelines for in-home rehabilitation therapy.

KEY CONCEPTS

- Representing patient interest in managed care
- Balancing beneficence and standards of care
- Justice in resource allocation

Managed care environments provide both opportunities and challenges to the provision of care for older persons. Opportunities for improved geriatric care arise from centralization of records, abilities to share information and coordinate care across the full range of providers, and, in some cases, payment for services not usually covered in the fee-for-service system. In some cases, HMOs and other managed-care organizations have enhanced information sharing regarding older clients, improved management of medications across providers, and widened the availability of preventive health interventions. In contrast, some managed care organizations have achieved efficiencies by limiting access to certain types of care.

In the case presented above, the nurse struggles between the conflicting values of beneficence and best interests on one side, and the rules and guidelines governing the provision of care in this organization on the other. This circumstance could be framed as a justice argument, in that the managed-care organization is making an effort to efficiently provide care to a **population** of clients, while the nurse in this case is primarily concerned with the well-being of an individual client. The most appropriate course of action in a circumstance such as this is for the nurse (1) to use existing practice guidelines and the community standard on state-of-the-art care to make an argument for the client's well-being, and (2) to fully understand and use the rules of the organization to the client's advantage. Unfortunately, these principles are often in conflict. Two specific ethical challenges for professionals working in managed-care environments are the question of representation (for whom does the professional act?) and authority (who is authorized to make policy for the organization?) (Thompson, 1999). Ethics of care has been identified as one of the core areas in which training is needed to prepare health care professionals to practice in a managed care environment.

SYSTEM-WIDE ETHICAL ISSUES

Sharon Wilson is a care manager who has just been advised that the new eligibility rules for the state Independent Seniors program will require her to inform several clients that they will no longer qualify for public payment for services they receive. In at least two cases, this may mean a move to a nursing home. She feels torn between her role as client advocate and her responsibility to apply state eligibility criteria fairly.

KEY CONCEPTS

• Justice and allocation of resources

• Advocating for client's best interest

• Supporting autonomy

Although clients and service providers experience ethical concerns and dilemmas on an individual basis, resources and constraints of a much larger system of care are at play. Factors that may limit or influence individual autonomy include financing and reimbursement mechanisms; private, state, local, and federal rules and regulations; limits in service availability; rules and practices of other professionals and agencies; limitations of the manpower pool; and family demands and values.

Public and private financing of services that constitute the system of care influence decision making for individual clients in a variety of ways. The autonomy of frail clients and the ability of care managers to develop optimal plans of care in the least restrictive environments are directly limited by client eligibility and funding mechanisms. Reimbursement caps and eligibility restrictions for community and in-home services may result in unnecessary or premature institutional placement, just as pressures of the hospital prospective payment system or managed-care models may result in early discharge to less-than-optimal service settings. Both managed-care and publicly funded services are constrained by eligibility criteria, spending caps, restrictions on types of services or providers, and payment limits for specific services. Moreover, many service agencies have minimal units of service (e.g., a minimum home visit of four hours) that limit flexibility in care planning and inflate daily costs of care. However, care managers who receive private payment directly

from family members report feeling additionally constrained in advocating for the client when the family disputes the client's choices or preferences. Capitated payment mechanisms covering populations of clients may pit one client's interests and preferences against those of another client or group of clients.

Fragmentation and gaps in the system of care in a particular individual's community may present value conflicts. State and federal agencies continue to implement new constraints in efforts to cut costs and balance budgets. Value considerations determine the distribution of resources within the health care system, influence the enactment of laws and enforcement of regulations, and provide the framework for policy making. Despite recent emphasis on home and community-based services, mechanisms for distribution of resources remain biased in several ways. Public monies are (1) more likely to be spent for medical/technical services than for social services, (2) more likely to pay for institutional services in hospitals and nursing homes than for services that keep people in their own homes, and (3) more likely to pay for later, more intrusive interventions than for earlier interventions that support the client, family, and other informal caregivers. An important ethical consideration is whether these allocation policies accurately reflect societal values or in fact save money in the long run.

On what basis do we distribute scarce health and social service dollars? How much do we hold the individual or family responsible to pay for or provide needed care? Health care professionals frequently find themselves in conflict with social policy. Physicians may be required by their hospitals to consider economic issues in the decisions to admit, treat, or discharge patients. Care managers for community-dwelling seniors may be forced to balance programmatic goals and funding constraints against the needs and wishes of clients (Gallagher, Alcock, Diem, Angus, & Melves, 2002). Nurses may find themselves trapped between residents' interests and the administrative or regulatory constraints of the nursing home in which they work. These ethical dilemmas are not easily resolved.

Two distinct yet closely related recent trends have

had substantial impact on long-term care systems. First, there is strong policy emphasis on providing necessary supports in the least restrictive setting possible. The Supreme Court's *Olmstead* decision of 1999 mandated that states and, by extension, health care providers, offer services to persons with disabilities in a setting that is as integrated into the community as possible, given their individual circumstances. A parallel movement, known as **consumer-directed care,** calls for a system that supports the client (or consumer) in making autonomous decisions regarding the nature and extent of the care he or she receives. The ethical challenges of these trends are only beginning to be explored. Key considerations include balancing safety and freedom, defining acceptable risks and associated responsibilities, assessing quality of care, and determining the respective roles of government, providers, and consumers (Moseley, 2001).

SPECIAL ETHICAL ISSUES IN CONTINUUM OF CARE SYSTEMS

Many of the ethical concerns raised throughout this chapter are relevant both to services provided independently and to those organized into a managed continuum of care. There are, however, ethical issues that are unique to, or are expressed differently in, an organized continuum of care. Such a continuum provides opportunities to more effectively address certain ethical concerns, but may, because of the very nature of its structure and coordination of care, raise others.

Opportunities for improved consideration or management of ethical concerns grow out of the more comprehensive and coordinated models of care, improved structures and processes for sharing information among providers regarding client wishes and advance planning, and increased consistency among providers regarding decision-making processes.

More comprehensive and better coordinated systems of care are more likely to provide individual clients a timely array of service and treatment alternatives, thus enhancing autonomous choice. Cost-efficient and appropriate services may enhance long-term autonomy by prolonging the period that the client is able to remain at home, and will facilitate movement among service settings as the client needs change. A care manager may also facilitate discussions of client preferences and ethical issues, particularly if that care manager is well known to and trusted by the client, and acts as the client's advocate. The shared (usually computerized) information systems common to coordinated continuums of care offer another opportunity to enhance client autonomy and reduce ethical conflicts. At any point in the system, a detailed discussion of issues and options and careful solicitation of client preferences can be accurately documented, shared with other providers, and remain in the record for efficient changes should the client's wishes change.

An integrated continuum of care may raise ethical concerns, and specific aspects of such a system of care may require special attention from an ethics perspective. As with other systems using care managers, there are potential role conflicts between gatekeeping functions and client advocacy functions. These conflicts may be exacerbated in a system for which the care manager is the key to accessing the entire continuum of services. Integrated information systems may require special vigilance to protect client privacy and to ensure that the client understands how information will be shared among various levels of care and providers of services. It is also important that all people and agencies among which information is disseminated share common understandings of the ethical implications and appropriate use of client information, including advance directives and advance care planning processes.

CONCLUSION

Autonomy—the right of an individual to make decisions for himself or herself—is a fundamental ethical premise to consider in service delivery. Familial rights, societal values, and cultural norms may all affect individual autonomy. External system influences affect the individual's autonomy as well. Older people and those with disabilities are at increased ethical risk for a number of reasons, including ageism, physical and cognitive impairments, and fragmentation of services.

Health professionals must balance the client's right to autonomy with professional obligations of beneficence and nonmaleficence, including ensuring safety across various settings. Structures and formal mechanisms are essential to support health professionals as they address ethical dilemmas in their daily work.

Effective attention to ethical issues requires proactive consideration and planning. Carefully developed policies and procedures that are well documented and disseminated are crucial. The organization of an ethics committee for purposes of system-wide education, promulgation of policies and procedures, and review of conflicts or difficult cases has been useful in many systems of care. An ethics committee with representation of various providers within the continuum can be a useful resource, particularly for agencies or organizations that may not yet have ethics committees of their own. Community-based resources may include faculty from local universities, clergy, senior law programs of the state bar association, volunteer and advocacy groups, and clients themselves.

A number of additional resources are available to health care professionals faced with ethical challenges in their work. Most professional associations have adopted codes of ethics that identify core ethical principles and guide decision making from a particular disciplinary perspective. Many professional societies also have special interest groups devoted to the study of ethical concerns. Educational institutions and advocacy organizations may provide helpful resources. Finally, continuing professional education and scientific conferences provide opportunities for further exploration of these issues, as well as the development and application of practical tools for use in difficult cases where the balancing of clinical, legal, and ethical considerations is particularly complex.

WHERE TO GO FOR FURTHER INFORMATION

American Association of Retired Persons (AARP)
Legal Council for the Elderly
601 E Street, NW
Washington, DC 20049
(202) 434-2135
http://www.aarp.org

American Bar Association
Commission on Legal Problems of Elderly
740 15th Street, NW
Washington, DC 20005-1019
(202) 662-1000
http://www.abanet.org

American Society of Law and Medicine and Ethics
765 Commonwealth Avenue
Boston, MA 02215
(617) 262-4990
http://www.aslme.org

Center for Bioethics
University of Pennsylvania
School of Medicine
3401 Market Street, Suite 320
Philadelphia, PA 19104-3319
(215) 898-7136
http://www.bioethics.upenn.edu

Center for Biomedical Ethics
Case Western Reserve University
Department of Bioethics
10900 Euclid Avenue
Cleveland, OH 44106-4976
(216) 368-6196
http://www.cwru.edu/med/bioethics

Institute for Ethics
American Medical Association
515 N. State Street
Chicago, IL 60610
(312) 464-5260
http://www.ife@ama-assn.org

Midwest Bioethics Center
1021-25 Jefferson Street

Kansas City, MO 64105
(816) 221-1100
http://www.midbio.org

National Reference Center for Bioethics Literature
Kennedy Institute of Ethics
Georgetown University
Box 571212
Washington, DC 20057-1212
1-888-BIO-ETHIX or (202) 687-3885
http://www.georgetown.edu

Office of Public Information
The Hastings Center
255 Elm Road
Briarcliff Manor, NY 10510
(914) 762-8500

Partnership for Caring, Inc.
1620 Eye Street NW, Suite 202
Washington, DC 20006
(202) 296-8071
http://www.partnershipforcaring.org

Promoting Excellence in End of Life Care
RWJ Foundation National Program Office
c/o The Practical Ethics Center
The University of Montana
1000 East Beckwith Avenue
Missoula, MT 59812
(406) 243-6601
http://www.promotingexcellence.org

U.S. Department of Health and Human Services
200 Independence Avenue, SW
Washington, DC 20201
(202) 619-368-6196
http://www.hhs.gov/ocr/hipaa/privacy

FACTS REVIEW

1. Identify system-level factors that may limit autonomy.
2. Describe the hierarchy of surrogate decision making.
3. Identify systemic biases in resource allocation.

4. Define several core ethical principles relevant to the delivery of health care across the continuum.

REFERENCES

Baker, M. E. (2002). Economic, political and ethnic influences on end of life decisionmaking: A decade in review. *Journal of Health and Social Policy, 14*(3), 27–39.

Benjamin, A. E., & Matthias, R. E. (2001). Age, consumer direction and outcomes of supportive services at home. *The Gerontologist, 41,* 632–642.

Cantor, M. D., & Pearlman, R. A. (2003). Advance care planning in long term care facilities. *Journal of the American Medical Association, 4*(2), 101–108.

Collopy, B. (1993). The burden of beneficence. In R. A. Kane & A. L. Caplan (Eds.), *Ethical conflicts in the management of home care.* New York: Springer.

Cornelison, A. H. (2001). Cultural barriers to compassionate care: Patients' and health professionals' perspectives. *Bioethics Forum, 17*(1), 7–14.

Ditto, P. H., Danks, J. H., Smucker, W. D., Bookwala, J., Coppola, K. M., Dresser, R., Fagerlin, A., Gready, R. M., Houts, R. M., Lockhart, L. K., & Zyzanski, S. (2001). Advance directives as acts of communication: A randomized controlled trial. *Archives of Internal Medicine, 1619*(3), 7–14.

Gallagher, E., Alcock, D., Diem, E., Angus, D., & Melves, J. (2002). Ethical dilemmas in home care case management. *Journal of Healthcare Management, 47*(2), 85–96.

Gostin, L. O. (2001). National health information privacy: Regulations under the Health Insurance Portability and Accountability Act. *Journal of the American Medical Association, 285*(23), 3015–3021.

Hochhauser, M. (1999). Informed consent and patient's rights: A right, a rite, or a rewrite? *Ethics and Behavior, 9*(1), 1–20.

Kane, R. L. (2003). Definition, measurement and correlates of quality of life in nursing homes: Toward a reasonable practice, research and policy agenda. *The Gerontologist, 43*(Special no. 2), 28–36.

Kane, R. L., & Kane, R. A. (2001). What older people want from long term care and how they can get it. *Health Affairs, 20*(6), 114–127.

Kapp, M. B. (2002). Decisional capacity in theory and practice: Legal process versus "bumbling through." *Aging and Mental Health, 6*(4), 413–417.

Lahn, M., Friedman, B., Bijar, P., Haughey, M., & Gallagher, E. J. (2001). Advance directives in skilled nursing facility residents transferred to emergency departments. *Academic Emergency Medicine, 8*(12), 1158–1162.

Moseley, C. (2001). *Balancing safety and freedom in consumer-directed systems of support.* Durham, NH: Institute on Disability, University of New Hampshire.

Naylor, M. D., Brooten, D., Campbell, R., Jacobson, B. S., Mezey, M. D., Pauly, M. V., & Schwartz, J. S. (1999). Comprehensive discharge planning and home followup of hospitalized elders: A randomized clinical trial. *Journal of the American Medical Association, 218*(7), 613–620.

Prendergast, T. J. (2001). Advance care planning: Pitfalls, progress, promise. *Critical Care Medicine, 29*(2), N34–N39.

Rawls, J. (1971). *A theory of justice.* Cambridge, MA: Harvard University Press.

Shawler, C., Rowles, G. D., & High, D. (2001). Analysis of key decisionmaking incidents in the life of a nursing home resident. *The Gerontologist, 41,* 612–622.

Smucker, W. D., Houts, R. M., Danks, J. H., Ditto, P. H., Fagerlin, A., & Coppola, K. M. (2001). Modal preferences predict elderly patients' life-sustaining treatment choice as well as patients' chosen surrogates do. *Medical Decision Making, 20*(3), 271–280.

The Support Investigators. (1995). A controlled trial to improve care for seriously ill hospitalized patients. *Journal of the American Medical Association, 274,* 1519–1598.

Thompson, D. F. (1999). The institutional turn in professional ethics. *Ethics and Behavior, 9*(2), 109–118.

Volicer, L., Cantor, M. D., Derse, A. R., Edwards, D. M., Prudhomme, A. M., Gregory, D. C., Reagan, J. E., Tulsky, J. A., & Fox, E. (National Ethics Committee of the Veteran's Health Administration). (2004). Advance care planning by proxy for residents of long term care facilities who lack decisionmaking capacity. *Journal of the American Geriatrics Society, 50*(4), 761–767.

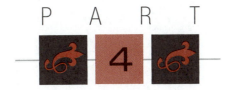

P A R T
4

Continuums for Special Populations

Continuums of care are organized around client needs. One organization may be part of several continuums, or it may offer several continuums in parallel or overlapping structures, each orchestrated around clients with a particular type of need. The chapters in this part describe continuums that focus on the needs of special segments of the long-term care population. Each continuum has its own funding streams, applicable public policies, and management challenges.

CHAPTER 17

Disability

Kathleen Tschantz Unroe and Ann Scheck McAlearney

People with disabilities access a wide range of services along the continuum of long-term care. According to the 2000 U.S. Census Bureau survey, which excludes institutionalized persons, almost 20 percent of the population, or 49.7 million persons, had some level of disability, including sensory losses, mobility impairments, difficulty learning, difficulty performing activities of daily living (ADLs), difficulty leaving the home, and an impaired ability to work (U.S. Census Bureau, 2003). In 1997, more than 2 million persons age 15 and older used a wheelchair, and another 6.4 million used a cane, crutches, or a walker (McNeil, 2001). The U.S. Census Bureau estimated that the costs of disability exceeded $340 billion in 2000, representing a doubling since 1990 (Hellwig, 1999).

People with disabilities are a heterogeneous group. They are often categorized by others and themselves into age- and condition-specific groups, such as deaf people, paralyzed war veterans, people with HIV/AIDS, elderly disabled, or people with mental illness. Disabilities can be obvious, such as a person using a wheelchair or sign language; however, most

are not apparent, including conditions such as heart disease or psychiatric disorders. People in the disability community sometimes describe people who are not disabled as "temporarily able-bodied" (Fleischer & Zames, 2001). This label demonstrates the reality that disability is a possibility for all people and a commonly occurring aspect of the human condition.

The medical and social support services available for people with disabilities are challenging to coordinate. Eligibility criteria for different programs can be confusing. Further, individuals may have vastly different needs, and coverage guidelines restrict what they can access. Discrimination and barriers to participation in society led to civil rights legislation for people with disabilities. It is important to be familiar with the public policy and legal issues surrounding this population.

This chapter provides an overview of disability and the issues surrounding disability and long-term care, with an emphasis on physical disabilities in the adult population. The special needs of children with disabilities and people with mental retardation and mental illness are discussed in separate chapters of this text (Chapters 23 and 20, respectively).

DEFINITION

Disability is defined in numerous different ways, and the way disability is defined can have important policy implications. Having a clear definition of disability is important to determine service need and eligibility, and to decide how to appropriately administer public programs, prevent discrimination, and conduct research. Agreement on a universal definition has not been reached, and the nature of this complicated concept may make a consensus impossible. However, discussion of some of the more common definitions, such as those used by the Social Security Administration, the Americans with Disabilities Act, the World Health Organization, and the Institute of Medicine, can help improve understanding of the perspectives and experiences that inform disability.

Social Security Administration Definition. To determine benefits eligibility for the financial assistance available through the Social Security Disability Insurance and the Supplemental Security Income programs, the federal Social Security Administration requires that a person must demonstrate an inability to work due to any physical or mental impairment expected to result in death or lasting continuously for at least 12 months (Wunderlich, Rice, & Amado, 2002).

Americans with Disabilities Act Definition. The 1990 Americans with Disabilities Act (ADA) broadly defines *disability* as a substantial limitation in a major life activity, such as walking, seeing, hearing, learning, breathing, caring for oneself, or working (Fleischer & Zames, 2001). Psychiatric disorders, alcoholism, and recovered drug addiction are included under this definition. Court cases continue to test this definition and have imposed some limits on it.

World Health Organization Definition. The World Health Organization (WHO) has an interest in defining disability in order to estimate its impact on global public health. The WHO created the International Classification of Impairments, Disabilities, and Handicaps (ICIDH) in 1980 to establish a common language for discussion of the consequences of disease from a biopsychosocial perspective. According to the ICIDH, *impairments* are functional losses, and *disability* is the resulting limitation of activity. *Handicap* refers to the performance of social roles and social participation (i.e., the disadvantage to the person caused by disability that prevents fulfilling normal social roles) (Council of Europe, 1999). In 2001, the WHO began using a revised paradigm, the International Classification of Functioning, Disability, and Health (ICF) to discuss disability, moving away from the "consequences of disease" model to a "components of health" classification. This newer WHO model considers the impact on participation due to disability and includes two major components: (1) functioning and disability, and (2) contextual factors (WHO, 2003). Examples of types of disabilities classified by this definition are shown in Table 17.1.

Institute of Medicine Definition. The Institute of Medicine (IOM) defines *disability* as requiring assistance with certain tasks normally accomplished independently. Developed by Saad Nagi of the Ohio State University, the Nagi model serves as the basis for the IOM definitions of *disability*. This conceptualization of disability considers that disability has a pathologic origin that causes impairment and leads to functional limitations and, thus, disability. Nagi emphasized that environmental factors, including physical and sociocultural barriers, are important in discussing disability. The IOM considers a person with an impairment or functional limitation as potentially disabled; however, the degree of disability is actually determined by the physical and social environment. Disability itself, rather than handicap or participation, as emphasized in the WHO models, is considered the outcome (Brandt & Pope, 1997).

Clearly, the way in which disability is defined has important policy implications. A 1991 Health and Human Services report stated: "Differences in programmatic definitions [of disability] result in wide

Table 17.1 International Classification of Functioning, Disability, and Health (ICF) Definition Used by the World Health Organization

	Components of Health	Examples of Disability
Functioning and disability	Bodily functions and structures	Loss of a limb
	Activities and participation	Ability to perform tasks such as self-care
Contextual factors	Environmental factors	Inaccessible buildings
	Personal factors	Age, health conditions

SOURCE: WHO, 2003.

variations in the number and characteristics of persons eligible to receive benefits and huge differences in how much programs cost" (Adler, 1991). Administrators and service providers must not only be familiar with the legal definitions of disability, but also be aware of the dynamic approaches to defining disability used by researchers, policymakers, and the disability community.

The Origin of Disability

Disability can originate from three different causes: congenital, developmental, and acquired. *Congenital* causes of disability are those disabilities due to genetic factors. Examples include cystic fibrosis and muscular dystrophy. Disabilities that occur from *developmental* processes are defined as those that occur before age 22. They may become more severe over time, and include conditions such as cerebral palsy or epilepsy. Disability may also be *acquired,* by causes such as brain injury and heart disease (Dell Orto & Marinelli, 1995).

Emphasis placed on these different origins of disability has led to the development of separate service systems for different disabled populations. This is problematic, however, because there is very wide variation in the functional abilities of people with different conditions. For example, many factors determine how disabling a stroke is for an individual, such as the part of the brain affected by the stroke and the type of treatment received. However, when determining actual service needs, many regard the

degree of functional limitation as more relevant than the actual origin of the disability. Figure 2.3 in Chapter 2 shows how these distinct causes of disability relate to paths of care.

PROFILE OF AMERICANS WITH DISABILITIES

Americans with disabilities are disproportionately older, impoverished, and female, compared to the general U.S. population. However, the profile of disability changes with age and varies by race. Younger, disabled Americans are more likely to be male, and blacks and whites are more likely to report disability than Asians or Hispanics. The 2000 Census found that nearly one in five noninstitutionalized persons over age five reported having a disability. These disabilities included sensory, physical, and mental conditions (see Figure 17.1). The census also looked at whether people had disabilities that affected self-care (performing ADLs), employment, or the ability to go outside the home (U.S. Census, 2003).

Across the U.S. population, the prevalence of disability increases with age (Figure 17.2). In 1997, 8 percent of the under-15 age group had a disability, and 4 percent of this age group was considered severely disabled (McNeil, 2001). For the 45- to 54-year age group, the proportion of the population with any disability increases to 23 percent, and 14 percent of this age group report having a severe

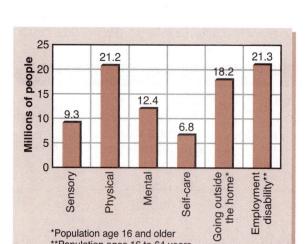

Figure 17.1 Types of Disability, Population Age 5 and Older, 2000
SOURCE: U.S. Census Bureau, 2003.

disability. The trend of increasing disability with age continues such that nearly three-quarters of the population age 80 and older report having a disability, with more than half of this age group describing a severe disability.

People with disabilities are much more likely to be impoverished than individuals who do not have disabilities. For the general U.S. population, about 8 percent of people between 25 and 64 years old lived in poverty in 1997. However, among those with a severe disability, more than one-quarter (28 percent) were reportedly poor (McNeil, 2001).

Gender differences associated with disability are also evident. In 1997, the prevalence of disability in the 15- to 24-year age group was higher among men (12 percent) than women (10 percent). However, in older age groups, a higher proportion of women had a disability. More women are disabled overall, with 28.3 million women having any dis-

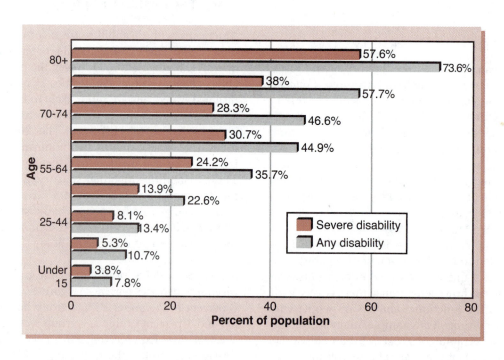

Figure 17.2 Percent of Population Reporting a Disability, by Age
SOURCE: McNeil, 2001.

ability, compared with 24.3 million men (McNeil, 2001).

There is also variation in the prevalence of disability by race. In 1997, among Asians and Pacific Islanders, 9 percent had a disability; among Hispanics, 10 percent had a disability. Disability among whites was 12 percent, and blacks had the highest rate of disability, at 16 percent of the population (McNeil, 2001).

DISABILITY RIGHTS AND INDEPENDENT LIVING MOVEMENTS

Historically, people with severe disabilities were expected to live their lives in chronic care institutions. However, in the late 1950s and early 1960s, a trend toward deinstitutionalization arose (Fleischer & Zames, 2001). When trying to reestablish themselves in the community, people with disabilities encountered many obstacles, especially in finding appropriate housing and jobs. The presence of these barriers led many people with disabilities to begin to advocate for the support they needed to live productive, independent lives in their own communities. Such early advocacy efforts became the inspiration for the disability rights and independent living movements (Switzer, 2003).

The core philosophy of these movements is that each person needs independent control over his or her own life. Language is seen as important, and the term *consumer* is preferred over the paternalistic term *patient*. Although independence in performing activities of daily living (ADLs) may never be possible for some, it is still possible to enable these individuals to have autonomy in decision making, if they receive appropriate support and information. Assuring this autonomy is empowering to individuals and is seen as a core principle of disability rights (Allen & Mor, 1998).

With respect to policy making, it has been difficult to organize the heterogeneous mix of disabled individuals to advocate for disability rights. However, coalitions of disability groups worked together

to support the passage of Section 504 of the 1973 Rehabilitation Act and the 1990 Americans with Disabilities Act (Fleischer & Zames, 2001). Collectively, the disability community remains focused on the goal of enabling people with disabilities to live in community-based settings, outside of institutions.

SERVICES NEEDED

Long-term care for people with disabilities requires many different services and depends on the type of disability, degree of impairment, co-morbid conditions, an individual's support network and resources, and an individual's personal goals. Although a person with severe disabilities may never be able to function without assistance, having control over services and care planning can still allow this individual to live independently. Long-term care in institutional settings is discussed in other chapters of this book. This chapter focuses on home and community-based services for people with chronic disabilities.

The components of long-term care for a person with disabilities include both health and social support services. Income support, accessible housing, access to health care, and personal support are all necessary to enable people with disabilities to achieve the goals of independence. These types of services are discussed in the following sections.

Income

Poverty often accompanies disability. In 1997, for people between the ages of 25 and 64, 28 percent of those with a severe disability, versus 8 percent of people with no disability, lived in poverty. Eighty percent of people with a severe disability had an income of less than $20,000 a year, compared with 44 percent of people with no disability (McNeil, 2001).

Two federal programs, Social Security Disability Insurance (SSDI) and Supplemental Security Income (SSI), provide cash benefits to eligible people with long-term disabilities. They use the same definition of *disability* to determine eligibility, as described earlier. Applicants for disability benefits must work with State Disability Determination Services offices, which decide whether applicants are disabled according to the defined criteria.

In 1956, the SSDI program was enacted to provide cash benefits to people who were unable to participate in substantial gainful activity. SSDI is financed through Social Security payroll taxes. To be eligible for benefits, the disabled person must have worked for a certain length of time, and this time varies by age. A person with disabilities often may also qualify for SSDI if he or she is the spouse, widow or widower, or dependent child of a worker. The amount of the benefit is based on previous earnings and varies widely among individuals. According to the Social Security Administration (SSA), claims for disability benefits take 60 to 90 days to process. Benefits are not paid until the sixth full month following the onset of disability. Persons receiving SSDI are not permitted to earn more than $800 per month (Wunderlich et al., 2002).

The SSI program for the aged, blind, and disabled was enacted in 1972. It was designed to guarantee a minimum level of income for this needy population. However, unlike SSDI, SSI applicants must apply for aid under all other programs, including SSDI, before they will be considered for SSI. SSI is funded through general tax revenues, and earnings limits for beneficiaries vary by state (Wunderlich et al., 2002). The monthly federal SSI benefit in 2003 was $552, but 15 states supplement that benefit amount with additional state funds (SSA, 2003).

Critical to the discussion of income is the topic of employment. People with disabilities are much less likely to be employed, for many reasons. A 2000 survey found that although 81 percent of nondisabled people ages 18 to 64 worked full- or part-time, only 32 percent of working-age people with a disability were employed full- or part-time (Switzer, 2003). People who are capable of performing in a job face discrimination in hiring, as well as many physical barriers (Iezzoni, 2003). People who do

find employment risk losing their public benefits, and this is an ongoing policy concern. Technological advances, including the increased capability of computers, coupled with repeated mandates to make workplaces accessible, can help support people with disabilities in the workforce.

Accessible Housing

Having accessible housing available is imperative to enable people with disabilities to live in the community. Several laws have been passed over the last 40 years that relate to discrimination against people with disabilities with respect to housing and that encourage housing to be made accessible (Switzer, 2003). Personal homes can be modified in many ways to increase accessibility. Modifications, such as adding entrance ramps or handrails, are relatively low-cost solutions to major physical access barriers to housing. Another option for people with disabilities, and especially those with mental disabilities, is to provide housing in group home settings. The concept of *universal design* describes an approach to creating environments that are broadly accessible to people with and without disabilities throughout the lifespan (Fleischer & Zames, 2001). Applying these concepts to the variety of individual and group home options can help make housing accessible to individuals with all types of disabilities. (See Chapter 9 for a more detailed description of housing.)

Access to Health Care

Access to care for people with disabilities requires consideration of both insurance coverage and barriers encountered in different health care settings. With respect to insurance, public financing is especially important. As discussed in Chapter 14, Medicare and Medicaid are important payers for services for those with disabilities. This insurance coverage is actually linked to income support: people who receive SSI are also eligible to receive Medicaid coverage, and people who receive SSDI support for two years become eligible for Medicare coverage. Despite the availability of public coverage, a substantial proportion of those with disabilities still remains uninsured. For those with severe disabilities in the 25 to 64 age group, 17 percent lacked health insurance coverage in 1997, compared to 15 percent uninsured in the general U.S. population (McNeil, 2001).

Managed-care plans also provide coverage for many people with disabilities. Because such persons often need coordinated care, managed-care plans may be more effective in meeting their needs. However, the addition of services such as effective case assessment, service planning, care coordination, and ongoing case management may increase the cost of providing care for these individuals, because of increased demand for needed services. Additional issues, such as access to specialists and coverage for durable medical equipment, are particularly problematic for the disabled population. Appropriate risk adjustment is necessary to ensure adequate reimbursement for managed-care organizations trying to provide optimal care for this population (Vladeck, 2003; Regenstein, Schroer, & Meyer, 2000).

For those with physical disabilities, access to care is also affected by the physical barriers that often exist in health care settings. However, relatively simple accommodations can help improve access. In ambulatory settings, options such as examination tables that can be lowered and raised can improve physical access. Similarly, people with visual impairments can benefit from modifications such as enlarged written information and tape-recorded instructions. Interpretation services should include sign language interpreters who can be available to translate during medical appointments and procedures (Fleischer & Zames, 2001).

Personal Support Services

Both personal assistance services and assistive technologies help people with disabilities to live independently in their homes, perform their jobs, and participate more fully in their communities. These types of personal support are described further in this section.

Personal Assistance Services

Personal assistance services encompass personal care and home maintenance needs of people with disabilities. Home health, assistance with performing ADLs, and homemaker services, such as doing chores, are considered personal assistance services. Most people who need personal assistance services receive them from informal caregivers, such as family members. Formal caregivers provide a variety of these services, from skilled nursing to low-skill domestic activities. Some of these services, especially homemaker services, are generally not covered by insurance.

In the traditional medical service delivery model, physicians approve a plan of care, and nursing aides, supervised by home health nurses, provide the care for the consumer. Home health care agencies, however, struggle with the same workforce issues as other sectors of the long-term care industry. Turnover is high among the direct care workers needed to provide services for people with disabilities.

Consumer-directed service is an emerging alternative model that involves the person with a disability more actively in her or his own care. The disabled person, with appropriate information and support, hires, trains, and (if necessary) fires her direct care workers. Consumer direction allows for customization of personal assistance services (Allen & Mor, 1998; Russell, 1998; Stone, 2001).

Many states now offer various forms of consumer-directed home care services. As opposed to care and services being coordinated by an agency, this model allows individuals to arrange and supervise their own personal assistance services. Multiple reasons have been cited for the growing popularity of these programs, including advocacy work by the disabled population seeking autonomy, the belief that such services are less costly because they reduce the need for agency participation, the implications of the *Olmstead* decision (described later), and the shortage of traditional direct care workers (Benjamin, 2001).

Assistive Technologies

Assistive technology refers to any device that helps a person with a disability perform an activity. Canes, raised toilet seats, wheelchairs, computerized voice synthesizers, and hearing aids are examples of such devices. Table 17.2 shows the widespread use of assistive technology in the United States (Russell et al., 1997). In the United States, 7.4 million persons use assistive technology such as canes, walkers, wheelchairs, and scooters for mobility impairments. Devices for orthopedic impairments, including back, neck, knee, and leg braces, as well as artificial limbs, are used by 4.6 million people. Further, to compensate for hearing impairments, about 4.5 million people use assistive devices such as hearing aids, amplified telephones, closed-captioned television, and signaling. For vision impairments, an estimated half-million people used a device such as telescopic lenses, Braille, white canes, or computer equipment.

WORK-RELATED DISABILITY

From the perspective of employers, disability within the workforce is a major problem. The Bureau of Labor Statistics (BLS) has reported that almost 7 of every 100 U.S. workers have a work-related illness or injury each year. Further, from these 5.9 million annual incidents, nearly half were associated with time lost from work (BLS, 1999; Fitzpatrick & King, 2001).

Work-related disability can be classified into three major categories: injuries, chronic conditions, and mental and behavioral problems. *Occupational injuries* often result in time lost from work, with nearly one in four injuries resulting in time lost of three days or more (Zolkos, 1998). **Chronic conditions** are also problematic at work, and the top five chronic conditions among workers—hearing impairments,

Table 17.2 Use of Assistive Technology in the United States, 1994

Type of Impairment	Number of persons* (in millions)
Mobility impairments	7.4
Orthopedic impairments	4.6
Hearing impairments	4.5
Vision impairments	.5

*Excludes institutionalized persons

SOURCE: Russell et al., 1997.

orthopedic impairments, hypertension, arthritis, and heart disease—affect more than half of the working population age 45 to 64 (National Academy on an Aging Society [NAAS], 1999). Research has shown that chronic conditions are generally associated with workers earning less money, being absent more frequently, and being more likely to retire early than workers who do not have chronic conditions (NAAS, 1999). *Mental and behavioral health problems* are also difficult issues for employers. In the private sector, more than 13 percent of the cost of all claims and 9 percent of group long-term disability insurance total claims are for mental disorders; in the public sector, 26 percent of SSDI beneficiary workers reportedly have mental disorders (Salkever, Goldman, Purushothaman, & Shinogle, 2000; Health Insurance Association of America [HIAA], 1995). This type of disability is also problematic because individuals with mental and behavioral health problems notably experience more trouble returning to work than their counterparts with other disorders (Rupp & Scott, 1995; Salkever et al., 2000).

Disability is extremely expensive, especially from an employer perspective. One study reported that the average cost associated with a single missed day of work due to a work-related illness or injury was $13,000 (Matthes, 1992). According to the Work Loss Data Institute (WLDI), in 2000 direct disability lost-time costs were $91,360 per 100 workers and total (direct and indirect) disability lost-time costs were $458,150 per 100 workers (WLDI, 2002). Workplace accidents and injuries exceeded a cost of $80 billion in 1996, with employers reportedly spending an average of 10 percent of payroll costs on direct and indirect expenses associated with worker disability (Johnson & Strosahl, 1998; Fitzpatrick & King, 2001). These costs estimates are even higher when they include the lost productivity and medical care costs associated with work-related disability.

Worker's Compensation

Worker's Compensation programs pay medical expenses of people injured in the course of performing their jobs. While the worker is considered disabled, he or she is also eligible to receive cash payments of a portion of his or her income. Some workers may not miss any time at work because of the work-related injury or illness; others may be permanently disabled. Benefits can be either short- or long-term, depending on the individual situation. Injured workers are classified in one of three categories to determine the types of payments they receive: temporary total disability, permanent total disability, or permanent partial disability (Pignone & Carey, 2003).

Worker's Compensation programs are state-regulated insurance programs. An important difference from the SSA programs is the availability of the category of partial disability. Worker's Compensation programs are based on a "whole man" concept that establishes a range of percentages that are assigned for different injuries (Pignone & Carey, 2003; Wunderlich et al., 2002).

Worker's Compensation is a no-fault system; a worker can still receive benefits even if his or her own negligence was a factor in the injury. Difficulty may arise, however, in determining the true cause of an injury. Distinguishing an injury that occurs because of work from one caused by outside activities can be challenging. Legal disputes may arise regarding Worker's Compensation claims, and case law varies from state to state (Pignone & Carey, 2003).

Disability Management

Disability management refers to an employer-based strategy of managing disability and health (McAlearney, 2003; McAlearney, 2002). Specifically, *disability management* is defined as "attempts to reduce the incidence of and costs associated with disability in the workplace" (McAlearney, 2003). Because of the considerable costs associated with disability and time lost from work, disability management strategies are important to help employers and society reduce this cost burden.

Disability management programs help to reduce the incidence and impact of worker disability. Programs are often employer-based, and may combine elements such as prevention, early intervention, case management, transitional work programs, ergonomics, employee assistance programs, on-site rehabilitation clinics, and absence management. Examples of these program components are shown in Table 17.3.

Disability management programs optimally follow certain basic principles, including: (1) prevention of exacerbation; (2) focus on functional ability; (3) establishment of realistic expectations for recovery and return to work; (4) specification of limitations and abilities; (5) assessment of medical and psychosocial issues; (6) effective communication with employers and employees; (7) inclusion of vocational rehabilitation when appropriate; and (8) work to prevent recurrence (Margoshes, 1998). Attention to program details and the needs of disabled workers can help employers devise approaches that are both comprehensive and proactive in the management of work-related disability.

Ergonomics is defined as "the science of designing jobs and tools to accommodate human capabilities" and is an important component of disability management strategies (Fitzpatrick & King, 2001). The principles of ergonomics can be applied to help enhance and improve human effectiveness,

Table 17.3   Sample Disability Management Program Components

Program Component	Intent	Approach	Example
Prevention	To reduce or avoid injuries, illnesses, and work-related disabilities	Train employees how best to perform functions of job	Program to control blood pressure among employees (Foote & Erfurt, 1991)
Early intervention	To intervene as quickly as possible after injury or illness	Help employees continue to see themselves as valued contributors to the organization	Program to provide timely and coordinated medical and rehabilitation services to ill or injured persons (Fitzpatrick & King, 2001)
Transitional work programs	To accommodate workers who have compromised physical capabilities to perform typical job functions	Maintain contact between workers and the employer and help employees return safely and quickly to work	Transitional-duty department created to provide productive work options for employees with temporary restrictions (Fitzpatrick & King, 2001)

SOURCE: McAlearney, 2003.

as well as to reduce the risk of injury from different activities (McAlearney, 2003). Ergonomic principles can enable disabled workers to best perform their jobs by helping employers to understand what accommodations are necessary and possible for those individuals. In addition, for employees who become permanently disabled while employed, ergonomics can be used to assess the residual work capacity of these individuals so that reasonable job accommodations can be made, as required by the Americans with Disabilities Act (Fitzpatrick & King, 2001). Successful ergonomics programs have proven effective in reducing the number of injuries occurring on the job, including cumulative stress injuries, upper limb disorders, and back injuries.

The benefits of implementing disability management programs can be seen from both employer and employee perspectives. In particular, programs can help employers save money, as reflected in lower costs for disability benefits and Worker's Compensation (Shrey, 2000; Gice & Tompkins, 1989; Bernacki & Tsai, 1996). Reducing employee absenteeism and reducing the time lost from work overall are also helpful to employers that are trying to im-

prove worker productivity (Shrey, 1998, 2000; Carruthers, 2000). From the employee perspective, programs are also associated with improvements in morale and health and wellness (Carruthers, 2000).

Disability management activities are not limited to those that occur in the workplace. As described in Chapter 10, many disability management tactics are used by payers and providers to help their members and clients prevent or reduce the problems associated with disability.

POLICY ISSUES

Legislation and court decisions regarding people with disabilities have helped to define the rights and responsibilities of individuals with disabilities and the organizations with which they interact. Two key legislative acts and one court case are presented in greater detail in this section: the Rehabilitation Act of 1973; the Americans with Disabilities Act of 1990; and the *Olmstead* decision of 1999. Public policy and legal issues must be considered by those providing services to people with disabilities.

The Rehabilitation Act

In 1973, the Rehabilitation Act expanded the rights of those with disabilities. Specifically, Sections 501 and 503 of the Act prohibit employment discrimination on the ground of disability. Section 502 concerns architectural and transportation barriers, and Section 504 reinforces the civil rights of people with disabilities who receive assistance from federal programs. The Act authorizes programs of vocational rehabilitation, supported employment, and independent living. At the federal level, the Rehabilitation Services Administration oversees the programs and administers grants. State bureaus work with people with disabilities to achieve vocational goals.

Disability advocacy groups were very active in promoting enforcement of the Rehabilitation Act. Several court cases narrowed the scope of the legislation, but legislative provisions also have been added to the Act over the last 30 years. Notably, the Rehabilitation Act of 1973 served as the precursor to the Americans with Disabilities Act of 1990 (Fleischer & Zames, 2001).

The Americans with Disabilities Act of 1990

The Americans with Disabilities Act (ADA) is also important civil rights legislation for people with disabilities. The ADA consists of five major sections:

- Title I deals with discrimination in the public and private sectors
- Titles II and III require state and local governments, and private entities operating public services, to give people with disabilities an equal opportunity to benefit from programs, activities, and services, including transportation
- Title IV requires telecommunication relay services and closed captioning
- Title V addresses additional issues, such as defining the relationship of the ADA to other statutes

Many different federal agencies have been given responsibility for portions of the ADA. Since the passage of the ADA, hundreds of court cases have refined various aspects of the law, including the definition of phrases such as *reasonable accommodation*. Switzer (2003) observed that "advocates for persons with disabilities seldom argue that the ADA is a cure-all for unemployment, lack of affordable housing, social isolation, or other problems faced by the population at large. They do believe, however, that the statute is the only way of starting to end patterns of discrimination that have persisted for decades."

The *Olmstead* Decision

In June 1999, the Supreme Court ruled on a case with important implications for people with disabilities who require long-term care. In *Olmstead v L.C.*, the Court ruled that, under certain conditions, states are required to provide services to people with disabilities in community settings rather than in institutions. The ruling is based on the requirements of the ADA.

The *Olmstead* case involved two Georgia women with mental retardation and mental illness. They were treated in institutions and kept there even though their physicians had determined that their conditions were stable and that their needs could be met in a community-based program. Responding to a lower court's mandate to provide services in a community setting, the state attempted at one point to discharge one of the plaintiffs to a homeless shelter. The Supreme Court ruled that a state can be required to provide community-based services to individuals for whom institutional care is inappropriate, if such services represent a reasonable accommodation and do not require the state to fundamentally alter its public programs.

The state's responsibility, however, is not unlimited. Recognizing budget constraints, the Court stated that the aggregate needs of all people with disabilities must be considered; states are permitted to demonstrate that they lack appropriate resources to care for a given person in the community. States are required to have a comprehensive plan to place qualified persons with disabilities in less restricted settings, and to have a waiting list for such services that moves at a reasonable pace (Rosenbaum, 2000). The implications of the *Olmstead* decision continue to be explored through the judicial system.

INTEGRATING MECHANISMS

No two people with disabilities use exactly the same set of services. Within the broad field of disability many public and private service programs exist. Creating cohesion from fragmentation is a major challenge. Because "disability" is not a single condition, the integrating mechanisms are not as well developed in the disability arena as in continuums for other population subgroups, but they are therefore all the more important. Achieving the ideal of a true continuum of care for persons with disabilities will require a commitment to strengthen integrating mechanisms for these services.

Integrating planning and management across service providers is challenging. For many people with disabilities, clinical and functional management of these conditions involves many different providers. Physicians, therapists, rehabilitation specialists, social workers, vocational trainers, and device specialists may all be involved in helping a single individual to function better in the community. Helping to address the needs of people with disabilities requires communication among acute and chronic care providers, as well as between public and private entities. Planning and management among these providers can help to ensure that care is coordinated and services are appropriately delivered.

Integrated financing may be difficult to achieve for individuals with disabilities. With multiple funding sources using various eligibility criteria potentially available, coordinating the requirements and benefits from each can be challenging. Problems can emerge because financing sources provide different levels and types of coverage, and negotiating how each service or device will be covered can be problematic. Gaps created by the use of multiple financing sources must also be addressed. For people with disabilities who are uninsured, the problem is especially troublesome, often requiring a patchwork system of coverage based on ability to pay for services and support. Developing strategies to coordinate the needs of disparate financing sources is critical to helping individuals with disabilities best manage their own care plans.

Exemplary information systems for disability management are rare. Because disability can be so multifaceted, information is recorded by health care providers, educators, public agencies, private payers, and employers. Currently there is no uniform information system in place to gather comprehensive client data.

Finally, for services to remain personalized and empower individuals, sustained case management is essential. Case managers serve as guides to help the person with a disability navigate the complex systems of care. Especially when supported by appropriate information systems, a case management program can be extremely effective at helping with the provider planning and management functions needed by persons with disabilities, and can also help individuals and families negotiate the complicated world of disparate financing sources.

CONCLUSION

Disability is both common and costly. People with disabilities are a heterogeneous population, but they are linked by their functional needs. Many, in fact, feel that functional status is more relevant than actual clinical diagnosis or cause of disability.

Goals for support services vary depending on the consumer. Some people with disabilities may need support to go to school or job training, whereas others may need assistance to be able to remain at home. To live in the community, social and health support services are necessary, including income support, accessible housing, access to health care, and personal support services. Dr. Bob LeBow, a physician activist who was disabled after an accident in 2002, states that the "most important thing is to find a way to integrate the person into the community and the community into the person. It means getting the community involved in more active outreach to the disabled person who is at the disadvantage" (LeBow, 2003). In addition, the disability rights movement continues to emphasize empowering people with disabilities to make decisions regarding their own care. The challenge for health care leaders and providers is to design services and benefits that can meet the needs of individuals in a way that is cost-effective for society and of high quality for the person and their family.

Work-related disability and its associated costs are major issues for both employers and society. Trying to reduce the incidence of work-related injuries and illnesses, while also trying to manage disabilities in the workplace effectively, can have a profound impact on institutional costs and personal lives.

Civil rights legislation has been enacted to protect persons with disabilities from some of the discrimination and difficulties that persist in using transportation, finding employment, and participating in other aspects of society. The judicial system continues to define the responsibilities of public and private entities, as well as the rights of persons with disabilities, as legislation is tested through court cases.

Advances in acute care have made it possible for people to survive severe injuries and accidents. Medical care and technology have also increased the lifespan of those with congenital and developmental disabilities. The chronic care and social support services that people with disabilities need are less well developed. The continuum of long-term care services needed varies for each person, but people who have coordinated, strong support systems are demonstrating that even those with severe disabilities can live, work, and play active roles in the community.

CLIENT EXAMPLE

Creative Living in Columbus, Ohio

Creative Living is a nonprofit organization that exists to provide an independent living setting for adults with severe physical disabilities (i.e., paraplegics and quadriplegics). Creative Living provides wheelchair-accessible apartment complexes adjacent to the Ohio State University campus. Creative Living opened in 1974 and now numbers 34 apartments. The apartments are designed with many important amenities, including accessible shower stalls, countertops, door handles, and an intercom system.

Creative Living is an example of a public/private, federal/local partnership; it is financed one-third through a Housing and Urban Development rent subsidy, one-third by resident rent and fees, and one-third from contributions from private donors and grants. Residents pay rent based on their incomes. The executive director of Creative Living interviews potential residents to determine whether they have the skills and the maturity to manage their personal care and finances on their own.

Creative Living has no medical personnel on duty, so residents must arrange for their own home care according to their needs. However, a unique aspect of Creative Living is its Resident Assistant (RA) program. An RA is on duty in each of the buildings 24 hours a day. RAs, mostly college students, are on call to assist with small tasks or to get help in emergencies. RAs help by putting away groceries, locking doors, removing jackets, and other tasks. Most residents of Creative Living are pursuing an education, vocational training, or are working in the community (Creative Living, 2003).

Creative Living Resident—Lee

During his freshman year of college, Lee's sixth cervical vertebra was shattered in an auto accident, leaving him a quadriplegic. Following an operation to repair the damage as much as possible, Lee went through three months of outpatient rehabilitation. He ended up spending about eight months total in the hospital that year due to multiple complications, including a staphylococcus infection of his surgical site and pneumonia.

Once his medical condition stabilized, Lee returned home to live with his parents. His hospital case manager enrolled him with the Bureau of Vocational Rehabilitation, which paid for home modifications at his parents' home and paid his college tuition when he returned to school. His case manager also helped him fill out paperwork for benefits from SSDI, SSI, Medicare and Medicaid.

Lee graduated from college with a double major in life science and psychology. He began to pursue his Ph.D. in psychology at Ohio State and lived in Creative Living. Because it is subsidized housing, Lee was able to afford the rent for his apartment on his limited income. He requires assistance with all of his ADLs and has an agency home aide come each morning to get him out of bed and help him with bathing and grooming. He had two nursing visits a day to assist him with medications and other personal medical needs. An aide came at night to help him back into bed. After 10 years of graduate study, Lee completed his doctorate and began to fulfill his career goal of being a licensed counselor.

Personal Preference in New Jersey

An example of a consumer-directed care program is the Medicaid National Cash and Counseling Demonstration and Evaluation Program, which took place in Arkansas, Florida, and New Jersey from 1999 through 2002. New Jersey's program is called *Personal Preference.* Personal Preference enrolls Medicaid recipients who require personal care services. They are given a cash benefit each month, based on the cost of traditional Medicaid benefits. People with cognitive impairment are permitted to participate if they have a representative decisionmaker to assist them. The program is administered by the New Jersey Department of Human Services' Division of Disability Services and the Division of Medical Assistance and Health Services.

The monthly amount offered to participants is based on the amount of money the state Medicaid program spent on personal care assistants for the individual (it is a federal requirement that the new program be budget-neutral compared to the tradi-

tional program). About 10 percent of the overall money provided is subtracted to cover the cost of the consultant and other administrative expenses. In New Jersey, the average monthly allowance was about $1,400 in 2002. The consumer can choose to have the amount deposited directly into his or her bank account, or into an account established by a fiscal intermediary, who then acts as the agent of the consumer. If the money is deposited into the consumer's bank account, the consumer has the responsibility to make all payments, including payroll responsibilities such as tax deductions and withholdings. The consumer can allow the cash to accumulate month to month for up to a year to enable bigger purchases.

Cash management plans are developed in cooperation with program consultants. Consumers can use their allowance to purchase home care agency services or to hire independent care providers, including friends or relatives. A study found that 99 percent of consumers who used their allowances to hire caregivers were satisfied with their relationships with those caregivers. The money can also be used for home modifications, such as ramps and chair lifts, or other equipment that increases independence (Phillips & Schneider, 2003).

Consumer Example

Gina, a resident of New Jersey, was diagnosed with multiple sclerosis 10 years ago. She uses a wheelchair and requires assistance with dressing, showering, getting up and down stairs, cooking, cleaning, and shopping. Gina is a 36-year-old single mother of three children, ages 16, 7, and 4. She is a recovered alcoholic. Before her disability, Gina was a retail store manager.

Gina received home care services through Medicaid, but was unhappy with the high rate of staff turnover at the agencies, especially considering the very personal nature of care that she needs. Medicaid did not cover many things she needed, such as a ramp to her front door or a chair lift to help her go up and down her stairs. Determined to stay at home and raise her children, she was often frustrated by her lack of control over her care.

Gina quickly signed up for the New Jersey Personal Preference program after receiving a letter from the state program office advising her of this new option. She uses her management skills to work with her monthly allowance of $1,015. About half of that amount covers payroll and taxes for two personal assistants that she hired herself—one is a neighbor and the second is an aide she found through advertising in the community. Gina is able to arrange for the aides to come at times that make sense for her lifestyle, rather than being restricted by the schedule of the agency. With the remaining money, she buys incontinence pads and other personal items, and she has purchased an air conditioner unit and touch lamps as well. Gina also uses her allowance to pay for transportation to weekly Alcoholics Anonymous meetings.

Gina commented that she saw the program "as an opportunity to take control; to decide for myself who walks through my front door. That's very important when you have young children in the house." New Jersey's Personal Preference program allows Gina to manage her own care and decide how best to use the Medicaid program to meet her needs (Burness Communications, 2002).

WHERE TO GO FOR FURTHER INFORMATION

The Council for Disability Rights
205 West Randolph, Suite 1645
Chicago, IL 60606
(312) 444-9484 / TTY (312) 444-1967
http://www.disabilityrights.org

Disability Resources on the Internet
http://www.disabilityresources.org

Disability Statistics Center
University of California–San Francisco
3333 California Street, Suite 340
San Francisco, CA 94118

(415) 502-5253
http://dsc.ucsf.edu

Federal Web site of government disability-related resources
http://www.disabilityinfo.gov

National Center for Chronic Disease Prevention and Health Promotion
United States Department of Health and Human Services
Centers for Disease Control and Prevention
4770 Bufford Hwy NE
Atlanta, GA 30341
(770) 488-5200
http://www.cdc.gov/nccdphp

National Council on Disability
1131 F Street, NW, Suite 850
Washington, DC 20004
(202) 272-2004 / TTY (202) 272-2074
http://www.ncd.gov

National Health Interview Survey on Disability (NHIS-D)
Center for Disease Control and Prevention
National Center for Health Statistics
Hyattsville, MD 20782
(301) 458-4000
http://www.cdc.gov/nchs/nhis

National Institute on Disability and Rehabilitation Research (NIDRR)
400 Maryland Avenue, SW
Washington, DC 20202-2572
http://www.ed.gov/about/offices/list/osers/nidrr

National Organization on Disability
910 Sixteenth Street, NW, Suite 600
Washington, DC 20006
(202) 293-5960
http://www.nod.org

World Institute on Disability
510 16th Street, Suite 100
Oakland, CA 94612
(510) 763-4100
http://www.wid.org

FACTS REVIEW

1. Identify four types of support services often needed by people with disabilities.
2. Identify at least four professionals who may be involved in providing services to people with disabilities.
3. Identify the types of personal assistance services often needed by people with disabilities, and list some common problems encountered in meeting these needs.
4. Describe barriers to accessing health care faced by people with disabilities and strategies for overcoming these barriers.
5. Define consumer-directed home services, and discuss reasons for their growing popularity.
6. Discuss public policy legislation and court decisions regarding people with disabilities, and give examples of relevant federal legislation.
7. Identify integrating mechanisms necessary to address the needs of persons with disabilities.

REFERENCES

Adler, M. (1991). *Programmatic definitions of disability: Policy implications.* Washington, D.C.: Department of Health and Human Services.

Allen, S. M., & Mor, V. (Eds.) (1998). *Living in the community with disability: Service needs, use, and systems.* New York: Springer.

Benjamin, A. E. (2001). Consumer-directed services at home: A new model for persons with disabilities. *Health Affairs, 20*(6), 80–95.

Bernacki, E. J., & Tsai, S. P. (1996). Managed care for workers' compensation: Three years experience in an "employee choice" state. *Journal of Occupational and Environmental Medicine, 38,* 1091–1097.

Brandt, E. N., & Pope, A. M. (Eds.) (1997). *Enabling America: Assessing the role of rehabilitation science and engineering.* Washington, D.C.: National Academy Press.

Bureau of Labor Statistics. (1999). *Survey of occupational illnesses: 1998.* Washington, DC: U.S. Department of Labor, Bureau of Labor Statistics.

Burness Communications. (2002). *Cash and counseling: Demonstration and evaluation program.* Washington, D.C.: Office of the Assistant Secretary for Planning and Evaluation, U.S. Department of Health and Human Services and The Robert Wood Johnson Foundation.

Carruthers, M. (2000, December/January). Disability Management Employer Coalition. *Rehab Management,* 12, 14.

Council of Europe. (1999). *The use and usefulness of the International Classification of Impairments, Disabilities, and Handicaps (ICIDH).* Germany: Council of Europe.

Creative Living. (2003, June). Available at *http://www.creative-living.com/*

Dell Orto, A. E., & Marinelli, R. P. (1995). *Encyclopedia of disability and rehabilitation.* New York: Simon & Schuster/Macmillan.

Fitzpatrick, M. A., & King, P. M. (2001, January). Disability management pays off. *American Society of Safety Engineers/Professional Safety,* 39–41.

Fleischer, D. Z., & Zames, F. (2001). *The disability rights movement: From charity to confrontation.* Philadelphia, PA: Temple University Press.

Foote, A., & Erfurt, J. C. (1991). The benefit-to-cost ratio of worksite blood-pressure control programs. *JAMA, 265*(10): 1283–1286.

Gice, J., & Tompkins, K. (1989). Return to work program in a hospital setting. *Journal of Business Psychology, 4*(2), 237–243.

Health Insurance Association of America. (1995). *Disability claims for mental and nervous disorders.* Washington, DC: Author.

Hellwig, V. (1999, Winter). Integrating disability management to help improve the bottom line. *Compensation and Benefits Management,* 43–50.

Iezzoni, L. I. (2003). *When walking fails: Mobility problems of adults with chronic conditions.* New York: Milbank.

Johnson. P., & Strosahl, K. (1998, December). The new direction in disability management: Tactical teamwork. *Business and Health,* 21–24.

LeBow, B. (Past President, Physicians for a National Health Plan). (2003). Personal communication.

Margoshes, B. (1998). Disability management and occupational health. *Occupational Medicine, 13*(4), 693–703.

Matthes, K. (1992, April). Companies have the ability to manage disability. *HRx and Healthcare,* 3.

McAlearney, A. S. (2003). *Population health management: Strategies to improve outcomes.* Chicago: Health Administration Press.

McAlearney, A. S. (2002). Population health management in theory and practice. In G. T. Savage, J. D. Blair, & M. D. Fottler (Eds.), *Advances in health care management,* vol 3 (pp. 117–158). New York: JAI Press.

McNeil, J. (2001). *Current population reports: Americans with disabilities, 1997.* Washington, DC: U.S. Census Bureau.

National Academy on an Aging Society. (1999). *Chronic conditions: A challenge for the 21st century.* Washington, DC: NCD. [On-line article retrieved February 18, 2002 from *http://www.agingsociety.org.*]

Phillips, B., & Schneider, B. (2003). *Enabling Personal Preference: The Implementation of the Cash and Counseling Demonstration in New Jersey.* Retrieved July 14, 2003 from *http://www.aspe.hhs.gov/daltop/reports/enablepp.htm.*

Pignone, M. P., & Carey, T. S. (2003). *Social Security Disability Insurance and Workers' Compensation.* UpToDate. Retrieved July 5, 2003 from *http://www.uptodate.com*

Regenstein, M., Schroer, C., & Meyer, J. A. (2000, April). Medicaid managed care for persons with disabilities: A closer look. Washington, D.C.: The Kaiser Commission on Medicaid and the Uninsured.

Rosenbaum, S. (2000, March). *The Olmstead decision: Implications for Medicaid.* Washington, D.C.: Kaiser Commission on Medicaid and the Uninsured.

Rupp, K., & Scott S. G. (1995). Trends in the characteristics of DI and SSI awardees and duration of program participation. *Social Security Bulletin, 59*(1), 3–21.

Russell, M. (1998). *Beyond ramps: Disability at the end of the social contract.* Monroe, ME: Common Courage.

Russell, N., Hendershot, G. E., LeClere, F., Howie, L. J., & Adler, M. (1997). Trends and differential use of assistive technology devices: United States, 1994. *Advanced Data from Vital and Health Statistics of the Centers for Disease Control and Prevention, National Center for Health Statistics* (No. 292).

Salkever, D. S., Goldman, H., Purushothaman, M., Shinogle, J. (2000). Disability management, employee health and fringe benefits, and long-term-disability claims for mental disorders: An empirical exploration. *The Milbank Quarterly, 78*(1), 79–113.

Shrey, D. E. (2000). Worksite disability management model for effective return-to-work planning. *Occupational Medicine, 15*(4), 789–801.

Shrey, D. E. (1998). Effective worksite-based disability management programs. In P. M. King (Ed.), *Concepts and practices of cccupational rehabilitation* (pp. 389–409). New York: Plenum Press.

Social Security Administration. (2003). *Disability benefits (Publication No. 05-10029).* Available at *http://www.ssa.gov/pubs/10029.html.*

Stone, R. I. (2001). Providing long-term care benefits in cash: Moving to a disability model. *Health Affairs, 20*(6), 96–108.

Switzer, J.V. (2003). Disabled rights: American disability policy and the fight for equality. Washington, DC: Georgetown University Press.

U.S. Census Bureau. (2003). *Disability status: 2000. Census 2000 brief.* Retrieved July 1, 2003 from *http://www.census.gov/prod/2003pubs/c2kbrt7.pdf.*

Vladeck, B. C. (2003). Where the action really is: Medicaid and the disabled. *Health Affairs, 22*(1), 90–100.

World Health Organization. (2003). Introduction: International Classification of Functioning, Disability, and Health. Retrieved July 1, 2003 from *http://www.who.int.*

Wunderlich, G. S., Rice, D. P., & Amado, N. L. (Eds.). (2002). *The dynamics of Disability: Measuring and monitoring disability for Social Security programs.* Washington, DC: National Academy Press.

Zolkos, R. (1998, April). Return-to-work underutilized: Key to lost time: Survey. *Business Insurance,* 2.

CHAPTER 18

The Aging Network

Alex A. Sripipatana

Many advocates for older adults in the United States contend that a strategy for facilitating quality of life in older ages is through the maintenance of independence and the ability to "age in place," (Cutchin, 2003). Most older adults prefer to live at home. In fact, fewer than 2 million older Americans are cared for in nursing homes (Administration on Aging, 2000). One infrastructure established by the federal government that facilitates the preference to age in one's own home and community is the Aging Network.

The *Aging Network* is an informal term used to describe the array of federal, state, and local government agencies established by the Older Americans Act (OAA) and the community-based agencies that affiliate with them in serving older adults. Although exact service arrangements vary by state and community, overall, the Aging Network offers an array of support services that enhance the ability of older adults to maintain their independence and lifelong well-being.

As noted in Chapter 2, older adults are major consumers of long-term care. Most older people have one or more chronic conditions. Approximately one in five persons age 65 to 74 has a major functional disability. Of those persons age 85 and older, one in five has a major functional impairment. As the older population expands from 35 million in 2000 to 70 million in 2030, the older population requiring long-term care will increase simultaneously (American Association of Retired Persons [AARP], 2003). Thus, the Aging Network is a critical component of the nation's long-term care system.

The Older Americans Act was originally signed into law by President Lyndon B. Johnson on July 14, 1965. It is recognized as one of the major pieces of legislation of President Johnson's Great Society movement, which also included the Medicare and Medicaid amendments to the Social Security Act. It is periodically renewed and modified, most recently in 2000. Understanding the basic structure and mandates of the OAA will facilitate access to the Aging Network. The OAA contains seven titles that

Table 18.1 Titles Contained in the Older Americans Act

TITLE I: OBJECTIVES OF THE ACT
TITLE II: THE FEDERAL ADMINISTRATION ON AGING
TITLE III: HOME AND COMMUNITY-BASED SERVICES
          Part A: General Provisions
          Part B: Supportive Services and Senior Centers coordination, advocacy, program development, and funding
          Part C: Nutrition Services
          Part D: In-Home Services
          Part E: Special Needs
          Part F: Disease Prevention and Health Promotion
          Part G: Supportive Activities to Caregivers
TITLE IV: TRAINING, RESEARCH AND DISCRETIONARY PROJECTS
TITLE V: SENIOR COMMUNITY SERVICE EMPLOYMENT PROGRAM
TITLE VI: GRANTS FOR NATIVE AMERICANS AND OLDER HAWAIIANS
TITLE VII: ALLOTMENTS FOR VULNERABLE ELDER RIGHTS PROTECTION

are relevant to long-term care. These are outlined in Table 18.1.

TITLE I: OBJECTIVES OF THE ACT

Title I sets broad objectives for the OAA. For example, one objective states, "the older people of our nation are entitled to . . . the best possible physical and mental health which science can make available and without regard to economic status." The other nine objectives relate to availability of adequate income, affordable housing, restorative services, employment, dignity, recreation, community services, research, and independence.

This title reflects the philosophy at the time the OAA was passed. It sets a broad mandate for federal actions on behalf of older adults, much of

which has not been implemented because of resource constraints.

TITLE II: THE FEDERAL ADMINISTRATION ON AGING

Title II creates, authorizes, and provides guidance to the federal agency responsible for the implementation of the OAA: the Administration on Aging (AoA). The AoA is located within the Department of Health and Human Services. Until 1993 it was headed by a Commissioner on Aging who reported to the assistant secretary for Human Development Services. In 1993, the commissioner position was elevated to an assistant secretary level and now reports directly to the secretary of the Department of Health and Human Services.

The main functions of the AoA are (1) to develop and promulgate regulations guiding implementation of the OAA at the state and local levels; (2) to distribute funding to the states and territories; (3) to monitor implementation of the OAA at the state level; (4) to coordinate with other federal departments; (5) to advocate for aging services at the federal level; and (6) to implement directly Title IV: Training, Research, and Discretionary Projects (see below).

The AoA maintains a central office in Washington, DC, and an office in each of the 10 federal regions: Boston, New York, Philadelphia, Atlanta, Chicago, Kansas City, Dallas, Denver, San Francisco, and Seattle.

TITLE III: HOME AND COMMUNITY-BASED SERVICES

Title III of the OAA has seven parts and provides for the majority of services at the state and local levels.

Part A: General Provisions

Under Title III, the AoA works closely with its nationwide network, composed of regional offices, state units on aging (SUA), and area agencies on aging (AAA), to plan, coordinate, and develop community-level systems of services that are designed to meet the unique needs of older adults and their caregivers. Title III supports services designed to assist older persons at risk of losing their independence, as well as active older adults. Through this title, AoA advocates for the needs of older persons in program planning and policy development, provides technical assistance, issues best practices guidelines, and initiates policy relative to funding the 57 state units on aging and territories to provide services to older Americans.

Part B: Supportive Services and Senior Centers

Part B of Title III creates the majority of the structure known as the Aging Network (Figure 18.1). If a state is to receive funds under the OAA, it must designate a single organizational unit as the state unit on aging (SUA). Each governor has the discretion of where to place the SUA within the government structure. Therefore, in some states the SUA is an independent department with direct access to the governor; in other states it may be buried within a large umbrella-type social or health services agency.

The SUA has a variety of responsibilities. Within state government, it is mandated to serve as the focal point and advocate for aging services. It must coordinate with other state agencies and review and comment on all issues affecting older adults within the state.

Each state also receives some funding under the OAA for a Long-Term Care Ombudsman program (LTCOP). The LTCOP has the responsibility to investigate complaints regarding care in long-term care facilities within the state. Federal funding for the LTCOP is limited, so most states have a salaried ombudsman only at the state level. Some states have used the monies to expand the program to the local level. In either case, most of the visits to long-term care facilities and complaint investigations are conducted by trained volunteer ombudsmen.

In addition, the SUA must divide the state into

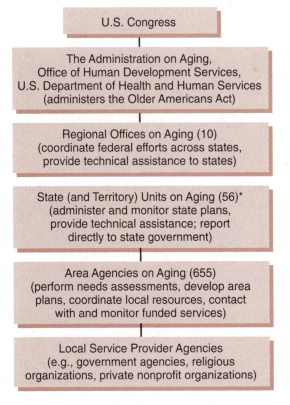

*Administer federal funds, report directly to state governments

Lines denote reporting relationships.

Figure 18.1   The Aging Network

geographic areas that logically serve as catchment areas for aging services. These substate geographic areas are known as planning and service areas (PSAs). Minimally they are one county in size, but they vary and can encompass 25 counties or more in rural areas. A few of the most rural and geographically small states (Alaska, Delaware, Nevada, New Hampshire, North Dakota, Rhode Island, South Dakota, and Wyoming) have designated the entire state as one PSA. In contrast, a few of the largest cities (e.g., Los Angeles, New York, and Chicago) have been designated as independent PSAs.

After dividing the state into PSAs, the SUA must designate one agency as the Area Agency on Aging (AAA) for each PSA. The AAA has the responsibility for implementing the provisions of the OAA at the local level, including the development of a community-based network of services for older adults. Approximately one-third of the AAAs in the country are located within county government, one-third within joint powers (multicounty) agencies, and one-third within private nonprofit agencies. At this time, there are 655 AAAs that blanket the nation to cover all older persons who reside in the country. To locate the AAA for a given county, call the national Eldercare Locator Number: 1-800-677-1116, or look at the Administration on Aging Web site: *http://www.aoa.gov.*

The SUA must also develop an intrastate funding formula for distribution of funds received under the Older Americans Act to the AAAs throughout the state. These formulas are at the center of much controversy. Each state receives its funding from the AoA based on the percentage of the nation's population age 60 and older in each state. Table 18.2 exemplifies how distributing OAA funds between states becomes complicated when the top five states with the highest *numbers* of people 60 years and older (California, Florida, New York, Texas, and Pennsylvania) are not necessarily the same top five states with the largest *proportion* of people 60 years and older (Florida, West Virginia, Pennsylvania, Iowa, and Maine).

When distributing the funds to the AAAs, the SUA is mandated to develop a different intrastate formula that takes into account the distribution of seniors throughout the state, with special attention to those in greatest social and economic need, especially low-income minority individuals. The controversy centers around how heavily to give preference to the target population. Generally the battle pits the large urban centers with a high number of minority seniors against suburban and rural AAAs with low numbers of minority seniors but growing numbers of Caucasian seniors. Although the concept of frailty is not dealt with clearly in the law, many AAAs attempt to address the issue by encour-

aging service providers to seek out persons who have difficulty with basic activities of daily living (ADLs).

One of the primary responsibilities of each AAA is to develop a comprehensive plan for services for the older adults within the PSA. Depending on the state, the plans are revised every one to five years. Each AAA conducts a needs and resource assessment of the older citizens within the PSA. The assessments may be conducted in a variety of ways, from distributing survey questionnaires to conducting community forums or public hearings. After the needs and resource assessment is completed, the AAA develops priorities for action on behalf of the older adults. Typically, priorities for action are stated in the form of measurable objectives in the plan. Each AAA is required by the OAA to establish an advisory council composed of members of which at least 51 percent are over the age of 60. An advisory council advises the AAA on the development and implementation of the plan and serves as a focal point for advocacy issues relative to the older population in the area.

AAAs tend to categorize their plan objectives into four activities: coordination, education/advocacy, program development, and funding.

Coordination. The AAAs strive to coordinate the organizations, public and private, that provide services to older adults. For example, within a given geographic area there may be a number of transportation services for the older adult, such as Dial-a-Ride. However, each service may provide transportation only within a limited service area, such as within the boundaries of a small city. An older person who lives in the city may not be able to travel to a hospital in another small city if the service areas do not overlap or abut. In the latter case, the trip could entail some inconvenient or even impossible transfers from one transportation system to another.

If this is the case, the AAA may establish a coordination objective calling for the coordination or integration of the multiple Dial-a-Ride systems into one system that is easier to use. If the services cannot be combined, the AAA might create an overlay,

Table 18.2 Population Age 60 and Over by State and the District of Columbia, in Rank Order of Highest Number to Lowest Number, 2000

Rank	State	Number	Percent of 60+/All Ages	Rank	State	Number	Percent of 60+/All Ages
1	California	4,742,499	14.0%	28	Oregon	569,557	16.6%
2	Florida	3,545,093	22.2%	29	Colorado	560,658	13.0%
3	New York	3,204,331	16.9%	30	Iowa	554,573	19.0%
4	Texas	2,774,201	13.3%	31	Arkansas	491,409	18.4%
5	Pennsylvania	2,430,821	19.8%	32	Mississippi	457,144	16.1%
6	Ohio	1,963,489	17.3%	33	Kansas	454,837	16.9%
7	Illinois	1,962,911	15.8%	34	West Virginia	362,795	20.1%
8	Michigan	1,596,162	16.1%	35	Nevada	304,071	15.2%
9	New Jersey	1,443,782	17.2%	36	Nebraska	296,151	17.3%
10	North Carolina	1,292,553	16.1%	37	New Mexico	283,837	15.6%
11	Massachusetts	1,096,567	17.3%	38	Utah	252,677	11.3%
12	Georgia	1,071,080	13.1%	39	Maine	238,099	18.7%
13	Virginia	1,065,502	15.1%	40	Hawaii	207,001	17.1%
14	Indiana	988,506	16.3%	41	New Hampshire	194,965	15.8%
15	Missouri	983,704	17.6%	42	Idaho	193,421	14.9%
16	Tennessee	942,620	16.6%	43	Rhode Island	191,409	18.3%
17	Wisconsin	907,552	16.9%	44	Montana	158,894	17.6%
18	Washington	873,223	14.8%	45	South Dakota	136,869	18.1%
19	Arizona	871,536	17.0%	46	Delaware	133,925	17.1%
20	Maryland	801,036	15.1%	47	North Dakota	118,985	18.5%
21	Minnesota	772,278	15.7%	48	Vermont	101,827	16.7%
22	Alabama	769,880	17.3%	49	District of Columbia	91,878	16.1%
23	Louisiana	687,216	15.4%	50	Wyoming	77,348	15.7%
24	Kentucky	672,905	16.6%	51	Alaska	53,026	8.5%
25	South Carolina	651,482	16.2%				
26	Connecticut	601,835	17.7%		TOTAL	45,797,200	16.3%
27	Oklahoma	599,080	17.4%				

SOURCE: U.S. Bureau of the Census, 2000.

such as taxi vouchers that would be accepted by any of the transportation services.

Coordination activities are political in that they often require the AAA to attempt to convince another agency to modify the way it provides services and expends its resources.

Advocacy. Many of the conditions affecting older people are converted into problems because of the lack of available services, fragmentation in services, or restrictive legislation. To address these problems, the AAA may develop objectives that call for education/advocacy activities. For example, an AAA may advocate with local elected officials for more affordable, accessible housing for seniors in safe and convenient neighborhoods. An AAA may advocate at the federal level for a lower Medicare co-payment for low-income seniors, or at the state level for a more integrated approach in policy development, service funding, and regulation.

Program Development. An AAA may have program development objectives in its plan that call for the development of services that do not currently exist within the PSA. In most, if not all, communities throughout the country, some services that do not yet exist are necessary for older people to maintain their independence. Respite care services are a prime example. Respite care provides time off for a family member or friend who provides significant care to an older person with disabilities. Respite care can be provided in the home by a volunteer or paid staff person or in an institution such as a nursing or congregate care facility. The AAA may sponsor the initiation of a respite program or encourage other agencies in the community to do so.

Funding. Each AAA receives some funding that can be used to provide services directly to senior citizens. Some services are mandated by the OAA (e.g., congregate and home-delivered meals and senior employment). Others, like in-home services, transportation, legal services, and information and assistance must be funded in an adequate proportion unless it can demonstrate that an adequate proportion of the services already exists within the PSA. The definition of adequate proportion is left to the discretion of each state. In addition, the AAA can choose to use its resources to fund a variety of other services, such as respite care, adult day services, case management, and home repair.

Typically an AAA funds services through contractual arrangements with community-based service agencies. The OAA prohibits an AAA from providing services directly unless it can demonstrate to the SUA that no other agency in the PSA can or is interested in providing the service, or that it can provide the service in the most efficient and effective manner. An AAA can contract for service with a for-profit corporation only with approval from the SUA, but contracts typically are with governmental and nonprofit agencies.

Perhaps the most important service required under Title IIIB is information and assistance (I&A), also called information and referral. This service must be available in every community and must have the capability to serve as a one-stop resource for persons inquiring about the availability of services for older adults. Typically the information is provided over the phone. Frequently a follow-up call is made to determine the success or failure of the referral. The service can be used by people of any age as long as they are requesting information about or assistance with services for people age 60 and older.

Case management services, sometimes called care coordination, are often associated with I&A. Case management provides assistance to people with multiple problems to access available services to support their continued residence in a community-based setting. Case management services usually include assessment (often in the home), care planning, service implementation, monitoring of the situation on a regular basis, and reassessment. In some cases case managers have access to funds that can be used to purchase services. In other instances the case managers act as brokers and advocates who arrange for the services to be provided through a third funding source.

By law, any service funded by the OAA is provided free of charge to any person over the age of 60 or to someone younger if she or he is married to someone who meets the minimum age requirement. Each individual receiving services must be provided with the opportunity to make a donation toward the cost of the service, but no individual may be denied service because of inability to pay.

Part C: Nutrition Services

As noted earlier, the AAA is mandated to provide congregate and home-delivered meals. Part C earmarks the funding for those services. Federal funding for nutrition services slightly exceeds funding for all other services in the OAA. Subpart 1 of Part C mandates congregate nutrition sites. Subpart 2 mandates home-delivered meals. Congregate and home-delivered meals must be served a minimum of once per day, five days per week, and each must meet one-third the daily Required Dietary Allowance as published by the American Dietetic Association. Furthermore, whenever possible and appropriate, meals must meet the special health, religious, ethnic, and cultural requirements of participants. Research trends indicate an increase in the need for home-delivered meals and a concomitant shift in resources.

Part D: In-Home Services

Part D of Title III mandates the provision of in-home services. Typically these services include, but are not limited to homemaker services, visiting and telephone reassurance, chore and maintenance services, in-home respite care and adult day care respite, minor modification of homes to facilitate continued occupancy by older persons, and personal care. However, its funding level has historically been very low—in some cases as little as one-tenth the amount available for in-home services for low-income individuals receiving Medicaid. As with Part B and C services, services under this part are typically provided through a subcontract with a community-based nonprofit agency.

Part E: Special Needs

The funding under Part E goes only to the state level for the SUAs to use to meet special or unique needs of older adults. The definition of *special needs* is left to the state.

Until recently, like Part D of Title III, the funding available under this title had been so limited that it rendered Part E symbolic rather than effective. However, as indicated earlier, the OAA is periodically renewed and modified.

As mentioned in Chapter 2, the aging of the U.S. population has heightened interest in designing efficient and effective systems for delivering health and related services to older people. Developing service networks to provide older people and their caregivers with a continuum of home and community-based long-term care has become especially important to better meet their support needs and preferences for independence.

Family caregivers are usually the overworked and underrecognized heroes that provide the vast majority of the assistance that enables older people to live independently or semi-independently in the comfort of their own homes and communities (see Chapter 3). However, family caregivers face substantial stresses and burdens as a consequence of caregiving obligations. Prolonged caregiving can adversely affect one's physical and psychological health, current and future employment status and earning capability, ability to balance the needs of older parents and younger family members, and ability to meet personal needs. Because caregivers play such an important role, services that sustain the caregiver role and maintain their emotional and physical health are an important component of any home and community-based care system.

In response to this need, the federal government established the National Family Caregiver Support Program (NFCSP) with the 2000 Reauthorization of the Older Americans Act. This program is also administered by the AoA. The AoA provides the SUAs with Title III-E formula grants to work in partnership with local AAAs and faith-based and community service providers, and Title VI-C formula grants to Native American tribes. These grants are used to provide direct support services that best meet the range of caregiver needs. These may include, but are not limited to information, assistance, individual counseling, support groups, and training, respite, and supplemental services to family caregivers of persons age 60 and older and to grandparents and relative caregivers of children not more than 18 years of age.

In fiscal year (FY) 2003, Title III-E funding for the NFCSP was $155.2 million (Carbonell, 2003). Formula grants were made available to all U.S. states and territories to run programs that provide critical support, including home and community-based services, to help families maintain their caregiving roles. Additionally, competitive caregiver program demonstration grants were awarded to 39 organizations, agencies, research institutions, and faith-based organizations to focus on systems development, service components, linkages to special populations and communities, field-initiated demonstrations to develop and test new approaches to support caregivers, and national projects that enhance the development of caregiver programs.

Part F: Disease Prevention and Health Promotion

Part F, also minimally funded at the national level, is relatively new. The funding, like that under Parts B, C, and D, flows from the AoA through the SUA to the AAA. The law allows a wide variety of disease prevention and health promotion activities, such as health screening, nutrition education, counseling, health promotion materials, and physical fitness programs. Some AAAs use this funding to purchase ongoing services, such as annual health screening clinics. Others conduct one-time events, such as a senior health fair at a shopping mall.

Part G: Supportive Activities to Caregivers

Part G is also minimally funded. The funding goes only to the state level. Each SUA uses the funding differently.

TITLE IV: TRAINING, RESEARCH, AND DISCRETIONARY PROJECTS

The Discretionary Funds Program, authorized by Title IV of the OAA, constitutes the major research, demonstration, training, and development effort of the Administration on Aging. Title IV is generally intended to build knowledge, develop innovative model programs, and train personnel for service in the field of aging. Twice annually the AoA releases a *Federal Register* announcement that delineates its priorities for funding. The priorities, length of project period, and funding levels vary with each announcement and administration. Generally, the priorities focus on applied research and demonstration efforts related to service issues.

TITLE V: SENIOR COMMUNITY SERVICE EMPLOYMENT PROGRAM

The very popular Title V provides funding to subsidize employment for low-income seniors in private nonprofit and public agencies. The funding flows to approximately 7 to 10 national contractors and to each SUA. Positions are allocated throughout the country. Although many agencies and organizations use Title V subsidized employees to increase their ability to provide service, the primary focus of the program is to provide the older individual with the experience and training needed to obtain a nonsubsidized position. This service is provided to people over the age of 55 who meet low-income guidelines.

TITLE VI: GRANTS FOR NATIVE AMERICANS AND OLDER HAWAIIANS

Under Title VI of the OAA, the AoA awards grants to tribal councils and Native Hawaiian organizations to provide supportive and nutrition services that are in accord with the unique cultural and other needs of these groups. Because of historical mistreatment of these two population groups, and other unique circumstances, they have warranted special attention. Furthermore, the U.S. Congress (1993) cites that older Native Americans (AIAN) receive less than adequate health care and are expected to live between three to four years less than the general population; Native Hawaiians have a life expectancy 10 years less than any other racial/ethnic group in the state of Hawaii, as well as ranking lowest on 9 of 11 standard health indices for all racial/ethnic groups in Hawaii. Funds allocated for this title may be used for the same purposes as identified under Title III. Of the amount appropriated for Title VI for each fiscal year, 90 percent is allocated to carry out Part A-Indian Program, and the remaining 10 percent to carry out Part B-Native Hawaiian Program.

TITLE VII: ALLOTMENTS FOR VULNERABLE ELDER RIGHTS PROTECTION

The funding under Title VII is earmarked for use in educating the public about elder abuse and providing ombudsman and legal services. The funding flows through the SUAs to AAAs at the local level.

The funding for elder abuse may be used for educational materials or events or for receiving and reporting complaints about elder abuse. The AAA is mandated to coordinate this service with the local adult protective services programs.

As noted earlier, the funding for ombudsman services is minimal and typically supports only a state-level office that receives and investigates complaints about abuse in long-term care facilities. In some states the program is locally operated and often relies heavily on the use of well-trained volunteers as ombudsmen.

The types of legal services provided under this title are usually defined locally, based on local needs and priorities. Like the other services funded under the OAA, these services are provided free, without regard to income, and are typically provided through a purchase-of-services contract with a community legal provider.

To illustrate the relative priority given to the several facets of the Older Americans Act and the Aging Network, Figure 18.2 shows how the Administration on Aging, under the auspices of the executive branch, allocated its FY2003 appropriation of $1.367 billion. Funds are allocated to programs, and thus may cut across titles.

POLICY ISSUES

Policy issues include (1) how to finance services; (2) whether to support categorical or needs-based (i.e., age-irrelevant) program eligibility criteria; (3) how to define *quality;* (4) how to measure outcomes; and (5) how to respond responsibly, as well as humanely, to population heterogeneity.

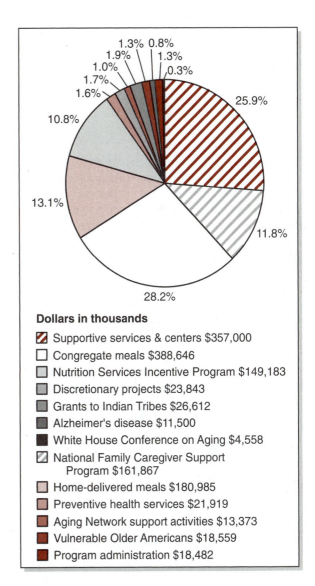

Dollars in thousands

- Supportive services & centers $357,000
- Congregate meals $388,646
- Nutrition Services Incentive Program $149,183
- Discretionary projects $23,843
- Grants to Indian Tribes $26,612
- Alzheimer's disease $11,500
- White House Conference on Aging $4,558
- National Family Caregiver Support Program $161,867
- Home-delivered meals $180,985
- Preventive health services $21,919
- Aging Network support activities $13,373
- Vulnerable Older Americans $18,559
- Program administration $18,482

Figure 18.2 Administration on Aging Fiscal Year 2003 Budget

SOURCE: AoA; *http://www.aoa.gov/about/legbudg/ current_budg/legbudg_current_budg.asp*

Quality is determined to be a function of availability, acceptability, accessibility, adequacy, and appropriateness.

Availability requires sufficient funding, expertise, space, and equipment to enable staff, volunteers, or peers to provide the service.

Acceptability requires service characteristics that attract and include clients rather than exclude them. Languages spoken and meal preparations must be compatible with client characteristics, and cultural differences must be respected. Providers' commitment to client autonomy is challenged when clients decide to reject services that professionals deem essential or when clients continue to practice self-destructive patterns of behavior.

Accessibility requires client awareness of the service, client eligibility, adequate transportation, and safe and effective program and environmental design. Literacy should not be a prerequisite for service, but promotional materials must be legible.

Adequacy requires that the right service be delivered at the time the client needs it and in a way that is acceptable to the client and supportive of the client's caregivers.

Appropriateness requires that services provided meet real client needs. An ethical dilemma arises for network personnel when their perceptions of clients' most serious needs fail to match clients' expressed needs.

Fees for Services

The OAA has historically provided free access to services for anyone over the minimum age (predominantly 60 years) with no consideration of income, either net or disposable. Because of the growing number of people over the age of 60, the increasing demands for services and the limited funding available, recent reauthorization debates have raised the question of the desirability of some type of means test to limit eligibility. Under debate is whether people over a certain income level should be required to pay for a portion or all of the cost of providing a service. Currently the law requires that all individuals who receive services under the OAA be given an opportunity, but not be required, to donate toward the cost of the service.

Financing

Currently public services for older adults are financed through a variety of laws that result in multiple funding streams and regulations flowing from the federal to the state and local levels. The result is often conflicting mandates, competing services, a high degree of fragmentation, and an almost complete lack of integration of services at the point of delivery. Recent debates have centered on the concept of integrating not only the titles of the OAA into one block-type grant for senior services, but also integrating the OAA with other funding streams such as Medicaid, Medicare, social services block grant, community services block grant, and Housing and Urban Development funds.

Age-Integrated Services

Debate also occurs about whether services funded by the act should be restricted to those over the age of 60 or be provided to people of all ages who have long-term or chronic care needs.

People of color tend not to live as long as Caucasians and also tend to develop chronic health problems at an earlier age. Currently, except as noted in Titles V, VI, and IIIC I and II, the OAA prohibits the provision of services to anyone under the age of 60. Rights advocates argue that the 60-plus age limitation thus discriminates against people of color.

Population Heterogeneity

As the numbers and life expectancy of individuals over the age of 60 increase, their characteristics diversify. Many maintain excellent health and an ability to function independently with little or no assistance; some people can function independently with minimal assistance; and a minority need significant assistance with social functioning and health maintenance. Some older adults reside with their spouses, others are recent widows or widowers. Some older adults are employed, some are retirees. Income levels range from more than adequate to very needy. Currently the OAA does not recognize this diversity and places services for more disabled seniors in competition with those for healthier seniors.

The mandate to provide *services for all over the age of 60* has contributed to the growing claim of intergenerational inequities in government programs. Advocates for children and younger-than-60 taxpayers claim that seniors are receiving more than their fair share of social benefits under the Older Americans Act.

Measuring Outcomes

Research trends at the national and state levels indicate a growing interest from funders in meaningful data on service outcomes. Traditionally, service providers have collected data on input and output processes. The challenge of measuring service outcomes will require measurable indicators on changes in client knowledge, attitudes, behaviors, and satisfaction. At this time standardized indicators have not been defined, and the interactive nature of the multiple services in the Older Americans Act is not readily measurable.

CONCLUSION

In establishing and reauthorizing the Older Americans Act, Congress has attempted to provide a mechanism for the creation of an integrated network of services for the nation's older adults at the local level. Over the years, the focus of the network has been redirected to give preference, but not exclusivity, to those individuals age 60 and older who are in low-income minority groups, people of color, and those in greatest social and economic need. This multiple mandate has resulted in a confusing array of available services within communities. The most nationally consistent services provided are nutrition,

employment, and information and referral. Congress has been slow to reauthorize the OAA at times and is easily distracted by the more pressing issues of Medicare and Medicaid reform. Extensive grassroots advocacy has been fundamental in keeping the OAA funded. Policy debates concerning future changes in the law center around the lack of a fee-for-services structure, the deletion of the age requirement, addition of disability and income requirements to access services, and increased flexibility at the state and local levels.

CLIENT EXAMPLE

Mr. Stone is dying of prostate cancer, paralyzed, and has been in bed at home over the course of five months. Because of his illness, his wife has taken over many of the chores he used to perform around the house. Her adult children come as often as they can to help from 50 and 1,000 miles away, but they have jobs and families of their own to take care of. Mr. Stone is receiving some hospice care, but Mrs. Stone is his primary caregiver.

One day as she carries groceries into the house, Mrs. Stone trips and falls, breaking her arm. With her arm in a cast, Mrs. Stone can no longer perform household tasks. Her daughter comes over to help, but cannot stay. Clearly, more assistance is needed.

The hospice nurse gives them the telephone number for information and assistance at the local senior center. The intake operator helps Mrs. Stone and her daughter determine which services are needed. Because she cannot cook with her arm in a cast, Meals on Wheels are arranged for her and Mr. Stone. Homemaker and choreworker services are also arranged.

Through the AAA, a case manager becomes involved. She interfaces with Mr. Stone's hospice team to coordinate social support services with the clinical services being received through hospice. She answers questions about long-distance caregiving for Mr. and Mrs. Stone's adult children.

Because the cast impedes Mrs. Stone's driving

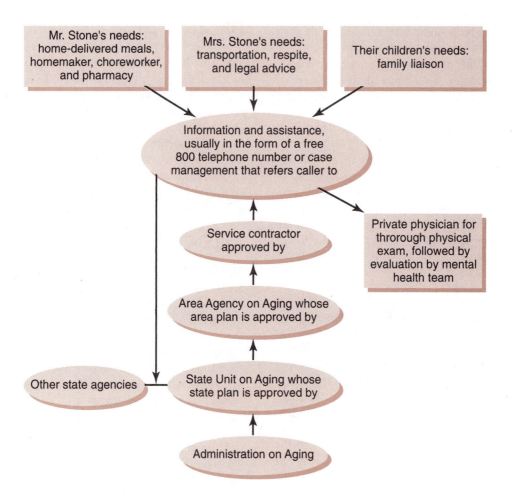

Figure 18.3   How the Aging Network Works

ability, transportation is arranged for her through Dial-a-Ride.

Her physician wants Mrs. Stone to begin rehabilitation on her arm. One of his prescriptions is for her to get more rest to facilitate the healing process. The local respite care program provides her with a much-needed break, and Mr. Stone enjoys having someone new to talk to.

With Mr. Stone's death imminent, the case manager arranges for legal services to make sure Mr. Stone's will and other legal affairs are in order.

Figure 18.3 illustrates how the Aging Network functions in cases like that of Mr. Stone and his family.

WHERE TO GO FOR FURTHER INFORMATION

Administration on Aging (AoA)
One Massachusetts Avenue
Washington, DC 20201

(202) 619-0724
http://www.aoa.gov

Eldercare Locator
1-800-677-1116
http://www.eldercare.gov

This is a nationwide public service referral agency that will assist private individuals in finding senior services in their location.

Appendix B lists a number of national organizations that deal with gerontology and aging services.

FACTS REVIEW

1. In what year and political context was the Older Americans Act passed?
2. What was the original intent of the OAA?
3. Describe the structure and financing of the Aging Network.
4. What do these acronyms stand for? OAA, AAA, SUA, AoA
5. List the seven titles of the Older Americans Act and what each covers in general.
6. How do the services of the Aging Network relate to the other services of the continuum of long-term care?

REFERENCES

Administration on Aging. (2000). *Caregiver support.* Available at *http://www.aoa.dhhs.gov/FactSheets/CaregiverSupport2000.html*

American Association of Retired Persons. (2003). *A profile of older Americans.* Retrieved October 1, 2003 from *http://www.aarp.org*

Carbonell, J. G. (2003, October). *Legislation and budget: Current budget information.* Retrieved October 5, 2003 from *http://www.aoa.gov/about/legbudg/current_budg/legbudg_current_budg.asp*

Cutchin, M. P. (2003). The process of mediated aging-in-place: A theoretically and empirically based model. *Social Science and Medicine, 57,* 1077–1090.

U.S. Census Bureau. (2000). *Summary File I (SFI) 100 percent data.* Retrieved October 1, 2003 from *http://www.factfinder.census.gov.*

U.S. Congress. (1993). *Compilation of the Older Americans Act of 1965 and the Native American Programs Act of 1974 as amended through December 31, 1992* (Serial No. 103-E). Washington, DC: U.S. Government Printing Office.

CHAPTER 19

HIV/AIDS

Marie F. Denis, Kathryn Hyer, Margaret Lampe, and Laurence G. Branch

The discovery in the early 1980s of the human immunodeficiency virus (HIV) and the acquired immunodeficiency syndrome (AIDS)—the most advanced stage of the HIV infection—alerted the world to a life-threatening disease that scientists have referred to as the "modern plague" and the "first plague in the globalization era." Since then, health care professionals from many disciplines have been working to develop effective treatments to prolong lives and alleviate the suffering from this dreadful disease. The development and implementation of anti-HIV drug therapies have enabled people with HIV infection to live longer by delaying the progression from HIV to AIDS. With these treatment advances, HIV is becoming a chronic rather than fatal disease, and its patients are becoming clients of the continuum of long-term care.

At the beginning of the HIV/AIDS pandemic, in the early 1980s, health care systems in developed and developing countries were not equipped to handle the many challenges involved in caring for people living with AIDS (PLWAs). Once HIV makes its entrance into a community, it causes havoc in the existing economic and health infrastructure. The scope of the overwhelming burden was unprecedented in modern times. Cumulative AIDS deaths, worldwide, by the end of 2002 were estimated to be 28 million (Kaiser Family Foundation, 2003). Although the U.S. health care system has made great progress in providing assistance to the nation's PLWA population, the trends of this disease are constantly changing. With anti-HIV drug treatments, mortality has declined. However, with this success comes a steady increase in the prevalence of AIDS. HIV/AIDS is no longer the disease of young adults, homosexual males, and/or those who get involved in what is referred to as "high-risk" behaviors. According to the U.S. Centers for Disease Control and Prevention (CDC), through December of 2001 11 percent of all reported AIDS cases in the U.S. were among people age 50 or older. CDC further reports that among the 90,513 AIDS cases in people over age 50, nearly 79,000 are in people between the ages of 50 and 64, and about 12,000 are 65 years and older.

DEFINITION

AIDS is an acronym for the most advanced stages of HIV infection. Progression from HIV infection to AIDS is measured by monitoring changes in indicators of immune functioning. Healthy adults usually have CD4 T-cell counts of 1,000 or more per cubic millileter of blood. The primary indicators are CD4 T-cell count, CD4:CD8 ratios, and measures of the amount of HIV virus in the system. During the course of HIV infection, a gradual decline in the number of CD4 T-cells will occur in HIV-infected persons. Though some may have abrupt and dramatic drops in their CD4 T-cell counts, a person with CD4 T-cells above 200 may experience some of the early symptoms of AIDS. Others may be asymptomatic even though their CD4 T-cell counts are below 200. The CDC developed official criteria for the definitions of *HIV* and *AIDS* and is responsible for tracking the spread of disease in the United States. The CDC's definition of AIDS includes all HIV-infected people who have fewer than 200 CD4 T-cells per cubic millimeter of blood. In addition, the definition includes 26 clinical conditions that affect people with advanced HIV disease. Most of these conditions are opportunistic infections that generally do not affect people with healthy immune systems. An HIV-positive person may live 14 to 20 years while displaying AIDS symptoms to a greater or lesser degree.

BACKGROUND

The origin of HIV is unclear. Scientists have proposed several hypotheses regarding its origin and the origin of HIV-like precursors in other species, as well its first detection in the human population. Two will be discussed here. One possible and accepted theory is that HIV was transmitted to humans from infected monkeys carrying a related virus, or through the common and frequent consumption of undercooked monkey meat in Africa. Another plausible explanation is a 1950s trial vaccine in the same region using monkey sera. The HIV-like virus (SIVcpz) found in these African monkey species

(*Pan troglodytes* from West Africa and *Pan troglodytes scheinfurthii* from East Africa) is believed to have evolved into HIV (Hirsch, Dapolito, Goeken, & Campbell, 1995). In retrospect, it has become apparent that the HIV chronology dates to a handful of cases:

1. Scientists traced the first known AIDS-infected blood-to-blood samples collected between 1959 and 1982 for the purpose of detecting malaria infection in Kinshasa, Republic of Congo. The HIV-infected individual, a Bantu man who most likely died of AIDS, became infected from an unknown source.
2. Evidence of AIDS was first reported in the United States in 1969, when a 15-year-old male prostitute developed Kaposi's sarcoma (KS) and died later that year; frozen tissue samples of the deceased were shown to contain HIV antibodies and details were first reported much later, at the 11th International Congress of Virology in 1999.
3. Evidence of AIDS in Europe was detected in a Danish surgeon who died in 1976 and is known to have worked in Zaire, Africa (Stine, 2003).

HIV/AIDS GLOBAL EPIDEMIC

According to the World Health Organization (WHO), in 2002 194 (95 percent) of 209 countries had documented diagnosed HIV/AIDS cases (Stine, 2003). The dissemination of HIV worldwide includes men, women, and children. Statistics on prevalence (total cases at a given point in time) and incidence (new cases in a defined interval) for the year 2002 were as follows:

1. 42 million people worldwide were living with HIV/AIDS. These cases included 19.4 million men, 19.2 million women, and 3.2 million children under 15 years of age.
2. Most of the people living with HIV/AIDS (95 percent) are inhabitants of developing nations: 29.4 million of these people live in sub-Saharan

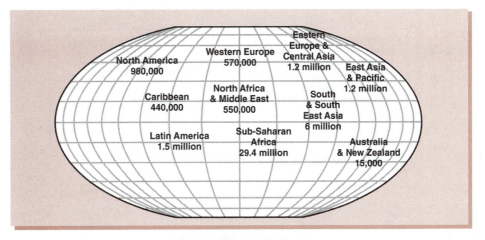

Total: 42 million

Figure 19.1   Adults and Children Estimated to Be Living with HIV/AIDS, 2002

SOURCE: UNAIDS; *http://www.unaids.org/html* (go to World Health Organization; the Joint United Nations Program on HIV/AIDS; "Epidemiology" topic; "Slides02"; slide 04).

Africa; 7.2 million live in Asiatic countries (see Figure 19.1).

3. 12 in every 1,000 adults aged 15 to 49 years worldwide are infected with HIV (1.2 percent); in sub-Saharan Africa, 9 percent of all adults aged 15 to 49 years are infected with HIV. The prevalence of HIV infection is highest in southern Africa, with an infection rate estimated as high as 40 percent (NIAID/NIH, 2003a; Stine, 2003).

4. WHO estimated that in 2002, there were 5 million new or incident HIV infections worldwide, affecting 4.2 million adults and 800,000 children under 15 years of age. These figures translate into 2,000 new HIV infections per day among children under 15 years old and 6,000 new cases per day in young adults between the ages of 15 and 24.

5. Approximately 90,000 new incident cases of HIV occur every year in developed nations. Worldwide, more than 80 percent of HIV transmission is attributed to heterosexual sex (NIAID/NIH, 2002b).

CLIENTS IN THE UNITED STATES

As Figure 19.1 indicates, approximately 1 million adults and children are infected with HIV/AIDS in the United States. Almost 500,000 people are documented to have died from AIDS-related deaths since this became a reportable cause of death. Of the people infected with HIV in this country, the CDC estimates that 25 percent are not aware of their HIV status (NIAID/NIH, 2003a).

Figure 19.2 contrasts the declining incidence of new AIDS cases and the rising prevalence of the disease in the United States. Prevalence provides a good picture of the overall state of the epidemic. The prevalence line begins when the first cases of AIDS were reported, in the early 1980s. When AIDS first surfaced in the United States, there were no effective medications to combat the underlying immune deficiency, and few treatments existed for the opportunistic diseases that resulted. However, in the mid-1990s researchers developed drugs to fight both HIV infection and its associated infections and

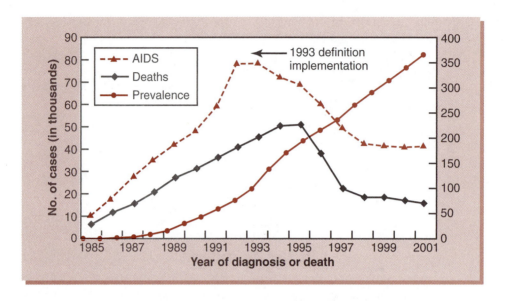

Figure 19.2   Incidence, Prevalence, and Deaths among Persons with AIDS, 1985–2001, United States
SOURCE: CDC AIDS Surveillance Trends Slide Series; *http://www.cdc.gov/hiv/graphics/Images/L207/L207-1.htm*

cancers. As a result, deaths from AIDS decreased and, consequently, the prevalence of PLWAs increased. The number of new cases, or the incidence of AIDS, rose dramatically until about 1994 and then began to fall and stabilize at approximately 40,000 cases per year in the late 1990s.

The Changing Face of HIV/AIDS in the United States

The face of the more than 300,000 Americans living with AIDS in the United States has changed. In the early 1990s, 60 percent of PLWAs were white, 25 percent were African American, and 15 percent were Hispanics. Although the first cases of AIDS in the United States were in white, homosexual men, today minorities are overrepresented in the incidence of new AIDS cases and in new HIV infections reported each year. For the first time in 2002, half of all persons reported with AIDS were African American (Jaffe, 2003). The prevalence rates of AIDS are nearly seven times greater among African Americans

and three times greater among Hispanics than among whites. According to the National Institutes of Health (NIH), more than 82 percent of the existing AIDS cases reported among women in the United States occurred among African American women and Hispanic women, even though they constitute only 25 percent of the U.S. population. Although AIDS deaths are declining in the United States, AIDS is still one of the leading causes of death among black men between 25 and 44 years of age and the third leading cause of death among black women in the age group 15 to 44 (NIAID/NIH, 2003a).

Minorities and adolescents are overrepresented in the 40,000 new HIV infections that occur each year in this country. African Americans represent 13 percent of the U.S. population but 54 percent of the new infections, whereas Hispanics represent about 12 percent of the population yet accout for 19 percent of new HIV infections. Half of the new HIV infections in the United States occur among young adults (under age 25). The gender distribution of new infections indicates that 70 percent occur among men and 30 percent among women (CDC, n.d.). Unlike the rest of the world, where 80 percent of new infections are from heterosexual contact, the CDC estimated the U.S. transmission modes of HIV among men as 60 percent through homosexual contact, 25 percent through drug injection, and 15 percent via heterosexual contact. Among U.S. women, 75 percent of new HIV infections were transmitted heterosexually; injection drug use accounted for 25 percent (CDC, n.d.).

All 50 states, the District of Columbia, and the U.S. territories report HIV/AIDS cases. The four states with the highest number of cases are New York, California, Florida, and Texas, respectively. Within these states, the large metropolitan areas have the highest number of cases.

People with HIV also face many coexisting challenges, including poverty, drug addiction, mental ill-ness, trauma, and incarceration. The people most at risk for HIV—including women, injection drug users, and men who have sex with men—often face similar challenges. In addition, those predominantly affected with HIV early in the epidemic were white, often middle-class, gay men; currently, the gay men at risk for HIV infections and AIDS are most frequently men of color.

Perinatally Acquired HIV

Perinatal acquired HIV infection is the transmission of HIV from mother to child during birth. Because of antiretroviral drug therapy (most notably zidovudine or AZT) administered to HIV-infected women during pregnancy, labor, and delivery, and to the newborns immediately after birth, pediatric AIDS cases have dropped. A public health success story for HIV/AIDS, perinatally acquired AIDS decreased

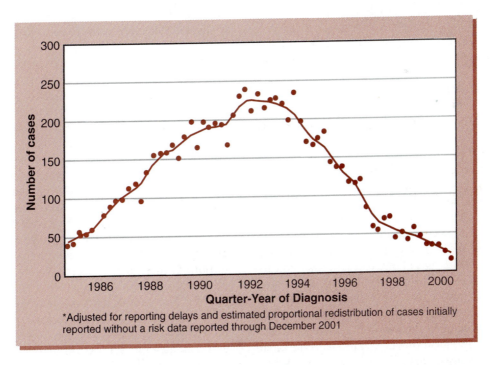

Figure 19.3 Perinatally Acquired AIDS Cases by Quarter-Year of Diagnosis,* 1985–2000, United States
SOURCE: CDC AIDS Surveillance Trends Slide Series; *http://www.cdc.gov/hiv/graphics/Images/L207/L207-1.htm*

89 percent from 1992 to 2001, as Figure 19.3 shows. The U.S. Public Health Service now recommends routine HIV testing of pregnant women, using an opt-out approach, and the use of antiretroviral medications and obstetric interventions by those infected. Although mother-to-child transmission has decreased, an estimated 280 to 370 cases of perinatal infection still occur each year (CDC, n.d.).

CASE MANAGEMENT

Given that there were no effective treatments for HIV/AIDS when it first surfaced in the United States, early HIV/AIDS case management services coordinated support for terminally ill patients and their families. Services focused primarily on organizing medical services and obtaining psychological support (Oregon Department of Human Services, 2003). During the past 20 years, however, researchers have developed drugs to fight both HIV infection and its associated infections and cancers. There are effective means of preventing complications and delaying, but not preventing, progression to AIDS.

Case management models reflect the evolving nature of the infections. Initial federal funding sources for HIV/AIDS case management services were from the Ryan White Comprehensive AIDS Resource Emergency (CARE) Act, approved by Congress in 1990. Ryan White, a 13-year-old hemophiliac, was barred from attending his local Indiana school in 1985 because he had AIDS resulting from a blood transfusion. His lawsuit highlighted the stigma of AIDS and the need for public education about transmission of HIV infection. When White died from AIDS at the age of 19, federal legislation to create a system of care for people with AIDS was named in his honor. Table 19.1 defines the sections or titles of the Ryan White CARE Act, summarizes the services included, and indicates how the 2002 federal appropriation of $1.9 billion was allocated across the services. This was the first federal bill to mandate case management services for people with HIV/AIDS.

The Centers for Disease Control (1997) identified the following six core HIV case management tasks: (1) client identification, outreach, and engagement; (2) medical and psychosocial assessment of need; (3) development of a service plan; (4) implementation of the care plan by linking with service delivery; (5) monitoring of the service plan and reassessment; and (6) advocacy on behalf of the client, including creating, obtaining, or brokering needed client resources. Although these case management services are required, the Ryan White CARE Act allows states a great deal of latitude in defining their case management programs and deciding what organizations will provide the services.

The Ryan White CARE Act has become the key link between medical and support services, even though states choose the model of case management: direct or brokered. In direct case management, the case manager coordinates activities around a network of support services. In brokered case management, case managers coordinate activities but frequently also manage the support services or "wraparound" services. Most HIV/AIDS case management has evolved as brokered case management because of the limited infrastructure of health care services, paucity of specialty health providers, limited housing, and poor access to transportation.

Working with HIV/AIDS clients also requires intensive education on the use of medications and adherence to the medication schedule; the schedule of doses of 20 or more pills must be taken at specific intervals to be effective. Although the new drug therapies are not a cure for AIDS, they greatly improve the health of many people with AIDS, as long as the patients adhere to the medication schedule and are under medical care to treat opportunistic infections as they develop and to ensure that the virus does not develop resistance to the antiretroviral therapy. For people with multiple medical, social and economic challenges, reducing risk behavior to prevent the spread of infection to others may be very challenging. With these patients, prevention case management (PCM) should be considered: it is an intensive intervention that combines individual HIV risk reduction with case management to provide

Table 19.1 Ryan White Act

Ryan White CARE Act Titles	Year Started	Purpose	Services	Funding Level in 2002 (in millions of dollars)
Title I: Grants to Eligible Metropolitan Areas	1991	Provides emergency assistance to the eligible metropolitan areas (EMAs) most severely affected by the HIV/AIDS epidemic. An EMA must have 2,000 AIDS cases during the previous 5 years and have a population of at least 500,000.	(1) Outpatient and ambulatory health services, including substance abuse and mental health treatment; (2) Early intervention that includes outreach, counseling, testing, and referral services designed to identify HIV-positive individuals who know their HIV status; (3) Outpatient and ambulatory support services, including case management, to the extent that these support services facilitate, enhance, support or sustain delivery, continuity, or benefits of health services; and (4) Inpatient case management services that expedite discharge and prevent unnecessary hospitalization.	$619.5
Title II	1991	Provides grants to all 50 states, the District of Columbia, Puerto Rico, Guam, the U.S. Virgin Islands, and 5 newly eligible U.S. Pacific Territories and Associated Jurisdictions. Title II also funds the AIDS Drug Assistance Program (ADAP) and grants to states for emerging communities.	(1) Ambulatory health care; (2) Home-based health care; (3) Insurance coverage; (4) Medications; (5) Support services; (6) Outreach to HIV-positive individuals who know their HIV status; (7) Early intervention services; and (8) HIV Care Consortia, which assess needs and contracts for services.	$997.4
Title II: Grants to States and Territories and AIDS Drug Assistance Program (ADAP)	1996	Awards grants to all 50 States, the District of Columbia, Puerto Rico, Guam, the U.S. Virgin Islands, the Marshall Islands, and North Marianas. Each state and territory establishes its own eligibility criteria, including income and CD4 cell count. Recipients must document their HIV status.	ADAP provides medications for the treatment of HIV disease. Program funds also may be used to purchase health insurance for eligible clients. Amendments to the Ryan White CARE Act in October 2000 added additional language allowing ADAP funds to be used to pay for services that enhance access to, adherence to, and monitoring of drug treatments.	Received $639 million from Title II funds

(continues)

Table 19.1 *(continued)*

Ryan White CARE Act Titles	Year Started	Purpose	Services	Funding Level in 2002 (in millions of dollars)
Title III: Capacity-Building Grant Program	1991	Funds public or nonprofit, including faith-based organizations that develop, enhance, or expand high-quality HIV primary health care services in rural or urban unserved areas and communities of color. Capacity-building grant funds are from 1–3 years and do not fund service delivery or patient care. Eligible applicants must intend to become comprehensive HIV primary care providers.	Some of the fundable activities include, but are not limited to: (1) Identifying, establishing, and strengthening clinical, administrative, managerial, and management information system (MIS) structures; (2) Developing a financial management unit of the organization; (3) Developing and implementing a clinical continuous quality improvement (CQI) program; (4) Purchasing clinical supplies and equipment for the purpose of developing, enhancing, or expanding HIV primary care services; (5) Developing an organizational strategic plan to address managed-care changes or changes in the HIV epidemic in the local community; (6) A package of activities that include the development of an organizational strategic plan for HIV care, education of board members regarding the HIV program, and staff training and development regarding HIV care.	$193.9 million (total for all Title III programs)
Title III: Planning Grant Program	1991	Funds eligible entities in efforts to plan for the provision of high-quality comprehensive HIV primary health care services in rural or urban underserved areas and communities of color. Planning grant funds are intended for a period of one year. Planning grants support the planning process and do not fund any service delivery or patient care.	Activities can include, but are not limited to: (1) Identifying key stakeholders and engaging and coordinating potential partners in the planning process; (2) Gathering a formal advisory group to plan for the establishment of services; (3) Conducting an in-depth review of the nature and extent of need for HIV primary care services in the community. This should include a local epidemiological profile, an evaluation of the community's service provider capacity, and a profile of the target population(s); (4) Defining the components of care and forming essential programmatic linkages with related providers in the community; (5) Researching funding sources and applying for operational grants.	$193.9 million (total for all Title III programs)

(continues)

| Title III: Early Intervention Services (EIS) | 1991 | Funds comprehensive primary health care for individuals living with HIV disease. Title III grants reached 108,945 patients in 1999; 67 percent were people of color. | Services include: (1) Risk-reduction counseling on prevention, antibody testing, medical evaluation, and clinical care; (2) Antiretroviral therapies; protection against opportunistic infections; and ongoing medical, oral health, nutritional, psychosocial, and other care services for HIV-infected clients; (3) Case management to ensure access to services and continuity of care for HIV-infected clients; and (4) Attention to other health problems that occur frequently with HIV infection, including tuberculosis and substance abuse. Two types of planning grants are also available: (1) Grants that prepare organizations to plan for the development of HIV early intervention services. These one-year grants are for $50,000. (2) Grants to provide capacity building for organizations to develop, enhance, or expand their capability to provide HIV primary care services. These grants may total up to $150,000 over a 3-year period. | $193.9 million (total for all Title III programs) |
| Title IV: Women, Infants, Children, & Youth | 1994 | Addresses the needs of women, infants, children, and youth living with HIV disease. Title IV enhances client access to care and to clinical trials and research. Participation in clinical research has increased among Title IV clients. In 2000, it grew to 7,992 clients. Clinical research helps ensure that all patients have access to the best treatments. From 1999 to 2000, the number of people served through Title IV increased 18 percent. In 2000, Title IV provided services to 53,051 clients, 54 percent of whom were HIV-infected. Of the clients with known race/ethnicity, the majority (88 percent) were | Title IV programs enhance client access to care and to clinical trials and research. Participation in clinical research has increased among Title IV clients; in 2000, it grew to 7,992 clients. Services provided include: (1) Primary and specialty medical care; (2) Psychosocial services; (3) Logistical support and coordination; and (4) Outreach and case management. | $71.0 |

Table 19.1 (continued)

Ryan White CARE Act Titles	Year Started	Purpose	Services	Funding Level in 2002 (in millions of dollars)
		minorities; of clients age 13 and older, 78 percent were female, more than one-half of whom reported exposure to HIV through heterosexual contact.		
Special Projects of National Significance (SPNS)	1996	Advances knowledge and skills in the delivery of health and support services to underserved populations diagnosed with HIV infection. SPNS grants fund innovative models of care and support the development of effective delivery systems for HIV care. The SPNS program is considered the research and development arm of the Ryan White CARE Act and provides the mechanisms to: (1) Assess the effectiveness of particular models of care; (2) Support innovative program design; and (3) Promote replication of effective models. Current priorities include: (1) Supporting the coordination and integration of existing services for Native Americans/Alaska Natives living with HIV and other co-morbidities; (2) Improving the quality of HIV care; (3) Developing methods to estimate unmet needs; (4) Collaborating with CDC on interventions for HIV-positive substance abuse users and continuity of care for incarcerated individuals; (5) Developing and evaluating end-of-life care and palliation models; (6) Assessing existing treatment education/	The SPNS program is an integral link to all CARE Act programs. Although it provides an opportunity to develop new services, the program places great emphasis on the legislative mandates to assess the effectiveness of models of care and promote their replication. As CARE Act grantees develop innovative services, the SPNS program will provide the funding and expertise for grantees to evaluate innovations and disseminate their findings to the HIV community.	

(continues)

adherence efforts; (7) Establishing and assessing HIV care networks; (8) Assessing innovations in serving those with chemical dependencies; (9) Continuing the U.S./Mexico border health effort; and (10) Assessing primary prevention strategies for HIV-positive persons.

| AIDS Education and Training Centers (AETC) | 1997 | Supports a network of 11 regional centers (and more than 70 associated sites) that conduct targeted, multidisciplinary education and training programs for health care providers treating persons with HIV/AIDS. The AETCs serve all 50 states, the District of Columbia, the Virgin Islands, Puerto Rico, and the six U.S. Pacific jurisdictions. The AETC program increases the number of health care providers who are effectively educated and motivated to counsel, diagnose, treat, and medically manage individuals with HIV infection, and to help prevent high-risk behaviors that lead to HIV transmission. Provider training: Training is preferentially targeted to providers who serve minority populations, the homeless, rural communities, incarcerated persons, and Ryan White CARE Act-funded sites. AETCs focus on training clinicians in primary health care (physicians, physician assistants, nurses, nurse practitioners, dentists, pharmacists); training activities are based on assessed local needs. | Provider training for professionals: National Resource AETC, National HIV/AIDS Clinicians' Consultation Center; "WARMLINE" (800) 933-3413 for information on treatment of individuals infected with HIV; PEPline (888) 448-4911 for information on possible health care worker exposure to HIV | $35.3 |

Table 19.1 *(continued)*

Ryan White CARE Act Titles	Year Started	Purpose	Services	Funding Level in 2002 (in millions of dollars)
Dental Reimbursement Program	1997	Supports access to oral health care for individuals with HIV infection by reimbursing dental education programs for nonreimbursed costs incurred in providing such care. By offsetting the costs of nonreimbursed HIV care in dental education institutions, the Dental Reimbursement Program addresses the dual goals of improving access to oral health care and training new generations of dental and dental hygiene students, and dental residents, to manage the oral health care of people with HIV. Eligible applicants are dental schools, postdoctoral dental education programs as described in §777(b)(4)(B) of the Health Professions Partnerships Education Act of 1998, and dental hygiene programs that are accredited by the Commission on Dental Accreditation. The Dental Reimbursement Program awards funds to support these institutions in providing comprehensive oral health care to individuals with HIV. This care includes diagnostic, preventive, oral health education and health promotion, restorative, periodontal, prosthodontic, endodontic, oral surgery, and oral medicine services.	Programs funded by the Community-Based Dental Partnership program are to be collaborative efforts between the eligible entity and community-based dental providers that propose to: (1) Provide oral health services for individuals with HIV; (2) Establish and manage clinical rotations for students and residents in community-based settings; (3) Collaborate and coordinate between the dental education programs and the community-based partners in the delivery of oral health services; (4) Collect, manage, and report data that will assess /describe the service delivery and educational components of the funded programs and; (5) Ensure patient confidentiality and the establishment and review of a system for control of records of HIV-positive patients.	$13.5

| Community-Based Dental Partnership grantees | 1997 | The Community-Based Dental Partnership program funds eligible entities' efforts to increase access to oral health care for unserved and underserved rural and urban HIV-positive populations. Funding will support oral health service delivery and provider training in community settings. Community-Based Dental Partnership grants are intended for a period of up to three years. Eligible applicants are dental schools, postdoctoral dental education programs as described in §777(b)(4)(B) of the Health Professions Partnerships Education Act of 1998, and dental hygiene programs that are accredited by the Commission on Dental Accreditation. | Initiatives funded by the Community-Based Dental Partnership program are to be collaborative efforts between the eligible entity and community-based dental providers that propose to: (1) Provide oral health services for individuals with HIV; (2) Establish and manage clinical rotations for students and residents in community-based settings; (3) Collaborate and coordinate between the dental education programs and the community-based partners in the delivery of oral health services; (4) Collect, manage, and report data that will assess/describe the service delivery and educational components of the funded programs; (5) Ensure patient confidentiality and the establishment and review of a system for control of records of HIV-positive patients. |
| HIV/AIDS Bureau (HAB) Office of Science and Epidemiology (OSE) Program Data and Evaluation | | Provides data and evaluation support to the Ryan White CARE Act, including bureau programs, grantees, and constituents. The multi-disciplinary data and research staff consists of epidemiologists, health services researchers, sociologists, statisticians, and ethnographers. Staff work in four areas: (1) CARE Act data collection; (2) Epidemiological studies of HIV services; (3) Evaluation of issues critical to HIV care; and (4) Research and demonstration projects to advance HIV care—Special Projects of National Significance (SPNS) | The bureau's data and evaluation activities reflect five broad questions that are critical to the successful delivery of HIV care in the United States today and are responsive to the priorities of a reauthorized Ryan White CARE Act: (1) Assessing unmet need; (2) Removing barriers to care; (3) Optimizing local service delivery systems; (4) Providing quality care; and (5) Adapting to change. |

SOURCE: Health Resources and Services Administration, HIV/AIDS Bureau Web site: *http://hab.hrsa.gov/programs.htm* (accessed on August 5, 2003)

intensive, ongoing support (Purcell, DeGroff, & Wolitski, 1998).

Given the need for medical care, many states, particularly those with rural communities, work through local health departments. Other states, especially those with well-developed community-based organizations and AIDS advocacy groups, use nonprofit groups to organize services. Still other communities have developed HIV/AIDS case management programs within community health centers. Consequently, while the Ryan White CARE Act can pay for services such as transportation, housing, support groups, mental health counseling, legal assistance, and substance abuse assistance, the ability to access these services and the amount of money available for them varies widely.

MEDICAL COVERAGE FOR HIV/AIDS CARE

HIV care is costly. The most effective treatments for HIV, as well as for people with AIDS, involve multiple medications or highly active antiretroviral therapy (HAART). Combination drug therapy costs alone ranged from $12,000 to $20,000 a year in 2000. In addition, physician visits, lab tests, and additional treatments or medications for opportunistic infections raise the total annual cost of HIV-related illness to approximately $20,000 per patient.

Gaining access to medical services is a challenge for people with HIV/AIDS. The major sources for financial coverage include private insurance, Medicaid, Medicare, and other publicly supported care, such as through the Ryan White CARE Act, the Veterans Administration, and community health centers. Estimates of people with HIV/AIDS who are in regular care vary from about one-third to about half of those who should receive care. Of those with access to regular medical care, the federal government pays for at least half the costs. The only representative study of people with HIV/AIDS in regular care, conducted in 1996, found that of those receiving regular care, 32 percent had private coverage, 20 percent were uninsured, 19 percent were

covered by Medicare, and 29 percent were covered by Medicaid (Bozzette, et al., 1998).

Medicaid

Medicaid is the largest source of public financing for HIV/AIDS care in the United States. In 1999 Medicaid paid $3.9 billion, which was half of all funding for AIDS health care in the United States. Fifty percent of all adults with AIDS and 90 percent of children with AIDS rely on Medicaid to pay for care. Although Medicaid covers HIV services, individuals with HIV must qualify for eligibility. Most states require a combination of low income, few assets, and poor health. States share Medicaid health care costs with the federal government, but state definitions of low income and limits on what services are covered vary widely. Furthermore, many states require adult Medicaid beneficiaries to be disabled, and thus these definitions of eligibility can undermine early diagnosis and treatment. One of the most important Medicaid benefits for people with HIV/AIDS is prescription drug coverage. All states provide this benefit, even though several states limit the number of prescription drugs covered each month and require that the drugs be purchased from specific vendors.

Medicare

A second federal program, Medicare, also covers HIV/AIDS care, but it is for working people who qualify as disabled through Social Security Disability Insurance (SSDI). Medicare is the second largest source of HIV/AIDS services and paid $1.7 billion for HIV/AIDS care in fiscal year (FY) 2000. Approximately 20 percent of those people with HIV/AIDS receive Medicare benefits. Funding from Medicare for HIV/AIDS services has increased 70 percent since FY1995, reflecting the increased longevity of those living with HIV/AIDS. To be eligible for disability under Social Security, as well as Medicare, requires a work history long enough to qualify for disability, application for disability status, a five-month waiting period after the disability determination to receive SSDI benefits, and then a 24-month waiting period to ensure that the disability is permanent. All this must transpire before an SSDI beneficiary can join Medicare. Thus, there is a 29-month waiting period after a person becomes disabled before he or she can receive Medicare health benefits. Although people with HIV/AIDS are living longer, the disease increases disability, and thus the prolonged waiting period is a barrier to accessing Medicare coverage. Once disability is established, the Medicare program will pay for Medicare-covered services; however, Medicare currently offers no prescription drug coverage, so most HIV/AIDS clients require additional resources. An estimated 13 to 17 percent of Medicare beneficiaries are "dually" eligible for Medicaid and use Medicaid services to supplement and cover non-Medicare covered services (Kaiser Family Foundation, 2003).

Ryan White CARE Act

The Ryan White CARE Act, the third largest source of federal funding, was initially designed to fill the gaps in financing of care for people with HIV/AIDS and to relieve the cost of care borne by large metropolitan areas. It is a discretionary program that requires annual appropriations from Congress; it is not an entitlement program like Medicare and Medicaid. Ryan White CARE Act beneficiaries receive services because they have no insurance or they are underinsured: there is no coverage for the care needed. Most states use CARE funds to cover outpatient care and support services rather than for hospitalizations and long-term institutionalization. As Table 19.1 indicates, the various titles of the Ryan White CARE Act cover different services and can provide for home health services, transportation, and housing benefits. By FY2000, Ryan White CARE Act federal spending totaled $1.595 billion, more than double the 1995 federal funding. As discussed in the case management section, Ryan White CARE Act programs vary significantly across the country. Drug coverage varies from a low of 20 medications covered in one state to more than 100

medications covered in other states (Kaiser Family Foundation, 2000). Many Ryan White CARE Act services use state Medicaid coverage as the base for medical care and supplement services or wrap services around Medicaid coverage. When Medicaid coverage is limited, as states struggle to control spiraling Medicaid costs, people with HIV/AIDS often are not able to obtain needed services.

The Ricky Ray Hemophilia Relief Fund Act of 1988 is another federal program administered by the Department of Health and Human Services (DHHS). The program provides compassionate payments of $100,000 to individuals with a blood-clotting disorder, such as hemophilia, who contracted HIV from contaminated antihemophilic factor between July 1, 1982 and December 31, 1987. Finally, the Substance Abuse and Mental Health Services Administration (SAMHSA), also part of DHHS, makes grants to states to provide counseling and treatment to individuals with HIV/AIDS.

People with HIV/AIDS face difficult circumstances as their ability to work (and therefore their income) declines and their health care expenses mount. Recognizing that homelessness threatens family stability as well as the health of persons with HIV/AIDS, the Department of Housing and Urban Development (HUD) developed Housing Opportunities for People with AIDS (HOPWA). HOPWA was designed to help low-income PLWAs and their families by providing funds for secure housing. States and localities must set long-term strategies to meet the housing needs of low-income PLWAs and their families, and communities must demonstrate efforts to better coordinate local and private efforts to serve PLWAs.

Although federal funds remain the major source of funding regarding the HIV/AIDS epidemic, many local governments, foundations, and charities also provide HIV/AIDS services. Public hospitals, for example, are usually supported by counties or cities and are often the sites of clinical HIV/AIDS care. Likewise, free clinics and specialized HIV/AIDS service organizations provide both care and prevention services. Several foundations have made substantial contributions to HIV/AIDS programs by funding demonstration projects, dissemination of best practices, advocacy groups, and research.

FEDERAL ROLE IN RESEARCH, PREVENTION, AND INTERNATIONAL SERVICES

Many branches of the federal government have responded to the HIV/AIDS epidemic during the past two decades. The following sections summarize the additional sources of financing from federal agencies for HIV/AIDS care (see Figure 19.4). The focus of this section is on federal activities in research, prevention, and international services, but the activities and programs may serve more than one purpose.

Research refers to the range of biomedical, epidemiological, behavioral, health services, and social science research activities. Research activities are conducted or supported by various federal agencies, including the National Institutes of Health (NIH), the Food and Drug Administration (FDA), the Agency for Healthcare Research and Quality (AHRQ), the Department of Defense, and the Department of Veterans Affairs. Included within this category are prevention research and international research activities at NIH and CDC.

Prevention refers to programs funded primarily by grants to states and to national groups for risk-reduction activities. The CDC funds most prevention programs. However, these programs are coordinated with other federal agencies, such as the FDA, Veterans Affairs, the Indian Health Service (IHS), the Department of Labor (DOL), the Department of Justice (DOJ), the Department of Education (DOE), and the Office of the Secretary for DHHS (OS). Spending for prevention research activities conducted by the NIH is included under the research category rather than the prevention category. In FY 2001, NIH estimated that it spent $862.1 million on combined domestic and international prevention research activities.

International refers to a range of international programs conducted primarily by the U.S. Agency for International Development and CDC. International prevention activities conducted by CDC in FY2001 totaled $104.5 million. The Departments of Defense, Labor, and Agriculture, and the Peace Corps, also conduct international programs. Included within this spending amount are U.S. contributions to the Global Fund to Fight AIDS, Tuberculosis, and Malaria (Global Fund). Created in 2001, the Global Fund is an independent, international, public-private partnership designed to garner additional support for global HIV/AIDS prevention, care, and research activities. In FY2001, the U.S. contribution to the Global Fund was $100 million.

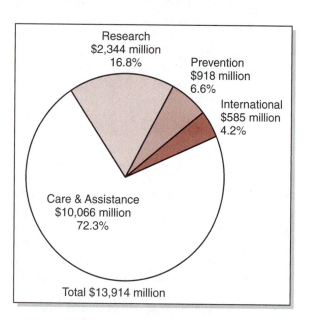

Figure 19.4 Total Federal HIV/AIDS Spending by Category, FY 2001

SOURCE: Kaiser Family Foundation, 2002, p. 18; *http://www.kff.org*

HIV/AIDS PREVENTION IN THE UNITED STATES

Efforts to prevent the spread of HIV infection in the United States have yielded mixed results. One area of success has been in the prevention of mother-to-child HIV transmission, through the implementation of universal, voluntary screening for HIV during pregnancy and, for women identified as HIV-infected, the use of antiretroviral medications by both the mother and the newborn. Increasing HIV screening as part of routine medical care is the most effective way to increase prevention. Recognizing this, CDC announced a new prevention initiative in 2003. The strategies to reduce risk behavior among the general population are all aimed at increasing the likelihood that people infected with HIV will be detected earlier. The strategies are: (1) make voluntary testing a routine part of medical care; (2) implement new models for diagnosing HIV infections, such as using rapid HIV testing for same-day results; (3) prevent new infections by working with persons diagnosed with HIV; and (4) further decrease perinatal HIV transmission.

Critics of current prevention strategies and care charge that efforts to fund HIV-related prevention and treatment programs do not fully appreciate the complexity of life and the disease for those with or at risk for HIV. Many people with HIV are coping with problems related to poverty and are already overwhelmed. Prevention efforts compete with issues of finances, housing, child care, transportation, employment, medical care, substance abuse, and crime (CDC, 2001). These factors suggest that prevention efforts, like care, must reflect the changing face of HIV/AIDS and work to develop culturally sensitive programs that fit the needs of those infected and at risk for infection.

CONCLUSION

As the HIV/AIDS epidemic enters its third decade, search for a vaccine or cure continues, but neither has yet been accomplished. The scientific community has made great strides in developing many potent treatment regimes to extend life. HIV/AIDS is now considered a chronic, rather than fatal, disease.

However, the cost of treatment is high. Furthermore, for treatments to be effective, drug regimens

must be adhered to faithfully and medical care must be accessible. Many in the United States have limited access to care, despite numerous public and private programs.

The high cost of anti-HIV therapies and overall care challenges the budgets of the federal government and all state governments. Thus, policymakers, service providers, and payers have begun to examine their initial approaches to HIV/AIDS. New state models of case managements, such as those used by Oregon and Massachusetts, are examining how to coordinate care more efficiently, including the introduction of managed care for Medicaid eligible HIV/AIDS clients (Oregon DHS, 2003; Massachusetts Department of Public Health, 2003).

Over the past 20 years, the long-term care needs of people living with HIV/AIDS have become a critical health policy issue internationally as well as nationally. AIDS was declared a development crisis by the World Bank in 2000. Fortunately, in the United States, a comprehensive, coordinated continuum of care is possible for HIV/AIDS victims—even if is not always obtained by each individual. The United States thus presents a model for the rest of the world, and will continue to do so as it refines its own HIV/AIDS comprehensive care delivery system.

CLIENT EXAMPLE

James is a 19-year-old African American who is HIV-positive. He left his family home in a blighted part of a large city when he was 17, and has basically been homeless ever since. He did not graduate from high school and survives by taking casual work when he can find it. His father has not been in touch with the family for years, and James seldom contacts his mother, who seems more concerned with his younger half-siblings than with him. He occasionally stays with a cousin or great-aunt, but primarily he lives on the street. He is not sure how or when he contracted HIV. He uses drugs when he can get them for free, but he has avoided becoming drug-dependent. He is not happy with his situation, but does not know how to change, nor does he have the resources (such as a mentor or support system) to change.

James becomes ill and ends up in the emergency room of the local hospital. He is diagnosed with walking pneumonia, given a prescription for antibiotics, instructions on caring for himself, and a referral to the HIV/AIDS program sponsored by the hospital, H-PAL (HIV/AIDS Persons Achieve Life). James has no way to pay for his treatment, so, although the hospital gives him a bill, both the hospital staff and James know that he will eventually be classified as a "bad debt."

H-PAL staff persuade James to enroll in the program. He is willing to do this only because it is the only way for him to get the medicine he needs. H-PAL arranges for its affiliated pharmacy to get James the antibiotics for the pneumonia. These emergency medicines are paid for from a state fund allotment for emergencies for low-income people. Meanwhile, the H-PAL staff member helps James submit an application to qualify for the state Medicaid program, which will take 60 to 90 days to process. The intake counselor tells him he will qualify as disabled because of the combination of being HIV-positive, having a history of drug abuse, and currently suffering from pneumonia and malnutrition.

The H-PAL counselor refers James to a facility for the homeless so he can get a bed and sleep indoors, as well as get a shower and one meal a day for up to 30 days. The counselor instructs him in the proper behavior so that he will not infect others with pneumonia. The price of the housing is $5 per day because it is subsidized by the city government. James can pay if he has a job, or he can work as maintenance staff at the shelter in exchange for free lodging and a $5 per day credit for extra meals. Because James is ill, the shelter grants him 10 days of credit so that he can allow the antibiotics to take effect before starting to work.

Before James leaves the H-PAL program office, the counselor refers him to a small room in the back of the building filled with used clothing. The counselor helps James find a set of clean clothes, including a jacket and an extra shirt. He also gives James a complimentary toiletry kit donated by the auxiliary of the hospital.

After two days, a member of the H-PAL program calls James to see if he obtained and is taking the medication. The counselor also suggests that James return the next evening to attend a support group of young men who are HIV-positive. Meanwhile, at the homeless shelter, James has been looking at ads for part-time jobs that do not require any special skills. He also notes an ad for a program that would give him training in auto mechanics, which he enjoys, and another that would enable him to complete his high school training.

When James returns to H-PAL to attend the support group, the counselor congratulates him for looking better, and asks how he is feeling. The counselor suggests that James come back the next week to learn about the services available to him through the Ryan White CARE Act. The counselor says that he will spend a hour or so with James talking about what he would like to do in the future; thereafter, the counselor helps James identify resources that will enable him to start on a path toward his future goal. The counselor tells James that there is no charge for his time, because he is paid through a combination of grant funds and he is there to help James. For the first time in two years, James feels like there is a place and a person he can turn to for help, and that perhaps there is indeed a way to change his situation for the future.

WHERE TO GO FOR FURTHER INFORMATION

AIDS Alliance for Children, Youth, and Families
1600 K Street, NW, Suite 300
Washington, DC 20006
(888) 917-AIDS
http://www.aids-alliance.org

Centers for Disease Control and Prevention (CDC)
Division of HIV/AIDS Prevention

National Center for HIV, STD, and TB
Prevention
Mail Stop E-49
Atlanta, GA 30333
(800) 342-2437 (AIDS)
http://www.cdc.gov/hiv

HIV/AIDS Bureau of the Health Resources and
Services Administration (HRSA)
U.S. Department of Health and Human
Services
Office of Communications
5600 Fishers Lane
Rockville, MD 20857
(301) 443-3376
http://www.hab.hrsa.gov

Kaiser Family Foundation
2400 Sand Hill Road
Menlo Park, CA 94025
(650) 854-9400
http://www.kff.org/

Offices of HIV/AIDS Policy
U.S. Department of Health and Human
Services
200 Independence Avenue, Room 736E
Washington, DC 20201
(202) 690-5560
http://www.surgeongeneral.gov/aids/ohaphome

FACTS REVIEW

1. Compare and contrast the transmission of
   HIV in the United States with transmission
   in the rest of the world.
2. How has the face of AIDS changed in the
   United States over the past 20 years?
3. Why does the comprehensiveness of HIV
   services vary across states?
4. What is the Ryan White CARE Act and what
   programs does it include?
5. What are the two largest insurers for HIV
   services?

REFERENCES

Bozzette, S. A., Berry, S. H., Duan, N., Frankel, M. R.,
Leibowitz, A. A., Lefkowitz, D., Emmons, C. A.,
Senterfitt, J. W., Berk, M. L., Morton, S. C., &
Shapiro, M. F. (1998). The care of HIV-infected
adults in the United States. *New England Journal of
Medicine, 339*(26), 1897–1904.

Centers for Disease Control. (2001). HIV incidence
among young men who have sex with men—Seven
U.S. cities, 1994–2000. *Morbidity and Mortality
Weekly Report, 50*(21), 440–444.

Centers for Disease Control. (1997, September).
*HIV prevention case management: Literature
review and current practice.* Retrieved August 14,
2003, from *http://www.cdc.gov/hiv/pubs/pcml/
pcml-doc.htm*

Centers for Disease Control. (n.d.) *A glance at the HIV
epidemic.* Retrieved August 14, 2003, from
http://www.cdc.gov/nchstp/od/news/At-a-Glance.pdf

Hirsch, V. M., Dapolito, G., Goeken, R., & Campbell,
B. J. (1995). Phylogeny and natural history of the
primate lentiviruses, SIV and HIV. *Current Opinion
Genetic Development, 5*(6), 798–806.

Jaffe, H. (2003, July). *HIV/AIDS in America today.* Paper
presented at the 2003 National HIV Prevention
Conference, Atlanta, GA.

Kaiser Family Foundation. (2003, June). *HIV/AIDS
policy fact sheet: HIV testing in the United States.*
Menlo Park, CA: Author.

Kaiser Family Foundation. (2002, June). *Report: Federal
HIV/AIDS spending.* Retrieved August 20, 2003
from *http://www.kff.org/content/2003/6076/
ChartPack2002.ppt*

Kaiser Family Foundation. (2000, October). *Financing
HIV/AIDS care: A quilt with many holes.* Menlo
Park, CA: Author.

Massachusetts Department of Public Health. (2003).
HIV case management: A review of the literature.
Boston: Author.

NIAID/NIH. (2003a). *HIV/AIDS statistics* (National
Institute of Allergy and Infectious Diseases and
National Institute of Health "Fact Sheet"). Retrieved
March 28, 2003, from *http://www.niaid.nih.gov/
factsheets/aidsstat.htm*

NIAID/NIH. (2003b). *How HIV causes AIDS* (National
Institute of Allergy and Infectious Diseases and
National Institute of Health "Fact Sheet"). Retrieved

March 30, 2003, from *http://www.niaid.nih.gov/factsheets/howhiv.htm*

Oregon Department of Human Services. (2003). *Ryan White Title II HIV/AIDS case management standards of service.* Salem, OR: Author.

Purcell, D. W., DeGroff, A. S., & Wolitski, R. J. (1998). HIV prevention case management: Current practice and future directions. *Health & Social Work, 23,* 282–289.

Stine, G. J. (2003). *AIDS update 2003: An annual overview of Acquired Immune Deficiency Syndrome.* Upper Saddle River, NJ: Prentice Hall.

CHAPTER 20

Mental Health and Mental Retardation Services

Ruth B. Pickard and James H. Swan

Functional limitations in self-care activities are the major reason people need long-term care services. These limitations can result from either physical or mental impairment. Mental illnesses, especially those that are severe and persistent in nature, and the more serious levels of mental retardation and developmental disabilities, interfere with the capacity for independent living and frequently require supportive services. Thus, mental health and long-term care policy are inextricably bound together.

Most mental illnesses (MI), mental retardation (MR), and developmental disabilities (DD) are chronic in nature, often spanning entire lifetimes of those affected. Treatments and services may be needed intermittently or continuously over many years and are often complicated by the presence of co-morbidities. The starting and usual endpoint in making public policy pertaining to the care of persons with disabling mental conditions is cost. According to the 1996 *Global Burden of Disease* study, which uses a measure of Disability Adjusted Life Years (DALYs) to compare the relative toll of different disease conditions, mental illnesses account for more than 15 percent of the burden of disease in countries with established market economies (Murray & Lopez, 1996). This is greater than the burden imposed by all forms of cancer taken together. In the United States, mental illnesses were estimated to cost $148 billion in direct and indirect costs for 1990, the last year for which total calculations are available (NIMH, 1999).

BACKGROUND

Mental illness, mental retardation, and developmental disabilities, although often blurred in public image, are distinct.

Mental Illness

Before World War II, there were few outpatient mental health facilities. People in the United States with serious mental illness frequently spent variable periods in institutional settings where behavioral controls were accomplished largely through structural and physical restraints. Once institutionalized, many never returned to community living.

Dismal conditions in mental institutions became a focus of growing concern, which led in 1946 to the creation of the National Institute of Mental Health (NIMH). The NIMH was charged with consolidating and better coordinating the oversight of federally funded research and program development addressing the needs of the mentally ill. Around the same time, the Veterans Administration (VA) hospitals began expanding their mental health services in recognition of the psychological problems being evidenced by many soldiers who had returned from World War II. Even with these reforms, most care continued to be delivered in inpatient hospitals, using the medical model.

During the 1950s changes began. With major advances in psychopharmacology providing chemical relief to long-intractable symptoms, the illnesses of many persons could suddenly be managed effectively on an outpatient basis. New outpatient treatment approaches developed slowly, though. In 1955, the National Mental Health Study Act was passed, authorizing a three-year study of the mental health system in the United States. Six years later, the resulting report focused heavily on the need to expand community-based services (Pasamanick, 1962).

This led to the passage of the Mental Retardation Facilities and Community Mental Health Centers Construction Act of 1964 (Pub. L. No. 88-164), which allotted construction dollars for community mental health centers (CMHCs) to be located in catchment areas of 74,000 to 200,000 people. The CMHCs were required to provide, regardless of the client's ability to pay, inpatient services, outpatient services, emergency care, day treatment, and education and consultation services. However, funds for staffing and operations of the newly built CMHCs continued to be scarce until 1967, when an amendment to the legislation provided what was intended to be "seed money," on a matching basis and in declining increments, for a period of eight years. The intent was for communities to gradually assume financial responsibilities for providing comprehensive services to those not requiring hospitalization

and those who had previously had no access to services.

However, the capability of many communities to generate matching funds and subsequently assume responsibility for the CMHCs was limited. This was most true in low-income communities, the very locales that demonstrated the greatest need. A later amendment to the 1967 law added an extra year of "distress" operational support for the struggling CMHCs but it also called for increasing the required number of services to 12. It was hoped that states would be able to realize enough savings from the downsizing of their costly mental hospitals to allow funds to be shifted in amounts sufficient to subsidize more appropriate community care.

Deinstitutionalization, then, was enabled by new treatments, a desire to reduce treatment costs, and a societal emphasis on civil liberties that called for placement of those with mental illnesses into the least restrictive settings in which they could function. Unfortunately, deinstitutionalization has largely been carried out with inadequate attention to issues of discharge planning and transfer to less restrictive environments, and community resources were never able to accommodate these demands fully (Duurkoop & van Dyck, 2003; Toward & Ostwald, 2002). Compared to hospital care, community care was necessarily more diffuse, with fewer specialists and services for severe mental illness in any one locale. The efficiencies of institutional consolidation for the most difficult and medically fragile clients were lost. Furthermore, people who had been coping through the use of informal supports that kept them out of institutions now began tapping into the new community resources.

Although continued deinstitutionalization does serve the cause of placing patients in the least restrictive environments, it is much less successful at ensuring freedom from risks of harm, particularly because of the lack of standards for community service delivery (Marty & Chapin, 2000). Not only did insufficient dollars follow former hospitalized clients into the community to underwrite the growing service needs, the necessary commitment to meaningful service integration was rarely attainable.

Treatment innovation was often resisted by providers and clients, as well as the ill-informed public. Thus, even high-functioning persons receiving outpatient care for mental conditions tended to remain segregated from community life.

By the mid-1970s, many CMHCs had already closed or were in serious financial trouble. A President's Commission on Mental Health was established in 1977 to investigate avenues for shoring up the floundering system. It greatly influenced the subsequent Mental Health Systems Act (MHSA). Passed by Congress in 1980, the MHSA would have authorized additional spending on new CMHCs and related initiatives. However, under the more conservative administrations that followed, the Act was never implemented. Provisions in the Omnibus Budget Reconciliation Act of 1981 (OBRA 81) withdrew support for a national system of CMHCs, thus returning the burden of community care to states and localities that had historically shouldered the major responsibility for care of the mentally ill.

At the federal level, even with considerable opposition, the Community Support Program (CSP), a NIMH demonstration program for persons with severe mental impairments, produced evidence of the benefits of community-based care. This led to the passage of the State Comprehensive Mental Health Services Plan Act of 1986. This Act encouraged states to work with their Medicaid agencies to make specific plans to serve the needs of individuals with serious mental illness.

In subsequent legislation, states have been invited to shift client venues in order to capture larger portions of matching federal funds or to seek fiscal relief through use of less costly services. For example, provisions of the Nursing Home Reform Act in 1987 offered incentives for states to provide long-term mental health care in nursing homes. The Mental Health Parity Act of 1996 required implementation by 1998 of a limited mental health parity in insurance coverage for mental disorders. Also, provisions of the Balanced Budget Act of 1997 provided some block grant monies to states for mental health benefits for children, as well as giving states

more flexibility in their payment methodology for nursing facilities. Finally, the 1999 Supreme Court decision in *Olmstead v. L.C.* held that unnecessarily keeping individuals with disabilities in institutions violates the Americans with Disabilities Act. Subsequently, President Bush, in Executive Order 133217, urged the mobilization of federal resources in support of the *Olmstead* decision. Nonetheless, many persons with mental illnesses continue to reside in institutions inappropriately (President's New Freedom Commission, 2003).

Overall, however, while the federal legislation has encouraged reforms, the government has been unwilling to establish incentives that might shift the burden of public funding for care of the most seriously ill and costly clients away from the state and local levels. States have attempted to cope with the increased cost pressures by privatizing various services or adopting managed-care strategies that appear to be further reducing resource availability. As a consequence, treatment for serious mental illness is deficient in the United States in several respects: woeful underfunding, lack of any treatment by up to half of those who suffer, and insufficient or incorrect treatment by large proportions of those who do receive treatment (Wang et al., 2002).

Mental Retardation and Developmental Disabilities

Although the two systems of care are often considered separately in clinical practice, most of the policy developments affecting services for the mentally ill include provisions regarding care for persons with mental retardation and developmental disabilities (MR/DD). Because various constituents among the two groups often must compete for dollars from the same politically controlled funds, benefits sometimes accrue to one group at the expense of the other. At times, policy patterns in the two spheres are so similar, if perhaps lagged in sequence, as to suggest the purposeful borrowing of successful strategy from one to the other. However, given important differences in the two populations, some policy affecting MR/DD services stands alone or is contained within broader measures on education, housing, or employment.

It is impossible to catalog the entirety of the policy fragments, but once again, there are clear indications of the cost-driven interplay between policy and service developments. When Medicaid was enacted in 1965, coverage excluded residents of public institutions and institutions for mental disease (IMD), except those in medical facilities. This prohibited the expenditure of federal dollars for institutionalized persons with MR/DD unless they resided in skilled nursing facilities (SNFs). Consequently, eligible MR/DD clients were shifted to private nursing homes and states set about converting public institutions into medical facilities, whether or not residents of these facilities actually needed skilled nursing care.

Two years later, Congress reacted by authorizing the Intermediate Care Facility (ICF) program to provide federal monies for less intensive care of persons with MR/DD. This move encouraged states to consider general nursing homes as a viable placement option to the more costly state institutions. Thus, at a time when persons with mental illnesses were being sent into community settings, those with MR/DD were increasingly diverted into ICFs, even when some of the latter might have done well in the community, given appropriate supports.

In 1971, Public Law No. 92-223 authorized Medicaid coverage of intermediate care facilities that would provide care specifically for the mentally retarded (ICF/MRs). The intent was to funnel federal dollars into less restrictive and more normalized residences for persons with MR/DD. However, when promulgation of the federal regulations was delayed, state policies at first failed to cover facilities with fewer than 16 beds. It was not until three years later that licensing of ICF/MRs as small as four beds was authorized. Thereafter, states gradually began to refocus their funds once again.

States use 1915 waiver programs, which waive provisions under the Social Security Act, to provide more flexible coverage for specific groups, such as stipulating a higher income eligibility level or a reduced benefit package for more costly populations.

In contrast to ICF/MR regulations, Home and Community-Based Care (HCBC) waivers allow considerable state discretion and use of a state's own program regulations in providing care. Nonetheless, all HCBC programs authorized under such waivers require the provision of appropriate services in the community for eligible persons who have been moved out of institutional settings. Services most frequently covered are habilitation (adaptive skills instruction) and respite care. Demand for these and other HCBC will likely increase as more clients are returned to community settings or diverted from institutionalization altogether. Federal participation in the coverage will remain essential, but the formulas for funding and administrative arrangements are likely to continue to evolve.

CLIENTS

Those using mental health services include both people with psychiatric and emotional illnesses and those with mental retardation and developmental disabilities.

Mental Illness

Indefinite boundaries make it difficult to specify the magnitude and scope of those who have mental illness. According to the 1999 Surgeon General's *Report on Mental Health in the United States* (U.S. Department of Health and Human Services, 1999), *mental illness* is used broadly to refer to all diagnosable mental disorders characterized by alterations in thinking, mood, or behavior (or some combination thereof) associated with distress or impaired functioning. The report distinguishes mental disorders from mental problems, which are distress-producing signs and symptoms whose duration and intensity do not meet standard diagnostic criteria. Bereavement is cited as an example of a mental problem that, in short duration, can cause great pain and sadness, but unless it proves unremitting over a long period of time, is not likely to reach the level of debilitation that would qualify as a mental

PREVALENCE OF MENTAL ILLNESS

Although no definitive count is available of those with mental illness, NIMH estimates that in any given year 28 percent of adults in the United States ages 18 to 54 (approximately 56 million people) will suffer:

- Some form of mental disorder   19%
- Substance abuse disorder   6%
- Both   3%

SOURCE: U.S. Department of Health and Human Services, 1999.

disorder. As is the case with other types of illness, the definitions of mental disorders can change as science improves or public beliefs and values shift.

Nonetheless, only about 15 percent of adults will actually use mental health services. Further complicating the picture, only slightly more than half of those users (8 percent) have specific mental or addictive disorders that meet established diagnostic criteria.

About 7 percent of adults have mental disorders that persist for at least a year, and 5 percent are considered to be afflicted with serious mental illness (SMI). *SMI* refers to mental disorders that interfere with social functioning. About half of those with SMI are further classed as having severe and persistent mental illness (SPMI), which includes schizophrenia, bipolar and other severe forms of depression, panic disorders, and obsessive-compulsive disorder (OCD). Individuals with SMI, SPMI, and co-occurring disorders are more likely to experience the chronicity that requires long-term care (U.S. Department of Health and Human Services, 1999).

Estimates for U.S. children and adolescents ages 9 to 17 indicate that approximately 21 percent will evidence diagnostically significant impairment in one year. Although this is approximately the same percentage of young people seeking treatment annually,

again the picture is more complex. Of the 21 percent receiving mental health services, only about 10 percent had diagnostically significant disorders. The remainder had less serious mental health problems. That means that about 11 percent of those with impairments meeting full diagnostic criteria failed to receive care for their conditions (U.S. Department of Health and Human Services, 1999).

Among adults, 5.4 million individuals annually are afflicted with the more severe and persistent forms of mental disease. According to the *Diagnostic and Statistical Manual of Mental Disorders (DSM-IV)* (1994), there are 16 major diagnostic classes, determined by positive and negative symptom configurations. Symptoms may include inappropriate anxiety, thought and perception disorders, cognitive disorders, and mood disturbances. Diagnostic criteria are set by professional convention that increasingly attempts to account for cultural differences. Over time, changes in definitions have resulted in major shifts in who is counted among the mentally ill. Rates of disease in the middle of the twentieth century were far higher than those at the end of the century, when more modern and restrictive definitions were used in prevalence and incidence studies. Table 20.1 shows the distribution of cases across the major categories of mental illness in adults between the ages of 18 and 54. Depression afflicts more adults than any other mental diagnosis, afflicting more than 19 million adults. Anxiety disorders are the second most frequently diagnosed mental disorder, afflicting more than 16 million adults. Among children, anxiety disorders are experienced by 13 percent, while 10 percent have disruptive disorders, 6 percent have mood disturbances, and 2 percent have substance use disorders.

The prevalence of mental illness among adults age 55 years and older is not as well documented as that among younger adults. Estimates indicate that in a given year, slightly less than 20 percent of this population experience a diagnosable mental condition. About 4 percent have SMI and slightly less than 1 percent have SPMI (Kessler et al., 1996). Additionally, approximately 8 to 15 percent suffer

Table 20.1   Prevalence of Mental Illness Among Adults in the United States

Category	Approximate Frequency (in millions)
Depression	>19
Anxiety disorders	>16
Social phobias	5.3
Post-traumatic stress disorder	5.2
Obsessive-compulsive disorder	3.3
Panic disorders	2.4
Manic-depressive illness	>2.3
Schizophrenia	>2.0
Suicide	0.03

SOURCE: National Institute of Mental Health, 1999.

from severe cognitive impairments, including Alzheimer's disease (Ritchie & Kildea, 1995).

Over the long term, very few persons will experience unremitting, acute mental illness across a lifetime. Even individuals with severe forms of disease may at times improve enough to fall outside the service census. With new treatment developments, some consumers and experts now speak of recovery in even the most previously persistent cases.

Certain populations are at increased risk of experiencing a mental illness, having difficulty accessing competent care, or both. Individuals with cultural or linguistic characteristics that differ from those of mainstream Americans in the United States often encounter societal barriers that predispose them to reactive disorders while decreasing their ability to find appropriate treatment. Others become more vulnerable as a result of living in highly congested, violent, or remote environments.

Poverty is a well-known co-variate of mental illness, but the relationship between the two is difficult to disentangle. Many studies suggest that the stress of living on the economic margins overwhelms the coping mechanisms of susceptible individuals. But it is also apparent that those who suffer from severe

and disabling mental disease are unlikely to find steady, well-paid employment. Among children whose parents live in poverty or who have suffered severe economic crises, the reported rates of depression, anxiety, and antisocial behaviors are increased. However, when socioeconomic status is held constant, the rates of these symptoms are relatively smallest among low-income Hispanics, African Americans, and Native Americans, suggesting a protective effect of cultural factors.

Homeless people, the vast majority of whom are among the poorest of the poor, have a particularly high risk of mental illness. About one-third of that population are thought by experts to be afflicted with severe mental problems.

Public perceptions often overestimate this risk of mental illness among the homeless, leading to inappropriate stigmatizing of all homeless individuals. Before the deinstitutionalization movement, many such persons would have resided in state mental hospitals. However, with the rise of the community-based movement, numerous individuals who have trouble self-managing their care arrangements have ended up outside any system of care. Freed from institutional routine and the constant watchfulness of staff, some former clients abandon their medications and slip into the anonymity of street life. Some find community in the street culture. Some fall victim to hard drugs and violence, the harsh consequences of which may, in turn, lead to their preying on others. Although living on the street is rarely conducive to longevity, homeless mentally ill age 65 and older are an especially challenging population because their complex needs overlap traditional service categories.

Mental Retardation and Developmental Disabilities

In 1999, the Administration on Developmental Disabilities (ADD), a federal agency that administers the Developmental Disabilities Act, estimated that nearly 4 million Americans have developmental disabilities (DD). *DD* refers to a "severe, chronic disability of an individual five years of age or older that (a) is attributable to a mental or physical impairment or their combination; (b) is manifested before the age of 22; (c) is likely to last indefinitely; (d) results in substantial limitations in three or more defined functional areas; and (e) reflects the individual's need for ongoing specialized services and supports throughout life." When applied to infants and children up to age five, the definition refers to individuals who have substantial developmental delay or specific congenital or acquired conditions that, without services, are apt to result in DD (Administration on Developmental Disabilities, 1999).

The term *mental retardation* is being replaced in many circumstances by the more general term *developmental disabilities*, although this change is resisted by some parties who fear it will weaken claims for the support of individuals with more severe and profound disabilities. Mental retardation is traditionally grouped into four diagnostic categories according to the determined source of impairment: (a) due to infection, intoxication, or trauma; (b) Down's syndrome; (c) functional or undifferentiated conditions; and (d) other diagnoses, such as gestational and metabolic disorders (Eyman, Borthwick, & Tarjan, 1984).

As with mental illness, incidence and prevalence of developmental disabilities vary by social groups. Variation may stem in part from factors external to the individual or his or her condition. As yet, there are no standard diagnostic criteria or definitive treatment protocols for developmental anomalies.

The schema used most frequently to quantify the degree of cognitive and adaptive impairment includes five levels of functional disability: borderline, mild, moderate, severe, and profound. Profound retardation is traditionally associated with IQ scores of 0 to 19; severe to moderate retardation falls in the IQ range of 20 to 49; mild retardation ranges between an IQ of 50 to 70 (Eyman, Borthwick, & Tarjan, 1984). In addition, many individuals with MR have related disabling conditions, including epilepsy, cerebral palsy, autism, spina bifida, blindness, or deafness. Compounding the problem of unduplicated counts, some residents in facilities in which persons with MR live have only the related

conditions, but the groups are often lumped together in reporting. Being labeled is usually a result of political or advocacy tactics employed by agents (family, provider, or payer) attempting to secure supportive resources.

One measure of this population is the approximately 146,000 Medicaid recipients reported in 1997 to be receiving covered services in ICF-MR facilities (HCFA, 1999). However, many additional individuals are likely to need such care. States often delay or refuse requests for facility placement in an attempt to steer clients to less costly community support services. According to a study by the ARC of the United States, in 1997 more than 218,000 persons with mental retardation were on waiting lists for community-based services (The Arc, 1997).

SERVICES

Mental Illness

Mental health services are delivered in diverse settings, by a variety of professional and support personnel, using a wide range of treatment and assistance methods. According to the National Center for Health Statistics (NCHS), nearly 32 million office visits for mental disorders are made to physicians annually (NCHS, 2000). There are no national databases containing complete records of these and no overarching coordination of the segments. Table 20.2 shows annual admissions to different types of mental health providers.

Practice variation, market dynamics, client preferences, and political considerations result in a disjointed set of arrangements that defy description as a true "system" of care. In general, these arrangements are classified in four sectors: specialty services, general medical services, human services, and voluntary support networks. All may be involved to some degree in both acute care and long-term care of chronic conditions. Services may be provided in institutional settings such as hospitals or nursing facilities, in a variety of community-based organizations, or in the home.

Table 20.2   Admissions to Mental Health Organizations According to Type of Service and Organization, United States, 1983, 1990, 1994, 1998 (in thousands)

	1983	1990	1994	1998
Inpatient and residential treatment				
All providers	**1,633**	**2,035**	**2,267**	**2,314**
State and county mental hospitals	339	276	238	206
Private psychiatric hospitals	165	406	485	481
Nonfederal general hospitals with separate psychiatric services	786	960	1,067	1,145
VA psychiatric services[1]	149	198	173	144
Residential treatment centers for children	17	42	47	49
All others[2]	177	153	257	288
Outpatient treatment				
All providers	**2,665**	**3,298**	**3,516**	**3,967**
State and county mental hospitals	84	48	42	42
Private psychiatric hospitals	78	163	214	226
Nonfederal general hospitals with separate psychiatric services	469	659	498	615
VA psychiatric services[1]	103	184	132	143
Residential treatment centers for children	33	100	167	153
All others[2]	1,360	2,145	2,464	2,788
Partial care treatment				
All providers	**177**	**227**	**236**	**216**
State and county mental hospitals	4	91	72	57
Private psychiatric hospitals	6	32	27	21
Nonfederal general hospitals with separate psychiatric services	46	38	36	37
VA psychiatric services[1]	10	18	18	11
Residential treatment centers for children	3	28	29	30
All others[2,3,4]	103	21	54	59

[1]Includes DVA neuropsychiatric hospitals, general hospital psychiatric services, psychiatric outpatient clinics.

[2]Includes multiservice mental health organizations with inpatient and residential treatment services not elsewhere classified.

[3]Beginning in 1986, outpatient psychiatric clinics providing partial care are counted as multiservice mental health organizations in all other categories.

[4]Includes freestanding psychiatric partial care organizations.

SOURCE: Adapted from USDHHS, Survey and Analysis Branch, Division of State and Community Systems Development, Center for Mental Health Services. Manderscheid, R. W., and M. A. Sonnenschein, *Mental Health, United States, 1996; Mental Health, United States, 2000,* Tables 3, 4, and 5.

Specialty mental health services are targeted toward specific types of disorder or at distinct client populations constituting the more clinically complex and severely afflicted cases. Professionals who assume the lead in providing these services usually hold specialized mental health credentials in psychiatry, psychology, psychiatric nursing, or psychiatric social work. They practice in settings such as hospitals, offices, or agencies designed and staffed to support the provision of specialized care. About 6 percent of the adult population and 8 percent of the child population receive specialty care services in one year.

Mental health services are also delivered in the general medical sector. Annually, about 5 percent of adults and 1 percent of children receive mental health care in this sector. Primary care physicians and medical specialists in such fields as internal medicine, endocrinology, neurology, and geriatrics often manage clients with mental disorders and problems. So, too, do physician assistants and nurse practitioners. The clients seen by these professionals and their ancillary personnel are typically less seriously ill, and the treatments are delivered in inpatient and outpatient settings designed to provide for a broad range of general medical and health care services. As is the case with the specialty sector, services provided in the general medical sector tend to reflect a medical model.

The human services sector includes a diversity of providers and settings. Mental health care delivered in this sector overlaps in various degrees with social welfare, criminal justice, religious, charitable, housing, and educational services. The providers of these services, who employ a diverse array of treatments and interventions, may or may not hold highly specialized credentials in mental health or related fields. The private and public settings in which they practice range from offices, clinics, or departments within government agencies, schools, hospitals, and penal institutions, to large and small charitable and religious organizations. For example, efforts to reach persons with mental illness among the homeless population can include mental health training for the staff of homeless shelters (Vamvakas

& Rowe, 2001). Annually, about 5 percent of adults use human services for mental health conditions. Children are more likely to receive mental health care in this sector than in any other. About 16 percent of children annually are given in-school services related to a mental health problem or disorder. About 3 percent of children receive mental health care from one of the other human services providers (U.S. Department of Health and Human Services, 1999).

The fourth sector, the voluntary support network, consists of self-help groups that cater to a wide range of client needs. The exact number of self-help groups is unknown, but evidence suggests the numbers of persons seeking their assistance are growing rapidly. Such groups are usually staffed by consumers who draw on their shared experience and vested interests to assist and educate one another, to mobilize public support, and to prompt desired responses from other service sectors. They are often sponsored by credentialed mental health professionals and frequently become part of formal referral networks. About 3 percent of adults participate in self-help groups in a year (U.S. Department of Health and Human Services, 1999).

Community-Based Outpatient Care

About two-thirds of the providers of mental health services are outpatient-based organizations. In general, these may be classed as one of three provider types: those exclusively offering outpatient services, those offering only partial care where the client spends some part of the day on campus, and multiservice organizations that offer both. Services geared toward acute illness and immediate postacute care offer short-term, episodic assistance. Others involve long-term interventions that may or may not include case management strategies. Case management, in turn, may range from cost controls that minimize service utilization to broad integrative programs that link clients with an array of rehabilitation services.

Which clients receive which community services depends on many factors, the most important being adequate funding to support the development and maintenance of a provider network. Purchaser demand and market incentives will influence the range and scope of available services. As funding streams ebb and flow and public policies continually redirect dollars in attempts to take advantage of more efficient or effective programs, the configuration of community resources will be repatterned. This was clearly seen in the changes that occurred in the last 30 years of the twentieth century.

In the late 1960s and the 1970s, promoting community mental health centers became a major federal initiative. State and local governments received federal assistance and incentives to develop the centers, but were expected to continue to provide the primary leadership and funding for mental health services. The federal role was reduced significantly when CMHC funding was rolled into one of a series of block grants created under the Omnibus Budget Reconciliation Act in 1981. Faced with increasing competition for the block grant funds, states used the budget pressures as an excuse to reduce their commitment to CMHCs. Throughout the 1980s, the number of CMHCs and other freestanding outpatient mental health organizations grew more slowly. The count of new clients in the CMHCs dropped from 2.2 million in 1979 to 2 million in 1988. During the same decade, the census of new cases treated in outpatient clinics attached to inpatient facilities doubled, from 476,000 to 955,000 (National Institute of Mental Health, 1992).

The 1990s saw increasingly varied service options, but as the decade neared its close, the spread of managed care and coverage restrictions created new barriers to access for many individuals. Most mentally ill persons must now navigate a community system whose vacillating fragments contain a confusing array of eligibility criteria and benefits. Even in metropolitan areas with adequate supplies of mental health providers, financial barriers and enrollment caps often impede service continuity for all but the most affluent.

The movement of Medicaid into managed care has had particularly severe effects on the mentally ill: "organizational changes affecting mental health providers have been so extensive that their ability to buffer patients has been constrained." This effect is particularly severe if the state's Medicaid managed-care policies do not exempt mental health services from general managed-care practices (Waitzkin et al., 2002, p. 599). Although providers were in fact able to buffer patients from many of the effects of the switch to managed care, rural users of mental health services were disproportionately affected, as were specialty providers, particularly mental health providers—major concerns being the authorization of lower-than-needed levels of care, low and delayed payment, and consequent provider reluctance to accept Medicaid patients. The problems altogether contributed to further erosion of the mental health system (Waitzkin et al., 2002).

For some populations, access to comprehensive, well-integrated services is difficult for other reasons. In smaller cities and rural communities, separate mental health services may be nonexistent. When this is the case, clients may take their mental ailments to their general physician, perhaps masking them as physical problems. Consequently, the number of mental conditions masquerading under somatic symptoms is unknown, as are any distortions in diagnosis and treatment that may result. This is not to suggest that clients with psychiatric problems can never be appropriately managed in the general medicine environment. In fact, there is an increasing reliance by all client populations on services from this sector. Still, there remains concern about the preparedness of general practice physicians to treat the more intractable cases. Increasingly, new programs are being developed to help primary care physicians better diagnose and manage the more common disorders they are likely to see.

This issue of provider appropriateness is particularly salient among older adults, who tend to feel more comfortable consulting their regular medical practitioner about mental or emotional symptoms. Conversely, when older persons attempt to seek help from CMHCs, they may not find services well adapted to the needs of their generation. Traditionally, CMHCs have focused on younger people who are comfortable with and skilled in the therapeutic use of talking therapies. In particular, older adults for whom mental or emotional problems first appear later in life, perhaps as a reaction to the various threats to identity that characterize passage into late life stages, may resist the expectations for intimate disclosure. They may even deny the possibility of psychiatric origins of their pain or resist the medicalization of their grief, thus aggravating their conditions and leading their providers to brand them as noncooperative and difficult. Because few CMHCs yet include experts in gerontological care, such clashes of beliefs are fairly common. The result can be assignment of the troubled older client to custodial care in a nursing facility without provision for the separable therapeutic mental health services.

For people of all ages, partial hospitalization can provide a cost-effective alternative to institutionalization for those needing long-term treatment but who are less impaired or have better social supports. *Partial hospitalization* refers to venues where a client routinely spends part of a day in hospital and part in another setting. Multiservice organizations house a majority of partial-hospitalization programs, especially those that cater to older adults.

Institutional Inpatient Care

Although the vast majority of mental health treatment is now delivered in outpatient settings, not all care can be accommodated in the community. Brief inpatient stays are often more effective in acute or crisis episodes. In appropriate cases, such admissions may involve intense, focused therapy under controlled conditions that facilitate the breaking of destructive patterns. Once that goal is achieved, the client may be transferred back to community care. Today most acute care is provided in special psychiatric units within general medical facilities or in dispersed general medical hospital beds that are designated for such clients. (See Table 20.3 for a breakdown of inpatient care by organization type.)

For clients with severe and persistent disorders, especially those whose conditions represent a danger to themselves or others, there continues to be a need for residential and institutional long-term care settings. More sustained inpatient treatments are provided in private psychiatric hospitals, residential pediatric treatment centers, and publicly funded state and county mental hospitals. About 1 percent of the U.S. population use inpatient services annually (U.S. Department of Health and Human Services, 1999), with one-third of these services delivered in the public sector. Clients cared for in public facilities are disproportionately in need of intensive, long-term treatments. Not surprisingly, such clients typically have fewer financial resources than do those utilizing private institutions, which rely on patient fees to cover costs of care.

One private care option chosen for by some clients is care in institutions for mental disease. *IMDs* are private hospitals or nursing facilities dedicated to the care of mentally ill individuals. States have the option of using Medicaid dollars to cover care in IMDs, but relatively few public dollars are spent for such services. In states that allow IMD coverage by Medicaid, utilization rates range from 0.03 to 230 users per 100,000 population (Swan, Harrington, Grant, Luehrs, & Preston, 1993).

In recent years, the proportion of aged residents of public mental hospitals has been shrinking. In state and local public hospitals, institutionalization rates for those age 65 and older are much lower than the rates for younger adults, although this varies widely by state. In seven states, the rates for older patients are less than one-half those of the general population (Harrington, Carillo, Thollaug, & Summers, 1999).

The nursing home industry has been particularly affected by the deinstitutionalization movement. Recent decades have seen dramatic increases in the numbers of mentally ill residing in nursing facilities. Data suggest that a high proportion of nursing home residents have mental disorders. One in five nursing home clients is classified with a primary psychiatric disorder while about three in five residents have some degree of dementia. As many as 80 percent have moderate or intense psychosocial problems (Fries, Mehr, Schneider, Foley, & Burke, 1993). Despite the high level of assessed

Table 20.3 Inpatient and Residential Mental Health Providers and Beds, by Type of Organization, United States, 1984, 1990, 1994, 1998

	1984	1990	1994	1998
Number of mental health providers				
All providers	**2,849**	**5,284**	**5,392**	**5,722**
State and county mental hospitals	277	273	256	229
Private psychiatric hospitals	220	462	430	348
Nonfederal general hospitals with separate psychiatric services	1,259	1,674	1,612	1,707
VA psychiatric services[1]	124	141	161	145
Residential treatment centers for children	322	501	459	461
All others[2]	647	2,233	2,474	2,832
Number of beds				
All providers	**262,673**	**272,253**	**290,604**	**261,903**
State and county mental hospitals	130,411	98,789	81,911	63,525
Private psychiatric hospitals	21,474	44,871	42,399	33,635
Nonfederal general hospitals with separate psychiatric services	46,045	53,479	52,984	54,266
VA psychiatric services[1]	23,546	21,712	21,146	13,301
Residential treatment centers for children	16,745	29,756	32,110	33,483
All others[2]	24,452	23,646	60,054	63,693
Beds per 100,000 civilian population				
All providers	**112.9**	**111.6**	**112.1**	**97.4**
State and county mental hospitals	56.1	40.5	31.6	23.6
Private psychiatric hospitals	9.2	18.4	16.4	12.5
Nonfederal general hospitals with separate psychiatric services	19.8	21.9	20.4	20.2
VA psychiatric services[1]	10.1	8.9	8.2	4.9
Residential treatment centers for children	7.2	12.2	12.4	12.4
All others[2]	10.5	9.7	23.2	23.7

[1]Includes DVA neuropsychiatric hospitals and general hospital psychiatric services.

[2]Includes multiservice mental health organizations with inpatient and residential treatment services not elsewhere classified.

SOURCE: Adapted from USDHHS, Survey and Analysis Branch, Division of State and Community Systems Development, Center for Mental Health Services. Manderscheid, R. W., and M. A. Sonnenschein, *Mental Health, United States, 1996; Mental Health, United States, 2000*, Tables 1 and 2.

need and the mandate to provide care for identified patients, the provision of appropriate medications and other mental health treatments remains lacking in nursing facilities. This is particularly problematic given the relationship between hospital readmissions and the lack of substance abuse by nursing facility residents (Anderson, Lyons, & West, 2001, p. 313).

Veterans Administration Medical Centers (VAMCs) have also become a major supplier of mental health care. Evidence suggests that more severely impaired clients fare better in VAMCs than in nursing homes (Timko, Nguyen, Williford, & Moos, 1993). Although the number of VAMC inpatient psychiatric beds dropped by half, and the number of residents fell by 60 percent between 1970 and 1988, turnover continued to fill the remaining beds. Thus, as the average length of hospital stay was shortened, the number of new cases increased during that time by 80 percent (National Institute of Mental Health, 1992). An exception was seen among aged clients with mental illness. For them, stays in VAMCs declined as they were increasingly admitted to care in general hospitals and nursing homes (Gatz & Smyer, 1992).

Finally, a type of short-term inpatient stay that provides respite for caregivers of difficult-to-manage clients living at home has become an important staple in the continuum of care for people with mental illness. These brief stays in residential settings offer full-time supervised care whose intensity is intermediate between that provided in a nursing facility and that typically available in the home. Such "relief service" is especially helpful to families caring for persons with severe disabilities, such as those in acute states of schizophrenia or having advanced dementia.

Mental Retardation and Developmental Disabilities

With assistance from modern facilitation strategies and technologies, people with MR/DD are frequently able to improve functionality and attain considerable independence in living. Some of the more highly functioning individuals go on to various levels of integration with society, taking their place in educational, social, and occupational settings with an ease that far surpasses clinical expectations of earlier eras. Such people are likely to seek most health and social services from providers undifferentiated from those who serve the needs of the general population.

Nonetheless, many individuals with more severe forms of MR/DD must depend on special services to meet their health and daily living needs. Until the

mid-1970s, the care of such persons was typically considered too difficult to manage at home, and many were placed in institutional settings where they remained throughout their lives.

By the mid-1980s, states were taking aggressive measures to reduce their inpatient census or close outright their large public institutions. As they had with hospitals for the mentally ill, states argued that institutional care of people with MR/DD was too costly, inefficient, and inhumane. Advocates with a more libertarian ideology celebrated the downsizing as a civil rights issue. However, many families warned that unless dollars followed the clients into the scattered communities where they were relocated, the vision of maximized independence and community integration would prove an unsupportable illusion.

Community-Based Outpatient Care

Given a trend toward deinstitutionalization, the need for the reallocation of dollars to expand community service capacity is critical. Many services needed by formerly institutionalized residents are so specialized that few communities have the providers or technology in place. This is particularly true in small or remote communities. Furthermore, many families of the residents returning to the community no longer have the resources or vitality needed to care for their relatives at home.

Some community returnees end up in small public or private residences, such as group homes, with various levels of supervision and bundled services. Supported living is one such alternative arrangement in which many persons with MR/DD who are unable to live with their families are now being placed. This option combines a variety of community services with residential care that is as restriction-free as possible.

Though much attention has been given to people returned to the community from institutions, these make up a relatively small segment of the MR/DD population. About 95 percent of children with MR/DD grow up at home with natural families (Stroman, 1989). Among the nonresidential services now offered in the community for both groups are advanced assessment and intervention strategies, case management, adaptive and assistance technologies, housing supports (including independent and assisted living), and a growing stock of effective pharmacotherapies. Also available in many locales are day care and work activity programs, such as sheltered employment, day habilitation, and supported competitive employment. Nonetheless, even while supported living and community complement services respond to the needs of many affected individuals, there continues to be a dearth of services available for those with more complex problems, including persons who also suffer some form of mental illness.

A fairly recent addition to disability policy is the concept of family support. Historically, the only means of receiving publicly funded services for a child with severe MR/DD was by placing the child in a state institution. With a conceptual shift in the early 1980s to a more family-centered approach, many states initiated family support legislation. This legislation was often the result of initiatives developed by the state developmental disabilities councils who, in turn, were responding to the increasingly well-organized consumer/patient movement. Currently, all states plus the District of Columbia offer some type of family support program. Such programs vary widely in their offerings. Services that fall within "family support" provisions include, but are not limited to, cash subsidy payments, respite care, family counseling, architectural adaptation of the home, in-home counseling, sibling support programs, education and behavior management services, and the purchase of specialized equipment. Chapter 23 describes in detail the service system for children with chronic conditions, including mental and developmental problems.

The federal government's involvement in family support began in 1982 with the "Katie Beckett Waiver." This is a Medicaid option, rarely exercised by states, which allows for the waiver of means testing for families of a child age 18 and under who is otherwise eligible for placement in a Medicaid-certified long-term care institution or hospital, ICF/

MR, or nursing home. The waiver permits parents who assume the care of such children to access an array of family, home, and community supports.

Although without state participation, few families benefited from the Katie Beckett Waiver, increasingly other federal disability policy began to reflect principles of family-centered, coordinated, community-based care. Some of the subsequent legislation that emphasized these principles included:

- Temporary Respite Care and Crisis Nurseries Act of 1986
- Part H provisions for infants, toddlers, and their families added in 1986 to the (then) Education of the Handicapped Act
- Reauthorization in 1989 of the Maternal and Child Health Care block grant, which initiated a Children with Special Health Care Needs program
- Developmental Disabilities Assistance and Bill of Rights Act of 1990

These developments have had strong support from groups advocating community integration, natural supports, case management, and articulated service networks. Many clients, families, and supporters celebrate such changes and work to expand the array and reach of community-based care, while ensuring the quality of services already in place.

The matter is less clear-cut to others. Many parents and other advocates of persons with profound disabilities scoff at care philosophies that claim all persons with MR/DD would fare better in community-based living arrangements. For example, they are quick to dispute the worth of offering independent living choices to a person with a mental functioning level of six months. Even families who might wish for more normalized living situations for higher-functioning relatives often fear that transition to the community risks erosion in service availability and quality of care. With the worst of the state institutions closed and many others having undergone massive refurbishment, such advocates are increasingly vocal in opposition to abolishing the institutional option, claiming that this fails to account for special needs of persons with profound retardation or severe behavioral problems. They also point to the failures of mental health deinstitutionalization and warn of similar disastrous results in MR/DD.

Institutional Inpatient Care

Hill and Lakin (1986) noted that one of the difficulties in developing uniform national data sets to capture cost and use information on services for people with MR/DD was the confusing variety of providers. To illustrate the problem, they published a "partial" list of 121 different types of residential facilities named on state licensing forms. They then proposed a now widely used taxonomy that groups facilities into five types:

TAXONOMY OF GROUP FACILITIES

- Special foster
- Group residence
- Semi-independent
- Board and supervision
- Personal care

Group residence facilities were further subdivided into categories by size and ownership type: small (1–6, 7–15), large private (16–63, 64–229, 300+), and large public (16–63, 64–299, 300+). Following by less than a decade the experience of deinstitutionalization in hospitals for the mentally ill, downsizing of large state hospitals for MR/DD clients began. The resident census in MR/DD institutions of 16 or more beds decreased by more than one-half in the 20 years preceding 1987. That rate of decline accelerated dramatically in the following 4 years, a time during which 60 institutions were closed nationwide. Lakin and associates note actual or planned closures of 47 additional facilities between 1992 and 1995, a trend particularly affecting the northeastern United States (Lakin, Braddock, & Smith, 1994).

In some locations, the proportion of persons with MR/DD who moved to less restrictive settings during downsizing was similar to the proportion moved to more restrictive settings. This net balance suggests that new clients continued to come into the affected institutions as others were being transferred to community settings. Without further information, it is impossible to verify that such shifts resulted in a better fit between client needs and services provided, but it is assumed that these were not merely capricious moves.

Residents who remain in MR/DD institutions tend to be more medically fragile or demonstrate the most difficult behavioral problems. Legal concepts of free will and "least restrictive environment" seemingly hold little relevance for a person who at, say, age 40 has never been able to roll over, hold a spoon, or drink from a straw, much less use speech or be toilet trained. In addition to any medically prescribed treatment, such people clearly have basic survival needs, including safety, as well as appropriate touch and stimulation needs. Evidence suggests that just moving such individuals from one facility to another can increase their chance of death.

LICENSURE, CERTIFICATION, AND ACCREDITATION

Licensing, certification, and accreditation of mental health service providers is quite complex. Facilities that care for people with mental conditions are licensed according to state laws and definitions. Inpatient facilities are licensed as hospitals but may be freestanding psychiatric hospitals or psychiatric units of general hospitals. Similarly, psychiatric outpatient programs may be freestanding mental health clinics, outpatient programs of a psychiatric or general hospital, or one component of a more comprehensive community health center. Thus, licensing varies, and, similarly, so does accreditation. The Joint Commission for the Accreditation of Healthcare Organizations (JCAHO) does offer distinct accreditation for psychiatric providers.

Certification of psychiatric service providers is

equally complicated. According to Linkins et al. (2001), Medicaid policy "is best characterized as a patchwork of laws, rules, and interpretations rather than as a seamless monolithic policy authorized by law, elaborated by regulations, interpreted by guidance, and executed by States." Under Medicaid law, states must designate a single state agency to administer the state Medicaid program. These agencies bear the ultimate responsibility for responsiveness to Title XIX provisions. Medicaid agencies may delegate to the state mental health authority (SMHA) the provision of, or arrangement for, specialized services to nursing facility (NF) residents with mental illnesses. However, Medicaid agencies may not claim reimbursement for any such NF services for residents with mental illness unless the expenditures are eligible for federal financial participation (FFP).

Reimbursement eligibility depends on compliance with the Preadmission Screening and Resident Review (PASRR) regulations. These PASRR statutes are themselves fragmented and difficult to understand. Nonetheless, an examination of their origin and development over time provides crucial insight into the role of federal policy regarding the provision for care of persons with mental disorders by state Medicaid agencies, SMHAs, and nursing homes.

Following recommendations from studies by the Institute of Medicine (IOM) and the General Accounting Office (GAO), Congress passed new Medicaid laws as part of the Omnibus Budget Reconciliation Act of 1987 (OBRA 1987). There was at the time widespread concern that the deinstitutionalization movement was resulting in inappropriate placements of many individuals with SMI or MR. Both the IOM and the GAO studies found evidence that more than one-third of all U.S. nursing homes were then operating with conditions that failed to meet federal standards for staff training, sanitation, food quality, and enforcement of safety regulations (Linkins et al., 2001).

OBRA 1987, subsequent statutory changes in 1990 and 1996, and interpretations published in 1992 by the Centers for Medicare and Medicaid Services (CMS), specified requirements regarding patients' rights, patient assessments, and criteria for staffing. Included were provisions regulating the use of antipsychotic medications and physical restraints. States were also instructed to implement new sanctions for noncompliance. The federal government was granted enforcement authority in the form of denial of reimbursements, leverage of fines, and a process to assume temporary management of facilities until improvements or proper closure occurred.

The new laws were intended to counter the existing financial incentive for states to use NFs rather than state hospitals to provide care for the mentally ill. Because Congress at that time prohibited Medicaid payment for care in IMDs of persons age 22 to 64 (this is now optional for states), moving hospitalized patients in that age range to Medicaid-certified nursing homes allowed states to shift approximately 50 percent of their costs to the federal sector. However, many NFs were unprepared to offer appropriate care to those with mental conditions who were being transferred from state institutions. Compounding the problem, the rules then in effect prohibited CMHCs from being reimbursed under Medicaid for any services offered elsewhere. Thus, NFs were left without access to vital community resources that might have provided care of the newly transferring residents (Linkins et al., 2001).

The nursing home reforms required all states to have a PASRR program, which is key to current regulatory policy. PASRR provisions carry the force of law, as do rules and regulations issued by the CMS under congressional mandate. In contrast, the state medicaid manual offers guidance in interpretation of law but does not carry statutory authority.

In regard to mental conditions, PASRR prohibits nursing homes from admitting individuals with SMI without a predetermination by the SMHA that the applicant needs the level of services provided by the facility. Additionally, it must be determined whether each applicant requires specialized services for his or her mental illness.

Under PASRR rules, a Level I screening must be conducted on all nursing home applicants to identify individuals suspected of mental illness. Exempt from this requirement are patients transferred directly from a hospital after receiving care for an acute condition, if they will require additional treatment of the condition for which they were hospitalized, and if the attending physician precertifies that their expected stay in the NF will be fewer than 30 days. The Level I assessments may be conducted by the state Medicaid agency, the NF, or any other agent the state specifies. If the screening identifies an individual as someone who may have a mental illness, a Level II screening is triggered and must be conducted within an annual average of seven to nine working days (U.S. Department of Health and Human Services [DHHS], 2001).

For the purposes of compliance with PASRR, a *serious mental disorder* is one that may lead to chronic disability and is diagnosable under the DSM-IV as other than dementia (unless the primary diagnosis is major mental disorder). The exclusion of dementia means that the identification and provision of specialized services for patients with Alzheimer's disease, organic brain disorders, and other types of dementia is the responsibility of the NF, which must cover the costs within the NF reimbursement.

To be deemed a serious mental disorder, the condition must have caused recent serious functional limitations and the patient must have experienced one or both of: (1) psychiatric treatment more intensive than outpatient care, and (2) significant disruption of normal life requiring intervention or support services from law enforcement or housing agencies. SMHAs are also required to review the needs of current NF residents with SMI to see if their level of care and requirements for specialized services remain appropriate. Prior to the 1996 amendments, such reviews were required annually, but current law requires NFs to promptly report significant changes in a resident's mental condition to the SMHA—and that triggers a Level II screen.

Within the federal minimum diagnostic requirements, states have great flexibility in the screening instruments used and the definition of what constitutes specialized mental health services. Not surprisingly, comparison among states is problematic. Likewise, the lack of consistency, completeness, and compatibility in the federal data sets used to capture NF information (Minimum Data Set and Medicaid Statistical Information System) renders results of program evaluations, and subsequent policy decision based on them, tentative at best (U.S. DHHS, 2001).

ADMINISTRATIVE CHALLENGES

System-Level

A completely coordinated and integrated state long-term care system is rare. Instead, a variety of models are used to administer loosely articulated sets of services for mental health, mental retardation, and developmental disabilities. In most cases, multiple state and local agencies divide responsibility for oversight of the patchwork of state and federal programs. However, due to runaway costs in recent years, states have become increasingly willing to tackle the difficult political barriers to consolidation of fragmented services and programs. By establishing single administrative entities, states can achieve efficiencies in dealing with various constituents, awarding and monitoring contracts, and ensuring service quality.

Theoretically, system consolidation should work to the benefit of the client by enhancing communication flow between various service providers and reducing gaps resulting from disarticulation of program boundaries. For example, state mental hospitals now have large numbers of younger clients, many of whom engage in dangerous behavior and are unsuitable for discharge to other facilities or to the community. However, they also pose risks for older hospitalized clients. The ability to draw on consolidated resources can permit the separation of incompatible client groups while still offering economies through coordinated sharing of those services and providers needed by each group.

Consolidated administrations are more apt to see and address gaps existing beyond traditional service boundaries. This is especially important as lengths of stay in inpatient settings continue to be reduced and people are returned to the community with more intensive needs. With dispersed purview over inpatient and outpatient care, no one agency may claim responsibility for assuring articulated resources or quality of care beyond their own service cluster.

Organization-Level

Even without administrative consolidation at the state level, some former service gaps are being closed through increasing elaboration of mental health care within general hospital systems. As organizations expand horizontally and vertically to increase efficiency and effectiveness, they often integrate or contract with providers of step-down services and therapies.

For chronic mental illness, however, general hospital care often complicates continuity and comprehensiveness, necessitating efforts to manage services across stays and settings. Integration with nursing home care can be particularly challenging, as nursing homes provide various mental health services. Burns and associates (1993) found that less than 5 percent of aged nursing home residents receive any mental health care, and of those who were getting such care, only half was delivered by mental health specialists. Receipt of mental health care in nursing facilities is greater with psychiatric diagnosis, mood disturbance, aggressive behavior, referral from a psychiatric hospital, and residence in a facility with low Medicaid funding; it is lower with older age, but transfer between nursing homes and general hospitals often disrupts treatment patterns.

Preadmission Screening

OBRA 1987 requires that inappropriate nursing home admissions (e.g., individuals with no physical dependencies) be screened out. Typically, activities of daily living (ADLs) are used to gauge nursing home eligibility based on functional status. ADLs, especially when used with ratings of instrumental activities of daily living (IADLs), generally identify those with cognitive impairments. However, better

targeting can be achieved when specific cognitive impairment measures are incorporated, and these have now become standard screening criteria.

One general approach to defining and diagnosing cognitive function employs the concept and measure of executive cognitive function (ECF). Fogel and associates (1994) define these as "mental functions necessary for organization, planning, insight, judgment, self-control, and self-regulation." Deficits in ECF appear in dementia. They may also contribute to physical disability and predict the need for supervision with ADLs and IADLs.

Staffing

Staffing in settings where care is provided to people with mental illness and/or DD is one of the most critical organizational issues. Mental health organizations employ more than half a million full-time equivalent (FTE) staff. Seventy-two percent of those are professional personnel: psychiatrists (5.3 percent), psychologists (4.8 percent), social workers (12.1 percent), registered nurses (23 percent), and other therapists, counselors, and teachers (26.3 percent). The distribution of professionals and other mental health workers varied by setting. Psychiatric services in nonfederal general hospitals employ the largest percentage of professional patient care staff (87.7 percent), largely explained by the large numbers of nurses (62.6 percent) in such organizations. At the other end of the continuum, state and county mental hospitals employ proportionately the fewest professionals (40.5 percent). Veterans Affairs psychiatric services have the second largest percentage of professionals and the largest percentage of psychiatrists (28.9 percent) on staff (Manderscheid & Sonnenschein, 1996).

Another concern is staff turnover. Turnover is much higher in community settings, and somewhat higher in public community-based facilities than in large public institutions. Turnover is strongly linked to wage and benefit levels. However, feelings of competency regarding the assigned tasks, degree of autonomy over work conditions, inclusion in communication channels, and respect shown by both peers and supervisors are also key to increased job satisfaction and reduced attrition.

POLICY ISSUES

Deinstitutionalism was the dominant public policy issue during the latter third of the twentieth century. Most states have completed massive downsizing or closure of their large institutions. At the beginning of the twenty-first century, policy concerns are focused on access, affordability, and appropriateness of care. The three domains overlap both conceptually and operationally. For discussion purposes, they are treated separately. Nonetheless, the reader should remain aware of the complex interconnectedness among service supply, funding availability, funding source, public mood, and political climate.

Access

Access to care depends on many factors, including adequacy of service supplies, the cost to make them available, the ability for potential clients to pay whatever is charged for their provision, and the willingness of providers and clients and their agents to invest in a given therapeutic modality. Although service gaps are most typically the target of discussions on access, unused or underused services present additional challenges from the demand side. Furthermore, third-party reimbursement greatly influences both supply and demand.

Bed Supply

Service utilization and cost to the payer are linked to resource availability. Experience shows that the greater the supply of a health resource, such as physician or bed census, the higher the demand for those resources. Among the options states use to restrain service costs is to limit resource growth. They frequently employ statutes to restrict the addition of inpatient beds and often place limits on the use of existing bed supply. Many states offer incentives to institutions, including nursing homes, for converting units to assistive living or other levels of residen-

tial care. Some encourage the banking of unfilled beds so that they are excluded from occupancy rate triggers in reimbursement formulas, but become available should need increase. Though such tactics benefit payers and may prove helpful to providers, the effect often inhibits client access.

Financing

For many years, Medicaid has been the predominant source of public funds for long-term care expenditures on mental illness. Medicaid dollars finance nearly three-fourths of the operating costs of state MR/DD systems. State Medicaid programs are mandated to pay for nursing home care and home health care for eligible persons. Optionally, they may also provide eligible beneficiaries with services under the Personal Care program and the HCBC program. The shift in public funds from inpatient to community settings has been striking. According to Burwell (1998), Medicaid spending between 1987 and 1997 for long-term care in nursing homes and ICF-MR facilities dropped from 90 percent to 76 percent of total Medicaid expenditures on long-term care. During the same period, spending on Medicaid HCBC services skyrocketed from $451 million in 1987 to $8.1 billion in 1997 (Burwell, 1998).

States use 1915(c) waiver programs, which grant exceptions to provisions of the Social Security Act, to provide more flexible coverage for specific groups. This can result in restrictions on especially vulnerable populations by stipulating a higher income eligibility level or a reduced benefit package for more costly illnesses or conditions. Of the 173 waivers in effect at the start of 1992, 64 were for MR/DD. In contrast to ICF/MR regulations, HCBC waivers grant states considerable discretion to apply their own service statues. Nonetheless, all HCBC waivered programs require the provision of appropriate services in the community for eligible people moved out of institutional settings. Services most frequently covered are habilitation (adaptive skills instruction) and respite care. Demand for these and other community-based services increase as more clients are returned to community settings or diverted from institutionalization altogether. Federal participation in the coverage remains essential, but the formulas for funding and administrative arrangements continue to evolve.

Rate Setting

The Balanced Budget Act of 1997 instituted a prospective payment formula for paying for care in SNFs. This replacement for Medicare's previous cost-based reimbursement system raised concerns about the adequacy of the new payment levels. The GAO found that although the new method produced adequate total Medicare payments for all SNFs, it was less capable of adapting nontherapy ancillary payments in response to differences in need across client groups (GAO, 1999).

Future Funding

Although such changes as the implementation of the Balanced Budget Act of 1997 were expected to influence Medicare and Medicaid funding, including that for mental health, they are likely to be overshadowed by the fiscal problems facing the states. In 2003 and 2004, many states made major cuts in Medicaid, including benefits cuts in some states that eliminate select mental health benefits (Smith, Ramesh, Gifford, Ellis, & Wachino, 2003). Reimbursement cuts to nursing facilities in a large number of states (Smith et al., 2003) may result in facility decisions to cut care, including mental health care provision. Although a GAO (2003) report downplays this, it does so by a "glass half full" interpretation of the same data shown in the Kaiser Family Foundation report (Smith et al., 2003). Thus, the uncertain outlook for major entitlement programs generally may have major impacts on mental health funding.

Carve-Outs

In the early 1990s, many states began to separate their Medicaid financing and administration of men-

tal health services from those of physical health services. To guard against the underprovision of services, the CMS requires states electing to use such mental health carve-outs to set service contract standards; allow beneficiaries choice of providers; and reduce requirements for prior authorization of outpatient services. States generally add their own monitoring measures to avoid inappropriate service limitations, through use of site visits, ombudsmen, and financial incentives for meeting performance goals.

Uninsured

In addition to those covered by private insurance and Medicaid, approximately 0.5 percent of the population receive disability benefits from the Social Security Administration for mental-health related reasons (Braddock, Hemp, Parish, & Westrich, 1998). Still, many people with mental illness or developmental disabilities lack health insurance. Those with incomes exceeding the eligibility threshold for public coverage often find out-of-pocket costs for needed services to be prohibitive. The number of uninsured persons in the United States continues to grow by about 1 million per year. More than 15 percent of the population is uninsured and thus at risk of lacking access to appropriate health and mental health services. Because of the high cost and moral hazard involved, few public decisionmakers have called for a universal fix to this problem. Nonetheless, in 1997, Congress took an important remedial step with the implementation under the Balanced Budget Act of the State Children's Health Insurance Program (SCHIP). The SCHIP program gives block grants totaling $24 billion to states for the provision of health insurance benefits to otherwise uninsured children. Some mental health benefits are included in the coverage.

Mental Health Parity

Most employers that offer health insurance coverage to their workers include at least some benefits for care of mental health problems. However, typically the mental health benefits have been far more limited than those covering other types of care. For years, mental health advocates have lobbied to close the gap between coverage of physical diseases and coverage of mental diseases.

In 1996, Congress passed the Mental Health Parity Act. Its impact was curtailed by provisions intended to limit costs to employers and insurance companies. Nonetheless, the Act mandated that employers of more than 50 people whose employee insurance coverage included mental health benefits must offer their employees mental health benefits that equal, on a dollar-to-dollar match, those provided for medical care. For example, if a health benefits plan capped lifetime medical benefits at $1 million, it was no longer permissible to put a lifetime limit on mental health coverage of anything less than $1 million. Though this was a significant breakthrough for mental health advocates, the Act did not require businesses to offer mental health benefits in the first place, nor did it prohibit them from dropping coverage altogether. Also, given the census of workers in companies employing 50 or less people, the small business exemption excluded some 80 million employees and their dependents from the mandated coverage. Furthermore, employers whose premium costs would increase more than 1 percent as a result of complying with the parity law were also exempted from the mandates (The Hay Group, 1998).

After passage of the national law, nearly all states considered some form of parity bills of their own. However, many have yet to be passed into law. As of April 1998, 18 states had enacted parity legislation. Both the enacted laws and the proposed bills that have so far failed passage vary with respect to the definition of mental illness and the scope of coverage mandates. Some states have opted to include all mental illnesses, whereas others choose to cover only serious, or biologically based, mental illnesses. Furthermore, many of those states that legislated broader coverage have inadequate provider pools; thus, would-be consumers remain without available services (Varmus, 1998).

Other access barriers failed entirely to be addressed in the parity laws. Among the most costly services to provide are those for substance abuse. The annual costs for the direct and indirect effects of substance abuse total hundreds of billions of dollars. With employers and insurers warning that inclusion of substance abuse coverage would lead to unacceptably high insurance premiums, Congress dropped it from the final version of the parity bill. Some states inserted various levels of substance abuse provisions into their own mandates, but in those states, companies that self-insure under the federal Employment Retirement Income Security Act of 1974 (ERISA) laws are still able to skirt parity altogether.

Affordability

Closely related to the access issue is affordability of care from the perspective of the payer. Estimates of the direct cost of mental illness totaled $69 billion in 1996, a figure accounting for 7.3 percent of all spending on health care in the United States. In addition, in 1996, $17.7 billion was expended to care for sufferers of Alzheimer's disease and $12.6 billion on treatment of substance abuse disorders (U.S. DHHS, 1999). Table 20.4 shows annual mental health expenditures by provider.

Singly, indirect costs of mental illness reflecting lost productivity were estimated by Rice, Kelman, and Miller (1992) to be $78.6 billion. About four-fifths of these indirect costs result from disability rather than death.

In 1993, for the first time, expenditures for community mental health programs exceeded spending on state and county mental hospitals. States use federal Medicaid and Older Americans Act funds as well as state general revenues to finance community-based services. Medicaid dollars account for almost half the funding for public mental health services. In 1994, total Medicaid reimbursement for mental health was $22.9 billion, while state and local governments spent $21.7 billion, Medicare $3.1 billion, and other federal government $2.8 billion. As seen in Table 20.4, 43 percent of mental heath expenditures in 1996 went to general service providers, while nearly 58 percent went to specialty providers (U.S.

Table 20.4 Estimate of Mental Health Expenditures and Average Annual Growth Rate by Provider, 1996

	$Millions	%	Growth Rate
Total General Service Providers	**28,195[1]**	**43.2**	**7.2**
Community hospitals[2]	10,774	16.2	8.9
Physicians	6,558	9.8	9.1
Home health	277	0.4	26.6
Nursing home	4,714	7.1	0.7
Retail prescription drugs	5,871	8.8	9.6
Total Specialty Providers	**38,509**	**57.7**	**7.3**
Psychiatric hospitals	11,083	16.6	4.4
Psychiatrists	3,682	5.5	7.4
Other professionals	9,475[3]	14.2[4]	8.5
Residential treatment centers for children	2,642	4.0	12.8
Multiservice mental health organizations[5]	11,627	17.4	8.8
Total Mental Health Expenditures	**66,704**	**100.0**	**7.3**

[1]Limited to treatment.

[2]Includes psychiatric units.

[3]Includes psychologists and social workers.

[4]Includes psychologists, social workers, and counselors.

[5]Includes a variety of providers such as community mental health centers, residential treatment centers, residential treatment facilities for the mentally ill, and partial care facilities.

SOURCE: Adapted from U.S. DHHS, 1998, 64, 66.

DHHS, 1999). Most home care is financed by sources other than Medicaid, much of its cost being paid out of pocket by the users and their families.

The field of mental health has tended to be less successful than general health care in capturing resources. Both private and public payers impose greater restrictions on mental health care (e.g., higher Medicare co-payment rates). Coverage is often limited to minimal short-term benefits, despite long-term need and the potential savings that might ensue from providing appropriate care of whatever length. Outpatient benefits may be more limited than inpatient benefits. For example, under some payment plans (but not Medicaid for persons under the age of 65), more diagnostic and therapy sessions may be covered for hospitalized clients than for similar services received in a CMHC outpatient clinic. When this is the case, the use of institutional care, with its associated higher overhead costs, is encouraged even if the same or better results might be gained in the outpatient arena. Nevertheless, some effective community-based care is covered. For example, Medicare pays for beneficiaries to receive psychiatric home health nursing (Kozlak & Thobaben, 1992). Medicare severely limits coverage of services in mental hospitals and covers only about 5 percent of partial hospitalization costs (Culhane & Culhane, 1993). The latter fact may explain why partial hospitalization services are so underused by the aged.

To date, the CMS has not allowed Medicaid to fund psychiatric care in nursing homes except that provided in IMDs. Under OBRA 1987, nursing homes are required to provide active mental health treatment for residents needing such care who also meet strict nursing home screening requirements, but much of this mental health treatment is not Medicaid-funded. Private insurers tend to avoid inclusion of long-term mental health care benefits. This is sensible from actuarial and financial perspectives, as service utilization is very sensitive to insurance coverage (Mechanic, 1987).

Nonacute care use has been determined to be a function of nursing home markets. Those who need some type of nonacute care may be admitted to psychiatric institutions, or, less appropriately, to nursing homes. Nursing home care may be employed when freely available; but with undersupply, such substitution is less likely. Substitution thus depends on nursing home supply relative to demand, especially Medicaid demand (Swan, 1987).

Insofar as individuals with mental disorders qualify for nursing home care, evidence suggests that such impairment is associated with higher resource use. This is a complex issue because other functional limitations and co-morbidities are most often involved. Requirement of initial and annual mental health screening itself entails considerable cost. Nursing home payment mechanisms can take into account such increased costs.

In the MR/DD field, Medicaid expenditures on nursing facilities and ICFs more than doubled between 1987 and 1997, from $19 billion to more than $40.8 billion. During the same period, Medicaid payments for home and community-based services for persons with MR/DD increased from $2 billion to $13.6 billion. In 1987, HCBC accounted for 10 percent of Medicaid long-term care expenditures; a decade later, that share had increased to about 24 percent. In 1997 alone, $56.1 billion representing 35 percent of the total Medicaid expenditures went to long-term care services. More than $7.6 billion of that was spent on care in ICF-MR and nearly another $35 billion on nursing homes. Understandably, states have been increasing their attempts to restrain these costs by expanding home and community-based services.

Managed Care

Managed care, including capitated systems, burgeoned in the 1990s. Its effectiveness is still in question, in part because rapid cost increases and health care industry instabilities limit proper evaluation. According to the National Advisory Mental Health Council (Varmus, 1998), at the end of the century, approximately 80 percent of all U.S. employees had some sort of managed-care coverage. Fee-for-service plans, which accounted for 62 percent of primary medical plans in 1992, dropped to only 20 percent of the market by 1997. During the same period, preferred provider organizations and health maintenance organizations increased market share from 13 percent to 34 percent and from 9 percent to 24 percent, respectively.

Most long-term care providers have little experience with risk contracting. It is questionable whether most are sufficiently capitalized to manage risk for large groups of clients. Outcomes for the mentally ill may be poorer in managed care. For example, depressed patients of prepaid plans were found by Rogers and associates (Rogers, Wells, Meredith, Sturm, & Burnam, 1993) to encounter greater role and functional limitations than those in fee-for-service plans. It is apparent that at the provider level, financial incentives and utilization review influence mental health treatment decisions. Providers who share financial risk are more likely to use collateral services that hold down their own costs, even if that results in higher costs for the client. Still, many argue that managed care, including capitated systems, is necessary to assure coverage of costly long-term mental health care.

Even managed-care firms with considerable experience in Medicare managed-acute care programs are cautious when it comes to entry in the long-term care market. Among the 41 firms interviewed by Weissert et al. (Weissert, Lesnick, Musliner, & Foley, 1997), most cited reluctance due to costs of assuming unlimited coverage responsibility, the lack of data needed for risk calculation, fear of adverse selection, and concerns about their ability to negotiate acceptable capitation rates with providers. A seemingly successful program is the Arizona Long Term Care System (ALTS). ALTS, the first statewide capitated long-term care Medicaid program in the country, was able to provide an expanded home care program while reducing nursing home use and lowering overall costs of long-term care. Program contractors receive a capitated rate for managing and paying for institutional and HCBC care, including acute and behavioral health care, for eligible older individuals with physical or developmental disabilities. The program's success appears to be due to the use of independent client assessment teams employed by a state agency, a cap imposed by the Health Care Financing Administration on the number of HCBC clients, an eligibility requirement that clients be in need of at least three months of nursing home care, and a blended capitated payment methodology that forced contractors to both hold down average HCBC costs and substitute HCBC for nursing home days (Weissert et al., 1997).

Appropriateness

Many factors affect service quality, including the appropriateness of care provided for any given client. *Appropriateness* generally refers to the fit between a diagnostically verifiable need and the remedy provided. Measure of such fit may account for client-provider agreement about the nature and seriousness of the condition, the prognosis for recovery given different treatment options, the availability and affordability of care alternatives, and the willingness of both client and provider to abide by the required regimen. The following discusses only two considerations that may affect appropriateness: cultural competency and small area variation.

Cultural Competency

Minority utilization of both institutional and community-based mental health programs has typically differed from that of white, middle-class clients.

Historically, people of color have been overrepresented in large public mental hospitals, CMHCs, and human services organizations, while they have been underrepresented in private residential facilities, specialty treatment settings, and community-based practices. Moreover, people with limited English skills are infrequent service recipients in any of the delivery sectors (U.S. DHHS, 1999; Mayberry et al., 1999). It is difficult to assess whether differences in mental health treatment by ethnicity are due to bias (Snowden, 2003), but at least some can be attributed to poverty status, which itself is related to ethnicity (Chow, Jaffee, & Snowden, 2003; U.S. DHHS, 2001).

These patterns of use have been associated with minority cultural, socioeconomic, or need factors. Sometimes they also appear to be related to discrimination in the delivery system. Given the underrepresentation of minorities among the decision-making ranks of mental health personnel, the potential is large for misinterpretation of culturally imbued diagnostic signs or treatment response. Some ethnic groups have no concept of mental illness. Others who recognize mental impairment but hold different beliefs regarding its meaning and treatment may refuse care from conventional mental health providers. In some cultural groups, standard practices, such as removal of a disturbed client from the family support structure for hospitalization may be strongly resisted by both client and family. Also, expectations of a regimen of talking therapy would bewilder someone from a culture that prizes self-reliance and inscrutability.

Cultural misunderstandings increase the chances that mentally ill minorities will be jailed rather than treated. In particular, homeless mentally ill minorities are often arrested and incarcerated for aberrant behaviors arising from their illness, whereas more fortunate sufferers would be taken to hospital for assessment and care (Wolff, 1998).

In recent years, awareness of the importance of providing culturally competent care has grown. Although research is still sparse, evidence is mounting that persons of color, those whose primary language is other than English, and those having other than western European heritage are far more likely to enter and succeed in treatment programs specifically designed to serve their needs.

Small Area Variation: Rural Residents

Provider practices vary from place to place. Much of this is due to who practices where and from which sources the practitioners receive their knowledge. However, market conditions further influence service offerings through their ability to attract and retain needed providers. Practitioners disproportionately prefer to work in resource-rich areas, creating an undersupply in many low-density locales. People living in rural and frontier areas encounter both geographic and cultural barriers to many amenities available to those in urban places, including health and mental health services.

Declining rural economies of the late twentieth century saw great social upheaval as many farm families left their failing homesteads to seek work elsewhere. Such wrenching transitions often increase mental health problems and service demand. But, the same erosion of the economic base in rural areas weakened the financial viability of service providers, and a growing number of small towns found themselves far removed from even a general practice physician. When care can be attained only at a great distance, many rural people elect to seek it only in crisis situations, relying instead on informal supports and indigenous healers. Those with severe and persistent illnesses requiring inpatient treatment or residential care are necessarily admitted to facilities far from familiar surroundings and supportive networks.

Service scarcity is not the only problem. Stigma against mental illness retains far more importance among rural residents than it does in other areas. Provider choice is limited or nonexistent and confidentiality is far harder to ensure in communities where everyone knows one another. Most mental health approaches are rooted in urban culture, with meanings and behavioral expectations that may be poorly suited to those found in rural lifestyles. Thus, when a rural person seeks care for a mental disorder

or problem, the chances of misunderstanding and inappropriate interventions are heightened.

Unlike their city counterparts, rural residents have shown little interest in the family support and advocacy movements that have become increasingly effective in shaping policy decisions. Nonetheless, rural mental health issues are now getting national attention, in part due to their reliance on public funding in an era when private services are expanding in urban markets. Strategies being proposed for improving the delivery of mental health care to rural residents include greater integration of mental health and primary care and the use of various telecommunication and computer technologies.

CONCLUSION

The current systems of care for people with mental illness and MR/DD lack integration and comprehensiveness. Although deinstitutionalization released many to more humane, less restrictive living arrangements, it also created enormous new pressures for the development of appropriate services in widely dispersed settings. Almost everywhere, these new market demands are outpacing service delivery due to the lack of adequate funding. Nonetheless, improvements in pharmaceutical products and assistive technologies continue to reshape service options. Not only are some conditions previously thought to be intractable now yielding to new therapies, but the availability of more effective medicines are, in some cases, resulting in greatly expanded demand for their use.

The definition of mental illness itself continues to evolve as a result of knowledge now rapidly being amassed in the field of mind-body connections. It is too early to know just how these changes will affect service delivery and financing, but it is likely that cost considerations will become even more central to decisions regarding resource allocation.

The field of developmental disabilities is similar. As with mental health, both the supply and adequacy of community-based services are of concern. Once again the central issue is cost. Fragmented benefit mandates have led to fragmented care systems. While some enjoy expanded access, others fall through breaches widened farther with the advent of cost-sensitive managed care.

Without predictable funding streams to ensure provider viability, the promise of a true continuum of care seems quite out of reach.

CLIENT EXAMPLE

Life had been kind to Lucy until she reached her late teen years. She did well in school, winning in her senior year a generous scholarship to attend the state university. At SU she met Ted, a bright, ambitious young man who was on his way to a successful career in international business. They dated a while and then moved in together into a small off-campus apartment.

Between classes and part-time jobs, the couple were constantly stressed. Both drank heavily on the weekends and sometimes used recreational drugs. Lucy began having bouts of depression during which she felt so tired and discouraged that she could hardly push herself out of bed. Unexpectedly, she became pregnant. Although her religion strongly opposed abortion, Lucy chose to terminate the pregnancy. For weeks afterward she cried uncontrollably and quit going to class altogether. She began seeing a therapist in the campus counseling center.

After a month, her mood lifted and her energy returned. She threw herself into her school work and was quickly able to regain her footing academically. She raced through her assignments, barely taking time to sleep. Never previously a shopper, she began buying new clothes, especially large numbers of sweaters, which she stacked neatly by color, often not bothering to remove the retail tags. When Ted mentioned her growing obsession with sweaters, Lucy became agitated and argumentative. Ted dismissed her emotional outbursts as end-of-semester pressure and assumed that things would stabilize when they married in the summer.

Throughout the next several years, Lucy's moods continued to make dramatic shifts. At times, she was so lethargic she seemed almost to vanish. Then she would swing into a frenzied excitement that made it impossible for her to sit quietly or to carry on a meaningful conversation. She sought help from a psychiatrist, who placed her on medications and referred her to a psychiatric social worker for ongoing counseling. Those measures seemed to help. She enrolled in graduate school and generally did well. Meanwhile, Ted was establishing his business. He stopped drinking and no longer had any interest in using recreational drug.

During Lucy's "up" periods, she began disappearing for days at a time. When she returned home, she seemed to have little recollection of where and how she had spent the missing hours. One night, long past midnight, Ted was called by the local police to come to the hospital. Lucy had slammed her car into a tree while driving approximately 85 miles an hour. Although badly hurt, she had survived the terrible crash, but the physicians were concerned about her raging delirium. Suspecting a brain injury, they consulted with a neurosurgeon. Extensive tests showed only minor brain trauma.

Within weeks, with her physical wounds healing nicely, Lucy was back in school preparing to take comprehensive exams. When informed that she had failed one section of the exams, she became enraged, throwing books through her office window and threatening to set fire to the homes of the reviewing professors. Then she lapsed into despondency, crying erratically and talking openly of killing herself. Ted, who was traveling in Europe, was contacted by university officials. He arranged for emergency admission and observation of Lucy in the local general hospital while he flew back home. By the time he arrived, Lucy was completely withdrawn and had been placed on 24-hour suicide watch.

Lucy's original psychiatrist took charge of the case. After a series of assessments, she was moved to a private inpatient facility. Although expensive, money was not a problem for this family. She was assigned a psychology assistant who stayed with her continually for the next 10 days. She participated in daily individual and group counseling sessions.

Once stabilized on new medications, Lucy was

released. She began to see a new therapist and soon returned to school. Within months she had successfully re-taken her qualifying exams. Feeling jubilant over her success, she decided she no longer needed her medication.

In a euphoric mood, she began a romantic relationship with a fellow classmate. That soon deteriorated, but she began drinking heavily and frequenting night spots with a group many years her junior. Her free spending and stories of having been involved in a satanic cult drew rapt attention from the party crowd. When he was called by police yet again in the middle of the night to retrieve her from the local jail, Ted had had enough. He filed for divorce, sending Lucy into a dark tailspin that landed her once again in the psychiatric ward of the local hospital.

From there, Lucy repeated the cycle through the private care facility, but this time, when she was released, Ted's lawyer informed her that Ted had changed his benefits package: she would now be enrolled in a managed-care program with steep co-pays and limited visits to mental health providers. Furthermore, given the assumed purchasing power of her advanced degrees, she was forewarned that she would need to take care of her own coverage once the divorce was final.

Fortunately for her, Lucy landed a teaching job in a nearby private college. She became known as a high-energy teacher whose dramatic renditions in the classroom soon led to teaching awards. For a while, the combination of medications, weekly therapy sessions, and meaningful work seemed to hold her demons in check. Lucy begin publishing and after some years achieved tenure. Then, gradually, she seemed to lose interest in her students. She began failing to show up for classes. After she missed several in a row, a colleague drove by her condo to check on her. She found Lucy darting among cars on the nearby freeway, ranting incoherently, her hair and clothes disheveled.

Lucy was again hospitalized. After the acute phase of the episode, she was transferred to a nursing facility offering mental health services. Fortunately, Lucy was able to take a leave of absence without los-

ing her health insurance, but it soon became clear that she would likely be permanently disabled on the basis of chronic mental illness.

Lucy applied for SDI and, after a wait of many months, this was granted. With the help of a case worker, she found an inexpensive apartment on the bus line, where she now lives largely as a recluse. There is no money for recreation, and even if there were, she lacks the initiative to get out socially among people she believes look down on her. Her psychiatrist enrolled her in a clinical trial for an experimental drug, and though her mind is no longer as sharp as it once had been, she has days when she is able to write. Nearly every week she attends a self-help group started by the local chapter of the National Alliance for the Mentally Ill (NAMI), where she socializes with others who have serious mental illness.

Although Lucy's current environment meets the intent of the 1999 *Olmstead* Supreme Court decision to "assure that persons with disabilities are served in the most integrated setting appropriate," in her case the rights granted by this decision have downsides that counter the benefits.

WHERE TO GO FOR FURTHER INFORMATION

Agency for Healthcare Research and Quality (AHRQ)
540 Gaither Road
Rockville, MD 20850
(301) 427-1364
http://www.ahrq.gov

Bazelon Center for Mental Health Law
1101 15th Street, NW, Suite 1212
Washington, DC 20005
(202) 467-5730
http://www.bazelon.org

Center for Mental Health Services (CMHS)
A Component of Substance Abuse & Mental Health Services Administration (SAMHSA)
(800) 789-2647
http://www.mentalhealth.org

Centers for Disease Control and Prevention (CDC)
1600 Clifton Road
Atlanta, GA 30333
(404) 639-3534 / (800) 311-3435
http://www.cdc.gov

Centers for Medicare and Medicaid Services (CMS)
7500 Security Boulevard
Baltimore, MD 21244-1850
(877) 267-2323 / (410) 786-3000
http://www.cms.gov

National Alliance for the Mentally Ill (NAMI)
Colonial Place Three
2107 Wilson Boulevard, #300
Arlington, VA 22201-3042
(703) 524-7600
http://www.nami.org

National Association of State Mental Health
Program Directors Research Institute, Inc.
(NASMHPD)
66 Canal Center Plaza, Suite 302
Alexandria, VA 22314
http://www.nasmhpd.org

National Center for Health Statistics (NCHS)
6525 Belcrest Road
Hyattsville, MD 20782-2003
(301) 458-4636
http://www.cdc.gov/nchs

National Institute of Mental Health (NIMH)
6001 Executive Blvd., Suite 8184, MSC 9663
Bethesda, MD 20892-9663
(301) 443-4513
http://www.nimh.nih.gov

National Mental Health Association (NMHA)
2001 N. Beauregard Street, 12th Floor
Alexandria, VA 22311
(703) 684-7722 / (800) 969-6642
http://www.nmha.org

National Mental Health Consumers' Self-Help
Clearinghouse
1211 Chestnut Street, Suite 1207

Philadelphia, PA 19107
(800) 553-4539
http://www.mhselfhelp.org

National Technical Assistance Center for State
Mental Health Planning (NTAC)
66 Canal Center Plaza, Suite 302
Alexandria, VA 22314
(703) 739-9333
http://www.nasmhpd.org/ntac

Substance Abuse and Mental Health Services
Administration (SAMHSA)
Room 12-105 Parklawn Building
5600 Fishers Lane
Rockville, MD 20857
(301) 443-8956
http://www.samhsa.gov

FACTS REVIEW

1. Approximately how many people suffer from mental illness? From mental retardation?
2. What effect did deinstitutionalization have on current mental health constituents?
3. Why is there a separation in public policy regarding mental health from that of developmental disabilities?
4. What are the most important policy issues in mental health?
5. How is the changing population demographic going to affect mental health policy in the years ahead?

Administration for Developmental Disabilities. (1999). *...... Children's health insurance program—Children with disabilities (ADD-IM-98-4, USDHHS, Administration for Children and Families). Washington, DC. *http://www.acf.dhhs.gov/programs/add/im-98-4.htm*
Anderson, R. L., Lyons, J. S., & West, C. (2001). The prediction of mental health service use in residential care. *Community Mental Health Journal, 37*(4), 313–322.

The ARC of the United States. (1997, November 10). *Community support services: State by state report.* Washington, DC: Author.

Braddock, D., Hemp, R., Parish, S., & Westrich, J. (1998). *The state of the states in developmental disabilities* (5th ed.). Washington, DC: American Association on Mental Retardation.

Burns, B. J., Wagner, R., Taube, J. E., Magaziner, J., Permutt, T., & Landerman, R. (1993). Mental health service use by the elderly in nursing homes. *American Journal of Public Health, 83*(3), 331–337.

Burwell, B. (1998). *Medicaid long-term care expenditures in FY 1997.* Cambridge, MA: The MEDSTAT Group.

Chow, J. C.-C., Jaffee, K., & Snowden, L. R.. (2003). Racial/ethnic disparities in the use of mental health services in poverty areas. *American Journal of Public Health, 93*(5), 792–797.

Culhane, D. P., & Culhane, J. F. (1993). The elderly's underutilization of partial hospitalization for mental disorders and the history of Medicare reimbursement policies. *Journal of Geriatric Psychiatry, 26*(1), 95–112.

Duurkoop, P., & van Dyck, R. (2003). From a "state mental hospital" to new homes in the city: Longitudinal research into the use of intramural facilities by long-stay care-dependent psychiatric clients in Amsterdam. *Community Mental Health Journal, 39*(1), 77–92.

Fogel, B. S., Brock, D., Goldschieder, F., & Royall, D. (1994). *Cognitive dysfunction and the need for long-term care: Implications for public policy* (American Association of Retired Persons, Public Policy Institute Publication No. 9309.) Washington, DC: AARP.

Fries, B. E., Mehr, D. R., Schneider, D., Foley, W. J., & Burke, R. (1993). Mental dysfunction and resource use in nursing homes. *Medical Care, 31*(10), 898–920.

Gatz, M., & Smyer, M. A. (1992). The mental health system and older adults. *American Psychologist, 47*(6), 741–751.

General Accounting Office. (1999). *Skilled nursing facilities: Medicare payments need to better account for nontherapy ancillary cost variation* (GAO/HEHS-99-185). Gaithersburg, MD: Author.

Harrington, C., Carrillo, H., Thollaug, S., & Summers, P. (1999). *Nursing home facilities, staffing, residents, and facility deficiencies, 1991–1997.* Department of Social & Behavioral Sciences, University of California–San Francisco.

Health Care Financing Administration. (1999). *Medicaid statistics: Program and financial statistics fiscal year 1997* (HCFA Pub. No. 10129). Baltimore, MD: Center for Medicaid and State Operations.

Hill, B. K., & Lakin, K. C. (1986). Classification of residential facilities for individuals with mental retardation. *Mental Retardation, 24*(2), 107–115.

Kessler, R. C., Nelson, C. B., McKinagle, K. A., Edlund, M. J., Frank, R. G., & Leaf, P. J. (1996). The epidemiology of co-occurring addictive and mental disorders: Implications for prevention and service utilization. *American Journal of Orthopsychiatry, 66,* 17–31.

Kozlak, J., & Thobaben, M. (1992). Treating the elderly mentally ill at home. *Perspectives in Psychiatric Care, 28*(2), 31–35.

Lakin, K., Braddock, D., & Smith, G. (1994). Trends and milestones. *Mental Retardation, 32*(1), 77.

Linkins, K., Robinson, G., Karp, J., Cooper, S., Liu, J., & Bush, S. (2001, July). *Screening for mental illness in nursing facility applicants: Understanding federal requirements* (SAMHSA Publication No. (SMA) 01-3543). Rockville, MD: Center for Mental Health Services, Substance Abuse and Mental Health Services Administration.

Manderscheid, R. W., & Sonnenschein, M. A. (2000). *Mental health, United States, 2000.* Rockville, MD: National Institute for Mental Health, U.S. Department of Health and Human Services.

Manderscheid, R. W., & Sonnenschein, M. A. (1996). *Mental health, United States, 1996.* Rockville, MD: National Institute for Mental Health, U.S. Department of Health and Human Services.

Marty, D. A., & Chapin, R. (2000). The legislative tenets of client's right to treatment in the least restrictive environment and freedom from harm: Implications for community providers, the need for trauma assessment and related clinical services in a state-funded mental health system. *Community Mental Health Journal, 36*(6), 545–556.

Mayberry, R. M., Mili, F., Vaid, I., Samadi, A., Ofili, E., McNeal, M., Griffith, P., & LaBrie, G. (1999). *Racial and ethnic differences in access to medical care.* Prepared by Morehouse Medical Treatment Effectiveness Center, Morehouse School of Medicine for The Henry J. Kaiser Family Foundation, Menlo Park, CA.

Mechanic, D. (1987). Evolution of mental health services and areas of change. In D. Mechanic (Ed.), *Improving mental health services: What the social sciences can tell us* (pp. 3–13). San Francisco: Jossey-Bass.

Murray, C. L., & Lopez, A. D. (Eds.). (1996). *The global burden of disease. A comprehensive assessment of mortality and disability for diseases, injuries, and risk factors in 1990 and projected to 2020.* Cambridge, MA: Harvard School of Public Health.

National Center for Health Statistics. (2000). FASTATS: Mental Health. Centers for Disease Control and Prevention, NCHS. Available at *http://www.cdc.gov/nchs/fastats/mental.htm*

National Institute of Mental Health. (1999). *The numbers count: Mental illness in America* (NIH Pub. No. NIH 99-4584). Washington, DC: U.S. Government Printing Office. Retrieved November 1, 2003 from *http://www.nimh.nih.gov/publicat/numbers.cfm*

Pasamanick, B. (1962, April). Action for mental health: Final report of the Joint Commission on Mental Illness and Health. *American Journal of Orthopsychiatry, 32,* 539–550.

The President's New Freedom Commission. (2003). *Achieving the promise: Transforming mental health care in America.* Final Report. Rockville, MD: USHHS National Institute of Mental Health, SAMSHA.

Rice, D. P., Kelman, S., & Miller, L. S. (1992). The economic burden of mental illness. *Hospital and Community Psychiatry, 43*(12), 1227–1232.

Ritchie, K., & Kildea, D. (1995). Is senile dementia "age-related" or "ageing-related"? Evidence from meta-analysis of dementia prevalence in the oldest old. *Lancet, 346,* 931–934.

Rogers, W. H., Wells, K. B., Meredith, L. S., Sturm, R., & Burnam, A. (1993). Outcomes for adult outpatients with depression under prepaid or fee-for-service financing. *Archives of General Psychiatry, 50*(July), 517–525.

Smith, V., Ramesh, R., Gifford, K., Ellis, E., & Wachino, V. (2003, September). *States respond to fiscal pressure: State Medicaid spending growth and cost containment in fiscal years 2003 and 2004: Results from a 50-state survey.* Washington, DC: Kaiser Commission on Medicaid and the

Underinsured, Henry J. Kaiser Family Foundation, September. Retrieved November 12, 2003 from *http://www.kff.org/*

Snowden, L. R. (2003). Bias in mental health assessment and intervention: Theory and evidence. *American Journal of Public Health, 93*(2), 239–243.

Stroman, D. F. (1989). *Mental retardation in social context.* Lanham, MD: University Press of America.

Swan, J. H. (1987). The substitution of nursing home for inpatient psychiatric care. *Community Mental Health Journal, 23*(1), 3–18.

Swan, J. H., Harrington, C., Grant, L. A., Luehrs, J., & Preston, S. (1993). Trends in Medicaid nursing home reimbursement: 1978–89. *Health Care Financing Review, 14*(4), 111–132.

Timko, C., Nguyen, A. Q., Williford, W. O., & Moos, R. H. (1993). Quality of care and outcomes of chronic mentally ill patients in hospitals and nursing homes. *Hospital and Community Psychiatry, 44*(3), 241–246.

Toward, J. I., & Ostwald, S. K. (2002). Exploring mental health service needs of the elderly: Results of a modified Delphi study. *Community Mental Health Journal, 38*(2), 141–149.

U.S. Department of Health and Human Services. (1999). *Mental health: A report of the Surgeon General.* Rockville, MD: USDHHS, Substance Abuse and Mental Health Services Administration, Center for Mental Health Services, National Institutes of Health, National Institute of Mental Health.

U.S. Department of Health and Human Services, Health Care Financing Administration. (2000). *A profile of Medicaid.* Baltimore, MD: Author.

U.S. Department of Health and Human Services, Office of Inspector General. (2001, January). *Younger nursing facility residents with mental illness: An unidentified population.* Washington, DC: Author.

United States Government Accounting Office. (2003). *Medicaid nursing home payments: states' payment rates largely unaffected by recent fiscal pressures.* Washington, DC: Author. Retrieved October 14, 2004 from *http://www.gao.gov/highlights/d04143high.pdf.*

Vamvakas, A. & Rowe, M. (2001). Mental health training in emergency homeless shelters. *Community Mental Health Journal 37*(3): 287–95.

Varmus, H. V. (1998). *Parity in financing mental health*

services: Managed care effects on cost, access, and quality (Interim Report to Congress by the National Advisory Mental Health Council, NIH 98-4322). Washington, DC: National Institutes of Health. Available at http://www.nimh.gov/research/prtyrpt/index.html

Waitzkin, H., Williams, R. L., Bock, J. A., McCloskey, J., Willging, C., & Wagner, W. (2002). Safety-net institutions buffer the impact of Medicaid managed care: A multi-method assessment in a rural state. *American Journal of Public Health* 92(4): 598–610.

Wang, P. S., Demler, O., & Kessler, R. C. (2002). Adequacy of treatment for the serious mental illness in the United States. *American Journal of Public Health* 92(1): 92–8.

Weissert, W. G, Lesnick, T., Musliner, M., & Foley, K. A. (1997). Cost savings from home and community-based services: Arizona's capitated Medicaid long-term care program. *Journal of Health Politics, Policy and Law, 22*(6), 1329–1357.

Wolff, N. (1998). Interactions between mental health and law enforcement systems: Problems and prospects for cooperation. *Journal of Health Politics, Policy and Law, 23*(1), 113–174.

CHAPTER 21

The Department of Veterans Affairs

Mark R. Levinstein

The Department of Veterans Affairs, with the nation's largest integrated health care system, offers the structure to provide comprehensive health care across the continuum of care and over time. Like all major government bureaucracies, the system's potential is not always realized. Efficiency and quality vary across sites.

BACKGROUND

In 1930, Congress consolidated a host of veterans' benefits that were provided through several agencies and organizations into the Veterans Administration (VA). In 1946, following World War II, Public Law No. 79-293 created the Department of Medicine and Surgery within the Veterans Administration. This department evolved into what is now called Veterans Health Administration (VHA). Within two weeks of its creation, the process for formal affiliations and working agreements between VA hospitals and medical schools had been established.

Today the VHA has affiliations with more than 1,000 educational institutions, including 105 medical schools. Approximately 100,000 students receive clinical training at VHA sites each year.

The VHA focuses on three main missions:

- Medical care
- Training and education
- Medical research

In 1982, Public Law No. 97-174 added a fourth responsibility, that of serving as the primary backup to the Department of Defense during war or national emergency for the care of injured military personnel.

In 1963, the VA formally entered into the provision of extended care when President Kennedy directed that 2,000 nursing home beds be created within the VA by modifying existing facilities. Next, in 1964, Public Law No. 88-450 provided for (1) the creation of 4,000 VA nursing home beds, (2) the VA to contract for the use of community nursing home beds at VA expense, (3) per diem payments to state veterans homes, and (4) matching grants to states for the construction of state veterans homes.

The availability of outpatient care was mandated by Congress in 1972. Since then, the VA has developed into a comprehensive health care delivery system that also provides education and training for all health care disciplines, as well as research. In recognition of the long-term health care needs of the rapidly aging veteran population, and for the purpose of identifying alternative modes of health care delivery, the Office of the Assistant Chief Medical Director for Extended Care was created in 1975. The Extended Care mission was expanded to include geriatrics by Public Law No. 96-330 in 1980.

In 1989, the Veterans Administration became the cabinet-level U.S. Department of Veterans Affairs. It has three main subdepartments:

- The Veterans Benefit Administration, which is responsible for socioeconomic assistance
- The Veterans Health Administration, which is responsible for health care
- The National Cemetery Service, which is responsible for burial services

In 1996, the Veterans Healthcare Eligibility Reform Act required veterans to enroll to obtain VA health care. However, once enrolled, veterans are eligible for a universal benefits package of services. This began the VA's entry into a managed-care approach. In 1997, in an effort to improve customer service, primary care was mandated for all clients. The VHA defines **primary care** as the provision of integrated, accessible health care services by clinicians who are accountable for addressing the large majority of personal health care needs, developing a sustained partnership with clients, and practicing in the context of family and community. This move to primary care was also designed to allow a decrease in inpatient beds by increasing the efficiency of outpatient care.

Public Law No. 106-117 of 1999, the Millennium Act, required that the VA continue to ensure 1998 levels of extended care, including nursing home, domiciliary, home-based primary, and adult day health care. It also expanded respite care revisions so that such care can be provided in the home or other community settings.

Within the VHA, *long-term care* is a system of primary care consisting of health care, personal care, and social services delivered over extended periods of time to individuals with multiple chronic medical, functional, cognitive, or social support system problems across the continuum of care by an array of institutional and noninstitutional VA and community-based programs and services.

NATIONAL PROFILE

The VHA is responsible for the largest health care organization in the United States, with 163 medical centers and 850 additional ambulatory care and community-based outpatient clinics. All VA medical centers provide inpatient long-term care either through VA or contract programs. More than 90 percent provide outpatient long-term care programs.

The veteran population is much older than the population in general. Of the 25.8 million veterans, nearly 9.6 were age 65 and older in 2001 (Meskin & Berkowitz, 2003). The veteran population is projected to decline from approximately 25.8 million to 20 million between 2000 and 2010, but over the same time period the number of those age 75 and older will increase from 4 to 4.5 million and the number of those age 85 and older will almost triple, from 510,000 to 1.3 million (Figure 21.1). This projected peak in older veterans will occur almost 20 years before that of the general population. Not all of these veterans seek care from the VA.

In 2002, 574,356 inpatients were discharged and 49,057,279 outpatient visits were provided. The budget for this clinical care, as well as training, education, and research, was more than $22 billion.

Programs under the auspices of the Office of Geriatrics and Extended Care include both institutional and community-based programs, as well as three other broad-based programs (Table 21.1).

Eligibility for VHA care was reformed in October 1996 to promote better client service. Veterans are classified into one of seven different priority groups

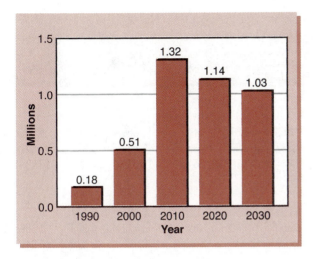

Figure 21.1 Veteran Population Age 85 and Older, 1990–2040
SOURCE: Meskin & Berkowitz, 2003.

based on their degree of service-connected disability, status as ex-prisoner of war, receipt of benefits from the VA, and requirement for co-payments. VHA allows enrollment for every priority group for which there are resources available on a yearly basis. As of October 1998, veterans were required to enroll annually to receive health care.

SERVICES

Geriatric Research Education and Clinical Centers

In the mid-1970s the VA, because of its demographic imperative, began to focus attention on increasing basic knowledge about aging, improving the quality of clinical care for older adults, and disseminating this information to health care providers. Key to this process are the 21 geriatric research education and clinical centers (GRECCs), each of which is a true center of excellence designed to advance and integrate research, education, and clinical care in geriatrics and gerontology into the VA health

Table 21.1 Veterans Administration Programs under the Auspices of the Office of Geriatrics and Extended Care

Institutional-Based
VA nursing home care units (NHCUs)
Contract community nursing homes
State nursing homes
VA domiciliary (residential care facilities)
State domiciliary
Respite care

Community-Based
Hospital-based home care
Community home health referrals
VA adult day health care
Contract adult day health care
Inpatient hospice referrals
Community hospice referrals
Hospice consultation teams
Community residential care
Pilot programs in health related services (homemaker/home health aide)

Other
Geriatric research and education clinical centers
Geriatric evaluation and management programs
Dementia/Alzheimer's special treatment programs

care system. Each has special research foci, including dementia, diabetes, falls, health care delivery, immunology, nutrition, osteoporosis, and sexual dysfunction. The number of GRECCs and their funding levels are mandated by Congress.

Geriatric Evaluation and Management Programs

A **geriatric evaluation and management (GEM)** program is a specialized inpatient or outpatient program in which an interdisciplinary health care team provides comprehensive, multidimensional assessments for targeted groups of older clients

Table 21.2 Long-Term Care, Average Daily Census 1998–2004

Census	Actual					Estimate	
	1998	1999	2000	2001	2002	2003	2004
Institutional Care:							
Nursing home care:							
VA nursing	13,391	12,653	11,812	11,672	11,969	9,900	8,500
Community nursing home	5,605	4,537	3,685	3,990	3,834	4,929	3,072
State home nursing	14,674	15,014	15,243	15,471	15,833	17,600	18,409
Residential Care (w/o Psych. Res. Rehab):							
VA domiciliaries	5,583	5,235	5,301	5,394	5,484	5,577	5,672
State home domiciliaries	3,626	3,680	3,684	4,042	3,772	4,323	4,389
Institutional Care Total	42,879	41,119	39,725	40,569	40,892	42,329	40,042
Noninstitutional Care (w/o Comm. Resid. Care):							
Home-based primary care	6,348	6,828	7,312	7,803	8,081	10,024	13,024
Contract home health care	1,916	2,167	2,569	3,273	3,845	3,959	4,070
VA adult day health care	442	462	453	446	427	442	458
Contract adult day health care	615	809	697	804	932	1,352	1,962
Homemaker/Home health aide services	2,385	3,141	3,080	3,824	4,180	4,247	4,315
Home respite	—	—	—	—	—	1,284	1,552
Home hospice	—	—	—	—	—	—	492
Noninstitutional Care Total	11,706	13,407	14,111	16,150	17,465	21,308	25,873
Total Census	54,585	54,526	53,836	56,719	58,357	63,637	65,915

who will most likely benefit from such resource-rich services. The assessment leads to an interdisciplinary plan of care that includes treatment, further assessment, rehabilitation, social service interventions, and preventative measures. Targeting criteria may vary from program to program. However, all exclude clients whose needs cannot be met by the GEM program, such as those with terminal illnesses; those whose needs for care in a skilled nursing facility will not be lessened by evaluation and management; and those who are unlikely to comply with the interdisciplinary evaluation and management recommendations.

Goals include:

- Improving the process and outcomes of care by improving diagnostic accuracy, optimizing drug use, assuring the most independent and least restrictive level of care by maximizing physical and psychosocial functional status, minimizing inappropriate use of resources (e.g., hospitalizations)
- Providing geriatric education for health care professionals and trainees
- Supporting geriatric research

In 2002 there were 57 inpatient GEM programs and more than 164,000 visits to GEM and geriatric primary care clinics.

Dementia/Alzheimer's Special Treatment Program

The Dementia/Alzheimer's Special Treatment program includes specialized inpatient and outpatient services provided by interdisciplinary teams. Three types of inpatient units have been established:

- Diagnostic units, with lengths of stay up to 30 days
- Behavioral units, which focus on problematic behaviors as well as physical problems, along with discharge planning, with lengths of stay of 30 to 90 days
- Long-term care units, with lengths of stay greater than 90 days, where the focus tends to be on comfort and supportive care

Outpatient units may focus on diagnosis and primary care. Caregiver education and support are key parts of all of these services.

VA Nursing Home Care Units

Nursing home care is provided to eligible veterans who do not require acute hospital care, but who need skilled care in an institutional setting. The 137 VA nursing home care units (NHCUs) are based at VA medical centers. They are designed and staffed to provide care for clients who can benefit from a comprehensive, interdisciplinary team-based system of health care delivery. Provided services include nursing, medical, psychosocial, rehabilitative, dietetic, recreational, dental, pharmacy, spiritual, radiologic, and laboratory. All VA NHCUs are accredited by the Joint Commission for Accreditation on Health Care Organizations.

Quality of life from the clients' perspective is a key consideration in the operation of NHCUs. Objectives include:

- Assisting each resident in attaining and maintaining the highest level of functional independence possible
- Providing for the greatest degree of autonomy, individuality, and dignity possible

- Designing administrative processes that enhance freedom of choice in the context of safe, health-promoting behaviors
- Involving clients and their significant others in the creation and revision of their interdisciplinary plans of care
- Promoting resident and family understanding of their rights as well as their responsibilities, in addition to the processes for their influencing the governance of the NHCU
- Facilitating the residents' return to a community setting if possible
- Developing and refining services based on continually evolving knowledge in long-term care, gerontology, and geriatrics

Admission and discharge criteria are based on needs for the level of skilled care that each NHCU can deliver and that each client can benefit from, as well as congressionally mandated eligibility criteria.

Community Nursing Homes

The community nursing home (CNH) program enables VA centers to place eligible veterans in 1 of approximately 2,500 nursing homes in the community at VA expense. Each facility may establish contracts with community nursing homes that meet predetermined criteria, including meeting Medicare and Medicaid standards. These contracts allow the placement of clients in CNHs at locally negotiated rates based on predetermined guidelines and formulas from the VA Office of Geriatrics and Extended Care. Veterans with service-connected disabilities that are related to their need for nursing home care may stay indefinitely. The contracts have provisions for returning the client to a VA facility if the client needs a higher level of care, or if the facility feels it cannot meet the client's care needs or tolerate the client's behavior while on contract.

Objectives of the community nursing home program include:

- Providing a mechanism for the delivery of nursing home care, including rehabilitative, mental health, and other special clinical services that can be provided in the contract facility, for veterans who do not need the level of care provided by the VA medical-center-based NHCUs

- Providing assistance with activities of daily living (ADLs) and medical needs for veterans who do not have the resources to meet their needs at home or in other community settings.

State Veterans Home Program: Nursing Home and Domiciliary

The 103 state veterans homes in 47 states are facilities approved by the VA for disabled veterans who, because of their disabilities, are unable to support themselves. State homes may include domiciliary (residential) or nursing home care. When provided in conjunction with such care, hospital services may also be included. Care may also be provided to veterans' family members.

Historically, the first state homes for disabled veterans were established at the close of the Civil War. These were created and operated at state expense with no federal assistance until 1888, when Congress authorized the payment of $100 per year for eligible veterans in state homes. Currently, funding from the VA for state homes is through two grant-in-aid programs:

- The VA may fund up to 65 percent of costs for the acquisition or construction of state nursing homes or domiciliaries or for remodeling of existing state homes. This program was first authorized in 1964.
- States may receive per diem funding from the VA for the care of eligible veterans in state homes. This program was first established in 1960. The rates may be adjusted as often as annually.

Since 1977, state home grant applications have exceeded the annual appropriations, and a backlog exists.

Objectives of the state home program include the provision of an economical alternative to provide safe, effective, quality care, as compared to more costly VA facilities. Current plans are for the VA to continue to fund at least one-fourth of state costs for providing nursing home care. Quality of care, as defined by VA standards, is assessed by annual inspections and audits performed by the VA health care facility of jurisdiction as mandated by Congress.

VA Domiciliary Care (Residential Care Facilities)

VA domiciliaries are residential care facilities that provide medical, mental, and rehabilitative care for veterans who do not need acute hospital or nursing home care, but who are not able to live independently because of medical or mental disorders, and who need a therapeutic structured environment. Congress first established this program in the early 1860s. In 2003, the VA had 43 domiciliary care homes. Health care is provided through the outpatient clinics of the medical center of which that domiciliary is a part. Objectives focus on attaining and maintaining the best possible level of function, autonomy, and health. The overall aim is to return as many veterans to the community as possible.

Within the VA domiciliary care program is the domiciliary care for homeless veterans (DCHV) program. The main objective of this program is to take seriously medically and psychiatrically ill veterans through a residential care program that will improve their health status as well as their employment and housing situations. Over time, more and more participants with substance abuse disorders have been admitted to this program.

Respite Care

A respite care program is designed to help the chronically ill and those with severe disabilities remain in their own homes by providing nursing home care or other VA medical center inpatient bed care on a short-term basis. This allows a predetermined period of relief for caregivers from the emotional and physical burdens of providing continuous care.

Admission is planned in advance according to the caregiver's needs. The participants are admitted to unoccupied beds for up to 30 days per year.

The primary objective of the respite care program is to support the caregiver. A respite program within the VA was first authorized by Congress in 1986. The program was initiated at 87 medical centers and has grown to include 136 sites.

The caregivers reported a high level of satisfaction with the program. The VA staff were found to be enthusiastic in the provision of care and in the opportunity to provide an empathetic response to the needs of hardworking caregivers.

Home-Based Primary Care

The 76 home-based primary care (HBPC) programs provide interdisciplinary primary care to homebound veterans for whom recurring travel to outpatient clinics is not reasonably possible. Disciplines involved include medicine, nursing, social work, rehabilitation therapy, dietetics, and others as needs and resources allow. The HBPC program serves clients with three types of conditions:

- Those with long-term multiple, chronic medical, psychosocial, or functional problems who require ongoing care to optimize and maintain health and to slow deterioration
- Those with terminal conditions who can benefit from ongoing interventions to help optimize the quality of their lives and assist in keeping them at home
- Those with relatively short-term needs for clinical services, and those for whom in-home training and home environment assessment and adaptation can be supported in the community.

The HBPC program was first established in 1970 as a demonstration project for the provision of outpatient follow-up services. Objectives include:

- Providing accessible, comprehensive, coordinated, continuous, accountable, and acceptable primary care services to homebound veterans

- Creating safe, therapeutic home environments
- Supporting caregivers in the care of clients
- Reducing the need for other health care services (especially unscheduled ones), such as emergency room and other outpatient program visits, nursing home placement, and acute hospitalizations, by providing a safe, acceptable alternative
- Facilitating timely discharge from inpatient settings
- Providing clinical and academic settings for education and training in the provision of interdisciplinary primary care in clients' homes

Community Home Health Referrals and Homemaker/ Home Health Aide Services

The community home health referral (CHHR) and homemaker/home health aide services (H/HHA) programs provide co-coordinated access to non-VA home health care and homemaker/home health aide providers for clients in need of such services. These services are paid for either by Medicare/Medicaid, for clients who are eligible for these resources, or by the fee-basis program that pays negotiated rates for specific services. The primary objective is to support veterans in their own homes while improving or maintaining their medical status and functional abilities, thus avoiding a higher degree of institutionalization.

VA Adult Day Health Care

For veterans who want to remain in their own homes, but whose caregivers cannot provide 24-hour-a-day, 7-day-a-week care, the 21 VA adult day health care (ADHC) programs offer an opportunity for veterans to remain in a safe, therapeutically oriented environment that offers health care, including rehabilitative services, and therapeutic activities in a congregate setting, during part of a day while the caregiver is gainfully employed or otherwise engaged. Health care professionals and supporting staff provide individualized interdisciplinary care.

ADHC was first established in the late 1970s

as an alternative to full-time institutionalization. The main focus is on maintaining or improving the health of frail older veterans with medically based disorders.

Contract Adult Day Health Care

The 81 contract adult day health care (CADHC) programs provide VA funding of adult day health services for veterans needing such care who cannot access VA ADHC programs. CADHC centers must meet published VA standards. When a CADHC agrees to accept a client from the VA, it does so at a previously established price. Eligibility criteria include the client having reliable transportation, dependence in two or more basic ADLs or in three or more IADLs, high use of medical services, clinical depression, living alone, recent discharge from a skilled nursing facility, or cognitive impairment. Provided services are similar to those available at VA ADHC centers and follow a more medical than a social day services model.

Hospice Care

VA hospice programs provide coordinated interdisciplinary supportive and palliative services across the continuum of care for veterans in the terminal stage of their incurable diseases. The focus is on providing these services in a compassionate manner to optimize the autonomy, dignity, and comfort of the patient. A medically directed team, consisting of at least a physician, nurse, social worker, and chaplain, along with volunteers, emphasizes the management of physical symptoms, including pain, psychosocial issues, and the spiritual comfort of the patient and the patient's family and friends. Bereavement care is also available following the patient's death. These services are available 24 hours a day.

All VA medical centers are required to have in place mechanisms to assure that hospice care is available to all eligible veterans who not only can benefit from this type of care, but select it. Hospice care requires the informed consent of the patient, the family, and the primary care physician. It is based on the mutual recognition that the illness is terminal and the mutual agreement that aggressive treatment should be discontinued.

Each VA medical center may choose the organizational models it uses to provide hospice care. These include:

- A designated hospice consultation team that consults with the patient's primary care team on terminal care issues, suggests policies to the medical center management team, conducts educational programs for the medical center and the community, and otherwise promotes hospice concepts of care
- Referral of Medicare- or Medicaid-eligible veterans to community-based hospice programs
- Purchase of community-based hospice care for eligible veterans who do not have Medicare or Medical benefits
- Provision of inpatient hospice care for eligible veterans who are without caregivers or homes
- Comprehensive hospice care with a dedicated inpatient unit, consultation team, home care possibly involving the HBPC program, and accessibility 24 hours a day

Community Residential Care Program

The Community Residential Care (CRC) program provides limited personal supervision, room and board at the veteran's expense, home visits by VA nurses and social workers, and outpatient care. The target population is veterans who are not able to live independently because of medical or psychosocial problems and who have no suitable significant others to help meet their needs. This program was introduced in the 1950s as an outplacement program for psychiatric patients. It may also be used for patients with mild basic ADL or IADL impairments. The residential care facilities must meet published VA standards. VA direct costs for this program are minimal, as they consist of administrative needs only.

Pilot Programs in Health-Related Services

In January 2002, the VA initiated a three-year pilot project, authorized by the Millennium Act, to contract for assisted living for up to six months. This requires another payment source, such as Medicaid, to assume responsibility for the cost when the contract ends.

The VA is also emphasizing new technologies, including telemedicine, with a focus on dementia. By using interactive technology to coordinate care and monitor veterans in the home environment, the VA hopes to advance its goal of significantly reducing hospitalizations, emergency room visits, and prescription drug requirements while providing veterans with a more rewarding quality of life and greater functional independence.

INTEGRATING MECHANISMS

Organization and Structure

The organizational and structural integration of all the aforementioned programs has been inconsistent and problematic. This has been, in part, due to legislative barriers, many of which have been eliminated.

In 1995 the VHA, as a part of a new vision for improved client service, restructured its headquarters and field operations. Headquarters was streamlined and refocused on supporting change in the field. The Office of Geriatrics and Extended Care became the Geriatrics and Extended Care Strategic Health Care Group. The field reorganization included the implementation of the Veterans Integrated Service Network (VISN) management structure. This divided the VHA medical centers and clinics into 22 geographically separate VISNs, each with its own management team and budget. This decentralized the day-to-day operations while enhancing the ability to

pool and align resources with local needs, thus facilitating the cost-effective provision of top-quality needed services for eligible veterans in the least restrictive environment while promoting the maximal level of autonomy and functional independence possible. Issues being addressed include:

- Designation of individual responsibilities
- Processes for assessing clients' needs and for assuring that the needs are being met
- Strategic planning
- Resource management
- Continuing education and research
- Development of long-term care partnerships with providers in the community

Case Management

In an effort to maintain the autonomy and dignity of veterans, the concepts of case management may be implemented by the VA through the use of care coordinators. Although there is no formal, system-wide case management program, a member of each interdisciplinary team is often given the role of coordinating the treatment plan for a given client. VA community health nurses follow veterans receiving their care from non-VA providers at VA expense to make sure that the contractors meet the clients' needs and to facilitate access to VA resources. A potential weakness in this system is at transition points from one team to another.

Information Systems

VA facilities all use the same software, which is under continuous development and refinement by national work groups consisting of representatives from different facilities. Thus, computerized clinical data are readily accessed throughout a given medical center. A patient has a single record for all services received. This means that different services can all access the same information and share information with each other. For example, when a patient enrolls in a VA hospice and is admitted to the hospital

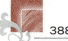

for an acute problem, both the hospital and the hospice have complete information about the care the patient received in both settings. Information may also be accessible from other VA health care facilities. This level of sophistication in integrating acute and long-term care patient records is extremely rare.

Financing

In 1997 the VHA began to use its new Veterans Equitable Resource Allocation (VERA) capitation-based system to distribute its congressionally appropriated medical care budget to the 22 VISNs. VERA has two levels of funding: Basic Care, which nationally averaged $3,121 per person a year in FY2002; and Special Care for clients with special needs, which averaged $41,667. Most extended-care clients are capitated at the Special Care rate. VERA was implemented in the context of an initiative to reduce per-client care costs by 30 percent.

Another source of funding is the mandated medical cost recovery program. There are three components:

- Billing and collection of payments from third-party health insurance carriers for nonservice-connected conditions
- Co-payments from certain veterans for treatment of nonservice-connected conditions
- Co-payments from certain veterans for medications related to nonservice-connected conditions.

Each VISN, and thus each medical center and freestanding clinic, is expected to collect a certain dollar amount. There are adverse financial consequences in subsequent budgets if this goal is not met. A key feature of the budgeting process is that each facility budget is based on data from two years past.

POLICY ISSUES

The VA, as a federal entity, is dependent on Congress, the president of the United States, and lobby-ists, including veterans and other providers of health care services and supplies.

As for health care reform, the VA has already made major efforts to become more responsive to the needs of its current clients by streamlining and focusing services to meet client needs in a cost-effective manner. This may well be an opportunity for the VA to expand its client population.

CONCLUSION

The U.S. Department of Veterans Affairs operates the largest health care system in the world. Although the system serves a wide range of clients, including many with acute illnesses, the VA has also been a leader in developing geriatric programs and a comprehensive scope of services for people with chronic conditions and disabilities. The VA has exemplary integrating mechanisms, with structure, financing, information systems, and case management that are all conducive to achieving continuity of care. The VA system continues to evolve to meet market and consumer demand. Further refinement of its integrated continuum of care can be expected as the VA rises to meet the needs of the burgeoning older and disabled veteran population.

CLIENT EXAMPLE

Mr. Dover is an 87-year-old retired veteran who lives with his wife of 59 years. His medical problems include diabetes mellitus, coronary artery disease, hypertension, and chronic obstructive pulmonary disease. He misses scheduled appointments at his nearby VA medical center, but uses its emergency room when he feels bad enough.

He suffers a stroke with resultant left-side paralysis. Shortly after completing his acute rehabilitation, he is hospitalized again with pneumonia. While in the hospital, he loses all the abilities he had regained through rehabilitative therapies.

He is transferred to the GEM team's inpatient unit, where he receives rehabilitative therapies and completes treatment for his pneumonia. His polypharmacy and noncompliance are also addressed, resulting in Mr. Dover taking only 4 different medications instead of the usual 12.

When discharged, he is followed by the HBPC, which closely monitors his condition, adjusts his medications, and assists his wife, as Mr. Dover could not remain in their home without her assistance.

His outpatient care is transferred back to the GEM team three months later. Mrs. Dover becomes exhausted caring for him. Mr. Dover is admitted to his VA's NHCU for two weeks' respite care so his wife can again take care of him in their home.

The Dovers pay $3 for each prescription and the VA covers the cost of the attendant.

WHERE TO GO FOR FURTHER INFORMATION

Contact your local VA medical center or the Department of Veterans Affairs, Veterans Health Administration, Office of the Assistant Chief Medical Director for Geriatrics and Extended Care.

Department of Veterans Affairs
810 Vermont Avenue, NW
Washington, DC 20420
(202) 273-5700 / (800) 827-1000
http://www.va.gov

VA Guide to Long-Term Care Programs and Services
http://www.va.gov/resdev/ps/pshsrd/ltcrguid/expage.htm

FACTS REVIEW

1. What is the Veterans Health Administration?
2. How many VA medical centers are there?
3. List five services available to veterans through the VA.
4. What does "GEM" stand for and what does it do?
5. What are the sources of funding for VA geriatric and extended care services?
6. Are all veterans entitled to all the services that the VA provides?
7. What is a "VISN"? How many are there?

REFERENCES

Meskin, S., & Berkowitz, A. (2003, January 24). Veterans population projections adjusted to Census 2000 and implications for CARES. Retrieved April 7, 2004 from *http://www.va.gov.*

CHAPTER 22

Rehabilitation

Debra J. Sheets and Louis Rubino*

Rehabilitation is recognized as an essential component of the continuum of long-term care.

DEFINITION

Rehabilitation (rehab) is an interdisciplinary approach to recovering function that is appropriate for individuals, regardless of age, who have sustained an injury, illness, surgery, or progressive disease. The purposes of rehabilitation are to maximize function, promote independence, and maintain quality of life, while recognizing that not everyone is able to achieve full functioning after a disability or injury.

Rehabilitation is a comprehensive service that can be provided in a variety of settings to a wide range of patients. The type of services offered include:

- Physical medicine
- Occupational therapy
- Physical therapy
- Speech therapy
- Cardiopulmonary conditioning
- Mental health services
- Complementary medicine
- Nutritional support

Treatment is provided only with an order from a physician or other licensed practitioner. Rehabilitation programs are individualized and are developed by a team of allied health care professionals who assess the patient; determine the type and intensity of treatment; set the level of intensity; and establish the goals for the individual's rehabilitation program. The benefits of rehabilitation for persons with disabilities and chronic conditions are well established in the research literature (DeJong, 1995; Liu, Gage, Harvell, Stevenson, & Brennan, 1999).

*The work for this chapter was supported, in part, by Grant 3 S06 GM048680-10S1 from the National Institute of General Medical Sciences, National Institutes for Health, Minority Biomedical Research Support (MBRS) Program, SCORE.

BACKGROUND

Prior to the injuries sustained by soldiers in World War I and the polio epidemics of the 1950s, rehabilitation was a relatively unknown area of health care. However, the field developed rapidly, reflecting advances in rehabilitation research and assistive technologies that provided new opportunities for intervention. The field of rehabilitation will likely continue to grow in future years in response to population aging, and increasing numbers of people with lifelong and significant disabilities.

Population aging has helped to drive a growing demand for rehabilitation services. In the United States, life expectancy has increased about one year every five years since 1965. Currently, life expectancy is more than 76 years (National Center for Health Statistics, 2000). Today, those age 65 and older account for 13 percent of the population. By 2030 this will increase to 20 percent (1 in 5 people) (National Center for Health Statistics, 2003).

Unfortunately, gains in longevity have come with an increase in the incidence and prevalence of chronic care conditions. Today, chronic conditions, such as heart disease, emphysema, stroke, cancer, and diabetes, are common and costly health problems. Most people live with chronic conditions for years, and chronic conditions are a leading cause of disability, particularly for older adults. Recent findings indicate that 20 chronic conditions account for almost 80 percent of all health care expenditures (Maguire, 2001) and account for 7 of 10 deaths among Americans (Centers for Disease Control & Prevention [CDC], 2003).

The demographics of the disability population are also changing, with growth occurring in both absolute numbers and the severity of impairment. Depending on how disability is measured, estimates of the population with disability range from 37 to 54 million people (McNeil, 1997). Like their nondisabled peers, persons with disabilities are experiencing increases in longevity and for the first time in history are achieving nearly normal life expectancies. Individuals with congenital or catastrophic injuries are surviving into mid- to later life. Many have significant disabilities (e.g., spinal cord injury, traumatic brain injury) that require intermittent but ongoing rehabilitation. New categories of disability are emerging as medical treatments transform what were once acute or even terminal illnesses (e.g., AIDS) into chronic disabling conditions that can benefit from rehabilitation.

CLIENTS

The profile of a typical rehabilitation patient and the most common rehabilitation diagnoses reflect the changing demographics of disability and the aging of the population. In the 1950s, rehabilitation programs were designed primarily for children and young adults. Today, 90 percent of rehabilitation patients are age 45 or older, the average age is 68 years, and women account for 58 percent of all rehabilitation patients (Fiedler, Granger, & Russell, 1998).

Fifty years ago, the most common rehabilitation diagnoses were post-polio or orthopedic conditions resulting from traumatic injuries. Today, stroke and hip fractures are responsible for the majority of days that older adults spend in rehabilitation, and account for the largest rehabilitation expenditures by Medicare (National Institute of Child Health and Human Development [NICHHD], 2001) (see accompanying box). In 1996, the average length of stay for rehabilitation provided in acute care hospitals ranged from 11.8 to 19.8 days.

In the past, the majority of rehabilitative services were provided in acute care settings, but today 90 percent of patients receive rehabilitation in postacute care (PAC) settings (e.g., skilled nursing facilities, outpatient rehabilitation). Specialized rehabilitation programs have been created to address the unique rehabilitation needs of certain age groups (e.g., geriatrics) or specific disabilities (e.g., stroke, cardiac). Reflecting the push to discharge earlier from acute settings to progressively lower levels of care, about one in three patients required more than one PAC setting (see Table 22.1).

MOST COMMON REHABILITATION DIAGNOSES*

Stroke

Congenital deformity

Spinal cord injury

Amputation

Brain injury

Major multiple trauma

Hip fracture

Neurological disorders

Burns

Polyarthritis (including rheumatoid)

* These diagnoses account for 75 percent of the population receiving rehabilitation through the Medicare program.

SOURCE: UB Foundation Activities, Inc., *IRG-PAI Training Manual*, UBFA Inc. (2002).

THE CORE REHABILITATION TEAM

The cardinal feature of rehabilitation is the interdisciplinary team approach. The team approach is necessary because clients typically have multiple and interacting problems that require input from several disciplines (Cole & Ramsdell, 1990). The "core team" typically includes the physician, nurse, social worker, physical therapist, and occupational therapist. Other disciplines, such as speech pathology, clinical psychology, pharmacology, and nutrition are called in for consultation as needed.

In a comprehensive rehabilitation program, the role of each team member is based on his or her expertise in the discipline (see Table 22.2). Occasionally a team meeting is held face-to-face to discuss urgent issues in providing care. However, in-person meetings have become rarer as they are replaced by other effective and more convenient ways of communicating. Team members typically update each other by routinely charting notes in centralized records, or leaving messages via e-mail or voice mail. These "virtual teams" discuss their assessment of the client and work together to develop an interdisciplinary plan of care that is placed with the client chart. Each individual team member gains an understanding of the contribution of each of the other disciplines to the client's overall plan of care by reading the chart and regularly updating other members. Each member of the team is assigned responsibility for the interventions appropriate to her or his skills and area of specialization.

Physicians

Rehabilitation teams are typically led by a physician with expertise in the specific type of injury or disabling condition that requires rehabilitation. The physician who provides rehabilitation is usually a physiatrist, orthopedic surgeon, or neurologist. **Physiatrists** are physicians who specialize in the field of physical medicine and rehabilitation. They focus on restoring function for clients who have experienced catastrophic events resulting in paraplegia, quadriplegia, or traumatic brain injury; and individuals who have suffered strokes, orthopedic injuries, or neurologic disorders such as multiple sclerosis or polio. Physiatrists also treat clients with acute and chronic pain and musculoskeletal problems, such as back and neck pain, tendonitis, pinched nerves, and fibromyalgia. **Orthopedic surgeons** may supervise the rehabilitation of clients with musculoskeletal problems that have been corrected by surgery, such as hip fractures, knee and other joint replacements, and broken backs. **Neurologists** may manage the rehabilitation of clients

Table 22.1   Hospital Discharge Destinations for Selected DRGs, 1996 and 2001

| | Percentage of Discharges to: | | | | | |
Year	No Post-Acute Care or Hospice	SNF Only	SNF + Home Health	Home Health Only	Other PAC Providers	Hospice
DRG 014 Stroke with infarction						
1996	33%	22%	7%	18%	19%	1%
2001	36	24	6	11	20	3
DRG 088 Chronic obstructive pulmonary disease						
1996	65	6	2	25	1	1
2001	74	8	2	12	2	1
DRG 127 Heart failure and shock						
1996	56	8	3	30	1	1
2001	68	12	3	14	2	2
DRG 209 Hip replacement						
1996	19	17	19	22	22	0
2001	17	20	16	17	29	0
DRG 475 Respiratory with ventilator support						
1996	42	18	6	26	6	2
2001	43	24	5	14	9	4

NOTE: DRG (diagnosis related group), PAC (postacute care), SNF (skilled nursing facility). Other postacute providers include long-term care, rehabilitation, and psychiatric facilities. These data show use of postacute care and hospice services by a 5 percent sample of beneficiaries enrolled in the traditional Medicare program. Totals may not add to 100 due to rounding.

SOURCE: Direct Research LLC analysis of 1996 and 2001 claims from CMS.

recovering from stroke, spinal cord injury, or traumatic brain injury.

Rehabilitation Nurse

The rehab nurse is in charge of coordinating the team members and ensuring that the care is appropriate for the client, who may have other medical problems as well. The nurse reinforces the goals and techniques of therapy, provides client and family education, and is responsible for ensuring continuity of care upon discharge. In the home health care setting, the nurse conducts the initial assessment of the client, determines what rehabilitative therapies are needed, and then monitors the course of treatment and charts the progress of the client.

Nurses are generally trained at the baccalaureate level, and many have graduate degrees. Registered nurses (RNs) are licensed by the state in which they work. Many take a comprehensive examination to obtain specialized certification in rehabilitation.

Physical Therapist

Physical therapists (PTs) evaluate and treat people with limitations in gross motor function. The goal

Table 22.2 The Core Rehabilitation Team

Health Care Professional	Typical Credential	Primary Responsibilities
Physiatrist/Rehabilitation physician	MD, four-year residency in Physical Medicine and Rehabilitation (PM&R), certifying written and oral examinations administered by the American Board of Physical Medicine and Rehabilitation	Leader of the team; responsible for assessment and establishment of goals
Rehabilitation nurse	Three-year diploma, baccalaureate, or post-baccaluareate (master's or doctoral) degree in nursing. Current license. May be designated as a Certified Rehabilitation Nurse (CRRN)	Executes medical treatment and coordinates the team; monitors the patient and progress toward rehab goals; instrumental in patient education
Physical therapist (PT)	Postbaccalaureate (master's or doctoral) degree, current license	Develops program to address goals that involve transfers, mobility, gait training, pain management, spasticity, and adaptive equipment
Occupational therapist (OT)	Bachelor or postbaccalaureate (master's or doctoral) degree in OT, current license. After Jan. 2007, all programs will be postbaccalaureate	Maximizes functional capacity for activities involving self-care, work, or leisure/play; prescribes adaptive devices and equipment
Speech-language pathologist	Postbaccalaureate (master's or doctoral) degree in Communication Sciences and Disorders; current license	Evaluates and treats speech and swallowing disorders; interventions focus on relearning language skills and maximizing ability to take foods orally

of treatment is to restore or maximize functional capacity by improving muscle strength, joint motion, and endurance. PTs use hot or cold compresses, ultrasound, or electrical stimulation to relieve pain, reduce swelling, or improve muscle tone. PTs also teach clients how to use crutches, prostheses, and wheelchairs for mobility. Currently PTs must complete an accredited graduate program, pass a registry examination, and receive licensure in the state in which they practice. In 32 states, physical therapists can provide services to clients without a physician referral.

Physical therapy assistants (PTAs) provide direct client care under the supervision of a physical therapist. The PTA assists the PT in implementing treatment programs by performing functions that include training clients in exercises and conducting therapeutic treatments. PTAs must complete a two-year associate degree program. About half of the states also require PTAs to be licensed, registered, or certified.

Occupational Therapist

Occupational therapists (OTs) evaluate and assess functioning in self-care, work, or leisure/play activities. Clients may have cognitive-perceptual difficulties, visual limitations, or social dysfunction that interfere with carrying out life skills. OTs teach clients how to perform essential daily activities, such as dressing, bathing, and eating. They help individuals develop skills important for living independently, obtaining an education, maintaining employment, and participating in leisure. OTs conduct home assessments and teach clients how to use adaptive equipment (e.g., splints, aids for eating and dressing) to perform activities of daily living. OTs must complete a graduate degree in an accredited OT program and pass a registry examination to receive licensure in most states

Occupational therapy assistants (OTAs) provide direct care under the supervision of an occupational therapist. OTAs must complete a two-year associate degree in an accredited program that includes supervised clinical experience.

Speech Therapist

Speech therapists, also called *speech-language pathologists,* are trained in the diagnosis of speech, voice, and language disorders. Speech therapists help clients relearn language skills. Disorders may result from hearing loss, stroke, cerebral palsy, mental disability, or brain injury. Speech therapists also help clients who have difficulty swallowing (i.e., dysphagia) to regain their ability to take foods orally. Speech therapists must complete a master's degree in an accredited speech and language pathology program and pass an examination to receive a license from the state. Speech therapy programs are moving toward requiring doctoral-level training. Table 22.3 shows the number of therapists as of 2001.

THE REHABILITATION SUPPORT TEAM

Rehabilitation teams add other disciplines as warranted by the individual case to achieve the goal of comprehensive and effective treatment. Other specialists (e.g., social workers, nutritionists) are called in as needed to consult on specific problems that require their disciplinary expertise. Table 22.4 lists other specialists who may participate on the rehabilitation team.

Social Worker

Social workers assess the client's social and psychological behaviors, living situation, financial resources,

Table 22.3   Allied Health Rehabilitation Professionals (2001)

Type	Number
Physical therapist	126,450
Occupational therapist	77,080
Speech-language pathology	83,110

SOURCE: Bureau of Labor Statistics, U.S. Department of Labor, 2001.

and availability of family support. They often function as case managers or discharge planners to help to ensure that the client's course of treatment is appropriate and cost-effective. Social workers work with the client, family, and health care team to arrange for necessary community-based services that will support the client's independence. Clinical social workers may provide counseling to clients and family members. Social workers may have a baccalaureate or master's degree. Clinical social workers (e.g., LCSWs) are licensed by the state. Some social workers have certification in case management.

Clinical Psychologist

Clinical psychologists assist the client in coping with behavioral and emotional issues that arise in adjusting to a disability. They are trained to assess intelligence, personality, cognitive skills, and perceptual-motor skill. Clinical psychologists play an important role in the rehabilitation of individuals with impaired cognitive ability and behavioral changes as a result of traumatic brain injury, stroke, or spinal cord injury. Psychotherapy can help individuals with a disability to cope more effectively during the course of the treatment process, and this can allow clients to gain the full benefits of physical, occupation, and speech pathology therapies. Clinical psychologists are trained at the doctoral level (receiving PhD or PsyD degrees), and are licensed by the state in which they work.

Table 22.4 Members of the Rehabilitation Support Team

Health Care Professional	Typical Credential	Primary Responsibilities
Social worker	Baccalaureate or postbaccalaureate (master's or doctoral) degree in Social Work; current license	Provides broad range of services, including discharge planning. Works closely with patient and family to assess adequacy of financial and social resources and to access community-based resources to meet needs.
Clinical psychologist	Doctoral degree (PsyD or PhD) and license	Identifies behavioral and emotional issues. Evaluates ability to cope with change and teaches new skill for adaptation. Counsels individual and family on one-on-one or group basis.
Pharmacist	Doctoral degree (PharmD) and license	Assesses effectiveness of drug therapy and evaluates response, looking for any untoward reactions. Recommends adjustments or changes in drug therapy.
Dietitian	Baccalaureate or postbaccalaureate (master's) degree. Complete 900 hours of practice and pass registration exam (RD)	Assesses nutritional needs to ensure sufficient nutrients. Determines whether nutritional supplementation is needed to maximize recovery.
Certified occupational therapy assistant	Associate degree	Provide direct care under the supervision of an occupational therapist.
Physical therapy assistant	Associate degree	Assists in implementation of treatment programs under the supervision of a physical therapist.
Driver rehabilitation specialist	Certification	Plans, develops, coordinates, and implements driver rehabilitation services for individuals with disabilities.
Orientation and mobility specialist	Certification	Instructs individuals with visual impairment in the skills necessary to determine position within the environment and to move safely from place to place.

REHABILITATION SETTINGS

The availability of rehabilitation services and programs in inpatient and outpatient settings grew rapidly during the 1980s and 1990s, driven largely by the payment system used by Medicare. Until the Balanced Budget Act (BBA) of 1997, Medicare reimbursed all allowable charges for rehabilitation services and programs, although payments to a facility were capped at an annual maximum. In contrast to the diagnosis-related group (DRG) reimbursement system used by Medicare in hospital settings, this payment system served as an incentive for growth. Between 1985 and 1999, the total number of rehabilitation facilities (i.e., rehab hospitals, rehab units, long-term care hospitals, and comprehensive outpatient rehab facilities) grew threefold, from 626 to 1,863 facilities (see Figure 22.1). By 2002, because of the 1997 change by Medicare in the payment system, which was phased in over time, the growth trend stalled. The total number of rehabilitation facilities dropped back to 1,737, with most of the loss accounted for by the closure of rehabilitation units (American Rehabilitation Providers

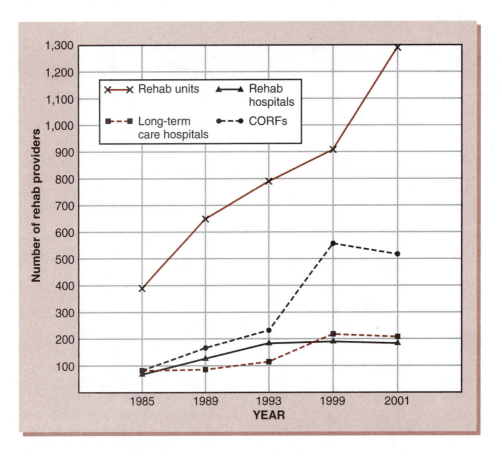

Figure 22.1   Number of Rehabilitation Facilities in the United States, 1985–1999
SOURCE: American Hospital Association, 2003.

Association, 2003). In addition, the following trends illustrate the dynamic nature of rehabilitation services and programs during this period:

- 1986 to 1993: The inpatient hospitalization rate for rehabilitation more than doubled, rising from 2.9 to 7.2 per 1,000 beneficiaries per year.
- 1990 to 1994: Medicare spending for services in rehabilitation hospitals doubled from $1.9 to $3.7 million (Gage, 1999).
- 1991 to 1994: Rehabilitation therapy increased from 15 to 31 percent of skilled nursing facility (SNF) expenditures (Prospective Payment Assessment Commission, 1996).

- 1992 to 1996: Average length of stay in rehabilitation hospitals decreased from 22.2 days to 18.5 days (Centers for Medicare and Medicaid Services, 1997).
- 1990 to 1996: The number of patients in rehabilitation hospitals climbed from 172,000 to 288,000 discharges (Gage, 1999).

Finally, there has also been an expansion in the types of settings in which rehabilitation is provided, which is not revealed in these trends. Across the continuum of inpatient and outpatient rehabilitation, service capabilities and client mix differ significantly. For example, rehabilitation hospitals/units and long-term hospitals are required to meet hospital certification standards (Medicare Payment Advisory Commission [MedPAC], 1999). Also, rehabilitation facilities are required to have 75 percent of their admissions in 1 of 10 specific diagnoses related to conditions requiring rehabilitation services if they are to qualify for Medicare payments (MedPAC, June 2003). The services provided in rehabilitation settings overlap. Patient placement is not always clear-cut; that is, patients with similar conditions may be found in the rehab hospital, SNF, long-term care hospital, or even at home. Where a rehabilitation patient is placed becomes a function of such conditions as location, availability, payer mandate, physician recommendation, family preference, and other factors. The criteria for these decisions are not always distinct and therefore make patient flow patterns unpredictable.

A study examining the amount of rehabilitation therapy provided in SNFs found that about one-half of new admissions received 90 or more minutes of rehabilitation therapy a day (Murray, Singer, Fortinsky, Russo, & Cebul, 1999). However, only 6.4 percent of SNF residents receive an amount of rehabilitation therapy that would qualify them for care on an acute rehabilitation unit.

Inpatient Rehabilitation

Inpatient rehabilitation settings include rehab hospitals, rehab units, long-term care hospitals, and skilled nursing facilities. Rehab hospitals usually have between 60 and 100 beds, whereas rehab units tend to be small, with 10 to 40 beds. Some rehab hospitals or units specialize in specific kinds of impairments, such as spinal cord injury or stroke. Generally, the clients in rehab hospitals or units are less functionally impaired than those in long-term care hospitals or skilled nursing facilities. Even though payments to inpatient rehabilitation facilities (about $4.2 billion in 2001) represent only a small part of total Medicare spending (about 1 percent), Medicare accounts for a large share of the revenue of inpatient rehabilitation facilities (MedPAC, March 2003).

Reimbursement. Until the enactment of the Balanced Budget Act (BBA) of 1997 rehab hospitals, long-term care hospitals, and comprehensive outpatient rehabilitation facilities (CORFs) were reimbursed by Medicare under the Tax Equity and Fiscal Responsibility Act (TEFRA) of 1982, which based payment on a per-episode system. The BBA significantly altered reimbursement for inpatient rehabilitation. Since October 1997, the BBA has required that clients who fall into 10 DRGs, who are discharged from an acute hospital to a postacute care setting, must be treated as transfers (Klein & Sugerman, 1997). This change forces providers of acute and postacute care services to share a capitated payment. Congress enacted legislation to add 19 additional DRGs to the postacute transfer policy beginning in fiscal year 2004 (MedPAC, March 2003).

The BBA implemented the Rehabilitation Prospective Payment System (RPPS), which took effect January 2003 (MedPAC, 2003). Under the RPPS, inpatient rehabilitation facilities (IRFs) are reimbursed by Medicare taking into consideration the patients' clinical characteristics and expected resource needs. An assessment called the IRF patient assessment instrument (IRF PAI) is completed on each patient upon admission and at discharge. This assessment instrument is derived from the Functional Independence Measure or FIM. The assessments are converted through a CMS formula to a case mix group (CMG) that has a rate attached. Each patient falls into a certain CMG, which will have a specific reimbursement rate regardless of what exact services the patient receives. This prospective payment is established for each facility and calculated nationally with local and facility-specific variations.

The long-term goal was to develop an RPPS that would predict resource utilization (i.e., length of stay) for clients regardless of whether they receive rehabilitation services in a rehab hospital, a long-term care hospital, an SNF, or a CORF. However, achievement of this goal has been complicated by significant differences in the client mix across settings and now in the payment mechanisms (Eilertsen, Kramer, Schlenker, & Hrincevich, 1998). CMGs are distinct from the DRGs used for acute care and the Resource Utilization Groups (RUGs) measures used for skilled nursing facilities, thereby delineating rehabilitation efforts as separate from other aspects of care. Since 1997, SNFs and home health agencies have been on a prospective payment system (PPS). However, as of 2003 inpatient rehabilitation and long-term care hospitals (LTCHs) remained on a cost-based payment system, and the delay in implementation of PPS contributed to a short-term rise in the use of inpatient rehabilitation and long-term care hospitals, as noted in Figure 22.2.

Also in an SNF, care of rehabilitation patients is reimbursed by a per diem payment model. This accomplishes two goals: to reimburse on the basis of case mix and to cap reimbursement. All SNF residents are placed into 44 categories (RUGs) utilizing the Minimum Data Set. Each RUG is associated with a market-based per diem level of payment (Warren, Wirtalla, & Leibensberger, 2001). There

are 14 rehabilitation RUG groups, which require a minimum amount of therapy utilization per week if payment is to be authorized (MedPAC, March 2003). In the first quarter of 2001, 78 percent of all Medicare residents were assigned to one of the rehabilitation RUGs at admission (Office of Inspector General, 2001).

The changes in payment method have significantly altered how therapy services (physical therapy, occupational therapy, and speech therapy) are used. One study found that freestanding SNFs, particularly for-profit ones, dramatically changed the services they provided in response to the new financial incentives (White, 2003). Another study compared care given to patients in an SNF with that in a rehab hospital, and demonstrated that the Medicare case mix treated in SNFs was less severe and the treatment less expensive (Buczko, 2001).

These types of variations show that the system is

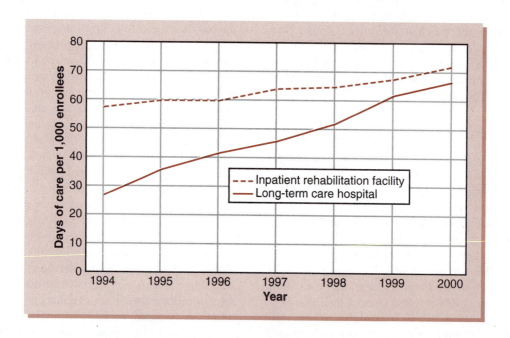

Figure 22.2 Medicare Utilization Rates for Inpatient Rehabilitation Facilities and Long-Term Care Hospitals, 1994–2000

SOURCE: CMS, Office of Information Services: Data from the Medicare Decision Support Access Facility; data development by the Office of Research, Development and Information.

still evolving. The last PPS applies to long-term care hospitals and began to be phased in by 2004. These LTCHs are the most expensive and have the highest mortality rate of the postacute care facilities (MedPAC, June 2003). Most LTCHs specialize in respiratory care or rehabilitation services (Liu et al., 2001). The changing reimbursement systems affect each type of service provider and the case mix distribution across providers. With so much change occurring throughout the first decade of 2000 to 2010, the ultimate impact of the financial status of rehabilitation providers, and on the differential case mix of each service, remains to be determined.

Outpatient Rehabilitation

Outpatient rehabilitation is provided in private practice (physical therapy, speech-language pathology, occupational therapy), CORFs, adult day health care, hospital outpatient departments, or home health agencies. Outpatient rehabilitation programs have traditionally served clients with orthopedic, neurological, or back conditions. More recently, outpatient rehabilitation services have broadened to include work-related injury, pain management, incontinence, and sports medicine cases. Many health care systems have recognized the profits that can be obtained from having outpatient rehabilitation centers. In 2002, there were 91 systems operating such outpatient centers, an increase of 5.8 percent over the previous year (Galloro & Reilly, 2003).

Reimbursement. The BBA of 1997 has affected outpatient rehabilitation providers since January 1999. The BBA imposes an annual payment limitation per Medicare beneficiary on all outpatient rehabilitation services provided under Medicare Part B (e.g., private therapy practices, clinics, rehabilitation agencies, SNFs, and home health agencies), *except* those provided in a hospital outpatient department, which were placed on a fee schedule.

The caps raised concern among rehabilitation professionals that Medicare beneficiaries with conditions requiring extensive rehabilitation, such as stroke or hip fracture, would receive only restricted access to rehabilitation because services would easily exceed the coverage limit. Congress twice delayed the implementation of this cap, implemented caps in September 2003, and then retracted them in December 2003. The payment mechanisms for outpatient rehabilitation thus remain fluid.

Home Care. Home care is a major setting for rehabilitation services, and home care agencies employ a significant number of rehabilitation professionals. Rehabilitation in the home is usually preferred by clients, particularly those with limited endurance, transportation difficulties, or restricted mobility. In addition, rehabilitation in the home is often more effective because the therapist can assess the individual's performance in the environment in which he or she actually lives. This makes it easier to determine the appropriate mix of home modifications (e.g., ramps, grab bars), assistive technology (e.g., walkers, shower chairs), and therapeutic exercise (e.g. strengthening activities). Studies suggest that home modification and assistive technology are generally more effective in improving the ability of frail and disabled seniors to do activities of daily living (ADLs) than therapeutic exercise delivered in a professional setting.

Most licensed home health agencies provide physical, occupational, and speech therapy services. Medicare authorizes physical therapy as a stand-alone service; however, occupational and speech therapy may be ordered in conjunction with nursing services.

The most common rehabilitation diagnoses seen by home health care providers include congestive heart failure, hip and knee surgeries, open heart surgery, and stroke. Since the BBA changed the way Medicare reimburses for home health services, utilization of home care has decreased. One study demonstrated a 22 percent decrease in the percentage using home health services post-BBA and a 39 percent decrease in the number of visits per user (McCall, Peterson, Moore, & Korb, 2003). For a fuller discussion of home health care, see Chapter 6 in this volume.

Adult Day Health Care. Adult day health care is a new setting for outpatient rehabilitation that targets services to those who have temporary or permanent limitations in daily functioning. Participants attending adult day health care arrive in the morning and participate in several hours of intensive rehabilitation therapy. At the end of the day they return to their homes. Some adult day health care programs qualify for reimbursement from Medicaid waiver programs that are designed to maximize the independence of those who are at risk for institutionalization.

QUALITY OF CARE OUTCOMES

All rehabilitation programs face increasing competition and a growing demand for evidence of quality. The growing interest in outcomes has led to the collection of data that can track trends in key indicators for quality such as average length of stay, total hospital charges, and functional status.

Institutional Outcomes. The Uniform Data Set for Medical Rehabilitation (UDSMR) has been used to collect national data since 1990. It provides a benchmark for average rehabilitation outcomes against which individual facilities can measure their effectiveness by comparing key indicators, such as length of stay (LOS) by impairment, functional status at admission, and functional status at discharge.

To receive payment, providers are required to submit information electronically regarding Medicare patients to the CMS, using the designated Functional Independence Measure-Function-Related Groups (FIM-FRG) patient assessment tool. The FIM-FRG measures independence in self-care, sphincter control, and social cognition. By adjusting for patients' primary impairments, medical complexity, and functional severity, payments based on CMGs will enhance access to care by providing greater levels of reimbursement to facilities caring for patients with greater clinical needs (Stineman, 2003).

REPRESENTATION, LICENSURE, AND ACCREDITATION

Representation. Representation for rehabilitation professionals is provided by discipline-specific as well as cross-cutting (e.g., medical rehab providers) associations. The rehab associations are a major force in furthering the development and evolution of rehabilitation as an important part of the health care continuum. Some of the more prominent organizations will be briefly described. Additional information is provided at the end of this chapter.

Professional Associations. Each discipline in rehabilitation has a professional association. For example, the American Academy of Physical Medicine and Rehabilitation (AAPM&R) is a national medical society representing physiatrists. The American Occupational Therapy Association represents occupational therapists and occupational therapy assistants. The American Physical Therapy Association represents physical therapists and physical therapist assistants. The American Speech Language and Hearing Association represents audiologists and speech-language pathologists.

Many of these professional associations are active at the national, regional, state, and local levels. Most of the associations have established standards of practice and a code of ethics for their discipline. Several associations provide accreditation for graduate degree programs in their discipline.

Cross-Cutting Associations. Cross-cutting associations include trade associations, research societies, and interdisciplinary organizations. There are several trade organizations that represent the field of rehabilitation. The American Medical Rehabilitation Providers Association (AMRPA) is the primary national organization and lobbying association for rehabilitation providers such as rehab hospitals, outpatient rehab facilities, and SNFs. Another national organization that attracts rehabilitation providers is the American Hospital Association (AHA). The AHA is a national lobbying organization that represents hospitals, health care networks, and clients. It has a section on long-term care and rehabilitation that is working to ensure adequate financing for postacute rehabilitation providers and to improve the continuity of care among acute, postacute, and long-term care services. The National Association for Home Care (NAHC) is a trade association representing home care agencies, hospices, and home care aide organizations that also offers individual memberships to professionals, such as nurses or physical therapists, who are involved in home care.

One of the leading organizations for rehab research is the American Congress of Rehabilitation Medicine (ACRM). Other specializations in rehabilitation are represented in interdisciplinary organizations such as the Rehabilitation Engineering Society of North America (RESNA), which represents individuals and organizations who are interested in technology and disability. Similarly, the National Rehabilitation Association is a national organization that represents rehab professionals who are involved in advocacy for rehab programs and services for people with disabilities.

Licensure. The authority and responsibility for establishing licensing requirements for hospital units, facilities, and outpatient programs is held, without exception, by the state. States have the right to expand on the federal regulations and accreditation standards and to establish additional requirements for practice, quality assurance, credentialing, and other areas. For example, a state may require that a program maintain a specific staff-to-client ratio when providing therapy, which accreditation organizations do not require. Some states require that a provider facility be accredited at regular intervals by the Joint Commission on Accreditation of Healthcare Organizations (JCAHO) and the Commission for Accreditation of Rehabilitation Facilities (CARF). Other states may accept accreditation in lieu of conducting their own survey. This limits the number of surveys a provider must undergo and saves states money.

As noted earlier in this chapter, professionals within each discipline (e.g. nursing, occupational therapy) must be licensed by their state. Many rehab professionals also seek additional certification in specialty areas from a professional association. Having appropriately licensed staff is often considered in the licensing and accreditation for the facility or provider organization.

Certification. To participate in the Medicare and Medicaid programs, the rehab provider must be certified. The provider must apply for a provider number and maintain licensure in the state, which may require the appropriate accreditation. (A facility that is accredited has *deemed* status—it has met the requirements of the federal government for participation in the Medicare program.)

Accreditation. Accreditation for acute and postacute care rehabilitation settings is shared by JCAHO and CARF. In 1997, JCAHO and CARF began offering a combined accreditation survey process to rehab hospitals. A year later, JCAHO expanded recognition of CARF accreditation to include medical rehabilitation programs that are units of larger entities, and no longer requires that they be included in JCAHO surveys.

CARF is an organization that develops specific programmatic standards for providing rehabilitation services to ensure quality. In 2003, CARF merged with the Continuing Care Accreditation Commission (CCAC). CARF, a not-for-profit organization founded in 1966, is the accrediting body for assisted living, behavioral health, employment and community services, and medical rehabilitation. The CCAC, a not-for-profit organization founded in 1985, is the accrediting body for aging services continuums, including continuing care retirement communities and other organizations.

CARF has responded to the rapid growth of inpatient rehabilitation services by developing specific program standards for Comprehensive Integrated Inpatient Rehabilitation Programs (CIIRP). A CIIRP is a "program of coordinated and integrated medical and rehabilitation services that is provided 24 hours per day" (CARF, 1996, p. 75). The CIIRP requires that SNFs provide at least one hour of rehabilitation therapy five days per week (CARF, 1996). Studies show that the average amount of rehabilitation therapy provided in most SNFs usually exceeds the CIIRP minimum (Murray et al., 1999).

Overall, CARF provides accreditation in more than 10 areas of rehabilitation, including Spinal Cord Rehabilitation Systems of Care, Outpatient Medical Rehabilitation Programs, Home and Community-based Rehabilitation Programs (for a fuller discussion of home care accreditation, see Chapter 6), and others. In the late 1990s, CARF developed standards for accreditation of adult day services programs, and began to accredit day care programs in 1999 (see Chapter 8).

INTEGRATING MECHANISMS

The interdisciplinary nature of rehabilitation makes integrating mechanisms particularly important for the effective delivery of services. The key mechanisms include case management and information systems.

Case Management

The rehabilitation team works together to plan the course of treatment for each client, to chart progress in reaching goals, and to plan for a successful discharge or transition. The team may have a specific person who functions only as a case manager, or the team member representing the primary services a client requires may assume the care coordinator/case management function. The case manager coordinates the functional assessment of the client, the evaluation of rehabilitation potential, and the availability of support systems. The case manager continues to monitor and evaluate client needs, and the team recommends and revises treatment protocols as the client moves through the rehabilitation continuum utilizing inpatient, outpatient, and home care services. Communication among the case manager and family, primary care and specialty physicians, insurance case managers, and employers contributes to the team effort that maximizes client outcomes.

Information Systems

The development of sophisticated intrahospital computer systems is helping to integrate rehabilitation into the continuum of health care delivery. Technological breakthroughs in security systems allow rehabilitation team members to share information more easily and quickly, although they must all comply with the Health Insurance Portability and Accountability Act (HIPAA). Because the rehabilitation provider depends on information from others in planning interventions, information systems are essential to maximizing function efficiently. As noted earlier, the MDS-PAC being required by GMS is helping standardize information across rehabilitation providers. The implementation of the new reimbursement system will also do so.

Complementary Rehabilitation Medicine

Complementary and alternative medicine (CAM) modalities are becoming more recognized and respected as part of the range of therapeutic options available to practitioners for treating rehabilitative patients. In fact, rehabilitative medicine has been a leader for many years in the application of alternative medicine to mainstream medical practice, as evidenced by the presence of so many alternative practitioners affiliated with academic departments of physical and rehabilitative medicine (Leskowitz, 2003). CAM provides another integrative method for enhancing the care provided in rehabilitation.

Finance Systems

The long-term care delivery system lacks an integrating financial system that spans the continuum of care. Unfortunately, as stated before, the system is very fragmented and there is little incentive to tie various financial systems into useful networks. Laws and regulations prohibit patient information from being shared without proper consent and privacy and security protections in place. Trying to integrate financial systems not owned by the same company can prove problematic and will be even more difficult to produce in the future.

POLICY ISSUES

Significant changes in the delivery and funding of rehabilitation will take place in the next few years. Whether rehabilitation is successful in positioning itself as part of the continuum of health care services in the emerging environment remains to be seen. Several important policy issues have yet to be resolved. These include accountability, ethics, and supply/demand.

Accountability

A primary policy issue is the growing demand for accountability in achieving specified outcomes while requiring that high standards of quality be maintained. The search for efficiency and streamlining is already consolidating management teams and blurring lines between acute and postacute care. Critical paths developed by interdisciplinary teams are helping clients move smoothly along the continuum while ensuring efficient use of resources and the achievement of client outcomes. Nevertheless, considerable changes are just around the corner.

In coming years, rehab providers will be asked to collect increasing amounts of data to provide evidence of effectiveness and efficiency. Outcomes will be measured at both the individual (e.g., MDS-PAC) and organizational (e.g., UDSMR) levels. However, "paper compliance" with the data requirements will require a significant time investment from rehab providers and may leave them with scant time for actual client therapy.

Ethics

Ethical issues in the rehabilitation setting are common and reflect both the dynamic nature of the health care environment and the team model of care. A recent survey of the most frequent ethical issues facing rehab clinicians in daily practice cited pressures relating from health care reimbursement changes (24 percent); conflicts among patients, physicians, team members, or families around goal setting (17 percent); and difficulty assessing decision-making capacity (7 percent) (Kirschner, Stocking, Wagner, Joye, & Siegler, 2001). Various ethical dilemmas from a more clinical perspective must also be addressed, with the patient always considered of foremost importance (Kornblau & Starling, 2000). Ongoing interactive educational interventions and good policy formation are warranted to address these issues.

Supply/Demand

Lastly, in another decade the baby boomers will begin entering later life, and the supply of rehabilitation services will probably fall considerably short of demand. Well-educated boomers are unlikely to accept disability and will demand access to rehabilitation services that maximize independence. At present, programs for PT and OT are overwhelmed with applicants for limited spaces. This has resulted in a bottleneck in the supply of rehab professionals. The resulting shortage of rehab professionals has reached a critical stage.

HIPAA

In April 2003, the new regulations imposed by HIPAA were implemented. This legislation has required significant technical and administrative changes to address the three areas of the regulations: (1) administrative simplification (electronic claims submission), (2) privacy of protected health information, and (3) security and electronic signatures.

CONCLUSION

In today's health care environment, the expectations of consumers and payers are high and rising, even as health care resources shrink. This is a challenging time for rehabilitation providers, who face pressures to improve services, provide more efficient treatments, and produce better outcomes—yet charge less. As the postacute care continuum shifts from a cost-based system to a prospective payment system, rehabilitation providers must begin to reshape their paradigms of care. Some view the shift to a PPS as impending doom, while others see these changes as an opportunity to integrate rehabilitation into the health care continuum of services. The ability to respond effectively in this new environment will determine the shape of the field in future years.

As our health care system becomes more vertically integrated, rehabilitation providers who want to survive must respond creatively, proactively, and strategically to ensure their place in the continuum of care. In many parts of the nation, the rapid penetration of managed-care organizations has had a tremendous impact on the pricing and delivery of health care services. Those who cannot successfully reposition themselves in the evolving health market are finding themselves locked out of their former referral networks.

Even those who are able to forge new relationships within the emerging health care networks are not guaranteed that rehabilitation will remain recognized as an essential service. Rehabilitation is frequently perceived as less essential than other specialties. When dollars are scarce, there is always the danger that rehabilitation will be perceived as an expendable component—making it the first service to be jettisoned. In an era of increasing accountability and reform, tracking outcomes will be a prime focus in the emerging dynamic between rehabilitation providers and managed care plans. Results must demonstrate that rehabilitation is the most affordable and efficacious treatment for recovery. The increasing availability of national rehabilitation data provides a benchmark against which an organization can gauge its performance.

Finally, it is the role of rehabilitation to be concerned with managing recovery rather than managing the bottom line. Rehabilitation expertise in managing clients is increasingly vital in the managed care environment. As rehab services continue to evolve, collaborative relationships will be critical to influence how, when, and where medical rehabilitation is provided.

CLIENT EXAMPLE

Mrs. Miller is a frail 70-year-old female who lives alone in a one-story apartment in Los Angeles. She is 5 feet tall and weighs about 95 pounds. She appears slightly older than her stated age and admits to smoking a pack of cigarettes a day for more than 50 years. Her medical history includes osteoporosis, arthritis, chronic bronchitis, and congestive heart failure. While standing on a step stool reaching for a can of soup, she falls and fractures her right hip.

Mrs. Miller is admitted to her local hospital for surgery to repair her hip. Her postoperative recovery is stormy and complicated by respiratory and cardiac complications, which force a transfer to the critical care unit for several days. During her stay in critical care, her health deteriorates and she is placed on an artificial ventilator to help her breathe. She is successfully weaned from the ventilator after two days and her condition stabilizes.

Now that Mrs. Miller is stable, she is transferred to a medical floor, where she is evaluated for rehabilitation. She is quite weak, and initially the rehab team focuses primarily on getting her up and out of bed. She still has an IV and foley catheter (i.e., a tube to drain urine from the bladder), and her appetite is poor. A dietitian is called in to assess her nutritional status, because she has lost seven pounds over the past two weeks. Based on the recommendations of the nutritionist, additional snacks are provided to help improve her health and increase her weight. Slowly, Mrs. Miller begins to improve. A week after her surgery her catheter is removed. Unfortunately, she has some difficulties with urinary incontinence and is often unable to make it to the bathroom in time. She finds this very embarrassing and expresses concern to the nurses that she might not ever be able to "control her water again." A program of bladder training is initiated and is successful in resolving the problem.

Two weeks after her surgery, Mrs. Miller is able to ambulate with a walker and one person assisting. The discharge planner comes by to see her to discuss transferring her to an SNF for additional rehabilitation. Mrs. Miller does not have sufficient endurance and strength to tolerate therapy in an acute rehabilitation hospital/unit, and she is still unable to manage sufficiently to live alone, so an SNF appears to be the most appropriate setting in which to continue her recovery. Mrs. Miller is terrified about the idea of going to a "nursing home." The discharge planner reassures her that it is only for a short-term stay so that she can get the rehabilitation she needs to return to her home.

Once at the nursing home, Mrs. Miller is seen by the rehabilitation team, who evaluate her functional capacity and mobility. The team meets to identify the goals and treatment plan for Mrs. Miller. She is assigned 30-minute sessions of physical therapy 3 times a day for a total of 90 minutes each day. Gradually Mrs. Miller becomes stronger and able to ambulate without assistance. She spends four weeks in the nursing home before being discharged home under the care of a home health agency.

On discharge, Mrs. Miller is able to ambulate alone with a walker, although she still tires easily. Within a few hours of her arrival home, a visiting nurse stops by her apartment to assess her needs. She determines that Mrs. Miller needs help with bathing, preparing meals, a home assessment, and additional physical therapy. She arranges for a home health aide to come in three times a week to help Mrs. Miller with her bath and for the delivery of home meals each day. She also orders an evaluation by occupational and physical therapists.

The OT assesses Mrs. Miller and makes sure that she has the necessary durable medical equipment (e.g., bath chair, raised toilet seat, grab bars) that she needs and that she knows how to use them. The OT also conducts a home safety check and finds several throw rugs, which she removes so that Mrs. Miller will not trip. The OT instructs Mrs. Miller not to go "climbing around" on her step stool, and places items that she could not reach on a lower shelf. The OT visits Mrs. Miller twice, and then OT services are discontinued.

The physical therapist assesses Mrs. Miller's ability to ambulate safely with her walker and makes sure that she can get out of her apartment. She continues to receive one hour of physical therapy three times a week in her home for another six weeks. Three months after her fall, she has finally regained much of her previous strength and mobility, and home health services are discontinued. Medicare paid for the majority of Mrs. Miller's care, although she had co-payments and deductibles.

WHERE TO GO FOR FURTHER INFORMATION

American Congress of Rehabilitation Medicine (ACRM)
6801 Lake Plaza Drive, Suite B-205
Indianapolis, IN 46220
(317) 915-2250
http://www.acrm.org

ACRM is a research and advocacy organization that promotes rehabilitation research. ACRM seeks to address issues that include outcomes, efficacy of treatment, managed care, best practices, and reimbursement for the field of rehabilitation.

American Medical Rehabilitation Providers Association (AMRPA)
1710 N Street, NW
Washington, DC 20036
(202) 223-1920 / (888) 346-4624
http://www.amrpa.org

AMRPA is the primary national organization and lobbying association for rehabilitation providers, including rehabilitation hospitals, outpatient rehabilitation facilities, and skilled nursing facilities.

National Center for Medical Rehabilitation Research (NCMRR)
Building 61E, Room 2A03 9000

Rockville Pike
Bethesda, MD 20892
(301) 402-2242
http://www.nichd.nih.gov/NCMRR

NCMRR is a component of the National Institute of Child Health and Human Development (NICHD) at the National Institutes of Health (NIH). NCMRR supports rehabilitation research that enhances the health, productivity, independence, and quality of life of persons with disabilities.

National Rehabilitation Association (NRA)
633 S. Washington Street
Alexandria, VA 22314
(703) 836-0850 / TDD (703) 836-0849
http://www.nationalrehab.org

The NRA is a national organization representing professionals in the field of rehabilitation—particularly vocational rehabilitation. The membership includes rehab counselors, physical, speech and occupational therapists, job trainers, consultants, independent living instructors, and other professionals involved in the advocacy of programs and services for people with disabilities.

National Rehabilitation Information Center (NARIC)
1010 Wayne Avenue, Suite 800
Silver Spring, MD 20910-5633
(301) 562-2400 / (800) 346-2742 /
TTY (301) 495-5626
http://www.naric.com

NARIC is a library service, funded by the National Institute on Disability and Rehabilitation Research (NIDRR), that collects and disseminates the results of federally funded research projects. NARIC's collection averages around 200 new documents per month and includes commercially published books, journal articles, and audiovisuals.

FACTS REVIEW

1. What are the goals of rehabilitation?
2. What are the five most common diagnoses calling for rehabilitation?
3. What are the primary sources of payment for rehabilitation?
4. Who are the core members of the rehab team?
5. How has the Balanced Budget Act of 1997 affected postacute rehabilitation services?
6. Which are the primary organizations that develop standards to assure quality and provide accreditation for the field of rehabilitation?

REFERENCES

American Hospital Association. (2003). *Hospital statistics 2003.* Chicago: Health Forum LLC.

American Rehabilitation Providers Association. (2003, July 10). Personal communication with staff.

Buczko, W. (2001, Summer). Effects of institutional services and characteristics on use of post-acute care settings. *Journal of Health and Human Services Administration,* 103–132.

Bureau of Labor Statistics. (2001). *2001 national occupational employment and wage estimates: Healthcare practitioners and technical occupations.* Retrieved October 13, 2003 from *http://www.bls.gov/oes/2001/oes_29He.htm*

Centers for Disease Control and Prevention, National Center for Chronic Disease Prevention and Health Promotion, United States Department of Health and Human Services. (2003). *Chronic disease overview.* Retrieved August 17, 2003 from *http://www.cdc.gov/nccdphp/overview.htm*

Centers for Medicare and Medicaid Services. (1997). *Statement of Barbara Wynn acting director bureau of policy development healthcare financing administration on rehabilitation and long-term care hospital payments house committee on ways and means subcommittee on health.* Retrieved October 13, 2003 from *http://www.cms.hhs.gov/media/press/testimony.asp?Counter=503*

Cole, K., & Ramsdell, J. (1990). Issues in interdisciplinary team care. In B. Kemp, K. Brummel-Smith, & J. Ramsdell (Eds.), *Geriatric rehabilitation.* Boston, MA: College Hill Press.

Commission for the Accreditation of Rehabilitation Facilities. (1996). *Standards manual and interpretive guidelines for medical rehabilitation.* Tucson, AZ: CARF.

DeJong, G. (1995, July/August). Rehabilitation has strategic prevention role in managed care. *Rehabilitation Report*, (14), 6–7.

Eilertsen, T., Kramer, A., Schlenker, R., & Hrincevich, C. (1998). Application of functional independence measure-function related groups and resource utilization groups-version III systems across post-acute settings. *Medical Care, 36*(5), 695–705.

Fiedler, R., Granger, C., & Russell, C. (1998). Uniform Data System for Medical Rehabilitation: Report of first admissions for 1997. *American Journal of Physical Medicine and Rehabilitation, 77*(5), 444–450.

Gage, B. (1999). Impact of the BBA on post-acute utilization. *Health Care Financing Review, 20*(4), 103–126.

Galloro, V., & Reilly, P. (2003). Trickling down. *Modern Healthcare, 33*(2), 26–31.

Klein, J., & Sugerman, A. (1997). The quake that rocked rehabilitation. The Balanced Budget Act of 1997: Business implications and survival strategies. *Rehabilitation Management, 10*(6), 108–111.

Kirschner, K., Stocking, C., Wagner, L. B., Joye, S. J., & Siegler, M. (2001). Ethical issues identified by rehabilitation clinicians. *Archives of Physical Medicine and Rehabilitation, 82*(2), S2–S8.

Kornblau, B., & Starling, S. (2000). *Ethics in rehabilitation: A clinical perspective.* Thorofare, NJ: SLACK, Inc.

Leskowitz, E. (2003). *Complementary and alternative medicine in rehabilitation.* St. Louis: Churchill Livingstone.

Liu, K., Baseggio, C., Wissoker, D., Maxwell, S., Haley, J., & Long, S. (2001). Long-term care hospitals under Medicare: Facility-level characteristics. *Health Care Financing Review, 23*(2), 1–18.

Liu, K., Gage, B., Harvell, J., Stevenson, D., & Brennan, N. (1999). Medicare's post-acute care benefit: Background, trends, and issues to be faced. Washington, DC: U.S. Department of Health and Human Services.

Maguire, P. (2001). Examining the quality "chasm" in health care. *CP-ASIM Observer* (American College of Physicians-American Society of Internal Medicine). Retrieved August 20, 2003 from *http://www.acponline.org*

McCall, N., Peterson, A., Moore, S., & Korb, J. (2003). Utilization of home health services before and after the Balanced Budget Act of 1997: What were the initial effects? *Health Services Research, 38*(1), 85–106.

McNeil, J. (1997). *Americans with disabilities: 1994–1995* (Data from the Survey of Income and Program Participation). Washington, DC: U.S. Department of Commerce, Bureau of the Census.

Medicare Payment Advisory Commission (MedPAC). (2003, June). *Report to Congress: Variation and innovation in Medicare.* Retrieved July 20, 2003 from *http://www.medpac.gov*

Medicare Payment Advisory Commission (MedPAC). (2003, March). *Report to Congress: Medicare payment policy.* Retrieved July 20, 2003 from *http://www.medpac.gov*

MedPAC's report to Congress raises concern. PPS system for rehabilitation hospitals and units. (1999). *Hospital Outlook, 2*(2), 6–8.

MedPAC's variation and innovation in medicare. (2003). Retrieved October 13, 2003 from *http://www.medpac.gov/search/searchframes.cfm*

Murray, P., Singer, M., Fortinsky, R., Russo, L., & Cebul, R. (1999). Rapid growth of rehabilitation services in traditional community-based nursing homes. *Archives of Physical Medicine and Rehabilitation, 80*(4), 372–378.

National Center for Health Statistics. (2003). Mortality data from the national vital statistics system. Retrieved October 13, 2004 from *http://www.cdc.gov/nchs/about/major/dvs/mortdata.htm*

National Institute of Child Health and Human Development. (2001). Clinical trial planning grants to guide timing, intensity, and duration of rehabilitation for stroke and hip fracture (RFA-HD-01-022). Retrieved July 10, 2003, from *http://grants1.nih.gov/grants/guide/rfa-files/RFA-HD-01-022.html*

Office of Inspector General. (2001, July). Trends in the assignment of resource utilization groups by skilled nursing facilities. Washington, D.C.: Department of Health and Human Services.

Stineman, M. (2002). Prospective payment, prospective challenge. *Archives of Physical Medicine and Rehabilitation, 83*, 1802–1805.

Warren, R. L., Wirtalla, C., & Leibensberger, A. (2001). Preliminary observations on reduced utilization in skilled nursing facility rehabilitation. *American Journal of Physical Medicine and Rehabilitation, 80*, 626–633.

White, C. (2003). Rehabilitation therapy in skilled nursing facilities: Effects of Medicare's new prospective payment system. *Health Affairs, 22*(3), 214–223.

CHAPTER 23

Services for Children with Special Health Care Needs

Janice E. Frates and Judith Connell

Children with special health care needs (CSHCN) have a variety of physical, mental, and behavioral conditions that may require complex configurations of long-term care services. The variety and complexity of these conditions make it difficult to provide a comprehensive system of care. Health care professionals must understand the complexity of this population and the service components necessary to provide a comprehensive and changing continuum of care throughout the child's lifespan. Children with special health care needs may outgrow the condition, stabilize with ongoing treatment, or continue to need intense support and extensive services through adulthood.

DEFINITION

Of the 70.4 million children under 18 years of age living in the United States in 2000, approximately 13 percent were children with conditions ranging from moderate health problems to severe disabilities (National Center for Health Statistics [NCHS], 2002).

Some studies suggest that children who have recurring ear infections and headaches should be included in the estimate, which would increase the number of children affected with chronic conditions to 24 million, or 1 in every 3 (Alliance for Health Reform, 2000). The federal Centers for Disease Control and Prevention (CDC) reports that 17 percent of U.S. children under 18 years of age have a developmental disability (Administration for Children and Families, 2003). *Developmental disabilities* are a diverse group of physical, cognitive, psychological, sensory, and speech impairments that begin anytime during development up to 18 years.

Definitions regarding CSHCNs vary tremendously. The most cited definition is that developed by the U.S. Maternal and Child Health Bureau (MCHB), Division of Services for Children with Special Needs (2000):

Children with special health care needs are those who have or are at increased risk for a chronic physical, developmental, behavioral, or emotional condition and who also require health and related services of a type or amount beyond that required by children generally.

Identification of special-needs children is essential for referral to public and private programs, monitoring quality, adjusting reimbursement amounts, and coordinating services. Substantial effort is currently being directed to developing efficient tools for identifying CSHCN in both the general population and managed care. There is no current national standard. One set of categories includes program eligibility, diagnostic, high cost, and low cost. Another set groups children according to the consequences and duration of their conditions. Other models apply a disease-specific classification. The National Association of Children's Hospital and Related Institutions (NACHRI) and 3M Health Information Systems developed Clinical Risk Groups (CRGs) to identify people with chronic conditions or those who are "at risk" (NACHRI, 2003). This system classifies children into a single category designed to capture the amount and type of health care services the child will use in the future. Their categories include healthy, single minor chronic, multiple chronic, malignancies, and catastrophic conditions. Within each category, there are severity levels associated with the condition.

Good data, when available, can provide much useful information for understanding and improving services to CSHCN. Methods for identifying CSHCN by health care organizations include surveys and analyses of administrative data such as those found in claims and encounter data or program enrollment files. There is a unique difficulty with children in that many of the severely disabling chronic conditions are rare. The diversity of identification methods in health care is compounded by different categorization methods in education, housing, and social services. A good example is that required under the federal Individuals with Disabilities Education Act (IDEA), through which millions of children receive special services designed to meet their unique needs. The IDEA provides definitions of the 13 disability categories. Most are disease-specific, such as autism, deafness, mental retardation; others are functional—orthopedic, speech or language, or visual impairment. Funding for public education services requires these classifications.

CLIENTS

A number of demographic and socioeconomic variables are positively correlated with chronic conditions. Chronic conditions tend to affect school-age children more than very young children. Boys are more likely to have a chronic condition than girls. Among minority populations, Asian and Pacific Islanders have some of the lowest rates (Family Voices, 2002a).

The most commonly occurring childhood chronic condition is asthma. Affecting nearly 5 million children nationwide, asthma is a major public health problem of increasing concern in the United States. It is the leading condition causing pediatric hospitalizations and school absences (American Lung Association, 2003). Low-income populations, minorities, and children living in inner cities experience disproportionately higher morbidity and mortality due to asthma (CDC, 2002).

Approximately 2 percent of school-age children in the United States have a serious developmental disability, such as mental retardation or cerebral palsy, and need special education services or supportive care (Administration for Children and Families, 2003). Attention deficit disorder is the most commonly diagnosed behavioral health disorder today, affecting between 3 and 5 percent of school-age children (American Psychiatric Association, 2003).

Approximately 150,000 babies each year are born with congenital abnormalities (such as cleft palate), more commonly known as *birth defects* (March of Dimes, 2003). Other major chronic conditions include AIDS, cerebral palsy, diabetes, and spina bifida. To make matters more difficult, children often suffer from a combination of conditions. Table 23.1 identifies typical characteristics of CSHCN.

Children lead very active lifestyles. Attending school, playing, socializing, and participating in sports are all normal activities for children growing

Table 23.1   Characteristics of Children with Special Health Care Needs (N=2220)

Child's mean age (in years)	9.02
Child's gender	
Male	58%
Female	42%
Child's race/ethnicity	
White/Caucasian	71%
Black/African American	10%
Asian/Pacific Islander/Southeast Asian	2%
Hispanic/Latino/Latina/Spanish	9%
Native American/American Indian/Aleut/Eskimo	1%
Multiracial	5%
Caregiver education level (Mother = 88% of respondents)	
Less than high school	9%
High school graduate	24%
Some college or associates degree	40%
Bachelor's degree	17%
Postgraduate degree	10%
Other special-needs children in family	23%
Community type	
City/urban	37%
Suburban	31%
Farming/rural	26%
Other	4%
Mean household pretax income (1997)	$34,337
Child is technology-dependent	17%
Average days of school missed because of condition	#
Child has primary health coverage	97%
Overall health of child	
Excellent	15%
Very good	32%
Good	33%
Fair	15%
Poor	4%
Overall stability of health	
Usually stable	34%
Changing once in a while	40%
Changing all the time	23%

SOURCE: Family Voices, 2000b; *http://www.familyvoices.org*

up. In 2000, 7 percent of children ages 5 to 17 were limited in their activities because of one or more chronic health conditions, compared with 3 percent of children younger than 5 (Federal Interagency Forum on Child and Family Statistics [FIFCFS], 2002). Older children have much higher rates of activity limitation than younger children, partly because some chronic conditions are not diagnosed until children enter school, and partly because the number of activities that children participate in increases with age. Figure 23.1 illustrates that children and youth in families of lower socioeconomic status (as measured by parental education and family income) have significantly higher rates of activity limitation than children of higher status families. Among children and youth ages 5 to 17, 8 percent of children whose parents had less than a high school education had activity limitations due to

chronic conditions in 2000, compared with 5 percent of children living with at least one parent who finished college (FIFCFS, 2002).

SERVICES

Long-term care services for CSHCN present a plethora of challenges to all involved in their care—parents, health care and human service professionals, and educators. Depending on the nature and severity of the condition, and the family and community resources available to handle it, there are typically numerous caregivers and organizations involved and often a confusing array of programs and funding sources.

Relationships in the Continuum of Care

Because CSHCN have complex problems, many need more services than those offered by the average health plan or pediatrician. The continuum of long-term care services for children is different than for adults because it typically involves the school system, often involves public social services, and may also involve the mental health system. Most of these children and their families will need, either permanently or intermittently, the following services (see Figure 23.2):

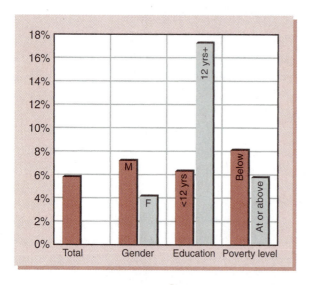

Figure 23.1 Percentage of Children Ages 0–17 with Any Limitation in Activity Resulting from Chronic Conditions: By Gender, Parental Education, and Poverty Level

NOTE: Education categories are for the level of the most educated parent in the household.

SOURCE: FIFCFS, 2002.

- Individual case management
- Extensive motor skills training
- Speech and language training
- Durable medical equipment, most of which must either be customized after purchase or custommade; because children grow, they may require new equipment annually
- Enabling services, such as transportation, home, and vehicle modifications
- Family support services, including respite care and family counseling
- Unusual procedures (e.g., a gait analysis to determine the need for orthopedic surgery)
- Frequent hospital stays and visits to primary

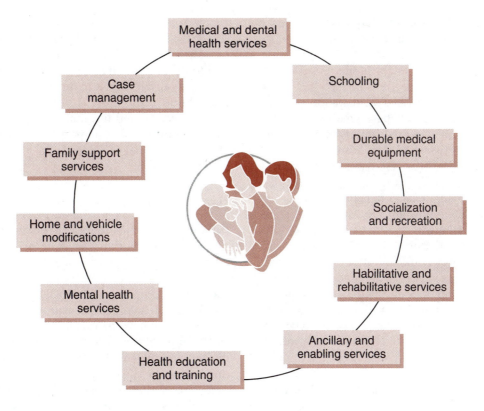

Figure 23.2   Delivery of Services in a Family-Centered Care System

care physicians, specialists, therapists, and labs that greatly exceed the norm (Family Voices, 1999)

Service Components

The principal long-term care service components for CSHCN include, but are not limited to, medical care, long-term residential care, ancillary and enabling services, education, and social support. These formal services are closely interrelated but, unfortunately, not always well coordinated—and none is as important as the family. With the family at the center, professionals from many disciplines form a care team to help each child develop and function at an optimal level.

Medical Care

At the primary care level, the pediatrician plays a central role in the care of CSHCN. The general pediatric practitioner is best suited to serve as the child's care manager, for several reasons:

- The pediatrician has a continuing relationship with the child and the family, which fosters trust and allows the development of a comprehensive client history.
- He or she is more likely to know the community resources and system participants.
- The generalist pediatrician's focus is on health of the whole child and on wellness, not just the disabling condition.
- Managed-care organizations are oriented toward

having a primary care provider serve as a client's care coordinator or "medical home."

Pediatricians need to establish office operational procedures and management structures for provision of efficient care to CSHCN. Extra time is often needed for discussion of these children's routine and special health care needs and for family counseling. Establishment and regular maintenance of a chronic disease client registry and a computer database with history, treatment, and care plan summaries can help ensure that these children receive appropriate follow-up care. Much of the coordination work can, and should, be delegated to the professional and administrative office staff. It is also vital to establish a communication structure with medical colleagues in the general practice who share coverage responsibilities and with specialist practitioners and other service providers (Desguin, Holt, & McCarthy, 1994). Too often, especially when referrals to many specialists and agencies are involved, children with special health care needs fall through the cracks in the health care system.

A 2000 survey of pediatricians found that most (71 percent) serve as the primary medical care coordinator for CSHCN, and 61 percent reported that they always assist families of special-needs children to set up appointments when referring to a specialist. However, the percentage of pediatricians who make it a regular practice to provide other care coordination services is much lower. Lack of time and lack of medical staff to provide such care services were the most frequently cited reasons for not providing them (American Academy of Pediatrics, 2001).

The American Academy of Pediatrics (AAP) emphasizes the importance of a medical home for all children, but especially those with special needs; *medical home* is defined as "[c]are that is accessible, family-centered, continuous, comprehensive, coordinated, compassionate and culturally competent." In 2002, the Maternal and Child Health Bureau of the U.S. Department of Health and Human Services (U.S. DHHS) established a national training

center in the AAP's Department of Community Pediatrics to fund educational programs and technical assistance for parents and caregivers of CSHCN and to develop and maintain a national network of experts to ensure access to quality care for CSHCN (AAP, 2000).

For specialty and hospital care, CSHCN receive treatment from pediatric specialists affiliated with a children's hospital or an academic medical center's pediatric staff.

Children's Hospitals

Children's hospitals represent less than 1 percent of all hospitals, but they account for 39 percent of admissions and 59 percent of costs for hospitalized children and train about 30 percent of all pediatricians in the United States (NACHRI, 2001).

Specialty rehabilitation institutions, such as the Shriners Hospitals, treat children with orthopedic and burn problems, as well as children with severely disfiguring congenital deformities. St. Jude's Children's Research Hospital in Memphis, Tennessee, specializes in the treatment of potentially fatal childhood diseases, including cancer and select genetic and immune deficiency disorders. However, not all families have access to them, because of either geography or restrictions imposed by their health insurers.

Providers and staff who deliver specialty and acute care services to CSHCN and their families have a critical role to play in explaining treatments and technology. Children's hospitals are designed with children and their families in mind, but many pediatric units in general acute care hospitals are not, so it is especially important for staff at all levels to proactively attend to the concerns and needs of both children and their families.

Long-Term Residential Care

Some children, usually those with both profound developmental and physical disabilities, require long-term institutional care. The majority of facilities

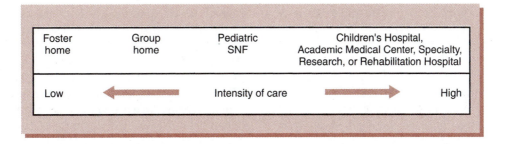

Figure 23.3 Long-Term Care Facilities for Children

serving profoundly disabled children are state institutions. There are also specialized residential and educational institutions for children with specific disabilities, such as blindness and deafness. Private facilities are differentiated mainly by size and service intensity. Pediatric subacute care or skilled nursing facilities primarily serve medically fragile, technology-dependent children. Their client population consists of children with severe congenital birth defects, head injuries, premature birth complications, seizure disorders; recipients of total parenteral nutrition (TPN) and continuous intravenous therapies; and those dependent on gastronomy or tracheostomy tubes. Children with severe disabilities requiring less intensive care may reside in community group homes or specialized foster homes. These facilities are smaller, generally serving from one to six children, and are often run by a family with some additional paid staff. Figure 23.3 shows the range of long-term care facilities for children.

In long-term care facilities, the staff are the primary caregivers for the resident children, so their responsibilities include attending to the children's emotional as well as physical care needs.

Ancillary and Enabling Services

Ancillary and enabling services include, but are not limited to, home health, respite care, transportation, equipment, and supplies. Nearly all families want to care for their child at home, but successful home care depends on the family's determination and resourcefulness and the quality of their support network. Physicians must initially recommend, periodically review, and request renewal of home care services (including equipment and supplies). Rehabilitation physicians are frequently called on to act as consultants in establishing home care treatment plans and recommendations for home-based physical therapy. Respite care is another essential service component; however, it is usually available only on a limited basis, such as when there is a high risk of parental abuse or caregiver burnout. It is seldom reimbursed by insurers and thus generally is not available to parents of modest means. Even for affluent families, the time and price of obtaining reliable respite care are often too high. For many families, obtaining these services from insurers or community agencies presents many financial, logistical, and bureaucratic challenges.

The real challenge to accommodating CSHCN is in the home. Rarely do public programs or insurers pay for physical modifications to the home, even though this is where the child will spend most of his or her time. Finding and obtaining appropriate clothing, school supplies, play equipment, and toys for children with severe physical and mental disabilities is another challenge—and an additional expense—for families. Organizations, such as Family Village and the National Lekotek Center, and publications such as *Exceptional Parent*, assist families of CSHCN with many of these issues (see *http://www.familyvillage.wisc.edu* and *http://www .lekotek.org*).

Education

School often involves medical care, training, and special accommodations. Most CSHCN do not need special education, and there is a strong trend toward educating all but the most severely disabled children in "mainstream" settings. Federal law mandates that transportation and corrective or developmental support services be provided for CSHCN to benefit from education. Children with special health care needs and their families need a plan for coordination of their educational and medical care needs, to foster both learning and socialization. The logistics can be quite formidable. They include administering medication, incorporating therapy into the educational schedule, frequent doctors' visits and thus absences, keeping up with schoolwork, physical accommodations for the disability, teacher training on how to handle likely crises, and facilitating social interaction. Parents are an integral component in the development of the child's education program and can appeal a school system's decision about a child's education plan.

Few schools have full-time nurses, and some have no nurse at all. This often means that school personnel with no medical training are asked to perform duties ranging from dispensing medications to monitoring insulin levels and administering injections, and to handle a challenging range of children's physical needs and behaviors.

Social Support

A child's chronic illness challenges families at several levels: cognitive, emotional, behavioral, and financial. The family has to learn about the condition, its prognosis, and their treatment options, and deal with a spectrum of feelings from shock and denial to sadness and guilt. Routines, tasks, and possibly roles change to accommodate the care of the child. Siblings as well as parents assume new physical and psychological caregiving responsibilities that foster

growth in some individuals and increase the risk of psychological problems in others (Desguin, Holt, & McCarthy, 1994). As previously mentioned, families of CSHCN often experience additional financial burdens. These family stress factors place CSHCN at high risk for abuse or neglect, especially when there are preexisting personal problems or the family is economically disadvantaged. Social support is thus extremely important.

Care coordination is an essential element of social support in the service continuum, but it is frequently difficult to achieve. Parents often find that they must assume the responsibility for integrating the various sources of care, but few have any training to perform this task. Skilled professionals can create sophisticated plans of care, but implementation of the plan takes place in the child's home and community. The Association for the Care of Children's Health (ACCH) emphasizes the importance of family-centered care, as the family is the foremost and most constant element in the child's life. As partners in a therapeutic alliance with health care professionals, and as the experts on the child's life outside the treatment setting, parents and other family members are essential to effective care management. The role of professionals is to support families as caregivers, respecting the family's values, preferences, priorities, and needs (ACCH, 1999).

The Multidisciplinary Health Care Team

Other key health professionals on the care team will vary according to the level, intensity, and site of care, but the most common are:

- *Nurses and nurse practitioners,* who provide a broad range of services, including case management, health education, and home health care. Nurses can also help families maintain information regarding the child's care and treatment.
- *Dietitians,* who play a vital role in the treatment plan for many children's chronic conditions. Nutrition is important for *all* children's general good health; for CSHCN, feeding difficulties

can erode therapeutic progress or undermine family morale. A dietitian can be invaluable as an educator in adaptive feeding techniques and monitoring intake. She or he can also provide help and advice in obtaining special equipment, foods, and supplements from insurers.

- *Social workers,* who guide families through the bureaucratic labyrinth of public programs, advocate with insurers, link families with community resources, and provide counseling services.
- *Physical, occupational, and speech therapists,* who each have professional expertise to offer in the continuum of care for CSHCN. Therapeutic camps for special-needs children provide opportunities for growth and development, formation of friendships, and respite care for families.
- *Mental health professionals,* who include social workers in their function as counselors/ therapists; psychologists for both diagnostic and therapeutic services; and psychiatrists for children with severe emotional illnesses (or their family members).
- *Dentists,* who are crucial but often overlooked members of the medical care team. Depending on the child's condition, there may be special treatment or considerations for oral health.

Nonprofit Organizations

Community-based organizations have played a strong role in providing services to CSHCN for more than a century. The first voluntary health organization dedicated to fighting a specific disease was the Pennsylvania Society for the Prevention of Tuberculosis, formed in 1892. This organization eventually developed into the American Lung Association. Today, hundreds of organizations exist whose efforts focus solely on the prevention and treatment of a specific condition. Agencies focusing on children address problems such as spina bifida, cerebral palsy, muscular dystrophy, diabetes, and asthma. Nonprofit organizations provide essential services to their communities, such as education and referrals to support programs; they also act as advocates for medical research and policy development. These organizations often are the strongest link for parents to learn how to obtain services from providers, other community agencies, and publicly funded programs. Hospital social workers and school health liaisons often refer families who have children with disabilities to community organizations to assist them with financial problems, social support, and programs that can help families cope with the condition.

FINANCING

Payment for services to CSHCN comes from both public and private sources. Many CSHCN receive services from both. Federally funded programs make up the greatest component of CSHCN services. The major program categories are income support, health care, and education. Commercial health insurance is the main funding source in the private sector.

Federally Funded Programs

The Social Security Act, enacted in 1935, was the first step the U.S. government took toward providing income security for its citizens. Title V of the Act was particularly important to the health of mothers and children. Title V authorized the development of the Maternal and Child Health Services programs, making federal grants available to state and local health departments to offer maternal and child health services, some specifically focusing on the needs of children with chronic illnesses. Title V funds are currently referred to as the Maternal and Child Health (MCH) Block Grant.

In 1965, Title XIX of the Social Security Act created Medicaid, a major federal government health program for the poor. Closely following in 1972 was the Supplemental Security Income program (SSI), another federal program that primarily provides additional income to individuals who are very poor, including those unable to work because of disabilities. This program extends to families who have CSHCN as well, to help cover the immense costs associated with the specialized care these children need. This program provided a standardized form of care, eligibility, and payment structure.

Social Security Administration

About 1 million children with disabilities receive benefits through the Social Security Administration (SSA), primarily through the Supplemental Security Income program.

Supplemental Security Income

Families with disabled children under 18 years of age can receive monthly payments from the SSA to assist with the costs of daily living. SSA standardizes medical eligibility for the program, although income eligibility is determined on a state-by-state basis. In most states, children eligible for SSI are entitled to medical assistance through Medicaid. To qualify for SSI benefits, a child needs to have a condition that "is so severe that it results in marked and severe functional limitations," and the family's income must meet their state's SSI requirements. Children can receive SSI benefits regardless of whether other family members are receiving other public assistance benefits (SSA, 1999).

In the early 1990s, the SSI beneficiary population grew dramatically. SSI added coverage after federal mandates broadened the list of medical conditions covered under the program to include learning disabilities, AIDS, and various other social and medical problems. By 1996, more than 965,000 children were eligible for SSI, a threefold increase from the 1990 number (SSA, 1999).

In 1996, the Welfare Reform Act (also known as the Personal Responsibility and Work Opportunity Reconciliation Act) changed the definition of children with disabilities. Prior to 1996, children with disabilities were rated on the same eligibility scale as adults for SSI qualification. The new definition states: "a child's impairment—or combination of impairments—will be considered disabling if it causes 'marked and severe functional limitations'"

(SSA, 1999). The definition narrowed eligibility standards for children receiving SSI, making it more difficult for these children to qualify and keep their benefits. Those most affected by the change include children with varying degrees of developmental disabilities or mental retardation, emotional and behavioral problems, or a combination of disabilities (Family Voices, 2000).

The Welfare Reform Act affects children's Medicaid coverage. When the eligibility criteria for SSI changed, the states where Medicaid and SSI were linked were obligated to provide Medicaid coverage to any children who lost SSI benefits. Unfortunately, the process of keeping medical coverage is not a smooth one. As a result, some children with disabilities lost their SSI benefits and their Medicaid benefits as well (Family Voices, 1998). Currently, there is no way to measure how these changes affect CSHCN. The SSA estimates that approximately 130,000 children throughout the United States lost their SSI benefits because of this change, but guidelines and accompanying evaluation protocols help ensure the careful evaluations of children today.

Approximately 882,000 children received about $456 million in federal SSI payments in 2001, with an average monthly payment of about $476 for each child plus Medicaid insurance coverage (SSA, 2002).

Temporary Assistance to Needy Families

Formerly known as Aid to Families with Dependent Children (AFDC), Temporary Assistance for Needy Families (TANF) is designed to provide time-limited cash assistance to families who need financial support to care for their children. Prior to 1996, qualifying for AFDC assistance automatically made poor families eligible to receive Medicaid, but changes made by the Welfare Reform Act terminated the automatic link between eligibility for cash assistance and eligibility for Medicaid. However, families are still eligible for Medicaid through TANF, including continued transitional coverage when parents go to work.

Medicaid

Medicaid is the primary source of health care payment for the low-income and disabled population. Both the states and federal government finance the Medicaid program in approximately equal proportions (although the federal share is higher for poorer states), and the federal government specifies mandatory and optional coverage "pathways" through which CSHCN may obtain Medicaid coverage. All states must cover SSI recipients, children in foster care, and those receiving adoption assistance under Title IV-E of the Social Security Act. States may also offer optional coverage through "medically needy" programs, in which the state sets an income standard and a family may "spend down" to achieve eligibility by deducting medical expenses, as well as through the Medicaid waiver programs.

Although children constitute more than half of the total Medicaid-eligible population, Medicaid spending on children accounted for only 15 percent of the total program expenditures in 2000. This is because the great majority of children on Medicaid are healthy dependents of TANF recipients.

Although Medicaid is administered by the states, federal guidelines mandate that states provide essential, medically necessary services, including hospital care; physician services; laboratory and x-ray services; nursing home and home health care; early screening, diagnosis, and treatment procedures for children under 21 years of age; and family planning. The states must also ensure the availability of mandated rural health clinics and federal health centers. The federal government reimburses states that provide a broad range of optional services, such as prescription drugs and transitional care for the mentally ill. Because states have such flexibility in managing the program, great variations in state-to-state coverage and spending exist (Guyer, 2001).

Typically, Medicaid eligibility is determined by the Department of Social Services of the county where the family resides. Social workers in health care settings and other human services agencies can also assist families with CSHCN to determine eligibility. CSHCN can receive Medicaid benefits in one of three ways: (1) if their disabilities and family income qualify them for SSI, (2) if family income is low enough, or (3) if they meet other requirements set by the states.

Special Programs Offered through Medicaid

Early and Periodic Screening, Diagnosis and Treatment Program

CSHCN can receive special benefits through Medicaid, such as the Early and Periodic Screening, Diagnosis and Treatment Program (EPSDT). This program, created in 1972, is designed to help prevent and manage, through early treatment, what could be costly long-term disabilities. Under this program, Medicaid must pay for any services needed to treat or prevent conditions in a child—not just services that treat a specific diagnosis, regardless of whether the service is included in the state Medicaid plan (O'Grady, 1996). EPSDT services include multiple therapies (e.g., speech or physical) that can help improve or correct a child's disability, as well as transportation and outreach services. EPSDT also mandates that children in Medicaid, in addition to receiving rehabilitative services, are entitled to case management, counseling, and long-term residential care when deemed necessary by the child's health care provider (O'Grady, 1996).

Medicaid Waiver Programs

Children who depend on technologies (e.g., ventilators or parenteral nutrition) and cannot be discharged from the hospital without requiring major health services such as skilled nursing may be eligible for the Medicaid Home and Community-Based Waiver program, commonly known as "Katie Beckett waivers." The purpose of this program is to reduce the cost of care to Medicaid and avoid institutionalization of CSHCN. Created as part of the Omnibus Budget Reconciliation Act in 1981, the program provides services such as case management, rehabilitative therapies, and homemaker services, as well as covering costs for home modifications. Because Katie Beckett waivers are part of a state's optional benefits, eligibility criteria and benefits vary by state.

Title V Maternal and Child Health Block Grant Funds

Maternal and child health (MCH) block grants to states focus on improving the health of all mothers and children in the United States, but pay particular attention to the needs of CSHCN. The program is meant to develop services systems within communities and provide comprehensive care for CSHCN, including coordination assistance with preventive programs (such as EPSDT), access to long-term care services, and rehabilitation services for children eligible for SSI. In addition, Title V programs must provide special diagnostic and rehabilitative services, as well as adaptive equipment and other care, to CSHCN that is not typically provided by other state programs (Feeney & Kaufman, 1994). A portion of the block-grant funding goes to grants for special projects of regional and national significance (SPRANS) and community integrated service systems (CISS). SPRANS grants focus on activities such as research, genetic services, and other maternal and child health improvement projects, whereas CISS grants strive to improve maternal and child health by funding projects that develop and expand integrated MCH services within the community (Maternal and Child Health Library, 2002).

In 2002, the Maternal and Child Health Bureau served 1,255,152 CSHCN, which represented 4.6 percent of its total service population and a volume severely limited by short budget funds. However, the dollars spent—$2,356 million—represented 51.8 percent of total expenditures, the highest percentage group. Those in the general children (1 to 22 years) cohort ranked second in expenditures (20.6 percent), or more than $934 million. Infants less than one year ranked third, at 11.3 percent or $513 million. Pregnant women ranked fourth in expenditures, at 8.9 percent or $402.8 million (Maternal and Child Health Bureau, 2004).

States are required to match the Title V funds received and are required to spend at least 30 percent of their funds to support programs for CSHCN. State health departments typically administer the block-grant programs and have the flexibility to decide what services will be provided. Also, as with other federal-state partnership programs, this often results in some children receiving excellent services in one state but not qualifying for services in another.

State Children's Health Insurance Program

The State Children's Health Insurance Program (SCHIP) was established in 1997 as part of the Balanced Budget Act. It is targeted at children without health insurance, including more than 1.4 million CSHCN. SCHIP provides health insurance for children under age 19 in families with incomes too high to qualify for Medicaid but who cannot afford private health insurance. Federal guidelines suggest an income limit for eligible families. Some states have raised the income level to 300 percent of the federal poverty level for a family of 4 in 2003 (300 percent = $55,200). SCHIP is considered to be the greatest step for children's health since Medicaid was enacted in 1965 (Lewitt, 1998). Under SCHIP, states receive federal funding through block grants to provide health insurance to uninsured children in low-income families. States have to contribute to the program, but the enhanced federal match rate reduces the states' share of costs by 30 percent of their regular Medicaid match rate (Lewitt, 1998). If states match and draw down all available funds, total federal and state expenditures are estimated at $56 billion over the 10-year life of the legislation's initial authorization period (U.S. General Accounting Office [GAO], 1999).

Congress has provided $24 billion for the SCHIP program since its inception, through allocations to states of about $4 billion annually. In fiscal 2001, SCHIP covered 6 million children (Alliance for Health Reform, 2002). States may select from among three options to create a program that addresses their unique needs: (1) expand the state's Medicaid program; (2) establish a separate child health insurance program; (3) develop a program that is a combination of Medicaid and a separate program.

Like Medicaid, SCHIP requires states to offer a defined benefits package, but optional benefits vary considerably among states. Most children are eligible for regular checkups, immunizations, eyeglasses, doctor visits, prescriptions drugs, and hospital care. Most SCHIP programs work within a managed-care structure and adhere to quality mandates.

Medicaid and SCHIP, because they are programs designed for low-income families and children, provide extensive benefits with no or low co-payment obligations. However, both Medicaid and SCHIP benefits vary considerably from state to state. To qualify for federal matching funds, states must provide a standard set of benefits for each program; however, under each program states have considerable discretion in funding he benefits defined as optional. Medicaid remains the most generous benefits package, but state SCHIP benefits are also typically more generous than most private plans. Still, there are some gaps for services that are vitally important for CSHCN in low-income families. For example, Colorado has a $2,000 benefit cap on durable medical equipment and does not cover diabetic supplies, and a number of states do not cover case management or nonemergency transportation (Hill, Lutzky, & Schwalberg, 2001).

Public School Programs

In 1973, federal civil rights legislation established that CSHCN have a constitutional right to publicly funded education in the least restrictive environment. The Education for All Handicapped Children Act mandated public school systems to provide medical services to disabled children. Amendments to this legislation in 1986 extended benefits to include early intervention services for infants and children up to five years of age who may have or be at risk for a disability. The amendments, along with the

1973 legislation, are now referred to as the Individuals with Disabilities Education Act (IDEA).

State education agencies are responsible for implementing the law, but receive federal funds to assist in providing the necessary programs. Figure 23.4 shows students served by IDEA. Federal grants to states in 2001 for IDEA programs totaled more than $7.1 billion (U.S. Department of Education, 2002). State and federal education departments spend about $36 billion annually on special education programs for developmentally disabled individuals ages 3 to 21 (Administration for Children and Families, 2003). In addition, schools can bill Medicaid for health services provided in educational settings to CSHCN who are eligible for program benefits.

Although the IDEA requires public schools to provide health support services to disabled children in all school settings, they often lack resources to do so. Teacher training, special education teachers, equipment and physical plan modifications, and accessible buses are all potential costs for schools. Local school officials are becoming increasingly concerned about the budgetary impact of these federal programs and the adversarial relationships that often develop between schools and families of children with special health care and educational needs.

Other Public Programs

- *Title IV Ryan White Care Act* provides comprehensive, community-based, and family-centered services to children and women with HIV and AIDS. Services include medical care, psychosocial services, outreach, and prevention, with the ultimate goal of providing a continuum of care for these populations. Title IV programs are designed to enhance access to and linkages with other publicly funded programs.
- *Special Supplemental Food Program for Women, Infants, and Children (WIC)* may provide assistance to children within the school system who have special diets and to younger children in the home.

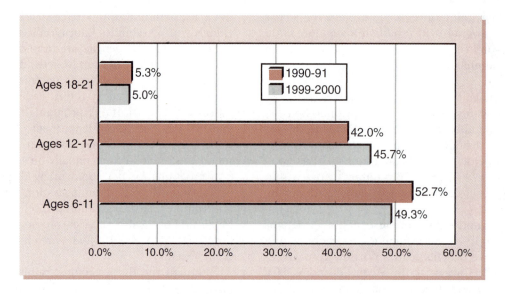

Figure 23.4   Percentage of Students with Disabilities Served by IDEA: By Age Group, 1990–1991 and 1999–2000
SOURCE: U.S. Department of Education, 2000.

- *Medicare's End-Stage Renal Disease Program* may be offered to children with this condition. The program provides health care benefits to cover the costs of dialysis and other services required in a health setting or at home (O'Grady, 1996).
- *Civilian Health and Medical Program of the Uniformed Services (CHAMPUS)* has a program under which CSHCN of military personnel may receive services such as home care, skilled nursing, provision of durable medical equipment, prescription medications, and occupational and physical therapy (O'Grady, 1996).

Private Health Coverage

Children with special health care needs in low-income families may receive coverage through Medicaid and SCHIP. Children with special health care needs in middle-class families typically obtain health insurance through the parents' health insurance programs. When a parent is self-insured or works for a company that does not offer health insurance,

the private health market offers individual policies for children as well as adults. Although comprehensive health insurance is available for children nationwide, choice and price vary considerably. Insurers may employ medical underwriting to deny coverage for specific or preexisting conditions, exclude treatments for certain parts of the body, or charge a higher premium based on health status. Some children's policies do not become effective until they reach a minimum age.

State and federal health insurance reform legislation mitigates the effect of medical underwriting for some, if not all, affected CSHCN. Some states require insurers to guarantee that they will issue policies to all applicants regardless of health status; others mandate guaranteed renewal of coverage. As of 2002, 30 states had created subsidized insurance pools for high-risk individuals (National Center for Health Statistics, 2004). However, even some of the subsidized products available through these pools are priced an average of at least 50 percent above the standard premium rate for an individual plan. The Kennedy-Kassebaum Health Insurance Portability and Accountability Act of 1996 (HIPAA) guarantees access to continuing individual market-rate coverage to individuals and their dependents who previously had group coverage. However, there are no restrictions on premium prices under HIPAA.

Insurance plans vary considerably as to covered benefits and payment levels. Even the most comprehensive health insurance packages exclude some items, so parents must either pay for the items themselves or petition their insurers for coverage. Insurers dictate payment methodologies for CSHCN. The shift to managed care and prepaid capitated payment systems has generated considerable criticism and controversy, as many providers feel that these systems do not adequately cover the costs of delivering care to children with special needs. Standard fee-for-service payment rates do not take into account the need for longer appointments, support and counseling to families, and care coordination with other providers or community agencies. The average cost of providing health care for these children is substantially higher than for children generally. Estimates of the annual cost difference range from a factor of 2 to 120.

A study of more than 300,000 children enrolled in managed-care health plans found that slightly more than ten percent of all child enrollees had special health care needs. Their service utilization was high compared to the overall child population, with an average monthly cost of $280 for all services to the health plan. Parents' out-of-pocket costs are also high, about 7 percent of total costs (Ireys et al., 2002). Thus, there are strong financial incentives for private managed-care plans to avoid enrolling CSHCN, because (unlike Medicaid) few such plans contain risk-adjustment mechanisms to reflect the higher costs of providing health care to these children.

Though accounting for only 13 percent of children, CSHCN account for 80 percent of all children's health care costs (Bethell, Read, Newacheck, Blumberg, & Wells, 2002). In addition to these children making more physician visits and requiring more hospitalizations, they are more likely to have mul-

Table 23.2   Secondary Health Benefits for CSHCN

Secondary Health Coverage and Source	
No secondary coverage	55%
Private secondary coverage	5%
Public secondary coverage	30%
Other secondary coverage	4%
Don't know/Not sure	1%
Does not apply, uninsured	3%
No response	2%
Other Benefits Received by the Children	
SSI	39%
Early Intervention	70%
Special Health Services in School	76%
Department of Mental Health services	9%
Department of Mental Retardation services	25%
Maternal and Child Health Service (Title V)	44%

SOURCE: NCHS, 2002.

tiple sources of health care. Nearly all (97 percent) CSHCN have a source of primary care (NCHS, 2002). Table 23.2 shows their use of secondary health benefits.

POLICY ISSUES

Public Awareness

The viewpoints of Americans toward children with special needs have changed dramatically, especially in the past 30 years. Years ago, a child born with a disability was considered a punishment, God's will, or even a reflection of the family's character. Children with disabilities were frequently put into institutions far from home and grew up within the confines of these facilities because of their conditions. Many parents put children up for adoption or in foster care when special conditions were diagnosed.

Many children died soon after birth, with only a few surviving into their teen years. Today, due to advances in medical technology in the past few decades, many childhood illnesses and disabilities can be substantially corrected, enabling children to lead productive lives. Such measures as in utero surgery, genetic screening, and corrective procedures immediately following birth, in conjunction with what health professionals now know about preventive measures that can be taken prior to and during pregnancy, provide a much greater chance of survival for children born with serious medical conditions.

These advances, along with the educational efforts of organizations such as the March of Dimes Birth Defects Foundation and the National Information Center for Children and Youth with Disabilities, have slowly changed the viewpoint Americans once held. Today families realize that many diseases and conditions often can be treated or managed effectively.

In some cases, however, a child's medical condition is so serious that treatment may be futile. However, a decision not to provide treatment is often highly problematic, because of the lack of professional policies on what constitutes medical futility and the enhanced rights of patient self-determination—especially when not providing treatment means allowing a child to die.

Federal

Federal policy with respect to right to life-and-death issues for CSHCN became a matter of national interest and controversy with the "Baby Doe" case of 1982. The parents of a child born with both Down's syndrome and a correctable congenital anomaly declined authorization of lifesaving treatment; the child died. The case generated amendments in 1984 to the Child Abuse Prevention and Treatment Act that require hospitals and states to establish infant care review committees and procedures for monitoring similar situations.

The "Baby K" case a decade later raised the issue again when the mother of a child with anencephaly (a congenital condition in which all or part of the brain is absent), insisted that her child receive mechanical breathing assistance, although attending physicians had recommended that the child receive only comfort care (food, water, and warmth). An ap-

pellate court in 1994 upheld the district court's decision to "err on the side of life," thereby requiring the hospital to continue providing treatment that it considered medically inappropriate (Garcia, 1996).

The debate over medical futility is likely to intensify in coming years as medical advances pose new ethical dilemmas for families and professionals. The lack of public and institutional policies about medical futility in pediatrics means that decisions about whether children with extremely serious conditions or severe congenital anomalies should be treated aggressively—or at all—are increasingly likely to be made by judges. Developing a public policy will provide the courts with some professional guidance for adjudicating these difficult and complex cases (Clark, 2002).

The federal government is responsible for articulating and implementing a national policy on services for CSHCN. The major federal agencies charged with implementing these policies are the Department of Health and Human Services, the Department of Education, and the Commission on Civil Rights. Within the U.S. DHHS's Maternal and Child Health Bureau, the Division of Services for Children with Special Health Needs (DSCSHN) has established a national agenda and progress indicators for children with special health care needs. The bureau uses these indicators, displayed in Table 23.3, to evaluate state programs for CSHCN. Within the Department of Education, the Office of Special Education and Rehabilitation Services (OSERS) supports programs that assist in educating children with special needs, provides for the rehabilitation of youth and adults with disabilities, and supports research to improve the lives of individuals with disabilities (see *http://www.ed.gov/offices/OSERS*). The U.S. Civil Rights Commission is the oversight agency for ensuring nondiscrimination and equal protection of the laws to disabled individuals.

State and Local

Among the critical operational policy issues for state governments is their responsibility to ensure

Table 23.3 Maternal and Child Health Bureau Indicators of Progress

Indicator of Progress	Description
Medical home	Once identified, CSHCN require a medical home: a source of ongoing routine health care in their community where providers and families work as partners to meet the needs of the children and their families. The medical home assists in the early identification of special health care needs; provides ongoing primary care; and coordinates with a broad range of other specialty, ancillary, and related services.
Insurance coverage	Families must have a way to pay for services. SCHIP has begun to address the issues of children who are uninsured, but the problem of underinsurance remains a major concern for CSHCN and their families. In addition, the range of wrap-around services needed by families requires the availability of private and/or public health insurance that covers a full range of needed services.
Screening	Infants and children with high-risk health conditions must be identified early to help ensure that they and their families receive the care and assistance needed to prevent future morbidity and promote optimal development.
Organization of services	For services to be of value to CSHCN and their families, the system has to be organized so that needs can be identified and services provided in accessible and appropriate contexts, and so there is a family-friendly mechanism to pay for them. Thus, effective organization of services is a key indicator of systems development.
Families' roles	Family members, including those representative of the culturally diverse communities served, must have a meaningful, enduring, and leading role in the development of systems at all levels of policy, programs, and practice. Family voices must be heard and families should be at each table in which decision making occurs. Thus, the involvement of families is a key indicator of systems development.
Transition to adulthood	Youth with special health care needs must be able to expect good health care, employment with benefits, and independence as adults. Appropriate adult health care options must be available in the community and provided within developmentally appropriate settings.

quality care for CSHCN who receive services from state programs. Congress requires state Title V programs to track and report on key maternal and child health indicators. They also have the data and analytical capacity to measure performance as required for federal reports and evaluations through such laws as the Americans with Disabilities Act (ADA) of 1990. Table 23.4 lists key federal laws affecting CSHCN.

Local governments serve principally as agents of the state in administering or operating state and federally funded programs. Local community organizations, especially those of a collaborative nature,

can assert leadership at the local or regional level to ensure that CSHCN have appropriate coverage and access to services.

LICENSURE, CERTIFICATION, AND ACCREDITATION

Providers of care to CSHCN are subject to the same regulations, licensing, and certification requirements applicable to providers of care to all children. Each state licenses and monitors its own institutions, although some states delegate responsibility to counties

Table 23.4 Legislative Landmarks

Year	Law	Key Provisions
1968	Architectural Barriers Act	Requires federally funded buildings designed, built, or remodeled after 1969 to be accessible to persons with disabilities.
1973	Rehabilitation Act of 1973	Revises state vocational rehabilitation grant program. Section 502 establishes a compliance board to enforce the Architectural Barriers Act of 1968. Section 504 prohibits discrimination against otherwise qualified persons with disabilities in any program or activity receiving federal funds.
1975	Education for All Handicapped Children Act	Mandates a free, appropriate public education for all children with disabilities in a state, regardless of the nature or severity of the child's disability.
1981	Omnibus Budget Reconciliation Act	Consolidated six programs under Title V of the Social Security Act into a single block-grant authority.
1985	Consolidated Omnibus Reconciliation Act	Authorizes state options to cover case management and home and community-based services to targeted groups under Medicaid, including ventilator-dependent children.
1989	Omnibus Reconciliation Act	Specified, among other things, that at least 30 percent of the Maternal and Child Health Block Grant under Title V of the Social Security Act must be used to improve services for CSHCN; EPSDT program.
1990	Americans with Disabilities Act	Prohibits discrimination against anyone who has a mental or physical disability, in the areas of employment, public service, transportation, public accommodations, and telecommunications.
1990	Individuals with Disabilities Education Act Amendments	Reauthorized programs to improve support services to students with disabilities, especially in the areas of transition and assistive technology.
1993	Family Medical Leave Act	Allows workers to take up to 12 weeks of unpaid leave to care for newborn and adopted children and family members with serious health conditions, or to recover from serious health conditions.
1996	Personal Responsibility and Work Opportunity Reconciliation Act	Establishes a new, more restrictive definition of *disability* for children under the SSI program; mandates changes to the evaluation process for claims and continuing disability reviews; requires redeterminations before a child turns 18.
1997	Balanced Budget Amendment	Establishes the SCHIP.
1998	The Assistive Technology Act	Continues federal funding for states to improve and expand access to assistive technology devices and services for people with disabilities.
1999	Ticket to Work and Work Incentives Improvement Act	Removes barriers that required people with disabilities to choose between health care coverage and work. Also increases consumer choice in obtaining rehabilitation and vocational services through the establishment of a Ticket to Work and Self-Sufficiency program.
2000	Developmental Disabilities Assistance and Bill of Rights Act	Enhances the Developmental Disabilities Councils, Protection and Advocacy Systems, University Affiliated Programs, and Projects of National Significance. Includes a provision creating training programs for early childhood education personnel that must be conducted in collaboration with programs such as Child Development Centers.
2000	Older Americans Act Amendments	Include a new National Family Caregiver Support Program, which provides funding to state and area agencies on aging, and other organizations they contract with, to provide systems of support services to family caregivers, including those of CSHCN.

for licensing small group and foster homes. Medicare and Medicaid providers are subject to federal regulation by the Centers for Medicare and Medicaid Services (CMS).

The Joint Commission on Accreditation of Healthcare Organizations (JCAHO) accredits hospitals, home health agencies, and long-term care facilities serving children as well as adults. Many children's hospitals are voluntary members of the NACHRI, and some states also have children's hospital associations with qualifying membership criteria.

The American Board of Pediatrics both certifies general pediatricians and verifies the credentials of pediatric subspecialists. As of December 31, 2002, a grand total of 77,328 general pediatricians were certified, as were 14,707 specialists in 16 specialty areas (American Board of Pediatrics, 2002). Though not a regulatory agency, the American Academy of Pediatrics proposed treatment guidelines that have been widely adopted by state Medicaid programs and major insurers as the standard of care for children.

At all levels of the continuum of care for CSHCN, the most critical issues are the competence and compassion of providers. In institutional and more formal settings, licensing, credentialing, certification, and accreditation serve as structural quality indicators of competence. Federal agencies have limited accountability for monitoring the quality of care for CSHCN in publicly financed programs (Szilagy, 2003). In many of the sites along the continuum, though, especially those where care is not so specialized, the principal indicator of quality from the client's and family's perspective is their perception of the provider's kindness and empathy.

INTEGRATING MECHANISMS

Children with special health care needs in the United States receive care through a larger health system that is highly fragmented, with neither a single entry point, a comprehensive integrating mechanism, nor consistent eligibility requirements

among public programs. A child eligible for Medicaid in one state may be ineligible in another. States have established maximum income eligibility levels for SCHIP, ranging from 100 to 300 percent of the federal poverty level. An injured child may not be eligible for the rehabilitative services provided to children with congenital deformities. To cope with this fragmentation, health care providers and organizations have developed a number of different integrating approaches. These approaches encompass and place varying degrees of emphasis on organization and structure, care coordination, and financing.

Organization and Structure

At the federal level, Title V funds the Maternal and Child Health Bureau. Its Division of Services for Children with Special Health Needs (DSCSHN) develops systems of care and services for state programs, as well as developing and promoting standards for such care. This division has two main branches. Genetic Services supports a number of Special Projects of Regional and National Significance (SPRANS) to facilitate the early identification of individuals with genetic conditions and integrate them into systems of care. The Integrated Services branch funds both state and local projects to enhance coordinated systems of care for CSHCN.

Children's medical centers frequently assume care-coordination responsibilities on a community level because they see more children with special needs and they play a leadership role in the community health care delivery system as the resident experts on children's health care needs.

Managed-care organizations (MCOs) serve as an integrating mechanism because they combine the insurance and service delivery functions of health care. Because they also emphasize coordinated systems of care, MCOs offer many benefits for CSHCN. As an increasing number of people become covered by managed care plans, state governments have developed legislation and regulations to ensure that CSHCN receive appropriate care. Most of the laws and rules apply to the general population, but a few are designed specifically for the protection of children. Some states have enacted access-to-care laws that allow health plan members direct access to specialist physicians or the right to select a specialist physician as a primary care provider.

Integrated Financing

A growing number of states are seeking to control Medicaid program costs and improve beneficiary access to care by implementing managed-care delivery systems. These state activities have increased the proportion of Medicaid managed-care enrollees from just under 10 percent in 2002 (CMS, 2003). After focusing their initial efforts on low-income families, states are now starting to use managed care for beneficiaries whose eligibility derives from the SSI program, including CSHCN. Aware of consumer and provider concerns about the suitability of managed care for disabled patients, Medicaid program officials are developing new, higher contracting standards for MCOs that serve beneficiaries with the most complex health care needs, such as provider network criteria to ensure that children with disabilities have access to qualified pediatric specialists and the nearest children's regional medical center.

SSI children with special health care needs and their families have much to gain from an effective managed-care system. As perhaps the most vulnerable client population of all, they also have the most to lose in a poorly run system if they lack access to appropriate and high-quality care.

Critical success factors for Medicaid managed-care programs serving CSHCN are provider payment rates, which need to reflect the higher costs of caring for CSHCN; service access, and the breadth to cover special services; and quality of care.

To address these concerns, state Medicaid programs have sought to structure managed-care contracts with "carve-outs" for both populations and services. Service carve-outs allow states to purchase a standard benefit plan from general managed-care plans while simultaneously ensuring that low-income children with special needs have access to services not typically available or considered medically necessary by commercial health plans. Most commonly carved-out services are mental health, health-related special education, and early intervention services (Fox, McManus, Almeida, & Lesser, 1997). Another alternative is to use specialized managed-care plans for individuals with particular conditions; many states have employed this approach for Medicaid mental health programs. Some states have exempted SSI children from mandatory Medicaid managed-care programs. State policies vary greatly with respect to enrolling CSHCN in Medicaid managed-care plans. Some require it for all groups; others mandate it for select groups (most commonly, SSI children); others exempt all groups (U.S. General Accounting Office, 2000).

ADMINISTRATIVE CHALLENGES

Managing an organization that serves CSHCN and their families can be deeply rewarding if the administrator can effectively understand and deal with the following types of administrative challenges:

- *Confusing eligibility criteria.* There are many different programs, each with its own qualifying requirements and application process.
- *Coordination of services.* Establishing a lead agency and clarifying roles and responsibilities of all the professionals involved in providing services to a child with chronic conditions is an important but often absent element in a comprehensive treatment plan. Too often, families are simply referred from one program to another.
- *Unmet needs and coverage gaps.* As noted earlier, CSHCN are disproportionately poor, and there can be many uncovered disability-related expenses. Geography also determines, to a considerable extent, the availability of services in the child's community.
- *Promotion of family-centered care.* It is important to respect parental preferences and cultural

differences, which sometimes conflict with professional recommendations and community standards of care.

- *Coordination with the educational, social services, and mental health systems.* Administrators usually must work with school officials and others to find creative and cost-effective ways to ensure that CSHCN receive the multiple services they need.
- *Evolving changes in health policy that affect CSHCN.*
- *Balancing resources for CSHCN versus other client groups.*

See Table 23.5 for a service integration matrix for several types of conditions.

CONCLUSION

Children with special health care needs present a wide spectrum of physical and mental health conditions. Care requires coordination of several complex systems: health care, education, and often social services and mental health. Families are essential to children's care, as they are often the coordinators of the services offered by these varying systems.

Financing and public policies pertinent to the health care of CSHCN are complicated, resulting in some children being eligible for duplicate services and some children falling through gaps.

Services for CSHCN have evolved as the many factors affecting access have changed. Moreover, as clinical understanding of children's health problems increases, new treatment modalities will become available that will continue to affect the financing, regulation, and structure of health and related services for children.

CLIENT EXAMPLE

Susan Allen's parents were perplexed by their seven-year-old daughter's behavior. She had always been a lively, inquisitive child with a good appetite and high energy. Her symptoms were rather vague, and not in themselves troubling: increased thirst, frequent urination, a slight weight loss, and complaints of fatigue—even when invited to do something fun.

The pediatrician administered a thorough examination. A blood glucose test confirmed her diagnosis of Type 1 juvenile diabetes, which occurs when the pancreas fails to produce enough insulin. The pediatrician explained the disease and the methods to control it, including injecting insulin several times a day. Diabetics must also carefully monitor their blood sugar levels, regulate their food intake to ensure that they eat frequently, and maintain a healthful diet, avoiding foods with high sugar content.

The Allens were shaken by the news, but determined to learn as much about the disease as possible and to help their daughter learn to manage it effectively. The pediatrician referred them to a pediatric endocrinologist on the medical staff of the local children's hospital. After an initial consultation with that physician, a clinical nurse specialist gave Susan and her parents detailed instructions and helped them practice the glucose monitoring and insulin injection techniques. She also provided information on the American Diabetes Association (ADA) recommended diet, as well as lists of foods produced especially for diabetics with reduced sugar content. The Allens were pleased to find that the ADA diet was not particularly restrictive, but emphasized healthy, low-fat foods; in fact, it was a wise choice for everyone in the family to follow.

Susan and her parents also began attending the hospital's educational and support sessions for children with diabetes and their families. It helped to know that they were not alone, and to learn from other families and children how to cope with the condition. They met with Susan's teacher and the school nurse and discussed how Susan would check her blood sugar and administer her injections there. The Allens also learned from other parents how to work with their physicians to obtain full coverage for the medical supplies and insulin that Susan needed. An added bonus was finding a wonderful

Table 23.5   CSHCN Service Integration

Condition	Services	Payer(s)	Key Provider(s)
Asthma	Disease management at home and school (monitoring diet, attack triggers, use of inhaler); special camps	Public or private insurer	Pediatrician, allergist, health educator
Attention deficit/ hyperactivity disorder	Physical and behavioral disease management at home and school; special education classes or programs; respite care; parental counseling and support group	Public or private insurer	Pediatrician, psychiatrist, psychologist
Cerebral palsy	Physical therapy; speech therapy; assistive devices; physical space modifications; special education classes or programs; assistance with activities of daily living at home and school; respite care	Public or private insurer	Pediatrician, neurologist, physical therapist
Developmental disability	Special education classes or programs; speech therapy; assistance with activities of daily living at home and school; respite care	Public or private insurer; SSI, depending on family income	Pediatrician, psychologist, child development specialist
Diabetes	Disease management at home and school (managing diet and insulin); special camps	Public or private insurer	Pediatrician, endocrinologist, health educator
Muscular dystrophy	Physical therapy; assistive devices; physical space modifications; special education classes or programs; assistance with activities of daily living at home and school; respite care	Public or private insurer	Pediatrician, neurologist, physical therapist
Spina bifida	Physical therapy; assistive devices; physical space modifications; special education classes or programs; assistance with activities of daily living at home and school; respite care	Public or private insurer	Pediatrician, orthopedic surgeon, physical therapist

babysitter, a teenager who was also diabetic and who, by example, showed Susan and her parents that diabetes was a complication but not as much of a limitation as they feared. Through the hospital's educational and support group, the family also ob-

tained a partial scholarship for Susan to attend a special summer camp for diabetic children.

An important element in Susan's babysitter's positive attitude was that she had an automated insulin pump, which eliminated the need for injections. Although insulin pumps are increasingly used for Type 1 diabetes, they are quite expensive (about $5,000, plus supplies) and require some rather careful handling, and so are typically not provided to children. When Susan was 11, Mrs. Allen raised the issue with the pediatric endocrinologist, and presented him with a carefully prepared statement and a letter from Susan's teacher attesting to her intelligence and maturity. When the insurance company attempted to delay authorization for payment because of Susan's youth, Mrs. Allen filed an appeal and the insurance company authorized payment.

Today, at age 16, Susan is a high-achieving student who participates fully in school and community life. She particularly enjoys swimming and in-line skating and is a member of the girls' volleyball team. She hopes to attend an out-of-state college, although her parents have some trepidation about this. They are concerned that without the supportive family and friends who can ensure that she is never alone for any significant length of time, she may risk becoming a "dead in bed" statistic. Every year, some people with diabetes die when they lose consciousness and no one is nearby to help them correct their insulin or obtain medical attention. They are also concerned that Susan be able to obtain employment with a firm that offers good health insurance benefits after graduation.

WHERE TO GO FOR FURTHER INFORMATION

The state Title V administering agency or local public health department can provide information about publicly funded programs for CSHCN. The nearest children's medical center is also an excellent source of information and often serves as a nexus and referral point for all types of community health resources for children. There are also hundreds of disease-specific organizations and support groups, an increasing number of which serve a national constituency through Internet Web sites. Appendix B contains a list of national, state, and trade organizations pertaining to an array of health conditions.

National Association of Children's Hospitals and Related Institutions (NACHRI)
401 Wythe Street
Alexandria, VA 22314
(703) 684-1355
http://www.childrenshospitals.net

Maternal and Child Health Bureau (MCHB)
Health Resources and Services Administration
5600 Fishers Lane
Parklawn Building, Room 18-05
Rockville, MD 20857
(301) 443-0767
http://www.mchb.hrsa.gov

Family Voices
3411 Candelaria NE, Suite M
Albuquerque, NM 87107
(505) 872-4780 / (888) 835-5669
http://www.familyvoices.org

U.S. Department of Education
Office of Special Education and Rehabilitative Services
400 Maryland Avenue, SW
Washington, DC 20202-0498
(202) 205-5465
http://www.ed.gov/about/offices/list/osers/index.html

National Information Center for Children and Youth with Disabilities (NICHCY)
P.O. Box 1492
Washington, DC 20013-1492
(800) 695-0285
http://www.nichcy.org

Federation for Children with Special Needs
1135 Tremont Street, Suite 420
Boston, MA 02120
(617) 236-7210 / (800) 331-0688
http://www.fcsn.org

American Diabetes Association (ADA)
1701 N. Beauregard Street
Alexandria, VA 22311
(800) 342-2383
http://www.diabetes.org

March of Dimes Birth Defects Foundation (MOD)
1275 Mamaroneck Avenue
White Plains, NY 10605
(888) 663-4637
http://www.modimes.org

FACTS REVIEW

1. Name five conditions to qualify a child as CSHCN.
2. List five major federal programs that assist CSHCN.
3. What are the obligations of public schools with respect to educating CSHCN?
4. What are the primary payment sources for the health services used by CSHCN?
5. What is the role of voluntary community agencies in the continuum of care for CSHCN?
6. Identify three health professionals that are the principal providers of services for CSHCN.
7. What special considerations are involved in delivering care to CSHCN in managed-care organizations?

REFERENCES

Administration for Children and Families, CDC. (2003). *ADD fact sheet.* Retrieved June 13, 2003 from *http://www.acf.dhhs.gov/programs/add/Factsheet.htm*

Alliance for Health Reform. (2002). Children's coverage: Key facts. Retrieved June 16, 2003 from *http://www.allhealth.org*

Alliance for Health Reform. (2000). *Covering health issues 2003.* Retrieved June 19, 2003 from *http://www.allhealth.org*

American Academy of Pediatrics. (2001). *Periodic survey of Fellows. Periodic survey #44: Health services for children with and without special needs: The medical home concept.* Retrieved June 6, 2003 from *http://www.aap.org*

American Academy of Pediatrics. (2000). *Improving care for children with special needs.* Washington, DC: Author. Retrieved June 14, 2003 from *http://www.aap.org*

American Board of Pediatrics. (2002). *Number of diplomats certified through December 2003.* Retrieved October 11, 2004 from *http://www.abp.org/abpfr.htm*

American Lung Association. (2003). Pediatric asthma: A growing health threat. Retrieved June 15, 2003 from *http://www.lungusa.org*

American Psychiatric Association. (2003). Fact sheet: Attention deficit/hyperactivity disorder. Retrieved June 15, 2003 from *http://www.psych.org/*

Association for the Care of Children's Health (AACH). (1999).

Bethell, C., Read, D., Newacheck, P., Blumberg, S. J., & Wells, N. (2002). *Measuring and reporting on the presence of a medical home for all children and CSHCN.* Retrieved June 17, 2003 from *http://www.facct.org*

Centers for Disease Control and Prevention (CDC), U.S. DHHS. (2002). *Asthma's impact on children and adolescents.* Retrieved June 19, 2003 from *http://www.cdc.gov/nceh/airpollution/asthma/default.htm*

Centers for Medicare and Medicaid Services (CMS). (2003). *Health care industry market update: Managed care.* Retrieved June 15, 2003 from *http://www.cms.gov*

Clark, P. (2002). Medical futility in pediatrics: Is it time for a public policy? *Journal of Public Health Policy, 23*(1), 66–89.

Desguin, B. W., Holt, I. J., & McCarthy, S. M. (1994). Comprehensive care of the child with a chronic condition. Part I: Understanding chronic conditions in childhood. *Current Problems in Pediatrics, 24,* 199–218.

Family Voices. (2002a). *National data on children and youth with special health care needs.* Retrieved June 20, 2003 from *http://www.familyvoices.org*

Family Voices. (2002b, February). *Your voice counts: Survey.* Retrieved October 11, 2004 from *http://www.familyvoices.org*

Family Voices. (2000).

Family Voices. (1999). *Important information about the SSI children's program.* Retrieved October 11, 2004 from *http://www.familyvoices.og/fs/ssinfo.html*

Family Voices. (1998). *SSI update.* Retrieved September 20, 1999 from *http://www.familyvoices.org/fs/ssiupdates98.html*

Federal Interagency Forum on Child and Family Statistics. (2002). *America's children: Key national indicators of well-being 2002.* Retrieved June 17, 2003 from *http://www.childstats.gov/americaschildren*

Feeney, D., & Kaufman, J. (1994). Children with special health care needs. *CARING, 13* (12), 12–16.

Fox, H. B., McManus, M. A., Almeida, R. A., & Lesser, C. (1997). Medicaid managed care policies affecting children with disabilities: 1995 and 1996. *Health Care Financing Review, 18*(4), 23–26.

Garcia, S. A. (1996). Sociocultural and legal implications of creating and sustaining life through biomedical technology. *Journal of Legal Medicine, 17,* 469–525.

Guyer, J. (2001). *The role of Medicaid in state budgets* (Policy Brief No. 4024). Washington, DC: Kaiser Commission on Medicaid and the Uninsured.

Hill, I., Lutzky, A. W., & Schwalberg, R. (2001). Are we responding to their needs? States' early experiences serving children with special health care needs under SCHIP. Washington, DC: Urban Institute. Retrieved June 6, 2003 from *http://www.urban.org*

Ireys, H. T., Humensky, J., Peterson, E., Wilkstrom, S., Manda, B., & Rheault, P. (2002). *Children with special health care needs in commercial managed care: Patterns of use and cost.* Washington, DC: Mathematica Policy Research, Inc. Retrieved June 6, 2003 from *http://www.mathematica-mpr.com/*

Lewitt, E. (1998). The state Children's Health Insurance Program (CHIP). *The Future of Children, 8*(2), 152–159.

March of Dimes. (2003). *Birth defects.* Retrieved June 15, 2003 from *http://www.marchofdimes.com*

Maternal and Child Health Bureau, Division of Services for Children with Special Needs, U.S. DHHS. (2000). *Title V, a snapshot of maternal and child health.* Retrieved June 10, 2003 from *http://www.mchb.hrsa.gov/programs/blockgrant/snapshot2000.htm*

Maternal and Child Health Bureau, U.S. DHHS. (2004). *Historic national totals for Title V expenditures and individuals served: Title V information system.* Retrieved April 24, 2004 from *http://www.performance.hrsa.gov/mchb/mchreports/Search/special/special_prgsch04_result.asp*

Maternal and Child Health Bureau, U.S. DHHS. (2000). *Achieving and measuring success.* Retrieved June 19, 2003 from *ftp://ftp.hrsa.gov/mchb/ach2000.pdf*

Maternal and Child Health Library. (2002). *MCH projects database.* Retrieved April 25, 2003 from *http://www.mchlibrary.info*

National Association of Children's Hospitals and Related Institutions (NACHRI). (2003). *Key issues: Children with special health care needs.* Retrieved June 20, 2003 from *http://www.childrenshospitals.net*

National Association of Children's Hospitals and Related Institutions (NACHRI). (2001). *All children need children's hospitals.* Retrieved June 6, 2003 from *http://www.childrenshospitals.net*

National Center for Health Statistics (NCHS). (2004). *National association of state comprehensive health insurance plans (NASCHIP).* Retrieved October 11, 2004 from *http://www.naschip.org*

National Center for Health Statistics (NCHS). (2002). *The state and local area integrated telephone survey (SLAITS).* Retrieved June 19, 2003 from *http://www.cdc.gov/nchs/slaits.htm*

O'Grady, R. (1996). Financing health care for children with chronic conditions. In P. Ludder-Jackson, & J. Vessey, *Primary care of a child with a chronic condition.* (2nd ed.). St. Louis, MO: Mosby-Year Book.

Social Security Administration (SSA). (2002). *Children receiving SSI, June 2002.* Retrieved June 20, 2003 from *http://www.ssa.gov/policy/data_sub12.html#sub15*

Social Security Administration (SSA). (1999). *Social security for parents: Benefits for disabled children.* Retrieved September 28, 1999 from *http://www.ssa.gov/kids/parent6.htm.*

Szilagy, P. G. (2003). *Care of children with special health care needs.* Retrieved June 6, 2003 from *http://www.futureofchildren.org*

U.S. Department of Education, Office of Special Education Programs. (2002). *Individuals with Disabilities Education Act (IDEA) program-funded activities fiscal year 2001.* Retrieved July 31, 2003 from *http://www.ed.gov/offices/OSERS/OSEP/Programs/PFA2001/PFA2001.doc*

U.S. Department of Education, Office of Special Education Programs, Data Analysis System (DANS).

(2000). *Twenty-third annual report to Congress on the implementation of the Individuals with Disabilities Education Act.* Washington, DC: Author.

U.S. General Accounting Office (GAO). (2000). *Medicaid managed care: States' Medicaid safeguards for children with special needs vary significantly* (GAO/HEHS-00-169). Washington, DC: Author.

U.S. General Accounting Office (GAO). (1999). *Children's health insurance program: State implementation approaches are evolving.* (GAO/HEHS 99-65). Washington, DC: Author.

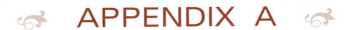

Major Federal Legislation Pertaining to Long-Term Care

Social Security Act	1935
Veterans Administration	1963, 1972, 1975, 1980
Mental Health Acts	1963, 1967, 1971, 1986
Title XVIII (Medicare), Social Security Act	1965
Title XIX (Medicaid), Social Security Act	1965
Older Americans Act	1965, latest reauthorization 2001
Housing and Urban Development Act	1965, 1974
Developmental Disabilities Services and Facilities Act	1970
Title XVI (Supplemental Security Income), Social Security Act	1972
Rehabilitation Act	1973
Title XX, Social Security Act	1974
Omnibus Budget Reconciliation Act	1987
Medicare Catastrophic Coverage Act	1988 (repealed 1990)
Americans with Disabilities Act	1990
Patient Self-Determination Act	1991
Family Medical Leave Act	1993

(continues)

Health Insurance Portability and Accountability Act	1996
Balanced Budget Acts	1997, 1999
National Caregiver Support Act	2000
Ryan White Act	1993, renewed 2000
Medicare Prescription Drug, Improvement, and Modernization Act	2003

APPENDIX B

National Organizations

*Information may have changed since printing

Administration on Aging (AoA)
One Massachusetts Avenue
Washington, DC 20201
(202) 619-0724
http://www.aoa.gov

Agency for Healthcare Research and Quality (AHRQ)
540 Gaither Road
Rockville, MD 20850
(301) 427-1364
http://www.ahrg.gov

AIDS Alliance for Children, Youth and Families
1600 K Street NW, Suite 300
Washington, DC 20006
(888) 917-AIDS
http://www.aids-alliance.org

Alzheimer's Association
919 N. Michigan Avenue, Suite 1000
Chicago, IL 60611-1676

(312) 335-8700 / (800) 272-3900
http://www.alz.org

American Academy of Hospice and Palliative Care
4700 W. Lake Avenue
Glenview, IL 60025-1485
(847) 375-4712
http://www.aahpm.org

American Association of Health Plans (AAHP)
1129 20th Street, NW, Suite 600
Washington, DC 20036-3421
(202) 778-3200
http://www.aahp.org

American Association of Homes & Services for the Aging (AAHSA)
2519 Connecticut Avenue, NW
Washington, DC 20008
(202) 508-9442
http://www.aahsa.org

American Association of Retired Persons (AARP)
601 East Street, NW
Washington, DC 20049
(202) 434-2300 / (800) 424-3410
http://www.aarp.org

American Association of Service Coordinators
919 Old Henderson Road
Columbus, OH 43220
(614) 324-5958
http://www.servicecoordinator.org

American Bar Association (ABA)
740 15th Street, NW
Washington, DC 20005-1022
(202) 662-1000
http://www.abanet.org

American Case Management Association
10310 W. Markham Street, Suite 209
Little Rock, AK 72205
(501) 907-2262
http://www.acmaweb.org

American College of Health Care Administrators (ACHCA)
325 S. Patrick Street
Alexandria, VA 22314
(888) 882-2242
http://www.achca.org

American Congress of Rehabilitation Medicine (ACRM)
6801 Lake Plaza Drive, Suite B-205
Indianapolis, IN 46220
(317) 915-2250
http://www.acrm.org

American Diabetes Association (ADA)
1701 N. Beauregard Street
Alexandria, VA 22311
(800) 342-2383
http://www.diabetes.org

American Health Care Association (AHCA)
1201 L Street, NW
Washington, DC 20005
(202) 842-4444
http://www.ahca.org

The American Health Information Management Association
233 N. Michigan Ave. Suite 2150
Chicago, IL 60601-5800
(312) 233-1100
http://www.ahima.org

American Hospice Foundation
2120 L Street, NW, Suite 200
Washington, DC 20037
(202) 223-0204
http://www.americanhospice.org

American Hospital Association (AHA)
One N. Franklin
Chicago, IL 60606
(312) 422-3000 / (800) 424-4301
http://www.hospitalconnect.com
http://www.aha.org

American Medical Association (AMA)
515 N. State Street
Chicago, IL 60610
(312) 464-5000
http://www.ama-assn.org

American Medical Information Association
4915 Elmo Avenue, Suite 401
Bethesda, MD 20814
(301) 657-1291
http://www.amia.org

American Medical Rehabilitation Providers Association (AMRPA)
1710 N Street, NW
Washington, DC 20036
(202) 223-1920 / (888) 346-4624
http://www.amrpa.org

American Public Health Association (APHA)
800 I Street, NW
Washington, DC 20001-3710
(202) 777-2742
http://www.apha.org

American Society of Law and Medicine and Ethics
795 Commonwealth Avenue
Boston, MA 02215
(617) 262-4990
http://www.aslme.org

American Society on Aging (ASA)
833 Market Street, Suite 511
San Francisco, CA 94130
(415) 974-9600
http://www.asaging.org

Assisted Living Federation of America (ALFA)
11200 Waples Mill Road, Suite 150
Fairfax, VA 22030
(703) 691-8100
http://www.alfa.org

Association for Gerontology in Higher Education (AGHE)
1001 Connecticut Avenue, NW
Washington, DC 20036
(202) 429-9277
http://www.aghe.org

Association of University Programs in Health Administration (AUPHA)
730 11th Street, NW, 4th Floor
Washington, DC 20002-4510
(202) 638-1448
http://www.aupha.org

Bazelon Center for Mental Health Law
1101 15th Street, NW, Suite 1212
Washington, DC 20005
(202) 467-5730
http://www.bazelon.org

Case Management Society of America (CMSA)
8201 Cantrell Road, Suite 230
Little Rock, AK 72227
(501) 225-2229
http://www.cmsa.org

Center for Bioethics
University of Pennsylvania
School of Medicine
3401 Market Street, Suite 320
Philadelphia, PA 19104-3319
(215) 898-7136
http://www.bioethics.upenn.edu

Center for Biomedical Ethics
Case Western Reserve University
Department of Bioethics
10900 Euclid Avenue
Cleveland, OH 44106-4976
(216) 368-6196
http://www.cwru.edu/med/bioethics

Center for Mental Health Services (CMHS)
A Component of Substance Abuse and Mental Health Services Administration
P.O. Box 42257
Washington, DC 20015
(800) 789-2647
http://www.mentalhealth.org

Center for Universal Design
North Carolina State University, School of Design
P.O. Box 8613
Raleigh, NC 27695-8613
(919) 515-3082
http://www.design.ncsu.edu/cud

Centers for Disease Control and Prevention (CDC)
1600 Clifton Road
Atlanta, GA 30333
(404) 639-3534 / (800) 311-3435
http://www.cdc.gov

Centers for Medicare and Medicaid Services (CMS)
7500 Security Boulevard
Baltimore, MD 21244-1850
(877) 267-2323 / (410) 786-3000
http://www.cms.gov
CMS OASIS Website
http://www.cms.hhs.gov/oasis

Commission for Case Management Certification
http://www.ccmcertification.org

Commission on Accreditation of Rehabilitation Facilities (CARF)
4891 E. Grant Road
Tucson, AZ 85712
(520) 325-1044
http://www.carf.org

Community Health Accreditation Program, Inc.
39 Broadway, Suite 710
New York, NY 10006
(800) 656-9656
http://www.chapinc.org

The Council for Disability Rights
205 West Randolph, Suite 1645
Chicago, IL 60606
(312) 444-9484 / TTY (312) 444-1967
http://www.disabilityrights.org

Department of Veterans Affairs
810 Vermont Avenue, NW
Washington, DC 20420
(202) 273-5700 / (800) 827-1000
http://www.va.gov

Disability-related government resource Web site
http://www.disabilityinfo.gov

Disability Resources Monthly (DRM) Guide to Disability Resources on the Internet
http://www.disabilityresources.org

Eldercare Locator
(800) 677-1116
http://www.eldercare.gov

Family Voices
3411 Candelaria NE, Suite M
Albuquerque, NM 87107
(505) 872-4780 / (888) 835-5669
http://www.familyvoices.org

Federation for Children with Special Needs
1135 Tremont Street, Suite 420
Boston, MA 02120
(617) 236-7210 / (800) 331-0688
http://www.fcsn.org

Foundation for Hospice and Home Care
228 7th Street, NE
Washington, DC 20003
(202) 547-7424
http://www.nahc.org

Gerontological Society of America (GSA)
1030 15th Street, NW, Suite 250
Washington, DC 20005-4006
(202) 842-1275
http://www.geron.org

GetCare
700 Murmansk Street, Suite 4, Bldg. 590
Oakland, CA 94607
(510) 986-6700
http://www.getcare.com

Growthhouse
(415) 863-3045
http://www.growthhouse.org

**Health Insurance Association of America
(HIAA)**
1201 F Street, NW, Suite 500
Washington, DC 20004-1204
(202) 824-1600
http://www.hiaa.org

**Health Insurance Portability and
Accountability Act of 1996 (HIPAA)**
http://www.cms.gov/hipaa

**Health Resources and Services
Administration (HRSA)**
5600 Fishers Lane
Rockville, MD 20857
(301) 443-2216
http://www.hrsa.dhhs.gov

**Healthcare Information and Management
Systems Society (HIMSS)**
230 E. Ohio Street, Suite 500
Chicago, IL 60611-3269
(312) 664-4467
http://www.himss.org

Healthy People 2010
200 Independence Avenue, SW, Room 738G
Washington, DC 20201
(800) 367-4725
http://www.healthypeople.gov

**HIV/AIDS Bureau of the Health Resources
and Services Administration (HRSA)**
U.S. Department of Health and Human Services
Office of Communications
5600 Fishers Lane
Rockville, MD 20857
(301) 443-3376
http://www.hab.hrsa.gov

Hospice and Palliative Nurses Association
Penn Center West One, Suite 229
Pittsburgh, PA 15276
(412) 787-9301
http://www.hpna.org

Hospice Foundation of America
2001 S Street, NW, #300
Washington, DC 20009
(800) 854-3402
http://www.hospicefoundation.org

Institute for Ethics
American Medical Association
515 N. State Street
Chicago, IL 60610
(312) 464-5260
http://www.ife@ama-assn.org

**Joint Commission on Accreditation of
Healthcare Organizations (JCAHO)**
1 Renaissance Boulevard
Oakbrook Terrace, IL 60181
(630) 792-5000
http://www.jcaho.org

Kaiser Family Foundation
2400 Sand Hill Road
Menlo Park, CA 04025
(650) 854-9400
http://www.kff.org

Long Term Care University
http://www.ltcuniversity.com/index.html

**March of Dimes Birth Defects Foundation
(MOD)**
1275 Mamaroneck Avenue
White Plains, NY 10605
(888) 663-4637
http://www.modimes.org

Maternal and Child Health Bureau (MCHB)
Health Resources and Services Administration
5600 Fishers Lane
Parklawn Building, Room 18-05
Rockville, MD 20857
(301) 443-0767
http://www.mchb.hrsa.gov

Medicare/Medicaid Integration Program
http://www.hhp.umd.edu/AGING/MMIP/index.html

Midwest Bioethics Center
1021-1025 Jefferson Street
Kansas City, MO 64105
(816) 221-1100
http://www.midbio.org

National Academy of Certified Care Managers
244 Upton Road
Colchester, CT 06414-0669
(800) 962-2260
http://www.naccm.net

National Adult Day Services Association (NADSA)
8201 Greensboro Drive, Suite 300
McLean, VA 22102
(866) 890-7357
http://www.nadsa.org

National Alliance for Caregiving
4720 Montgomery Lane, 5th Floor
Bethesda, MD 20814
http://www.caregiving.org

National Alliance for Infusion Therapy
1001 Pennsylvania Avenue, NW
Washington, DC 20004
(202) 624-7225

National Alliance for the Mentally Ill (NAMI)
Colonial Place Three
2107 Wilson Boulevard, #300
Arlington, VA 22201-3042
(703) 524-7600
http://www.nami.org

National Association for Home Care and Hospice
228 Seventh Street, SE
Washington, DC 20003
(202) 547-7424
http://www.nahc.org

National Association of Area Agencies on Aging (NAAAA)
927 15th Street, NW, 6th Floor
Washington, DC 20005
(202) 296-8130
http://www.n4a.org

National Association of Children's Hospitals & Related Institutions (NACHRI)
401 Wythe Street
Alexandria, VA 22314
(703) 684-1355
http://www.childrenshospitals.net

National Association of Housing & Redevelopment Officials (NAHRO)
630 Eye Street, NW
Washington, DC 20001
(202) 289-3500
http://www.nahro.org

National Association of Professional Geriatric Care Managers (NAPGCM)
1604 N. Country Club Road
Tucson, AZ 85716-3102
(520) 881-8008
http://www.caremanagers.org

National Association of State Mental Health Program Directors Research Institute, Inc. (NASMHPD)
66 Canal Center Plaza, Suite 302
Alexandria, VA 22314
(703) 739-9333
http:www.nri-inc.org

National Association of State Units on Aging (NASUA)
1201 15th Street, NW, Suite 350
Washington, DC 20005
(202) 898-2578
http://www.nasua.org

National Center for Health Statistics (NCHS)
6525 Belcrest Road
Hyattsville, MD 20782-2003
(301) 458-4636
http://www.cdc.gov/nchs

National Center for Medical Rehabilitation Research (NCMRR)
Building 61E, Room 2A03 9000
Rockville Pike
Bethesda, MD 20892
(301) 402-2242
http://www.nichd.nih.gov/NCMRR

National Center on Caregiving
Family Caregiver Alliance
690 Market Street, Suite 600
San Francisco, CA 94104
(415) 434-3388
http://www.caregiver.org

National Council on Disability
1131 F Street, NW, Suite 850
Washington, DC 20004
(202) 272-2004 / TTY: (202) 272-2074
http://www.ncd.gov

National Home Infusion Association
205 Daingerfield Road
Alexandria, VA 22314
(703) 549-3740
http://www.nhianet.org

National Hospice and Palliative Care Organization (NHPCO)
1700 Diagonal Road, Suite 625
Alexandria, VA 22314
(704) 837-1500
http://www.nhpco.org

National Information Center for Children & Youth with Disabilities (NICHCY)
P.O. Box 1492
Washington, DC 20013-1492
(800) 695-0285
http://www.nichcy.org

National Institute of Mental Health (NIMH)
6001 Executive Boulevard, Room 8189
MSC 9663
Bethesda, MD 20892-9663
http://www.nimh.nih.gov

National Institutes of Health (NIH)
9000 Rockville Pike
Bethesda, MD 20892
(301) 496-4000
http://www.nih.gov

National Institute on Aging (NIA)
31 Center Drive, MSC 2292
Building 31, Room 5C27
Bethesda, MD 20892-2292
(301) 496-1752 / (800) 222-2225
http://www.nia.nih.gov

National Institute on Disability and Rehabilitation Research (NIDRR)
(A Component of the Office of Special Education and Rehabilitative Services)
U.S. Department of Education
400 Maryland Avenue, SW
Washington, DC 20202-2572
(202) 205-8134
http://www.ed.gov/osers/nidrr

National Mental Health Association (NMHA)
2001 N. Beauregard Street, 12th Floor
Alexandria, VA 22311
(703) 684-7722 / (800) 969-6642
http://www.nmha.org

National Mental Health Consumer's Self-Help Clearinghouse
1211 Chestnut Street, Suite 1207
Philadelphia, PA 19107
(215) 751-1810 / (800) 533-4539
http://www.mhselfhelp.org

National Organization on Disability
910 Sixteenth Street, NW, Suite 600
Washington, DC 20006
(202) 293-5960
http://www.nod.org

National PACE Association
801 N. Fairfax Avenue, Suite 309
Alexandria, VA 22314
http://www.natlpaceassn.org

National Reference Center for Bioethics Literature
Kennedy Institute of Ethics
Georgetown University
Box 571212
Washington, DC 20057-1212
(202) 687-3885 / (888) BIO-ETHX
http://www.georgetown.edu

National Rehabilitation Association
633 S. Washington Street
Alexandria, VA 22314
(703) 836-0850
http://www.nationalrehab.org

National Rehabilitation Information Center (NARIC)
1010 Wayne Avenue, Suite 800
Silver Springs, MD 20910-5633
(301) 562-2400 / (800) 346-2742 /
TTY (301) 445-5626
http://www.naric.com

National Resource Center on Supportive Housing & Home Modification
Andrus Gerontology Center
University of Southern California
Los Angeles, CA 90089-0191
(213) 740-1364
http://www.homemods.org

National Technical Assistance Center for State Mental Health Planning (NTAC)
66 Canal Center Plaza, Suite 302
Alexandria, VA 22314
(703) 739-9333
http://www.nasmhpd.org/ntac

Offices of HIV/AIDS Policy
U.S. Department of Health and Human Services
200 Independence Avenue, Room 736E
Washington, DC 20201
(202) 690-5560
http://www.surgeongeneral.gov/aids/ohaphome

Partners in Caregiving: The Adult Day Services Program
Wake Forest University School of Medicine
Medical Center Boulevard
Winston-Salem, NC 27157-1087
(800) 795-3676
http://www.wfubmc.edu

Partnership for Caring, Inc.
1620 Eye Street NW, Suite 202
Washington, DC 20006
(202) 296-8071
http://www.partnershipforcaring.org

Partnership for Prevention
1015 18th Street, NW, Suite 200
Washington, DC 20036
(202) 833-0009
http://www.prevent.org

Pharmaceutical Research & Manufacturers Association
1100 15th Street, NW
Washington, DC 20005
(202) 835-3400
http://www.pharma.org

Programs of All-Inclusive Care for the Elderly (PACE)
http://www.cms.hhs.gov/pace/default.asp

Promoting Excellence in End of Life Care
RWJ Foundation National Program Office
c/o The Practical Ethics Center
The University of Montana
1000 East Beckwith Avenue
Missoula, MT 59812
(406) 243-6601
http://www.promotingexcellence.org

Steps to a HealthierUS
U.S. Department of Health and Human Services
200 Independence Avenue, SW
Washington, DC 2001
http://www.healthierus.gov/steps/

Substance Abuse and Mental Health Services Administration (SAMHSA)
Room 12-105
Parklawn Building
5600 Fishers Lane
Rockville, MD 20857
(301) 443-8956
http://www.samhsa.gov

U.S. Census Bureau
4700 Silver Hill Road
Washington, DC 20233-0001
(301) 457-4608
http://www.census.gov

U.S. Department of Education
Office of Special Education and Rehabilitative Services
400 Maryland Avenue, SW
Washington, DC 20202-0498
(202) 205-5465
http://www.ed.gov/about/offices/list/osers/index.html

U.S. Department of Health and Human Services (USDHHS)
200 Independence Avenue, SW
Washington, DC 20201
(202) 619-0257
http://www.dhhs.gov

U.S. Department of Housing and Urban Development (HUD)
451 Seventh Street, SW, Room 6116
Washington, DC 20410
(202) 708-1112
http://www.hud.gov

U.S. House of Representatives
Washington, DC 20515
(202) 224-3121
http://www.house.gov

U.S. Senate Special Committee on Aging
G31 Dirksen Senate Office Building
Washington, DC 20510-6400
(202) 224-5364
http://www.senate.gov/~aging

WebMD
(877) 469-3263
http://www.webmd.com

World Institute on Disability
http://www.wid.org

INDEX